ANESTHESIA *for* OPHTHALMIC *and* OTOLARYNGOLOGIC SURGERY

ANESTHESIA *for* OPHTHALMIC *and* OTOLARYNGOLOGIC SURGERY

Kathryn E. McGoldrick, MD

Associate Professor of Anesthesiology
Yale University School of Medicine
Medical Director
One Day Surgery
Yale New Haven Hospital
New Haven, Connecticut

W. B. SAUNDERS COMPANY
Harcourt Brace Jovanovich, Inc.   Philadelphia   London   Toronto   Montreal   Sydney   Tokyo

W. B. SAUNDERS COMPANY
Harcourt Brace Jovanovich, Inc.

The Curtis Center
Independence Square West
Philadelphia, Pennsylvania 19106

Library of Congress Cataloging-in-Publication Data

McGoldrick, Kathryn E.

Anesthesia for ophthalmic and otolaryngologic surgery/
Kathryn E. McGoldrick.

p.   cm.

ISBN 0–7216–2837–0

1. Anesthesia in otolaryngology.   2. Anesthesia in
  ophthalmology.   I. Title.   [DNLM: 1. Anesthesia.
  2. Eye—surgery.   3. Otorhinolaryngologic Diseases—
  surgery.   WW 168 M478a]

RF52.M34 1992   617.9′6751—dc20

DNLM/DLC   91–17559

Editor: Richard Zorab
Designer: Bill Donnelly
Production Manager: Bill Preston
Manuscript Editors: Pamela Wight and Amy Norwitz
Illustration Coordinator: Lisa Lambert
Indexer: Helene Taylor
Cover Designer: Risa Clow

Anesthesia for Ophthalmic and Otolaryngologic Surgery   ISBN 0–7216–2837–0

Printed in Mexico

Last digit is the print number: 9   8   7   6   5   4   3   2   1

To my loving family

Contributors

Martin A. Acquadro, MD, DMD
Clinical Instructor, Anaesthesiology, Harvard Medical School; Associate Director of Education, Department of Anesthesia, Massachusetts Eye and Ear Infirmary, Boston, Massachusetts
> *Recovery Room Care and Problems Following Ophthalmic and Otolaryngologic Surgery*

Alexander W. Gotta, MD
Professor of Clinical Anesthesiology, State University of New York Health Science Center at Brooklyn; Director of Anesthesiology, Kings County Hospital Center, Brooklyn, New York
> *Anesthetic Management of Maxillofacial Trauma*

Michael D. Ho, MD
Resident in Anesthesiology, Yale University School of Medicine, Yale New Haven Hospital, New Haven, Connecticut
> *Endoscopy Procedures and Laser Surgery of the Airway*

Jonathan Mardirossian, MD, FACS
Chief of Ophthalmology, Saint Agnes Hospital; Director, Fluorescein Angiography Laboratory, White Plains Hospital Center, White Plains, New York
> *New Technology: Understanding Ophthalmic Procedures and Their Anesthetic Implications*

Kathryn E. McGoldrick, MD
Associate Professor of Anesthesiology, Yale University School of Medicine; Medical Director, One Day Surgery, Yale New Haven Hospital, New Haven, Connecticut
> *The Larynx: Normal Development and Congenital Anomalies*
> *Managing Difficult Intubations*
> *Endoscopy Procedures and Laser Surgery of the Airway*
> *Anesthesia for Elective Ear, Nose, and Throat Surgery*
> *Pediatric Airway Emergencies: Foreign Body Aspiration, Epiglottitis, Laryngotracheobronchitis, and Bacterial Tracheitis*
> *Anesthesia for Ear, Nose, and Throat Emergencies*
> *Anesthesia for Otologic Surgery*
> *Complications Associated with Otorhinolaryngologic Anesthesia and Surgery*
> *Anatomy and Physiology of the Eye*

Anesthetics and Intraocular Pressure: Management of Penetrating Eye Injuries
Pediatric Ophthalmic Surgery: Anesthetic Considerations
Ocular Pathology and Systemic Diseases: Anesthetic Implications
Anesthetic Ramifications of Ophthalmic Drugs
Ophthalmic Procedures Performed on an Outpatient Basis
New Technology: Understanding Ophthalmic Procedures and Their Anesthetic Implications
Ophthalmologic and Systemic Complications of Surgery and Anesthesia

Francis X. McGowan, MD
Assistant Professor of Anesthesiology, Pediatrics, and Critical Care Medicine, University of Pittsburgh School of Medicine; Staff Anesthesiologist, Children's Hospital of Pittsburgh, Pittsburgh, Pennsylvania
Anesthesia for Major Head and Neck Surgery

John G. Muller, MD
Assistant Professor of Anesthesiology, Yale University School of Medicine; Associate Attending in Anesthesiology, Yale New Haven Hospital, New Haven, Connecticut
Anesthesia for Otologic Surgery

Lloyd R. Saberski, MD
Assistant Professor of Anesthesiology, Yale University School of Medicine; Clinical Director, Yale Center for Pain Management, New Haven, Connecticut
Regional Anesthesia for Surgery of the Nose, Sinuses, Throat, and Neck

Mary M. Stenger, MD
Staff Anesthesiologist, Sierra Vista Regional Medical Center, San Luis Obispo, California
Anesthesia for Outpatient Ear, Nose, and Throat Procedures

Colleen A. Sullivan, MB, ChB
Clinical Professor of Anesthesiology, State University of New York Health Science Center at Brooklyn; Clinical Director of Anesthesiology, University Hospital of Brooklyn, Brooklyn, New York
Anesthetic Management of Maxillofacial Trauma

Kenneth Zahl, MD
Assistant Professor of Anesthesiology, College of Physicians and Surgeons, Columbia University; Medical Director, Ambulatory Surgery, St. Luke's–Roosevelt Hospital Center, New York, New York
Selection of Techniques for Regional Blockade of the Eye and Adnexa

Foreword

The year 1884 marked an important milestone in the history of medicine. Dr. Karl Koller, an Austrian ophthalmologist, made the pivotal observation that cocaine used as a local anesthetic facilitated eye surgery. Although more than 100 years have passed since his initial report, the anesthesia literature has remained essentially without a definitive text on the perioperative management of patients undergoing ophthalmologic and otolaryngologic surgical procedures. This is all the more remarkable considering the fact that ophthalmologic operations are the most commonly performed surgical procedures for the elderly. It is also remarkable in that the management of a shared airway during procedures involving the respiratory tract represents a significant clinical challenge. In addition, many of these procedures are performed in an ambulatory surgical center where speed is essential in assessing the patient and developing a prioritized anesthetic management plan. Developing a textbook focused primarily on these issues provided a challenge that Dr. Kathryn McGoldrick is uniquely qualified to meet and master. She is a highly skilled senior clinician who daily faces the problems confronted by anesthesiologists managing ophthalmologic and otolaryngologic patients.

Working in an academic environment allows Dr. McGoldrick to identify those areas of the subspecialty that present the greatest challenge to trainees, both clinically and intellectually. Her observations form the basis of the clinical and educational approach used in this textbook. While a handbook would most certainly have required a less complicated approach, Dr. McGoldrick chose the greater challenge of uniting an extensive body of knowledge in a textbook. Indeed, *Anesthesia for Ophthalmic and Otolaryngologic Surgery* facilitates not only the "how-to-do," but more importantly the "why-we-do-it." Its style is in accord with Kathy McGoldrick's characteristic collegial facilitative manner and serves as a vehicle to increase communication among members of the anesthesia care team, surgeons, nurses, and other health care providers for perioperative patient management.

In summary, Dr. McGoldrick and her contributors have provided the reader with a comprehensive reference on the perioperative management of ophthalmologic and otolaryngologic procedures. In so doing, they have set a standard for a reference text that can be utilized in daily clinical practice.

Paul G. Barash, MD
Professor and Chairman
Department of Anesthesiology
Yale University School of Medicine
New Haven, Connecticut

Preface

In recent times, anesthesiology has shared with otorhinolaryngology and ophthalmology a stimulating relationship that has been remarkable for its productivity. During the past 3 decades, developments in antibiotic therapy and refinement of surgical techniques made possible by the operating microscope and the manufacture of exquisitely delicate surgical instruments have revolutionized ear surgery. Concomitant advances in anesthesia, including methods to minimize bleeding, have further improved operating conditions and resulted in improved surgical outcomes. Likewise, ophthalmologic advances have proceeded at a staggering pace during the past few decades. Vitrectomy surgery, intraocular gas injections, and intraocular lens implants were unheard of as recently as 25 years ago. Better understanding by anesthesiologists of the determinants of intraocular pressure and how anesthetic techniques can be modified to manipulate intraocular pressure have facilitated successful surgery.

Indeed, anesthesiology has more than kept pace with the new surgical technology. Contemporaneous additions to our anesthetic armamentaria have included pharmacologic advances and sophisticated monitoring equipment that have encouraged optimal operating conditions and improved patient care. It is now possible to operate safely on fragile premature infants and neonates with conditions such as congenital glaucoma, cataracts, and retinopathy of prematurity, in which optimal visual outcome is closely linked with early surgical intervention. Heretofore, the risk of general anesthesia in these vulnerable infants was considered too great for surgery to be contemplated for anything other than a life-threatening condition. Moreover, advanced age *per se* is no longer considered a contraindication to anesthesia. Many nonagenarians with cataracts are now reaping the benefits of improved anesthetic care.

There is a dearth of recent texts that specifically address the varied aspects of perianesthetic care for eye and ENT patients. *Anesthesia for Ophthalmic and Otolaryngologic Surgery* has been conceived and written to fill the void. This book is intended to be an accessible resource for anesthesiologists and anesthetists, both in practice and in training, as well as for nurses and other health care professionals involved in caring for patients with ophthalmic or otolaryngologic disease. Moreover, since operations in the head and neck region frequently find the surgeon and the anesthesiologist in competition for the upper airway space, it is crucial that each appreciate the other's problems and concerns. This book should be helpful not only to the anesthesia provider but also to the otorhinolaryngologist and the ophthalmologist.

This volume is a reference book rather than a primer. Those seeking a cookbook approach may be disappointed. However, it is hoped that readers interested in formulating an anesthetic plan for a particular patient will find sufficient background information to integrate concepts of applied physiology, pharmacology, and anatomy with clinical practice and thereby design the best strategy. Because anesthesiology is a constantly evolving field, we have attempted to avoid dogma and have sought instead to present objective data in an informative fashion. Considerable attention has been devoted to the lifelong and humbling task of becoming competent in both elective and emergency airway management. In addition, we have sought to explore a variety of vital issues including preoperative assessment, choice of anesthesia, perioperative monitoring, and postoperative complications that may be unique to ophthalmic and otolaryngologic patients and that receive but cursory mention, at best, in major standard textbooks. Discussion of the special problems of pediatric and geriatric patients is extensive and deliberate, because demographic and technical variables influence perioperative risk and surgical outcome. Emphasis has been placed on potential complications in the belief that the prudent anesthesiologist must anticipate the worst-case scenario and be prepared to intervene promptly with whatever routine or extraordinary measures are required.

Perhaps more than in any other anesthetic subspecialty, unabated vigilance is mandatory. Airway emergencies kill quickly, coughing during intraocular surgery can produce extrusion of intraocular contents and vision loss, and even a relatively common or "minor" extraocular procedure such as strabismus surgery may be associated with cardiac arrest once in every 2200 cases. However, mastering the real anesthetic challenges presented by eye and ENT operations can be extremely gratifying, for there is perhaps no other sphere of surgical endeavor in which the anesthesiologist can so dramatically influence the ultimate surgical result.

Kathryn E. McGoldrick, MD

Acknowledgments

Many sources have played a part in the genesis of this book. The extraordinary efforts of all the outstanding contributing authors are acknowledged with deep admiration and appreciation. In addition, over the years, I have had the good fortune of being taught by such distinguished individuals as Drs. Alan Van Poznak, Joseph Artusio, Leroy Vandam, and Robert Moors Smith; their influence permeates these pages. Moreover, my current chairman, Dr. Paul Barash, has been an invaluable and unfailing source of encouragement, support, and inspiration. His profound commitment to educational excellence in anesthesiology has served as both an impetus and a template for residents and faculty alike. Dr. Jonathan Mardirossian, my husband, deserves special commendation for his loyalty, understanding, technical advice, and moral support throughout this lengthy and, at times, seemingly endless endeavor.

Miss Jacki Fitzpatrick, my incredibly efficient secretary, spent many diligent hours at the word processor, typing manuscripts with expertise and alacrity. Her devotion to this project, along with the gracious help of Marion Mangino and Kristina Knobelsdorff, is gratefully acknowledged. Virginia Simon and Wendy Hill are responsible for the majority of the beautiful illustrations contained herein. Drs. Charlotte Bell, Jan Ehrenwerth, Burton Epstein, Dorothy Gaal, Caleb Gonzalez, Tatsuo Hirose, Margaret Kenna, Barbara Kinder, Tae Oh, David Walton, and the late Ron Michels generously donated helpful photographs. Lastly, I should like to thank all the professionals at W. B. Saunders for their excellence and dedication. Special gratitude is due Richard Zorab and his assistant, Dolores Meloni, for their editorial expertise and energetic efforts in bringing this book to fruition.

Contents

CHAPTER **1**

The Larynx: Normal Development and Congenital Anomalies **1**
Kathryn E. McGoldrick

CHAPTER **2**

Regional Anesthesia for Surgery of the Nose, Sinuses, Throat, and Neck **15**
Lloyd R. Saberski

CHAPTER **3**

Managing Difficult Intubations **24**
Kathryn E. McGoldrick

CHAPTER **4**

Endoscopy Procedures and Laser Surgery of the Airway **37**
Kathryn E. McGoldrick
Michael D. Ho

CHAPTER **5**

Anesthesia for Major Head and Neck Surgery **64**
Francis X. McGowan

CHAPTER **6**

Anesthetic Management of Maxillofacial Trauma **90**
Alexander W. Gotta
Colleen A. Sullivan

CHAPTER **7**

Anesthesia for Elective Ear, Nose, and Throat Surgery **97**
Kathryn E. McGoldrick

CHAPTER **8**

Pediatric Airway Emergencies: Foreign Body Aspiration, Epiglottitis, Laryngotracheobronchitis, and Bacterial Tracheitis **112**

Kathryn E. McGoldrick

CHAPTER **9**

Anesthesia for Ear, Nose, and Throat Emergencies **124**

Kathryn E. McGoldrick

CHAPTER **10**

Anesthesia for Otologic Surgery **133**

Kathryn E. McGoldrick
John G. Muller

CHAPTER **11**

Anesthesia for Outpatient Ear, Nose, and Throat Procedures **144**

Mary M. Stenger

CHAPTER **12**

Complications Associated with Otorhinolaryngologic Anesthesia and Surgery **156**

Kathryn E. McGoldrick

CHAPTER **13**

Anatomy and Physiology of the Eye **176**

Kathryn E. McGoldrick

CHAPTER **14**

Anesthetics and Intraocular Pressure: Management of Penetrating Eye Injuries **183**

Kathryn E. McGoldrick

CHAPTER **15**

Pediatric Ophthalmic Surgery: Anesthetic Considerations **190**

Kathryn E. McGoldrick

CHAPTER **16**

Ocular Pathology and Systemic Diseases: Anesthetic Implications **210**

Kathryn E. McGoldrick

CHAPTER **17**

Anesthetic Ramifications of Ophthalmic Drugs **227**
Kathryn E. McGoldrick

CHAPTER **18**

*Selection of Techniques for Regional Blockade of the Eye
and Adnexa* **235**
Kenneth Zahl

CHAPTER **19**

Ophthalmic Procedures Performed on an Outpatient Basis **248**
Kathryn E. McGoldrick

CHAPTER **20**

*New Technology: Understanding Ophthalmic Procedures
and Their Anesthetic Implications* **260**
Kathryn E. McGoldrick
Jonathan Mardirossian

CHAPTER **21**

*Ophthalmologic and Systemic Complications of Surgery
and Anesthesia* **272**
Kathryn E. McGoldrick

CHAPTER **22**

*Recovery Room Care and Problems Following Ophthalmic and
Otolaryngologic Surgery* **291**
Martin A. Acquadro

Index **303**

1

The Larynx: Normal Development and Congenital Anomalies

Kathryn E. McGoldrick

ANATOMY AND PHYSIOLOGY OF THE LARYNX

Evolutionally, the larynx is a protective valve at the cephalic end of the respiratory passages. It developed into an organ of phonation long after serving its initial function of protecting the respiratory tree from aspiration. As the eminent British laryngologist V. E. Negus so eloquently stated: "Much has been written about the larynx, its anatomical structure, its physiology and the diseases which affect it. And yet this small organ performs its work enshrouded in mystery. It is generally known as the organ of voice, and yet it takes but a moment's reflection to observe that thousands of species which have a larynx, never (or practically never) make use of voice."[1]

Several investigators[2-7] have reviewed aspects of laryngeal anatomy and physiology as they pertain to airway management, laryngoscopy techniques, difficult oral intubations, and nasal intubation. Two classic works by Fink[6] and Vandam[5] should be read by all students of anesthesiology.

The larynx is a framework of articulating cartilages, joined together by ligaments, that move in relation to one another by the action of the laryngeal muscles. In the adult, the larynx is positioned opposite the fourth, fifth, and sixth cervical vertebrae. It commences at the superior laryngeal opening and terminates below the cricoid cartilage, where it is attached to the trachea by the cricotracheal membrane (Fig. 1–1).

Discussions of laryngeal anatomy focus on the cartilages, ligaments, muscles, and innervation. Nonetheless, the anesthesiologist must be able to identify the aryepiglottic folds, false cords, true cords, vallecula, arytenoids, and posterior commissure (Fig. 1–2). The aryepiglottic folds join the apices of the arytenoid cartilage to the sides of the epiglottis. The false cords lie proximal to the true vocal cords and stretch from the base of the epiglottis to the tips of the arytenoid cartilage. The vallecula area is formed by the junction of the base of the tongue and the anterior aspect of the epiglottic body. The posterior commissure is between the arytenoids at the base of the true vocal cords.

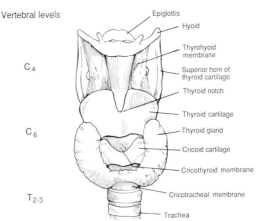

FIGURE 1–1. *Anterior view of the larynx and neighboring structures.*

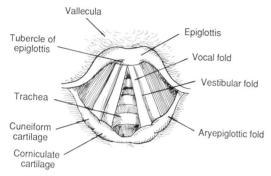

***FIGURE 1–2.** View of the larynx at laryngoscopy.*

LARYNGEAL CARTILAGES

The largest of the laryngeal cartilages is the thyroid, so named because it is shaped like a shield. Its broad laminae meet anteriorly to form the "Adam's apple" and provide attachment to some of the strap muscles of the neck (thyrohyoid, sternothyroid) that control laryngeal movement during swallowing and coughing. These muscles are innervated from the ansa hypoglossi with elements contributed by the hypoglossal nerve and branches of the cervical plexus. The thyroid attaches to the hyoid bone, superiorly, through the hyothyroid membrane.

The cricoid is the only complete cartilaginous ring of the airway. Its posterior signet portion affords a broad attachment to various intrinsic muscles of the larynx. The cricoid is attached to the thyroid through the cricothyroid membrane, the site of puncture or penetration during resuscitation in the presence of obstruction at the glottic level. The cricothyroid membrane is also the locus of needle insertion for administration of transtracheal (more properly, translaryngeal) topical anesthesia.

The last cartilages of functional significance are the paired arytenoids, located on top of the cricoid cartilage. All the laryngeal intrinsic muscles, both adductor and abductor, attach to the arytenoids. The presence of arthrodial joints between the arytenoids and the cricoid enables these cartilages to move. Rheumatoid arthritis may attack the arytenoids and the cricothyroids, as well as other joints throughout the body, resulting in a narrowed, fixed glottis and markedly restricted cervical spine mobility.

The remaining cartilages are of relatively slight functional significance. The fibrocartilaginous epiglottis is attached through the hyoepiglottic ligament to the interior of the thyroid cartilage and to the base of the tongue. Contrary to popular opinion, the epiglottis in humans does not act as a cover to close the glottis. Instead, during swallowing, the larynx is approximated to the base of the tongue by the extrinsic muscles, which receive their nerve supply from the ansa hypoglossi. The oral surface of the epiglottis is innervated by the glossopharyngeal nerve, and the laryngeal surface by the vagus.

The other cartilages of the larynx, the paired cuneiforms and corniculates, are primarily of evolutionary interest.

LARYNGEAL MUSCLES

The intrinsic muscles of the larynx lie entirely within the larynx and are responsible for moving the cartilages of the larynx against one another. The extrinsic muscles connect the larynx to surrounding structures. All the laryngeal muscles are striated, allowing temporary paralysis in time of need with neuromuscular blocking agents.

The intrinsic group contains seven paired muscles: posterior cricoarytenoids, lateral cricoarytenoids, vocalis, thyroarytenoids, aryepiglottics, oblique arytenoid and transarytenoid, and the single cricothyroid muscle. The cricothyroid muscle, a vocal cord tensor, is innervated by the external branch of the superior laryngeal branch of the vagus. All other intrinsic muscles of the larynx are innervated by the inferior laryngeal nerve. Contraction of the aryepiglottic and oblique arytenoid muscles brings the aryepiglottic folds together and narrows the laryngeal inlet. The cricoarytenoids are the only dilator muscles.

The extrinsic muscles of the larynx are the sternothyroid, thyrohyoid, and inferior constrictor of the pharynx. In addition, a few fibers of stylopharyngeus and palatopharyngeus reach forward to the posterior border of the thyroid cartilage. Other muscles indirectly play an important role in movements of the larynx, through the larynx's close attachment with the hyoid bone by ligaments and muscle. These muscles assist in elevating and depressing the larynx. The mylohyoid, stylohyoid, and geniohyoid are the indirect elevators, whereas the sternohyoid and omohyoid are the indirect depressors.

NERVE SUPPLY

The glossopharyngeal (IX) nerve, through its pharyngeal, tonsillar, and lingual branches, supplies sensory innervation for the pharynx, tonsil, and posterior one third of the tongue. However, the larynx in its entirety—both motor and sensory components—is supplied by the vagus (X) nerve, although elements of the glossopharyngeal nerve may be involved through the nucleus of cranial nerve X in the hindbrain.

A branch of the vagus, the mixed motor and sensory superior laryngeal nerve, departs from the parent nerve at the nodose ganglion located at the skull base. An internal branch pierces the hyothyroid membrane to give sensation to the glossopharyngeal plexus and that part of the larynx situated above the level of the vocal cords. The superior laryngeal nerve, through its external branch, also innervates one intrinsic laryngeal muscle, the cricothyroid. The remainder of the mucous membranes of the larynx, the true vocal cords, and the upper trachea receive sensory innervation from the inferior laryngeal nerve. In addition, the inferior laryngeal nerve supplies all the intrinsic muscles of the larynx, with the one exception noted previously. On the left side, the inferior laryngeal nerve is "recurrent," in that it passes around the arch of the aorta, near the ligamentum arteriosum, to reach its objective. Hence, the left (or recurrent) nerve is more vulnerable to injury or paralysis. Such damage may occur during ligation of a patent ductus arteriosus, secondary to aortic aneurysm formation, or because of left atrial enlargement associated with tight mitral stenosis.

Because the inferior laryngeal artery lies close to the inferior (or recurrent) laryngeal nerve, damage to the nerve may occur with attempts to achieve hemostasis during thyroidectomy. This damage is said to be the most common cause of vocal cord paralysis. Vocal cord paralysis may be partial or complete, depending on the number of branches damaged. Which branches are injured determines the variable positions of the cords in paralysis.

In addition, the inferior (or recurrent) laryngeal nerve can be injured by the trauma of endotracheal intubation and by stretching the neck.[8] The resultant vocal cord position and the patient's quality of voice depend on whether the injury is unilateral or bilateral and on whether the external branch of the superior laryngeal nerve, which innervates the vocal cord tensors, is involved. (Vocal cord paralysis also may occur as a congenital condition, usually secondary to central or peripheral nervous system pathology. Among the causes of laryngeal paralysis related to the central nervous system are intracerebral hemorrhage, cerebral agenesis, myelomeningocele with Arnold-Chiari malformation, and hydrocephalus.[9, 10] Peripheral motor nerves may be injured by birth trauma or congenital lesions in the mediastinum and neck.[11])

Fortunately, vocal cord paralysis following tracheal intubation is uncommon. Not surprisingly, it usually occurs when direct or indirect injury to the inferior or recurrent laryngeal nerves has occurred during head and neck surgery. However, vocal cord paralysis has followed various other types of procedures,[12, 13] and in these situations it seems reasonable to attribute the damage to endotracheal intubation rather than to the surgical procedure. Neuropraxia is thought to occur from pressure on the recurrent laryngeal nerve by the cuff of the tracheal tube.[14] Injury may be either unilateral or bilateral. The more benign unilateral injury may be associated merely with self-limiting hoarseness. (In addition to damage to the recurrent laryngeal nerves, voice changes can result from damage to the external laryngeal nerve.) However, bilateral vocal cord paralysis causes signs of escalating upper airway obstruction in the postextubation period. The patient manifests increasing difficulty in vocalizing the letter "E." Auscultation over the larynx reveals inspiratory and expiratory vibrations.[15] As complete obstruction supervenes, the usual methods of ameliorating respiratory obstruction, such as neck extension or insertion of an oropharyngeal airway, are ineffective. However, reinsertion of an endotracheal tube immediately rectifies the situation. Although most patients with bilateral vocal cord paralysis recover within a few months, a tracheostomy may be necessary in the interim.

NERVE BLOCKS

A superior laryngeal nerve block in conjunction with topical anesthesia of the pharynx and larynx can be highly effective for direct laryngoscopy, awake endotracheal intubation, and bronchoscopy. The glossopharyngeal (IX) nerve may be anesthetized by infiltration just posterior to the palatopharyngeal fold at its midline, 1 cm deep to the mucosa of the lateral pharyngeal wall.[16] This block should effectively eliminate the gag reflex.

The internal branch of the superior laryngeal nerve may be blocked from an intraoral approach, in the pyriform fossa, where it traverses just beneath the mucosa. Using the intraoral approach, the tongue is held forward, and lidocaine-soaked gauze is held for at least 2 minutes in the depth of each pyriform fossa. This should provide excellent analgesia all the way down through the level of the false vocal cords. Alternatively, the superior laryngeal nerve may be blocked from an external approach as it passes near the greater cornu of the hyoid bone.[17] (Contraindications include a full stomach or the presence of malignancy or infection in the area of the block.) The superior laryngeal nerve is anesthetized by inserting the needle anterior to the fingertip placed between the cornu of the hyoid bone and the superior cornu of the thyroid. Not unexpectedly, paresthesias may be referred to the external auditory canal, which also receives some of its sensory innervation from the vagus nerve. Then 4 mL of 2% lidocaine may be directly injected, using a 25-gauge needle, into the cricothyroid membrane to anesthetize the upper trachea of an adult. (To preserve the cough reflex, and in the presence of a full stomach, this block should not be performed.) In addition, the inferior laryngeal nerve can be anesthetized close to the inferior cornu of the thyroid. Blocks of the superior and inferior nerves, in conjunction with superficial cervical plexus blocks, permit laryngectomy with regional anesthesia alone.[5]

LARYNGEAL PHYSIOLOGY

There is still no consensus as to the precise definition or mechanism of laryngospasm. Rex[18] defines laryngospasm as an occlusion of the glottis by the action of the intrinsic laryngeal muscles. However, Suzuki and Sasaki[19] redefined laryngospasm on the basis of neurophysiological studies. They claimed that laryngeal spasm is separate from the glottic closure reflex and is solely mediated by the superior laryngeal nerve, resulting in firm approximation of the false cords. However, Fink[6] defined laryngospasm as a prolonged glottic closure persisting well beyond the triggering stimulus. He thought that laryngospasm is maintained primarily by the *extrinsic* muscles of the larynx. Thyrohyoid muscle action truncates the larynx and creates a ball-valve mechanism. The pre-epiglottic body is the ball and is pushed down into the "valve" formed by the approximated false cords. Regardless of the mechanism(s) involved, in clinical practice laryngospasm implies that either the true vocal cords or both the true and false cords have become approximated in the midline to close the glottis and prevent air flow.

Stimuli that may trigger laryngospasm include chemical irritation of pharyngeal or laryngeal mucosa by blood, secretions, or vomitus; visceral pain reflexes; and attempts at intubation with insufficient anesthetic depth. Prevention of laryngospasm involves assuring adequate anesthetic depth prior to instrumentation, use of muscle relaxants, and use of a complete laryngeal block. Treatment of laryngospasm involves removal of the triggering agent, lifting the mandible up and out, and if indicated, administration of a rapidly acting muscle relaxant, such as succinylcholine. Some advocate the use of gentle positive pressure with 100% oxygen by mask, but others maintain that positive pressure may occasionally exacerbate the laryngospasm by causing the pyriform fossae to bulge.

The larynx functions as a respiratory tract valve, an organ of phonation, and a device that improves the efficiency of alveolar ventilation.[5] In order to increase intrathoracic pressure, as in Valsalva's maneuver, coughing, or sneezing, the larynx must close before intrathoracic pressure is raised. Moreover, to increase intra-abdominal pressure, the diaphragm must first be stabilized by laryngeal closure before the abdominal muscles can function effectively to assist defecation or the bearing-down efforts of childbirth. In addition, during inspiration, the glottis and tracheobronchial tree dilate to afford smooth airflow and constrict during expiration, perhaps resulting in the reflux of dead-space air into the alveoli. Consider the postlaryngectomy patient and his or her tracheal stoma. Clearly, the patient with a tracheostomy is unable to cough effectively, needs assistance to remove secretions, and may not "bear down" well. Additionally, although anatomical dead-space is reduced, alveolar ventilation may not be as efficient.

COMPARISON OF THE INFANT AND ADULT LARYNX

The differences between the adult and infant larynx are many. Just as a baby is not merely a tiny adult, so is the infant larynx far from being a miniature version of the adult larynx. The main differences are in size, location, configuration, and tissue consistency.[20] Moreover, not all causes of pediatric upper airway obstruction are laryngeal. Pathology involving the nasal cavities, the nasopharynx, the oral cavity and pharynx, and the neck may all contribute to airway compromise in the young patient (Table 1–1).

SIZE

The infant larynx is approximately 2 cm in breadth. The absolute dimensions of the neonatal larynx are approximately one third those of the adult. The vocal cord length is 6–8 mm. In the infant, approximately one half of the vocal cord length is cartilaginous. In contrast, two thirds of the adult's vocal cord length is membranous. At birth, the subglottic anteroposterior diameter, which represents the critical dimension in the infant larynx, is approximately 5–7 mm. The average diameter is 6 mm, and subglottic stenosis is defined as 4 mm or less. Because the narrowest area of the infant's airway is in the cricoid region,[21] and because the cricoid is a complete, circular cartilaginous structure and consequently nonexpansile, an endotracheal tube may pass easily through an infant's vocal cords but be tight at the cricoid. Hence, the limiting factor is the cricoid ring. In the adult airway, however, the narrowest area is between the vocal cords, and the mature subglottic larynx more closely approximates the maximum dimensions. Thus, it is said that the infant larynx is funnel-shaped, whereas the adult larynx is cylindrical.

LOCATION

The larynx is located higher in the infant. In the 42-day embryo, the larynx is located at the base of the skull. The inferior margin of the cricoid cartilage descends during prenatal life from the second to the fourth cervical vertebra. During the latter part of childhood, another descent to the level of the fifth to the sixth cervical vertebra occurs. At adulthood, the larynx may further descend to the level of the seventh cervical vertebra. Thus, the larynx and the carina commonly descend two to three vertebral levels during life.

Also subject to change with normal growth and development is the relationship of the hyoid bone to the thyroid cartilage. A much closer approximation of the larynx to the hyoid bone exists in the infant than in the adult, whose thyrohyoid membrane is greatly elongated. This high position of the larynx is especially marked in the Pierre Robin syndrome, in which the larynx resembles the larynx in the fetus and is at the level of and posterior to the hyoid bone. The resultant lack of mobility of the hypopharyngeal-lingual-laryngeal complex creates an uncomfortably close approximation of the base of the tongue with the larynx, complicating normal airway function (Figs. 1–3 and 1–4).

The high position of the larynx tends to

TABLE 1–1. Some Nonlaryngeal Causes of Pediatric Upper Airway Problems

  I Nasal Cavities
     Nasal atresia or agenesis
     Choanal atresia
     Nasal encephaloceles
     Tumors
 II Nasopharynx
     Tumors
        Juvenile angiofibroma
        Sarcoma
III Oral Cavity and Pharynx
     Macroglossia
     Micrognathia
        Pierre Robin syndrome
        Treacher Collins syndrome
        Oculoauriculovertebral dysplasia
        Fetal alcohol syndrome
     Marked lymphatic hypertrophy
     Cysts or neoplasms
        Thyroglossal duct cyst
        Lymphangioma (cystic hygroma)
        Lymphosarcoma
     Abscesses
 IV Neck
     Congenital goiter
     Neoplasms

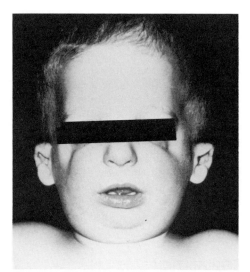

FIGURE 1–3. *Treacher Collins syndrome is associated with notching of the lower eyelids with antimongoloid obliquity of palpebral fissures, flattening of malar bones, and mandibular and aural defects. These children may be difficult to intubate because of micrognathia. (Photograph courtesy of Margaret A. Kenna, M.D., Department of Otolaryngology, Children's Hospital of Pittsburgh, University of Pittsburgh School of Medicine.)*

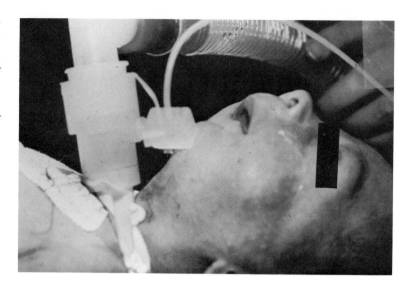

FIGURE 1–4. *Patients with Pierre Robin syndrome have micrognathia and a high anterior larynx. They may be extremely difficult to intubate. (Photograph courtesy of Margaret A. Kenna, M.D., Department of Otolaryngology, Children's Hospital of Pittsburgh, University of Pittsburgh School of Medicine.)*

make the child an obligate nasal breather during the first 9 months of life. The epiglottis, positioned so high in the pharynx, almost meets the soft palate, making oral ventilation difficult. However, the high position of the epiglottis and larynx allows the infant to breathe and swallow simultaneously.[22] (Teleologically, this is propitious for the nursing infant.) Because young infants are obligate nasal breathers, it is essential to clear the nose of an infant before, during, and after the administration of an anesthetic. If nasal obstruction does occur, it can usually be resolved by stimulating the baby to cry.

Because of the newborn's unique anatomical features, the technique of endotracheal intubation appropriate for an adult must be modified.[21] The baby's large head obviates the need for a pillow to achieve the "sniffing position" so favorable for intubation. The epiglottis is more omega-shaped and protrudes over the larynx at a 45-degree angle. Because the larynx of the infant is so high, causing an acute angulation of the base of the tongue to the larynx, a straight laryngoscope blade is preferred rather than a curved blade. Moreover, external pressure on the larynx, pushing it posteriorly, may greatly enhance the view.

CONFIGURATION

As mentioned, the infant larynx has a funnel-shaped lumen. In addition, the angle of the thyroid cartilage is wider in the child than in the adult male, measuring approximately 110 degrees. At puberty, the angulation changes to 90 degrees, with the vocal cords lengthening and the thyroid notch becoming more prominent in the adult male. In the female, however, the angulation remains essentially unchanged from childhood. Indeed, in the child and adult female the anterior cricoid ring may be the most prominent and easily palpable external laryngeal structure.

The trachea in the infant is directed downward and posteriorly, whereas in the adult it is straight downward. Hence, cricoid pressure is more efficacious in facilitating passage of an endotracheal tube in the infant. The distance between the bifurcation of the trachea and the vocal cords in the newborn is 4–5 cm. Therefore, an endotracheal tube must be positioned and secured with meticulous care. Because the tip of the tube can move about 2 cm during flexion or extension of the head, it is imperative that the anesthesiologist check the position of the endotracheal tube by auscultation of the lung fields every time the head is moved.

TISSUE CONSISTENCY

A child has softer and more pliable cartilage, muscle, mucous membranes, and submucosal tissue than does an adult. Because the airway submucosal tissues are looser and less fibrous, they are more "reactive," and one sees a more significant loss of lumen size with inflammatory and traumatic conditions in the pediatric population. This loss of lumen size is exacerbated by the fact that pediatric airway diameter is so small. For example, the newborn's trachea has a diameter of 4–5 mm. Airflow resistance is inversely related to the fourth power of the radius. Consequently, 1 mm of edema in the trachea of the newborn reduces its cross-sectional area by about 75% and augments the resistance to airflow 16-fold. The same amount of edema in an adult would reduce the cross-sectional area by merely 44% and increase the flow resistance only threefold.

STRIDOR

Noisy breathing, or stridor, is a cardinal symptom of airway obstruction and is due to turbulent airflow through narrowed passages. However, stridor is simply a symptom associated with many different conditions,[23] not an entity or diagnosis in itself.

Recognizing the timing of stridor in the respiratory cycle and some pertinent descriptive characteristics may be helpful in locating the affected area and establishing the proper diagnosis. The presence of stridor does not mean a priori that respiratory distress will inevitably occur, but stridor along with signs of respiratory distress is an indication that airway support will probably be necessary. Signs of tachypnea, retractions, tachycardia, flaring of the alae nasi, restlessness, and cyanosis add urgency to the need for a definitive diagnosis of stridor.

As mentioned, the quality and type of stridor may identify the location of pathology. Inspiratory stridor is suggestive of obstruction at the glottic or supraglottic level, whereas the addition of an expiratory component suggests a level below that of the glottis. Expiratory wheeze alone suggests there is no laryngeal obstruction, but rather that the location is more distal, e.g., in the bronchi, such as may be seen with asthma, foreign body, or external compression of a bronchus. A biphasic, "to-and-fro" stridor indicates an intermediate area of involvement, such as the trachea, with compression by an obstructing or constricting great vessel or a mediastinal mass (Fig. 1–5). Whereas a low-pitched, heavy, stertorous respiration suggests pharyngeal obstruction, a high-pitched inspiratory stridor with crowing respirations suggests laryngeal pathology. An audibly hoarse voice or cry suggests cordal or glottic pathology, or obstruction in the immediately adjacent conus elasticus area.

It is important to realize that not all laryngeal abnormalities are congenital. Table 1–2 outlines the wide spectrum of lesions that may cause laryngeal obstruction in the pediatric population.

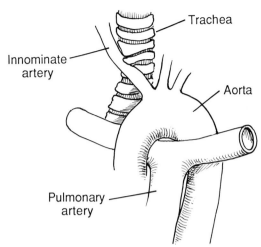

FIGURE 1–5. *Compression of the trachea by the innominate artery may be associated with biphasic, "to-and-fro" stridor.*

CONGENITAL ANOMALIES OF THE LARYNX

LARYNGEAL ATRESIA

Because only about 40 cases of true laryngeal atresia appear in the literature, this entity is thought to be a rare condition that may be considered an extreme case of laryngeal webbing, marked by total fusion or atresia of the larynx. Unless quickly diagnosed at birth, laryngeal atresia is uniformly fatal. However, a few cases have been reported in which forceful rigid bronchoscopy or immediate tracheostomy have been successful in resuscitating these neonates. Moreover, laryngeal atresia probably caused the occasional stillbirths in which the respiratory obstruction went undetected. Cundy[24] makes the point that even following autopsy (in which the larynx is often only

TABLE 1–2. Some Causes of Laryngeal Obstruction in Children

Congenital causes (see Table 1–3)
Infections
Epiglottitis
Laryngotracheobronchitis
Diphtheria
Trauma
Inhaled foreign body
Edema
Chemical or thermal injury
Postintubation
Cervical trauma
Acquired subglottic stenosis
Neoplasms
Juvenile laryngeal papillomatosis

cursorily inspected), laryngeal atresia may be unrecognized, so the true incidence of this entity may be greater than usually reported (Table 1–3).

Smith and Bain[25] reviewed 26 reported cases in the literature and added nine of their own. All nine cases were associated with other major congenital anomalies, which most probably in themselves were incompatible with life. The authors further classified laryngeal atresia into three types according to whether the site of the atresia was supraglottic, infraglottic (subglottic), or glottic. The infraglottic and glottic types were mainly associated with a solid dome-shaped cartilaginous deformity of the cricoid cartilage. However, in all three types, a small pharyngotracheal duct was present.

LARYNGOMALACIA

Laryngomalacia is a somewhat inappropriate term because it connotes a pathological process, such as softening seen in chondromalacia and osteomalacia. However, laryngomalacia is merely a retardation of development and involves no underlying tissue pathology. This most frequent cause of congenital laryngeal obstruction is variously known as the "flabby larynx," the "exaggerated infantile larynx," or "inspiratory laryngeal collapse."

In so-called laryngomalacia, high-pitched, crowing, inspiratory stridor becomes apparent 2 weeks–1 month after birth.[26] The stridor is usually worse in the supine position[27] and improves when the baby is placed prone. Often it can be completely, albeit temporarily, eliminated simply by extending the head and holding the jaw forward. In Holinger's impressive study of 866 infantile laryngeal problems, 75% were cases of laryngomalacia.[28]

Although the clinical picture is usually typical (Table 1–4), diagnosis is confirmed by direct endoscopy. Indeed, the number of infants coming to the operating room with this problem has declined markedly in recent years

TABLE 1–3. Congenital Laryngeal Pathology

> Laryngeal atresia
> Laryngomalacia
> Congenital laryngeal paralysis
> Congenital subglottic stenosis
> Laryngeal web
> Laryngotracheoesophageal cleft
> Laryngoceles and congenital laryngeal cyst
> Laryngeal neoplasms
>   Congenital hemangioma
>   Lymphangioma

TABLE 1–4. Features of Laryngomalacia

> Most frequent cause of congenital laryngeal obstruction
> Developmental delay rather than pathological process
> Characterized by high-pitched, crowing, inspiratory stridor
> Exacerbated by supine position; improves when infant is placed prone
> Usually resolves by age 2 years, when involved cartilages mature

with the advent of the flexible nasopharyngoscope.

Using the instrument, the endoscopist can examine babies satisfactorily without the need for anesthesia. One sees an unstable, long, narrow-based, thin, infolded epiglottis. This abnormally flaccid epiglottis and the aryepiglottic folds are sucked into the glottis during inspiration. Because the laryngeal cartilages are abnormally soft, during inspiration the supraglottic structures—devoid of inherent rigidity—fold in toward the glottis. These folds often become quite edematous, further exacerbating the obstruction. The prognosis for uncomplicated laryngomalacia is excellent, and the problem usually disappears spontaneously within 12–20 months. Rarely is an artificial airway required, although occasionally tracheostomy may be necessary. Moreover, in those patients in whom the epiglottis is mainly responsible for the obstruction, long-term relief can sometimes be achieved by suturing the epiglottis to the base of the tongue.[29]

Various etiologies, including nutrition and other factors, have been suggested but not confirmed. As stated, laryngomalacia is best considered a slowing of normal development that will resolve with maturation of the involved cartilages.

A much less common form of congenital laryngeal cartilage dystrophy is complete absence of the epiglottis. Although this condition *per se* does not cause respiratory obstruction, nonetheless it has its own morbidity. The resultant insufficient protection of the glottis that occurs during swallowing leads to symptoms of choking and chronic recurrent bouts of aspiration pneumonia.

CONGENITAL LARYNGEAL PARALYSIS

Second only to laryngomalacia as the most common cause of congenital laryngeal obstruction, paralysis of the vocal cords is frequently associated with a variety of lesions of the central or peripheral nervous system and some-times with anomalies in other organs. Among the central causes of laryngeal paralysis are hydrocephalus,[9] myelomeningocele with Arnold-Chiari malformation,[10] intracerebral hemorrhage, and cerebral agenesis. Birth trauma may cause significant peripheral nerve injury, leading to vocal cord paralysis. In addition, congenital lesions in the neck and mediastinum may cause damage also to the peripheral nerves.[11] In many instances, a definite etiology cannot be determined. Moreover, recurrent laryngeal nerve injury may also be secondary to surgery for other congenital anomalies such as patient ductus arteriosus ligation[5] and esophageal lesions.

Congenital laryngeal paralysis is not always manifest at birth. Depending on the etiology of the condition, there may be a delay of weeks to months before the patient becomes symptomatic. However, according to Cohen's extensive study, the average age at onset of symptoms was 38 days.[11]

Symptoms are proportional to the degree of obstruction, which seems to correlate with whether the vocal cord paralysis is unilateral or bilateral. Unilateral paralysis is more common than bilateral paralysis, and the left side is afflicted more frequently than the right because of the longer course of the recurrent laryngeal nerve on the left. Unilateral paralysis is also associated with a better prognosis; half of these patients will eventually have a full recovery. Infants with unilateral lesions commonly have some stridor and difficulty with feeding. The stridor tends to be position-related and may be alleviated by laying the infant on the affected side. However, it is possible for those babies with unilateral involvement to be almost asymptomatic or demonstrate only slight hoarseness.

Whereas unilateral paralysis is usually due to a peripheral lesion, bilateral vocal cord paralysis is usually secondary to disease involving the central nervous system. Respiratory obstruction and distress are more marked with bilateral involvement. Dysphagia and aspiration are also common, but dysphonia is difficult to discern. Indeed, it should be noted that the voice (cry) of an infant with bilateral recurrent and inferior nerve paralysis may not be especially remarkable, but inspiration is definitely stridorous.[28] Diagnosis is established by awake laryngoscopy. Prognosis is less favorable than with unilateral paralysis; only about one third of patients with bilateral damage have a full recovery.

Treatment depends on the degree of respiratory obstruction. In some mild cases of unilateral paralysis, no treatment is required, and the condition resolves with time. However, tracheostomy is necessary if there is persistent, serious respiratory obstruction or recurrent aspiration. Indeed, tracheostomy is commonly required with bilateral lesions. Arytenoidectomy should be postponed for many years to allow for spontaneous recovery. In addition, some surgeons have worked with innervated muscle pedicle grafts in an attempt to restore function.[30]

CONGENITAL SUBGLOTTIC STENOSIS

Although it accounts for only about 6% of all congenital laryngeal anomalies, congenital subglottic stenosis is responsible for the majority of tracheostomies performed in infants under 1 year of age.[9–11, 24–31] This anomaly is commonly associated with Down's syndrome and occasionally with other congenital afflictions, such as tracheoesophageal fistula.

Narrowing is usually most marked about 2–3 mm below the true vocal cords. Infants with only a slight degree of subglottic stenosis may be essentially asymptomatic, but those with a greater degree of narrowing will have stridor and other symptoms of respiratory obstruction, such as retractions or even cyanosis, present from birth.

Approximately 1 in 1000 infants has a larynx that is smaller than normal for her or his age owing to thickening of the anterior and lateral parts of the cricoid cartilage.[32] This narrowing often goes unnoticed until the infant is presented at 2 or 3 months of age with a history of recurrent episodes of respiratory infection similar to laryngotracheobronchitis and a characteristic "brassy" stridor. Mild stenosis usually disappears with growth of the larynx. However, those infants with excessive thickening of subglottic soft tissue are especially vulnerable to a critical loss of necessary airway. The least amount of laryngeal inflammation precipitates the need for a tracheostomy, because the limiting cricoid cartilage does not allow swelling of tissues in any direction other than inwardly, at the expense of the airway.

Diagnosis is established by bronchoscopy following normal laryngoscopy. Treatment depends on the severity of obstruction. Infants with a mild degree of stenosis may require little other than careful observation. However, the more severely affected infants may require repeated dilations. Those infants most severely afflicted require tracheostomy.[27] Indeed, laser excision of the stenosis and laryngotracheoplasty are frequently necessary.

It is essential to underscore that most cases of subglottic stenosis are iatrogenic—secondary to prolonged endotracheal intubation—and not congenital.[33] Indeed, the acquired lesions are generally more severe and more difficult to remedy owing to the dense type of scar tissue formation associated with acquired subglottic stenosis. Unless treated by early reconstructive surgery, the vast majority of patients with acquired subglottic stenosis will require tracheostomy, in contrast to less than 50% of those with congenital subglottic stenosis. Therefore, the mortality and morbidity rate is higher with the acquired variety. Indeed, mortality rates in infants with acquired subglottic narrowing and long-term tracheostomy are said to be as high as 24%.[34]

LARYNGEAL WEB

Membranous webs (partial fusion of the cords) are a rare cause of laryngeal obstruction and stridor in infants. In the series by Holinger and Brown,[28] laryngeal webs accounted for less than 5% of the congenital laryngeal anomalies they studied. Seventy-five percent of webs are located at the level of the vocal cords. Webs may be incomplete, thin, and membranous; they may be composed of thick, dense, fibrous tissue; or they may represent a partial fusion of the cords. Infraglottic webs also occur. The least common of the laryngeal webs, the supraglottic web, consists of a partial fusion of the false cords. As previously discussed, in the most extreme cases there may be total fusion or atresia of the larynx.

Infants with laryngeal webs have obstructive symptoms proportional to the degree of airway narrowing. Diagnosis is confirmed by laryngoscopy. The results of therapy seem to correlate with the thickness and nature of the web rather than with the particular type of treatment selected. For example, membranous webs often respond to endoscopic division with scissors. However, if thicker webs are treated in this fashion they tend to recur, and repeated endoscopic dilations become necessary. Some webs may be amenable to endoscopic lysis by laser. Not uncommonly, a tracheostomy is needed with thick, fibrous webs. In such instances, eventually laryngofissure with insertion of a keel will be required, or else endoscopic reconstruction of the larynx and insertion of Silastic keels may be attempted.[35] Phonation tends to be better with the latter procedure.

LARYNGOTRACHEOESOPHAGEAL CLEFT

This is a rare group of conditions characterized by incomplete separation of the larynx from the esophagus. In the mildest cases, there is merely absence of the interarytenoid muscle. The severest cases involve complete fusion of the larynx, trachea, and esophagus into one tube.[36] Other intermediate degrees of malformation also occur.

The clinical picture is not unlike that of a tracheoesophageal fistula, which may coexist, incidentally, in about 20% of these patients. Stridor is not always noted. The most obvious symptoms are copious pharyngeal secretions, respiratory distress triggered by attempts at feeding, and aspiration pneumonia.

Endoscopic and radiographic findings are difficult to interpret and often fail to provide a definitive diagnosis. The anomaly is best detected by probing the posterior laryngeal wall during endoscopy, when separation of the mucosal folds may disclose the cleft. Indeed, one should have a high index of suspicion if an infant has symptoms of a tracheoesophageal fistula but examination reveals an intact, patent esophagus.

Tracheostomy is relatively ineffective because of the proclivity of the tracheostomy tube to penetrate through the defect and find its way into the esophagus. Usually, nasotracheal intubation is elected, followed by early reconstructive surgery.[37] In some instances, a simple intraluminal, endoscopic suturing of the mucosal defect will suffice. Usually, however, the repair is more technically difficult, involving a lateral pharyngotomy incision and laryngeal reconstruction over the endotracheal tube, which is left in place to serve as a stent. Postoperative complications include surgical breakdown as well as eventual stenosis of the larynx or esophagus.

LARYNGOCELES AND CONGENITAL LARYNGEAL CYSTS

These epithelium-lined, cystic laryngeal lesions are rare causes of congenital respiratory obstruction. A laryngocele is an aberration of the saccular appendage of the laryngeal ventricle. Laryngoceles tend to protrude from between the true and false cords or to bulge within the aryepiglottic folds. The free communication of the laryngocele with the laryngeal lumen explains the great variation in size that can occur rapidly with fluctuations in intralaryngeal pressure. However, although congenital laryngeal cysts also originate from the saccular appendage, they are fluid-filled rather than air-filled, and they do not communicate with the laryngeal lumen.

Once again, respiratory symptoms are proportional to the degree of obstruction. Diagnosis is usually determined by laryngoscopy, which unfortunately can trigger severe respiratory obstruction secondary to an expansion of the lesion. This can be temporarily alleviated by aspirating the cyst. However, recurrence following aspiration is common. It is generally better to unroof the cyst endoscopically and strip its epithelial lining, but even with this maneuver recurrence rates are high.[38] Another approach is to wait several months while the baby grows, securing the airway by tracheostomy, and then eventually do an open neck operation.[27]

CONGENITAL HEMANGIOMA AND LYMPHANGIOMA

Although rare, laryngeal and subglottic hemangiomas frequently occur in association with similar cutaneous lesions on the face, neck, or scalp; they are decidedly more common in females than males. Indeed, any child with a strawberry nevus in the head or neck region who develops stridor may have laryngeal or subglottic hemangiomas. Because the lesion frequently is situated below the cords, phonation is usually not compromised.

Symptoms of obstruction tend to worsen as the hemangiomas grow slowly over several months. Typically, affected babies have a history of variable respiratory obstruction but a normal cry. Endoscopy and radiographic studies of the airway and the esophagus help to establish the diagnosis. However, endoscopic diagnosis is not always straightforward, because the overlying mucosa is normal, and the angioma blanches as pressure is applied to it. Growth of the tumor is limited, and most laryngeal hemangiomas regress spontaneously by the age of 2 years. Fortunately, these hemangiomas do not have a proclivity to bleed, either spontaneously or with manipulation. Hence, endotracheal intubation is not usually a problem in these infants. Treatment tends to be conservative, because the lesions usually regress spontaneously. If possible, tracheos-

tomy should be avoided to prevent tracheal seeding. Recurrent, partial endoscopic laser resection or cryoresection, in conjunction with systemic steroids,[39] is the currently popular therapy should relief of respiratory obstruction be required. Radiation therapy was previously in vogue but is now in disfavor for fear of permanent scarring, chronic laryngeal stenosis owing to loss of laryngeal growth potential, and eventual thyroid carcinoma.[40] In a tiny fraction of patients, the hemangiomas continue to grow for years despite appropriate therapeutic interventions. These rare individuals may come to require laryngofissure and open excision.[40]

In 1843 Adolph Wernher published a monograph on cystic hygroma.[41] Later, pathologists postulated a lymphatic origin for these lesions, but even today considerable controversy regarding their true nature remains. Cystic hygromas are variously thought to be the result of lymphatic congenital dysplasia, but possibly they may more properly be classified as hamartomas or neoplasms. Regardless of their true nature, lymphangiomas (Fig. 1–6) may be neatly described according to three general classes: (1) simplex, composed of small lymphatics, generally confined to mucous membranes or skin; (2) cavernous, composed of larger lymphatics, with deep, widespread extension; and (3) cystic hygroma, involving multilocular collections of fluid-filled cysts.

In approximately 70% of cases, cystic hygroma occurs in the neck, usually in the posterior triangle. Less commonly, a hygroma presents high in the anterior triangle and is linked with intraoral lymphangiomas. This variety is frequently associated with airway compromise, sometimes exacerbated by mediastinal extension of the hygroma. These lesions are usually noted at birth or shortly thereafter and have a predilection for rapid, often alarming, growth.[42]

Clearly, the anesthesiologist must appreciate the extent of the disease.[43] Radiological evaluation of the chest may be helpful in this regard. History is also extremely important, because any suggestion of respiratory difficulty or feeding problems may warn of intraoral or mediastinal pathology. In addition, visible cysts in the oral cavity should alert the anesthesiologist to the possibility of supraglottic extension of the pathology. For the neonate, an awake intubation should be gently performed, lest unsuspected epiglottic cysts rupture. Alternatively, a careful inhalation induction with N_2O, O_2, and halothane may be selected for the older infant, taking care to preserve spontaneous ventilation. It is mandatory to have adequate venous access, because substantial losses of blood and fluid usually occur during resection of the cysts. Bradycardia may occur secondary to carotid sinus manipulation or to dissection near branches of the vagus nerve. However, as always, hypoxia must be ruled out when bradycardia occurs in an infant. Postoperative airway management is determined primarily by the extent of the surgical procedures. If significant airway edema is anticipated, performing elective tracheostomy at the time of surgery is probably wise, rather than delaying and having to perform a tracheostomy under less than ideal circumstances. Postoperatively, one must also be alert for possible vocal cord weakness as well as for hypovolemia secondary to translocation of intravascular volume into the neck.

LARYNGEAL PAPILLOMAS

Although not really a congenital entity, laryngeal papillomas are the most common benign tumor of the pediatric larynx (Fig. 1–7). Multiple papillomas are seen in young children, usually between the ages of 3 and 15 years. These papillomas commonly regress at or before puberty and are thought to have a viral etiology.[44] They have a propensity for frequent recurrence and may spread to any location in the larynx, pharynx, or trachea. Fortunately, these pediatric papillomas do not undergo malignant transformation. (In adults, papillomas tend to be solitary rather than multiple, and a small percentage of them have been known to undergo malignant change.)

Children with laryngeal papillomas initially present with hoarseness, which progresses to aphonia and respiratory obstruction. Severe airway compromise by these growths may result in chronic hypoventilation, eventually causing pulmonary hypertension, right ventricular hypertrophy, and cor pulmonale.[45]

Endoscopic laser resection with the CO_2 laser is used to ablate the papillomas. However, multiple, frequent operative resections are usually required to maintain an adequate airway. No definitive cure is currently available. Autogenous vaccine prepared from the patient's own tumors has given ambivalent results.[45, 46] Great care is taken to avoid tracheostomy in these patients, because it may predispose to spread of the lesions into the tracheobronchial tree.[47] However, in some instances, the disease is so extensive that trache-

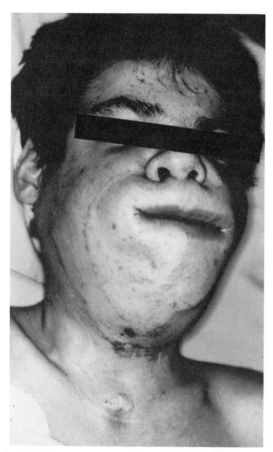

FIGURE 1–6. *A patient with lymphangioma. (Photograph courtesy of Margaret A. Kenna, M.D., Department of Otolaryngology, Children's Hospital of Pittsburgh, University of Pittsburgh School of Medicine.)*

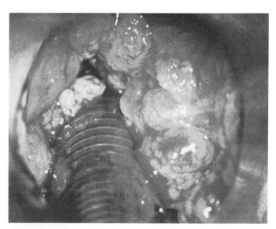

FIGURE 1–7. *Laryngeal papillomas. (Photograph courtesy of Margaret A. Kenna, M.D., Department of Otolaryngology, Children's Hospital of Pittsburgh, University of Pittsburgh School of Medicine.)*

ostomy is required to establish and protect the airway.

Anesthetic management of laser microsurgery of the airway is thoroughly discussed in Chapter 4. However, it is important to appreciate that in pediatric patients, laser microsurgery has an increased risk of anesthetic complications (approximately 15%), especially in those under 3 years of age with extensive disease who do not have the airway secured through tracheostomy.[48]

DIAGNOSTIC LARYNGOSCOPY IN NEONATES AND INFANTS

Although some pediatric laryngologists are satisfied with the visualization of periglottic anatomy obtained with transnasal use of small, flexible fiberoptic bronchoscopes, others prefer rigid endoscopes to study the pediatric upper airway. Because the usual indication for laryngoscopy in this age group is stridor, proper endoscopic examination requires assessment of vocal cord mobility as well as thorough investigation of supraglottic, glottic, and subglottic anatomy.

Newborns generally tolerate awake laryngoscopy extremely well, so general anesthesia is not usually necessary. However, because of the omnipresent threat of possible airway obstruction, the awake examination is performed in the operating room with an anesthesiologist prepared to intubate and ventilate the baby if necessary, or to administer anesthesia should a tracheostomy or other surgical procedure become necessary. All sedative premedication is omitted, but the newborn is given 0.1 mg atropine intravenously (IV) immediately prior to the examination in order to obtund salivation and to prevent the reflex bradycardia so common during laryngeal stimulation. Moreover, it is important to insert the tip of the laryngoscope blade in the vallecula rather than on the epiglottis. Direct blade application on the epiglottis may inadvertently fix the right cord of the neonate, resulting in an incorrect diagnosis of right-sided vocal cord palsy. Throughout the procedure the newborn is monitored fully and meticulously with a precordial stethoscope, temperature probe, electrocardiogram blood pressure device, and pulse oximetry.

In older infants and children, it is usually necessary to induce general anesthesia for diagnostic laryngoscopy. Once again, sedative premedication is omitted in patients with signs of respiratory obstruction, and IV atropine is administered in a dose of 0.02 mg/kg. With full monitoring, anesthesia is induced with halothane, oxygen, and if appropriate, nitrous oxide. When a sufficiently deep level of anesthesia has been achieved, the glottic area is sprayed with lidocaine, in a dose not to exceed 4 mg/kg. Should airway obstruction or ventilatory inadequacy ensue, the airway should be established through intubation or insertion of a rigid bronchoscope. If endoscopy discloses the indication for immediate tracheostomy or another surgical procedure, the patient is likewise intubated with anesthesia conducted according to the mandates of the particular operation involved. Ventilation is continuously monitored to ascertain, among other information, that the endotracheal tube does not become kinked, obstructed, or dislodged by surgical instrumentation. The incidence of postoperative laryngeal edema is high following operative intervention in this area. However, its incidence may be reduced by gentleness in performing all manipulations and instrumentation. Moreover, its effects may be minimized by routine administration of humidified gases by either mask or tent postoperatively. Occasionally, racemic epinephrine may be indicated; this is administered by intermittent positive-pressure breathing (IPPB) after diluting 1 mL of 2.25% racemic epinephrine with 5 mL of normal saline.

REFERENCES

1. Negus VE: The Comparative Anatomy and Physiology of the Larynx. New York, Grune and Stratton, 1949.
2. Hochman RA, Martin JT, Devine KD: Anesthesia and the larynx. Surg Clin North Am 1965;43:1031.
3. DeWeese DD, Saunders WIT (eds): Textbook of Otolaryngology, 5th ed. St. Louis, CV Mosby, 1977, pp 89–101.
4. Roberts J: Functional anatomy of the airway. In Roberts J (ed): Fundamentals of Tracheal Intubation. New York, Grune and Stratton, 1983, pp 9–34.
5. Vandam LD: Functional anatomy of the larynx. Weekly Anesth Update 1977;1:1–10.
6. Fink BR: The Human Larynx: A Functional Study. New York, Raven Press, 1975.
7. Danzl DF, Thomas DM: Nasotracheal intubation in the emergency department. Crit Care Med 1980;8:677.
8. Salem MR, Wong AY, Barangan VC, et al: Postoperative vocal cord paralysis in pediatric patients. Br J Anaesth 1971;43:696.
9. Bluestone CD, Delerme AN, Samuelson GH: Airway obstruction due to vocal cord paralysis in infants with hydrocephalus and meningomyelocele. Ann Otol Rhinol Laryngol 1972;81:778.
10. Holinger PC, Holinger LD, Reichert TJ, et al: Respiratory obstruction and apnea in infants with bilater-

ial abductor vocal cord paralysis, meningomyelocele, hydrocephalus, and Arnold-Chiari malformation. J Pediatr 1978;92:368.

11. Cohen SR, Geller KA, Birns JW, et al: Laryngeal paralysis in children. A long term retrospective study. Ann Otol Rhinol Laryngol 1982;91:417.

12. Hahn FW, Martin JT, Lillie JC: Vocal cord paralysis with endotracheal intubation. Arch Otolaryngol 1970;92:226.

13. Cox RH, Welborn SG: Vocal cord paralysis after endotracheal anesthesia. South Med J 1981;74:1258.

14. Gibbin KP, Eggiston MJ: Bilateral vocal cord paralysis following endotracheal intubation. Br J Anaesth 1981;53:1091.

15. Holley HS, Gildea JE: Vocal cord paralysis after tracheal intubation. JAMA 1971;215:278.

16. Barton S, Williams JD: Glossopharyngeal nerve block. Arch Otolaryngol 1971;93:186.

17. Calcaterra TC, House J: Local anesthesia for suspension microlaryngoscopy. Ann Otolaryngol 1976;85:71.

18. Rex M: Review of the structural and functional basis of laryngospasm. Nerve pathways and clinical significance. Br J Anaesth 1970;42:891.

19. Suzuki M, Sasaki CT: Laryngeal spasm: A neurophysiologic redefinition. Ann Otol Rhinol Laryngol 1977;86:150.

20. Tucker JA, Tucker GF: A clinical perspective on the development and anatomical aspects of the infant larynx and trachea. In Healy GB (ed): Laryngotracheal Problems in the Pediatric Patient. Springfield, CC Thomas, 1979, pp 3–8.

21. Eckenhoff JE: Some anatomic considerations of the infant larynx influencing endotracheal anesthesia. Anesthesiology 1951;12:401.

22. Crelin ES: Functional Anatomy of the Newborn. New Haven, Yale University Press, 1973, pp 1–40.

23. Maze A, Bloch E: Stridor in pediatric patients. Anesthesiology 1979;50:132.

24. Cundy RL, Bergstrom LB: Congenital subglottic stenosis. J Pediatr 1973;82:282.

25. Smith II, Bain AD: Congenital atresia of the larynx. Ann Otol Rhinol Laryngol 1965;74:338.

26. Marshak G, Grundfast KM: Subglottic stenosis. Pediatr Clin North Am 1981;28:941–948.

27. Cotton RT, Richardson MA: Congenital laryngeal anomalies. Otolaryngol Clin North Am 1981;14:203.

28. Holinger PH, Brown WF: Congenital webs, cysts, laryngoceles and other anomalies of the larynx. Ann Otol Rhinol Laryngol 1967;76:744.

29. Fearon B: Laryngeal surgery in the pediatric patient. Ann Otol Rhinol Laryngol (Suppl) 1980;89:146.

30. Tucker HM: Human laryngeal reinnervation. Laryngoscope 1976;86:769.

31. Smith RJH, Catlin FI: Congenital anomalies of the larynx. Am J Dis Child 1984;138:35–39.

32. Morrison JD, Mirakhur RK, Craig HJL: The larynx. In Anesthesia for Eye, Ear, Nose and Throat Surgery. London, Churchill Livingstone, 1985, p 25.

33. Hawkins DB: Glottic and subglottic stenosis from endotracheal intubation. Laryngoscope 1977;87:339.

34. Fearon B, Cotton R: Surgical correction of subglottic stenosis of the larynx in infants and children. Ann Otol Rhinol Laryngol 1974;83:428.

35. Hardingham M, Walshe-Waring GP: Treatment of a congenital laryngeal web. J Laryngol Otol 1975; 89:273.

36. Armitage EN: Laryngotracheo-oesophageal cleft. A report of three cases. Anaesthesia 1984;39:706.

37. Kingston HGG, Harrison MW, Smith JD: Laryngotracheoesophageal cleft—a problem of airway management. Anesth Analg 1983;62:1041.

38. Holinger LD, Barnes DR, Smid LJ: Laryngocele and saccular cysts. Ann Otol Rhinol Laryngol 1978;87:675.

39. Cohen SR, Wang C-I: Steroid treatment of hemangioma of the head and neck in children. Ann Otol Rhinol Laryngol 1972;81:584.

40. Saenger GL, Silverman FM: Neoplasia following therapeutic irradiation for benign conditions in childhood. Radiology 1960;74:889.

41. Wernher A: Die angeborenen Zysten-Hygrome und die ihnen verwandten Geschwulste in anatomischer, diagnostischer und therapeutischer Beziehung. Giessen, GF Heyer, 1843;76.

42. Pounds L: Neck masses of congenital origin. Pediatr Clin North Am 1981;28:841.

43. Evans P: Intubation problem in a case of cystic hygroma complicated by a laryngotracheal haemangioma. Anaesthesia 1981;36:696.

44. Szpunar J: Juvenile laryngeal papillomatosis. Otolaryngol Clin North Am 1977;10:67–70.

45. Hawkins DB, Udall JN: Juvenile laryngeal papillomas with cardiomegaly and polycythemia. Pediatrics 1979;63:156.

46. Oleske JM, Kushnick T: Juvenile papilloma of the larynx. Am J Dis Child 1971;121:417.

47. Donlon JV: Anesthetic management of patients with compromised airways. Anesth Rev 1980;7:22.

48. Leon DA, Hirshman CA: Pediatric laser airway microsurgery: Some problems and solutions. Anesthesiology 1980;S53:344.

Regional Anesthesia for Surgery of the Nose, Sinuses, Throat, and Neck

————————————————— Lloyd R. Saberski —————————————————

Regional anesthesia of the nose, sinuses, throat, and neck provides an alternative to general anesthesia and allows the anesthetist to indirectly monitor the patient's cerebral perfusion by assessing consciousness. It also provides postoperative analgesia.[1] Moreover, regional or local anesthesia is well suited to patients with severe cardiorespiratory disease and to patients having outpatient surgery.[1]

SENSORY NERVE SUPPLY OF THE NOSE, SINUSES, THROAT, AND NECK

The majority of structures involved in anesthesia are supplied by the trigeminal, glossopharyngeal, and vagus nerves (Figs. 2–1 through 2–3).

The trigeminal nerve has three major branches: the ophthalmic (V_1), maxillary (V_2), and mandibular (V_3) nerves. The ophthalmic nerve's three branches are the lacrimal, nasociliary, and frontal nerves (see Fig. 2–2).

The skin of the external nose is supplied by the terminal branches of the ophthalmic nerve and by the maxillary nerve. The ophthalmic nerve gives rise to the infratrochlear nerve from the nasociliary tract and the external nasal nerve from the frontal nerve system, and the maxillary nerve gives rise to the infraorbital nerve (see Fig. 2–2).

The nasal cavity receives its innervation

from the olfactory nerve and from branches of V_1 and V_2 (Fig. 2–4).

The maxillary sinus is innervated directly from branches of V_2 and from branches from the sphenopalatine ganglion. Both the frontal and the ethmoidal sinuses are innervated from branches of V_1.

Sensory innervation of the pharynx is supplied by the maxillary, glossopharyngeal, and vagus nerves (see Fig. 2–3).

The cutaneous innervation of the neck is provided by sequential cervical dermatomes (see Fig. 2–1).

OPERATIONS ON THE NOSE, SEPTUM, AND SINUSES

BLOCKADE OF THE EXTERNAL NOSE

Anesthetic blockade of the external nose is accomplished by blocking the infratrochlear, external nasal, and infraorbital nerves. This is done simply with a field block.

For the field block, the needle is inserted subcutaneously at the base of the alae and directed along the lateral wall of the nose, with 4–5 mL of local anesthetic injected on each side. Then the needle is directed from the same insertion site toward midline in the subcutaneous tissues below the naris, bilaterally.[2] Each side is injected with 2–3 mL of local anesthetic (Fig. 2–5). The field block can be

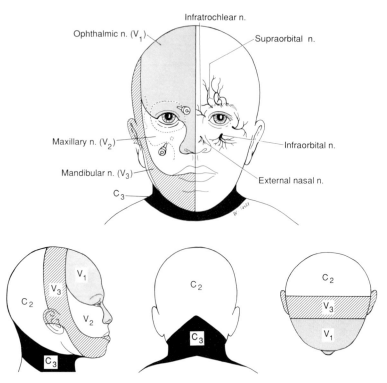

FIGURE 2–1. *Dermatomes of the head and neck.*

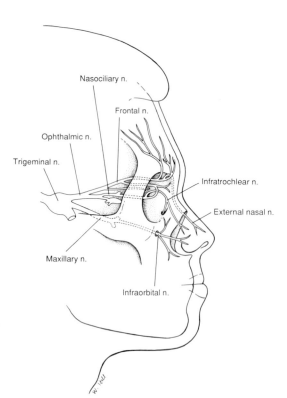

FIGURE 2–2. *Distribution of V₁ and V₂ branches of the trigeminal nerve.*

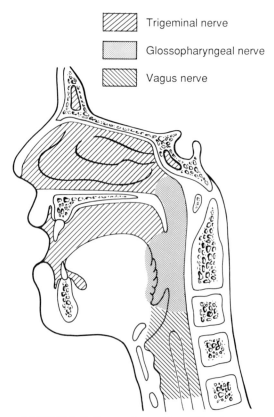

FIGURE 2–3. *Sensory innervation of the pharynx.*

FIGURE 2–4. *Innervation of the nasal septum and lateral wall.*

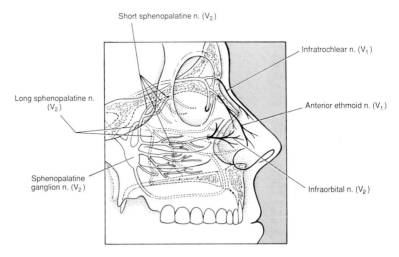

Short sphenopalatine n. (V₂)

Infratrochlear n. (V₁)

Long sphenopalatine n. (V₂)

Anterior ethmoid n. (V₁)

Sphenopalatine ganglion n. (V₂)

Infraorbital n. (V₂)

supplemented with regional blockade of the infratrochlear, external nasal, and infraorbital nerves.

Infratrochlear Nerve Block (Medial Orbital Nerve Block)

The needle is placed superior to the inner canthus of the eye and lateral to the medial wall of the orbit to a depth of about 2 cm (see Fig. 2–1). After a negative aspiration for blood, 2–3 mL of local anesthetic is injected. The infratrochlear nerve and anterior ethmoidal nerve are effectively blocked.

External Nasal Block

The external nasal block is performed by the injection of 2–3 mL of local anesthetic at the junction of the nasal bone and cartilage (see Fig. 2–1).

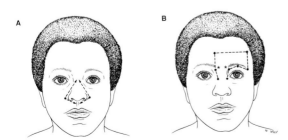

FIGURE 2–5. (A) *Field block for the nose.* (B) *Regional block for the frontal sinus. Asterisks indicate sites for medial orbital block.*

Infraorbital Nerve Block

The needle is positioned 1 cm below the orbital rim directly below the pupil. After negative aspiration, 2–3 mL of local anesthetic is injected. This anesthetizes the infraorbital nerve as it emerges from the foramen (see Fig. 2–1). Hence, analgesia is provided to the side of the nose and to the mucous membrane lining the nasal vestibule.

ANESTHETIC BLOCKADE OF THE NASAL CAVITY AND SEPTUM

The nasal cavity is supplied by branches from V_1, the anterior ethmoidal nerve, and from V_2 through the sphenopalatine ganglion. Both can be easily blocked by packing gauze soaked in local anesthetic with epinephrine. The gauze should be left in place for 10 minutes. Alternatively, cotton pledgets soaked in local anesthetic with epinephrine can be inserted to block the sphenopalatine ganglion and the branches of the anterior ethmoidal nerve (Fig. 2–6). The pledget should remain in place for 10 minutes. Direct injection of local anesthesia, 1–2 mL, into the membranous septum is often necessary. If septal anesthesia is still inadequate, the septum can be injected submucoperichondrially on both sides with local anesthetic.[3] If significant scar tissue is present, the anterior ethmoidal nerve and the terminal branches of the sphenopalatine ganglion (nasal palatine nerve) can be injected directly.[2]

LOCAL ANESTHETICS USED IN NASAL SURGERY

For skin infiltration of the external nose, 1% lidocaine and 0.25% bupivacaine are good

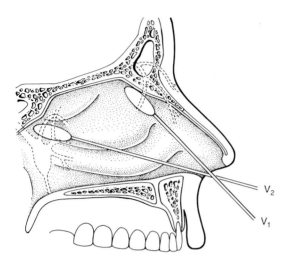

FIGURE 2–6. *The sphenopalatine ganglion block.*

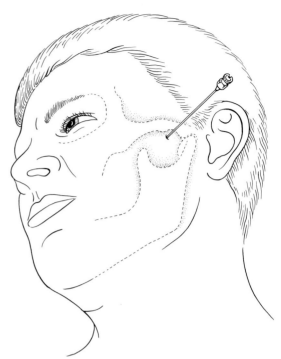

FIGURE 2–7. *The maxillary nerve block.*

choices. For anesthesia of the nasal cavity and septum, it is often advantageous to shrink the mucous membranes by vasoconstriction. This can be done with 4% lidocaine with 1:200,000 epinephrine, 0.75% bupivacaine with 1:200,000 epinephrine, or 10% cocaine solutions. If vasoconstriction is not preferred, 4% lidocaine, 1% tetracaine, or 0.75% bupivacaine can be used.

MAXILLARY SINUS SURGERY

Simple puncture into the maxillary sinus through the nasal cavity is easily done after a local anesthetic packing is supplemented at the puncture site with 10% lidocaine aerosol spray. More extensive operations into the maxillary antrum, e.g., for drainage of empyema, require bilateral maxillary nerve blocks. A medial orbital nerve block can make insertion of the cannula through the nasal cavity more tolerable (see Fig. 2–1). The maxillary nerve is easily blocked using the lateral approach (Fig. 2–7). The coronoid notch of the mandible is identified. A 22-gauge, 10-cm block needle is inserted into the center of the coronoid notch directly below the zygomatic arch. At a depth of 4–5 cm, the needle will strike the pterygoid plate. The needle is moved anteriorly 0.5–1.0 cm, until it slips into the pterygopalatine fossa. After careful aspiration, 5 mL of local anesthetic is injected. Because the area is highly vascular, a hematoma can extend back to the orbit. The hematoma is usually self-limited and requires symptomatic treatment only. Transient blindness as a complication of local an-

esthetic spreading to the optic nerve also can occur.[1]

CALDWELL-LUC OPERATION

The Caldwell-Luc operation involves intraoral drainage of the maxillary sinus. The inferior margin of the maxillary sinus and the dental plexus from the infraorbital nerve must be anesthetized. The naris on the ipsilateral side is packed with gauze soaked in lidocaine with epinephrine. This effectively blocks the sphenopalatine ganglion and gives good analgesia along the inferior margin of the maxillary sinus. The dental plexus is anesthetized by spraying lidocaine on the gingiva above the ipsilateral premolars. Subsequently, a 25-gauge needle is inserted down to the bone, and 8–10 mL of local anesthetic with epinephrine is injected. Additional local anesthetic can be injected into the mucous membrane of the maxillary sinus after it is entered. Alternatively, the maxillary nerve can be blocked (see Fig. 2–7). If the ethmoidal sinus is entered, block of the anterior ethmoidal nerve is necessary (see Fig. 2–6).

FRONTAL SINUS SURGERY

Although the frontal sinus is innervated from branches of V_1, a more comfortable analgesic state is achieved by also blocking adjacent structures. A maxillary nerve block (see Fig. 2–7) and a medial orbital nerve block (see Fig. 2–1) in conjunction with a frontal nerve block provide excellent analgesia.

The frontal nerves are easily blocked by drawing the needle from the infratrochlear nerve block (see Fig. 2–1) and directing it deep to the midpoint of the eyebrow. Upon contact with bone, the needle is withdrawn slightly, and approximately 2 mL of local anesthetic solution containing epinephrine is injected. The entire operative field is encircled with local anesthetic with epinephrine for better hemostasis (see Fig. 2–5). Because the frontal sinus often crosses the midline, bilateral infratrochlear nerve blocks should be performed in conjunction with the ipsilateral maxillary nerve block, frontal nerve block, and field block.[2]

OPERATIONS AND PROCEDURES INVOLVING THE PHARYNX AND LARYNX

Because structures in the pharynx tend to have multiple innervations, selective neural blockade is difficult. Biopsies and other pharyngeal procedures can frequently be done with infiltration anesthesia using an epinephrine-containing local anesthetic solution.

TONSILLECTOMY

The tonsils have a triple innervation from V_2 (lesser palatine nerve), V_3 (lingual nerve), and the glossopharyngeal nerve. Thus, it is easier to provide anesthesia by infiltration (Fig. 2–8). First, the throat and the palatal arches are sprayed with local anesthetic in preparation

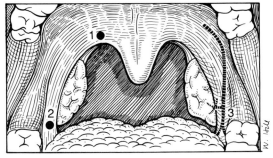

FIGURE 2–8. *Field block for tonsillectomy. 1 and 2, Needle insertion sites at the tonsillar poles. The anterior pillar (between the poles) is infiltrated next. 3, Glossopharyngeal nerve.*

for the infiltrative field block. Injection into the mucous membrane is begun at the posterior palatal arch and peritonsillar tissues.[3] Approximately 10–15 mL of local anesthetic will be required on each side. Lidocaine 0.5% with 1:200,000 epinephrine is an excellent choice for the local anesthetic. (See Chapter 12 for a discussion of local anesthetic toxicity.)

LARYNGOSCOPY

The sensory innervation of the larynx is through two branches of the vagus nerve. The superior laryngeal nerve provides sensation to the larynx above the vocal cords, including the laryngeal inlet and the epiglottis. The recurrent laryngeal nerve provides sensory innervation to the larynx below the cords and to the trachea.

Laryngoscopy is the most common procedure performed on the larynx. Tolerance to this procedure can be improved with a spray of local anesthetic. A tongue depressor can displace the tongue laterally and facilitate the application of local anesthetic to the hypopharyngeal tissues.

GLOSSOPHARYNGEAL NERVE BLOCK

A traditional glossopharyngeal nerve block is generally reserved for the management of intractable cancer pain. However, blocking the terminal branches of the ninth cranial nerve can facilitate various endoscopic procedures, especially if combined with superior and recurrent laryngeal nerve blocks.

The terminal branches of the glossopharyngeal nerve can be blocked easily by injecting the middle of the posterior pillar of the fauces (see Fig. 2–8).[4] This provides hypopharyngeal analgesia.

The traditional glossopharyngeal nerve block involves placement of a 22-gauge needle just posterior to but at the same depth as the styloid process, approximately 3 cm. A local anesthetic (2 mL) injected here blocks the glossopharyngeal, vagus, and accessory nerves. An effective block provides anesthesia to the pharynx and posterior two thirds of the tongue as well as anesthesia to the larynx with paralysis of the ipsilateral vocal cord. In addition, blockade of the accessory nerve leaves the ipsilateral sternocleidomastoid and trapezius muscles weakened. Because the internal carotid artery and internal jugular vein are just medial to the glossopharyngeal, vagus, and accessory nerves, during aspiration the needle must not be intravascular. Also, the anesthetic solution chosen, frequently 1% lidocaine, should not contain epinephrine, which could cause vasoconstriction of the internal carotid artery.

INTUBATION OF THE TRACHEA

To facilitate tracheal intubation, the pharynx, larynx, and trachea should be anesthetized.

As outlined earlier, the pharynx can be desensitized by spraying with lidocaine or by performing an intraoral glossopharyngeal nerve block (see Fig. 2–8).

To provide adequate anesthesia above the level of the vocal cords, the cords can be sprayed under direct visualization using a local anesthetic atomizer or a multiluminal laryngeal catheter. In lieu of spraying the laryngeal inlet and cords, a bilateral superior laryngeal nerve block can be performed (Fig. 2–9). This is done easily by inserting a short 25-gauge needle into the thyrohyoid membrane just inferior to the distal end of the hyoid bone. Palpation of the hyoid bone can be facilitated by pushing the larynx toward the side to be injected. This maneuver makes the hyoid bone and thyroid cartilage more prominent. Only 3–4 mL of local anesthetic is needed on each side. If concentrations greater than 1% lidocaine or 0.25% bupivacaine are used, motor blockade of the crycothyroid muscle ensues.

Branches of the recurrent laryngeal nerve can be blocked with a transtracheal injection of local anesthetic. This provides satisfactory analgesia to the area below the level of the vocal cords. A 22-gauge needle attached to a

5-mL syringe containing 4 mL of 4% lidocaine is inserted through the cricothyroid membrane. Upon entering the trachea, the syringe is aspirated. Air bubbles percolate through the local anesthetic in the syringe. Subsequently, the 4 mL of local anesthetic is injected rapidly. The patient will cough and thereby distribute the local anesthetic.

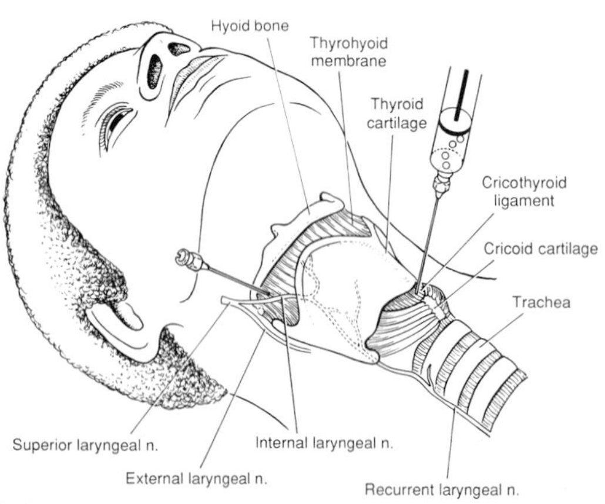

NECK SURGERY

TRACHEOSTOMY

Adequate anesthesia for a tracheostomy can be achieved by injecting the operative site with a field block or with regional blockade in conjunction with recurrent laryngeal nerve block through a transtracheal injection.

Possible regional blockades include segmental cervical epidural anesthesia and bilateral superficial and deep cervical plexus blocks. The usefulness of the cervical epidural and deep cervical plexus blocks may be limited to those patients who are already being ventilated mechanically, because potentially the diaphragm could be paralyzed by blocking of the phrenic nerves. However, the degree of motor block obtained is a function of the concentration of the local anesthetic solution. Dilute concentrations of local anesthetic may give a partial sensory blockade with less risk of motor block. One study found the incidence of phrenic nerve blockade to be low and reported unimpaired spontaneous ventilation with C2 epidural blocks utilizing 0.5% bupivacaine and 1% mepivacaine.[5]

CERVICAL EPIDURAL ANESTHESIA

Patients with severe cardiovascular disease or chronic obstructive pulmonary disease may be appropriate candidates for cervical epidural anesthesia. Reports in the literature have demonstrated the utility of cervical epidural anesthesia in patients undergoing carotid endarterectomy, breast and upper thoracic surgery, and neck dissection.[6] Cervical epidural block has been used alone or in combination with light general anesthesia.[7]

The patient is placed in the lateral decubitus position. After the skin is meticulously prepared and draped, a 17-gauge Tuohy needle is inserted into the interspinous ligament near C6–C7. Proper midline placement enhances the sensation of lack of resistance when the epidural space is entered. (The hanging drop

FIGURE 2–9. Superior laryngeal nerve block and transtracheal injection technique.

technique, although effective for finding the cervical epidural space, must be performed with the patient in the sitting position). The needle is slowly and carefully advanced 1 mm at a time. Each time, resistance must be confirmed by pressing the barrel of an air-filled or saline (preservative-free)-filled glass syringe. As long as a resistance is felt, the needle is superficial to the epidural space. Frequently, a "pop" is felt when the ligamentum flavum is entered. A definite loss of resistance confirms penetration into the epidural space. (The needle should not be inserted farther, lest the subarachnoid space be entered or the spinal cord be violated.) A catheter is then threaded into the epidural space approximately 3–4 cm. Following careful aspiration, a test dose of 3 mL of 1% lidocaine with 1:200,000 epinephrine is injected through the catheter. Tachycardia indicates an intravascularly placed catheter that must be repositioned. Bradycardia may indicate blockade of the cardioaccelerator fibers. Motor block of the upper extremity or respiratory paralysis may indicate improper placement of the catheter into the subarachnoid space. The position of the catheter can be confirmed with a lateral radiograph after injection of 1–3 mL of contrast medium (Fig. 2–10).

THE CERVICAL PLEXUS

The cervical plexus leads to deep branches that are primarily motor fibers to neck musculature and the diaphragm and superficial fibers that provide sensation to the head and neck.

Superficial Cervical Plexus Block

Blockade of the superficial cervical plexus provides adequate cutaneous analgesia for neck surgery through blockade of the anterior cervical and supraclavicular nerves (Fig. 2–11).

With the patient in the supine position with head tilted slightly in the contralateral direction, the posterior border of the sternocleidomastoid muscle is palpated. This can often be facilitated by asking the patient to raise his or her head. The midpoint of the sternocleidomastoid muscle is then identified. After aseptic skin preparation and draping, a 22-gauge block needle is inserted from the midpoint of the posterior border of the sternocleidomastoid muscle and advanced in a caudad direction until the "pop" of the fascia is felt. Following negative aspiration, 5 mL of local anesthetic solution is deposited. As the needle is with-

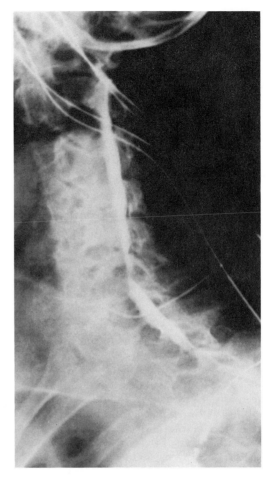

FIGURE 2–10. *Contrast in the cervical epidural space, lateral projection.*

drawn, an additional 5 mL of local anesthetic is injected. Subsequently, the needle is directed cephalad and the technique is repeated.[8] Lidocaine 1% and bupivacaine 0.25% are good choices for local anesthesia. With the exception of possible intravascular injection, generally few major complications are associated with this procedure.

Deep Cervical Plexus Block

Deep cervical plexus block can be used as an adjunct to superficial cervical plexus block for surgery confined to one side of the neck. Bilateral deep cervical plexus block should be reserved for patients who require mechanical ventilation, because bilateral blockade can cause bilateral phrenic nerve paralysis. Because the deep cervical plexus provides primarily motor innervation to neck muscles,

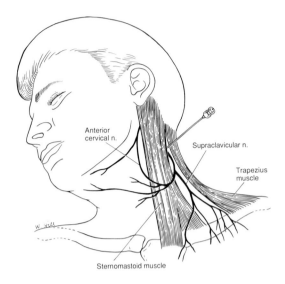

FIGURE 2–11. The superficial cervical plexus block.

blockade of this plexus relaxes the musculature and provides improved operating conditions.

The patient is placed in the supine position, and the head is turned slightly away from the side of the block. Chassaignac's tubercle and the mastoid process are identified, and a line is drawn between them (Fig. 2–12). The level of cervical blockade is determined from anatomical markers (see Fig. 2–12). Following aseptic skin preparation, a 22-gauge block needle is introduced through the skin along a line between the mastoid process and Chassaignac's tubercle at the appropriate level, maintaining a slight caudad direction. The tip of the transverse process will be contacted at

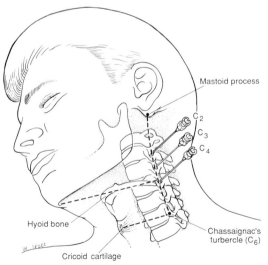

FIGURE 2–12. The deep cervical plexus block.

a depth of approximately 3 cm. The procedure is repeated at each of the desired levels. Frequently, paresthesias are elicited in the distribution of the cutaneous sensory branches. After careful aspiration, 3 mL of local anesthetic is injected at each level.

Complications of this procedure include inadvertent injection into the vertebral artery, extension of the local anesthetic into the epidural or subdural space, and, if the needle is superficial to the prevertebral fascia, a cervical sympathetic block.[1]

THYROID SURGERY

Thyroid surgery can easily be performed with regional anesthesia in conjunction with sedation. The operative site obtains its innervation from the superficial cervical plexus and from the sensory nerves that accompany the superior thyroid artery.

A bilateral superficial cervical plexus block is performed as outlined previously (see Fig. 2–10). Sensory fibers accompanying the superior thyroid artery are best blocked after the thyroid is exposed. A local anesthetic solution (2–3 mL) is injected above the superior pole of the thyroid. If discomfort occurs during traction on the thyroid, 2–3 mL of local anesthetic can be injected under the capsule of the thyroid.[3] Care must be taken during the intracapsular injection lest the recurrent laryngeal nerve be inadvertently blocked and the ability to check vocal cord activity during surgery be lost. Worse, bilateral paralysis of the recurrent laryngeal nerve can result in airway obstruction.

Anesthetic solutions containing epinephrine are preferred unless the patient has thyrotoxicosis. With the latter condition, addition of exogenous catecholamine can precipitate a thyroid storm.[3]

LARYNGECTOMY

Laryngectomy can be performed with regional anesthesia by blockade of the sensory fibers of the recurrent laryngeal and superior laryngeal nerves (see Fig. 2–9) as well as of the superficial cervical plexus (see Fig. 2–11).

ACUPUNCTURE ANESTHESIA

For centuries, traditional healers from China have used acupuncture for analgesia. More recently, circa 1957, Chinese researchers have found acupuncture capable of providing satisfactory anesthesia for head and neck surgery. Successful acupuncture anesthetics have been reported for tonsillectomies and thyroidectomies. Limited data are available regarding its associated hemodynamic stability, but systolic blood pressure is commonly reported to increase only 20% or less.

Not all patients respond well to acupuncture anesthesia. Patients with a high pain tolerance do best. Medications such as metoclopramide, droperidol, and fentanyl typically improve the effectiveness of acupuncture anesthesia. In contrast, ketamine and diazepam appear to decrease the effectiveness of acupuncture anesthesia. In the future, acceptable candidates—estimated as 70% of the general population—might be found by testing to see if the psychogalvanic reflex can be blocked with acupuncture.[9]

Additional information concerning acupuncture anesthesia can be obtained by writing to Xiao-Ding Cao, M.D., Ph.D., Professor of Neurobiology and Director of the Institute of Acupuncture Research, 138 Yi Xue Yuan Road, Shanghai 200032, People's Republic of China (FAX 0086-021-330543).

REFERENCES

1. Cousins MJ, Bridenbaugh PO: Neural Blockade in Clinical Anesthesia and Pain Management. Philadelphia, JB Lippincott, 1988, pp 533–558.
2. Adriani J: Labat's Regional Anesthesia: Techniques and Clinical Applications, 3rd ed. Philadelphia, WB Saunders, 1969, pp 150–151.
3. Eriksson E: Illustrated Handbook in Local Anaesthesia, 2nd ed. London, Lloyd-Luke Medical Books, 1979, pp 36–45.
4. Cooper M, Watson RL: An improved regional anesthetic technique for peroral endoscopy. Anesthesiology 1975; 43:372–374.
5. Wittich DJ, Berny JJ, Davis RV: Cervical epidural anesthesia for head and neck surgery. Laryngoscope 1984; 94:615–619.
6. Kainuma M, Shimada Y, Matsuura M: Cervical epidural anesthesia in carotid artery surgery. Anaesthesia 1986; 41:1020–1023.
7. Ullman DA, Schmitt L: Tracheostomy performed under epidural anesthesia. Anesthesiology 1989; 71:161–162.
8. Raj P: Handbook of Regional Anesthesia. New York, Churchill Livingstone, 1985, p 106.
9. Cao Xiao-Ding: Acupuncture anesthesia. Yale China Society Lecture, Yale University, November 29, 1990.

3

Managing Difficult Intubations

Kathryn E. McGoldrick

The importance of maintaining a patent airway has been recognized for millennia. Indeed, the first documented relief of a potentially fatal airway obstruction dates back to the second century A.D., when Antullus performed a tracheostomy. However, systematic approaches to the management of difficult airways or of airway obstruction were not well developed until the twentieth century.

Airway management demands much more than mere technical proficiency with traditional methods of intubation. The anesthesiologist must be highly skilled in assessing the adequacy of the airway and must be familiar with the implications of various forms of airway pathology. Clearly, patients with certain congenital, inflammatory, neoplastic, or traumatic disease processes may have imperfect airways. In addition to being adept at identifying patients in whom airway management may be challenging, the anesthesiologist must possess the knowledge and flexibility to formulate and implement alternative plans in the context of various clinical situations. As Shakespeare wrote in *King Lear:* "Readiness is all." The best way to prevent complications is to anticipate them.

ASSESSING THE AIRWAY: CAUSES OF DIFFICULT INTUBATIONS

The incidence of difficult intubation has been reported to range between 0.13[1] and 5.9%.[2] Although some data suggest that a high percentage of problem intubations are predictable,[3] other data conclude that many problem cases cannot be anticipated.[2] In their prospective study of 778 patients, Wilson and colleagues[2] were able to detect in advance 75% of complicated laryngoscopies. However, the false-positive rate associated with their criteria was unacceptably high.

A variety of factors may complicate laryngoscopy and intubation. Depending on the case, the larynx may be completely normal but inaccessible and difficult to expose (Fig. 3–1). Alternatively, the larynx may be distorted, narrowed, or displaced by a pathological process that impedes visualization. Moreover, disease or deformity of the tongue, mouth, jaw, tonsils, pharynx, or neck may hamper the performance of laryngoscopy and intubation.

A thorough preoperative history and physical examination are essential for accurate assessment of the airway. Indeed, this evaluation is the first step in the management of difficult airway problems.

The patient should be questioned about hoarseness or any recent voice change, shortness of breath, hemoptysis, dysphagia, and history of airway trauma or neoplasia, as well as about prior anesthetic experiences. Inquiry should be made concerning a history of radiation to the head or neck, because this can cause edema and induration of oropharyngeal soft tissue. Whenever feasible, previous anesthesia records should be studied. These may provide helpful information about techniques employed, the type of laryngoscope blade selected, and the size of the endotracheal tube used.

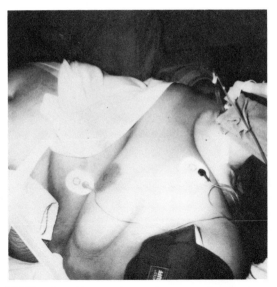

FIGURE 3–1. Obesity is frequently associated with difficult airway management. Intubation of this 550-pound woman was accomplished with the patient awake. (Photograph courtesy of Jan Ehrenwerth, M.D., Professor of Anesthesiology, Yale University School of Medicine.)

Physical examination is invaluable. Cass and associates[4] described prognostic signs of the difficult airway. These included a short, muscular neck with a full set of teeth; micrognathia with obtuse mandibular angles; protruding maxillary incisors owing to relative overgrowth of the premaxilla; poor mobility of the mandible owing to temporomandibular arthritis or trismus; a long, high-arched palate associated with a long, narrow mouth; and increased alveolomental distance. Others have mentioned the difficulties encountered with limited extension of the lower cervical vertebrae, increased posterior mandibular depth, and decreased (less than 3 fingerbreadths) distance from the symphysis of the mandible to the thyroid notch with the head fully extended.

Inability to open the mouth adequately may be due to a variety of causes, including microsomia, temporomandibular joint dysfunction, or trismus owing to pain rather than a structural deformity. Microsomia may be congenital, or it may be the result of contractures following burns. In addition, decreased mouth opening and neck mobility may be associated with a rare disease, such as myositis ossificans progressiva, or with a more common condition, such as rheumatoid arthritis. Although trismus associated with an acute process often disappears once the patient is anesthetized, trismus is not invariably improved by anes-

thesia and muscle relaxants, especially if it is severe and has existed for more than 24 hours.[5]

Cleft or high-arched palates may interfere with laryngoscopy and can be isolated findings or components of a malformation syndrome. Similarly, a large tongue may be associated with conditions such as acromegaly, Beckwith's syndrome, or trisomy 21 (Fig. 3–2). One can assess the probable degree of difficulty that will accompany intubation by asking the seated patient to open his or her mouth and maximally protrude the tongue. Mallampati and associates[6] determined that if the soft palate, fauces, uvula, and pillars are visible, an easy intubation should be expected. If, however, not even the soft palate is seen, extreme difficulty with intubation should be expected (Fig. 3–3).

Detection of micrognathia should be done viewing the patient in profile as well as frontally. A hypoplastic mandible or very short neck is characteristically associated with larynxes that are extremely anterior and difficult to visualize during conventional laryngoscopy. Syndromes associated with these problems include arthrochalasis multiplex congenita, arthrogryposis, Cornelia de Lange's syndrome,

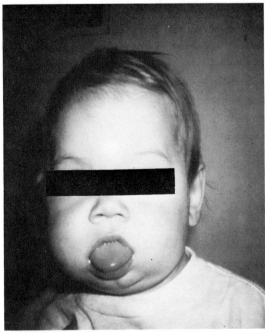

FIGURE 3–2. A large tongue, as seen in this child with Beckwith-Wiedemann syndrome, is commonly associated with challenging airway management situations. (Photograph courtesy of Burton Epstein, M.D., Professor of Anesthesiology, George Washington University School of Medicine.)

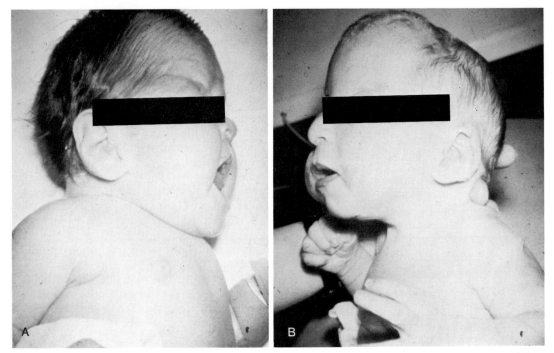

FIGURE 3–3. *Patients with craniofacial dysostosis, as seen with Apert syndrome* (A) *and Crouzon's disease* (B), *are frequently difficult to intubate. (Photographs courtesy of Burton Epstein, M.D., Professor of Anesthesiology, George Washington University School of Medicine.)*

cri du chat syndrome, DiGeorge's syndrome, Goldenhar's syndrome, Klippel-Feil syndrome, Noonan's syndrome, Pierre Robin syndrome, Treacher Collins syndrome, and Turner's syndrome (Fig. 3–4).

Although not all anterior larynxes can be appreciated in advance, the Schwartz-hyoid maneuver may be useful in identifying the anterior larynx. If the anteroposterior depth from the mentum to the hyoid bone is less than 3 cm, visualization of the larynx may be difficult. The probable ease of intubation can be predicted also by measuring the distance between the lower border of the mandible and

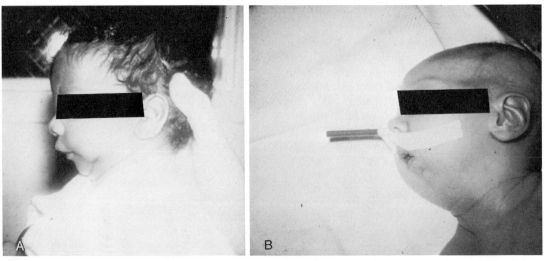

FIGURE 3–4. *A hypoplastic mandible is characteristic of individuals with Treacher Collins syndrome* (A) *and Pierre Robin syndrome* (B). *(Photographs courtesy of Burton Epstein, M.D., Professor of Anesthesiology, George Washington University School of Medicine.)*

the thyroid notch with the neck fully extended. Normally in adults, this distance is 6.5 cm or more. If the measurement is less, difficulty visualizing the larynx should be anticipated.[7, 8] It should be mentioned, moreover, that the term "anterior larynx" is somewhat of a misnomer. Certainly all larynxes are anterior in the sense that they are anterior to the esophagus. However, the term suggests that the position of the larynx has been displaced forward from the normal anatomical relationship. Although in some circumstances such may be the case, the term may sometimes be misleading in that other abnormal variants of the head and neck anatomy may give the false perception that the larynx is displaced anteriorly. For example, a large tongue, a truncated mandible, or a short neck modifies anatomical and spatial relationships such that the larynx is *perceived* to be displaced anteriorly. Under these circumstances, visualization of the larynx is difficult because the strategic position of the laryngoscope has been displaced posteriorly, not because the larynx has been displaced anteriorly.

Tumors or abscesses of the pharynx, hypopharynx, or larynx can displace and distort landmarks in addition to narrowing the airway. Use of the accessory muscles for respiration can suggest ominous airway obstruction. Indeed, stridor at rest implies that the airway diameter of an adult has been narrowed to less than 5 mm.[9]

The neck should be inspected carefully for length, thickness, and the presence of an old tracheostomy scar that might be indicative of previous airway problems. In addition, the neck should be palpated to detect masses and tracheal deviation. Moreover, the mobility and stability of the neck should be ascertained as well as the presence of vertebral artery compression.

Evaluation of cervical spine mobility is essential, because endotracheal intubation typically involves flexion of the lower cervical spine and extension of the neck at the atlanto-occipital joint to properly align the oral, pharyngeal, and laryngeal axes. Although the normal range of neck flexion-extension varies from 165 to 90 degrees and decreases somewhat with age, patients with ankylosing spondylitis[10] or rheumatoid arthritis may have almost no neck mobility as well as possible vertebral instability.[11] In addition, patients with facial, neck, and upper chest burns, those who have had radiation therapy to the head or neck, and individuals with critically placed fractures will also have markedly impaired range of motion of the cervical spine.

Any movement that triggers paresthesias or sensory or motor deficits must be avoided during intubation. External fixation devices may be necessary to protect against neurological damage. At the least, the head should be maintained in neutral position during intubation; neck manipulation must be avoided. Radiological demonstration of a distance from the anterior arch of the atlas to the odontoid process in excess of 3 mm confirms the diagnosis of atlantoaxial subluxation in the adult.[12] Its significance is that the displaced odontoid process can compress the cervical spinal cord or medulla, in addition to occluding the vertebral arteries. Even minimal trauma, as may be associated with movement of the neck during tracheal intubation, may cause further displacement of the odontoid process and damage to the underlying spinal cord. In addition to rheumatoid arthritis, ankylosing spondylitis, and cervical trauma, other conditions that predispose to atlantoaxial subluxation include pharyngeal infections and tumors, chondrodystrophia calcificans congenita, chondrodysplasia punta, spondyloepiphyseal dysplasia, and mucopolysaccharidosis.[13] Syndromes associated with atlantoaxial subluxation include Down's, Klippel-Feil, Kniest's, and Larsen's. The flexibility of the transverse ligament of the cervical spine of young children, combined with immaturity of the odontoid process, may place children at risk for atlantoaxial subluxation, at least until the odontoid fuses to the atlas at approximately age 4.[13]

Of interest is a retrospective investigation by Hogan and associates[14] reporting a 32% incidence of difficult laryngoscopies in diabetic patients having renal transplantation. The authors speculate that the stiff joint syndrome (SJS), a condition seen in some type I insulin-dependent diabetic patients in association with rapidly progressive microangiopathy, nonfamilial short stature, tight waxy skin, and limited joint mobility, might contribute to the technical difficulty encountered. Because SJS first involves the small joints of the digits and hands, failure to approximate the palmar surfaces of the interphalangeal joints (the "prayer sign") is highly correlated with SJS. Bedside examination of the neck can be misleading, however, because normal cervical mobility masks limited atlanto-occipital extension. Thus, cervical radiography, demonstrating inability to extend the atlanto-occipital joint, is essential for accurate diagnosis. Therefore, Hogan and associates recommend flexion-extension radiography of the cervical spine in diabetics with physical findings suggestive of SJS.[14] However, others have failed to demonstrate such a high incidence of difficult intubations in diabetic patients undergoing kidney transplantation.[15] Perhaps a prospective study from multiple institutions is needed to clarify this issue.[16]

Trauma to the cervical spine may be associated with significant prevertebral soft tissue swelling (PSTS).[17, 18] Indeed, its radiographic presence may indicate occult fracture of the adjacent vertebrae.[17-19] A more recent case report[20] describing sudden loss of airway patency from massive post-traumatic PSTS during placement of halotraction for cervical spine injury should be of interest to anesthesiologists, trauma surgeons, and radiologists.

In addition to a thorough history and physical examination as outlined earlier, other valuable aids to airway evaluation include anteroposterior and lateral radiographs of the neck and chest. Computed tomography is helpful in locating and quantitating both intrinsic and extrinsic airway aberrations. Moreover, both indirect laryngoscopy with a laryngeal mirror and flexible fiberoptic nasopharyngoscopy can be extremely useful in evaluating the pharynx and larynx.

ANTICIPATED DIFFICULT INTUBATIONS

GENERAL PRINCIPLES

Upper airway problems can be divided conveniently into three categories[21]:

1. Patients with an unobstructed airway for whom the mask airway may be easily manageable. However, intubation is made difficult by physiognomical or pathological anomalies or factors.

2. Patients with an obviously obstructed airway.

3. Patients in whom impending obstruction of the airway is compensated or concealed on presentation but occurs on induction of anesthesia, administration of muscle relaxants, or extubation. Such situations may occur with certain supraglottic neoplasms, pedunculated intralaryngeal lesions, extremely large tonsils and adenoids, or various congenital deformities for which the patient ordinarily compensates by muscular effort. Although extensive lesions of the oropharynx, tongue, or larynx may not cause clinically obvious obstruction when the patient is awake, the loss of pharyn-

geal muscle tone associated with general anesthesia may precipitate respiratory obstruction.

When problems are anticipated, a carefully conceived and detailed plan of management should be formulated in advance. This thoughtful strategy should include contingency planning and alternative techniques, in case the primary course of action fails.

Preparation in the operating room involves meticulous assembly of prearranged emergency airway equipment and experienced personnel. If the airway is compromised, it is essential to apprise the surgeon of the airway management plan and to have him or her physically present and prepared for emergency tracheostomy or other emergency surgical intervention.

Common signs of airway obstruction include stridor, tachypnea, cyanosis, anxiety, retractions and nasal flaring, diaphoresis, tachycardia, drooling, a muffled voice, and aphonia. Unlike cases of difficult intubations in patients with normal airways, patients with compromised airways must not be given muscle relaxants until the airway is secure. Moreover, "blind" awake intubations should not be attempted. Acceptable options for patients with compromised airways include awake direct laryngoscopy after topical anesthetization of the airway, spontaneous breathing of an inhalational agent (a plan frequently selected for children and uncooperative adults), awake fiberoptic intubation, and tracheostomy under local anesthesia.[22] In emergency situations, transtracheal oxygenation through cricothyrotomy and a 14-gauge needle can be accomplished. Each case must be assessed in context, and decisions should be based on the individual clinical picture, the available ancillary facilities, and the judgment and skill of the anesthesiologist.[5]

When the airway is normal and unobstructed, there is more flexibility in dealing with these Category 1 patients. An awake inspection is usually selected when it is anticipated that intubation of an adult patient will be technically challenging. If the initial preoperative evaluation suggests that intubation may be difficult, a more definitive examination can be performed in the operating room in the awake, but sedated, patient prior to the induction of anesthesia. Following administration of antisialagogues, the patient can be comfortably and safely sedated with combinations of tranquilizers and narcotics. The application of topical anesthesia to the mouth, tongue, and posterior pharynx permits gentle laryngoscopic examination. Not infrequently, such an examination may provide a view of the epiglottis and arytenoids. If it seems that endotracheal intubation will not be as challenging as previously suspected, then usually general anesthesia can be induced with conventional drugs prior to securing the airway. However, if examination reveals that intubation will be extremely difficult, awake intubation is the safest course of action.

PATIENT PREPARATION

Intubation with the patient awake must be performed in a gentle, deliberate fashion. Patient cooperation is essential for success. Special care should be devoted, therefore, to delivering a lucid explanation of the reasons for using an awake technique, stressing its increased safety, and outlining what the patient should expect to experience. The patient should be calmly and firmly reassured that discomfort will be minimized with local anesthesia and sedation. If, however, possible respiratory obstruction or severe respiratory depression is an issue, sedatives should be withheld until the patient is in the operating room, receiving supplemental oxygen, and properly monitored. Various combinations of narcotics and tranquilizers, such as fentanyl, midazolam, and droperidol, are carefully titrated intravenously (IV) in small amounts until the desired effect is achieved.

If possible, H_2 receptor blockers, such as cimetidine 300 mg or ranitidine 150 mg, should be given orally the night before surgery and again 90 minutes prior to the procedure to reduce the acidity of gastric contents.

Antisialagogues, such as atropine, scopolamine, or glycopyrrolate, are tremendously helpful, because secretions not only hinder visibility during laryngoscopy but also impair the efficacy of topically applied local anesthetics by their dilutional and barrier effects.[5] Appropriate dosages of these drugs should be administered intramuscularly (IM) 1 hour prior to airway manipulation and may be supplemented IV after the patient has arrived in the operating room.

The patient should be optimally positioned on the operating table equipped with a headpiece capable of flexion and extension. Folded towels should be readily available for insertion under the patient's head, neck, or shoulders as needed. Monitors, including an electrocardiogram (ECG), an automated blood pressure cuff, a precordial stethoscope, and a pulse oximeter, are applied. A capnometer or capnograph is especially valuable once intubation has been accomplished, but it can be adapted into nasal prongs delivering supplemental oxygen prior to intubation.

EQUIPMENT

An assortment of equipment must be available for airway management. This equipment must include a Magill forceps, widebore suction, oropharyngeal and nasopharyngeal airways of different sizes, and endotracheal tubes of various sizes, into which lubricated stylets have been inserted. Both straight and curved laryngoscope blades must be available in a wide array of sizes. A straight blade can be especially valuable in the setting of glottic or supraglottic cysts or tumors, because it can be used to displace obstructing tissue. Moreover, in cases of epiglottic pathology it may be impossible to insert a curved blade in the usual intended fashion.

A variety of laryngoscope blades have been designed for use in patients with an anterior larynx, a restricted mouth opening, or a short, obese neck. These include the curved Bijarri-Griffrida and the Siker blades. The Siker has a mirrored surface, allowing visualization of the extremely anterior larynx; however, it has the disadvantage of reversing and inverting the image. In patients in whom the distance from thyroid cartilage to mandible is particularly truncated, it may be advisable to attach Huffman prism clips directly onto the number 3 MacIntosh blade. Unlike the Siker blade, Huffman prism clips neither invert nor reverse the image.[21] Many anesthesiologists find a Bullard laryngoscope to be helpful in cases involving difficult laryngeal exposure (Fig. 3–5).

Fourteen-gauge needles or cannulae, a 3-mm endotracheal tube adapter, cannulae for cricothyroidotomy, and equipment for emergency transtracheal ventilation should be available (Fig. 3–6). In addition, a rigid bronchoscope, a flexible fiberoptic endoscope, "lighted stylet," and equipment for retrograde intubation should be accessible. For cases involving tracheal stenosis, a rigid pediatric bronchoscope should be included. Many institutions have a Difficult Intubation Cart to ensure that this special equipment is readily accessible when needed.

TOPICAL ANESTHESIA

After the patient and the necessary equipment have been prepared appropriately, the anes-

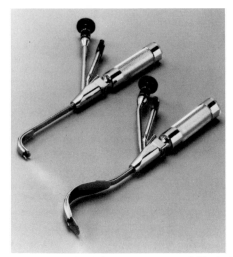

FIGURE 3–5. Bullard laryngoscopes, available in both pediatric and adult sizes, may facilitate difficult intubations.

thesiologist may proceed with topical anesthetization of the airway to facilitate awake intubation. Expertise in this phase of practice can greatly enhance both the smoothness and the safety of difficult airway management. Ineffective application of local anesthesia, for example, can foster agitation and gagging, which in turn can exacerbate obstruction in patients with airway compromise.

If nasotracheal intubation is planned, topical application of 4 or 10% cocaine to the nasal mucosa provides both satisfactory analgesia and vasoconstriction. Ribbon gauze or cotton-tipped applicators soaked with cocaine are inserted into the nostril for 5 minutes. The amount of cocaine must be carefully titrated and should not exceed 3 mg/kg. Moreover,

cocaine is contraindicated in severe hypertensives and in those patients receiving such adrenergic-modifying drugs as guanethidine, reserpine, tricyclic antidepressants, or monoamine oxidase inhibitors.[23]

Anesthesia of the tongue, epiglottis, and glottis is necessary for smooth laryngoscopy; anesthesia of the vocal cords, endolarynx, and trachea greatly facilitates tracheal intubation. Numerous techniques are available to accomplish these objectives.

Benumof[24] recommends a spray system that creates a fine, dense, deeply penetrating mist of local anesthetic. He furthermore suggests 0.5% tetracaine with 1:200,000 epinephrine as the agent of choice.[24] The system that best produces this type of mist consists of a high-flow oxygen source connected by oxygen supply tubing (with a hole in it) to the back of an atomizer.[25] When oxygen is flowing through the tubing and a finger is placed over the hole, a penetrating mist of local anesthetic is produced. Short spray intervals should be alternated with rest intervals (10–15 seconds), and sufficient time should be allowed to adequately topicalize the patient. Usually, a minimum of 10 minutes is required. Spraying can be discontinued when the operator can touch the epiglottis with the spray end of the atomizer without patient reaction. Nebulizers that produce a mist of topical anesthetic solution for inhalation by mouthpiece have been described also.[26, 27]

Another popular method involves placing a 5% lidocaine ointment on the tongue and allowing it to slowly melt and spread posteriorly. This should allow insertion of the laryngoscope blade. If this is inadequate, additional

FIGURE 3–6. Nu-trake sets are potentially valuable in situations requiring emergency airway establishment.

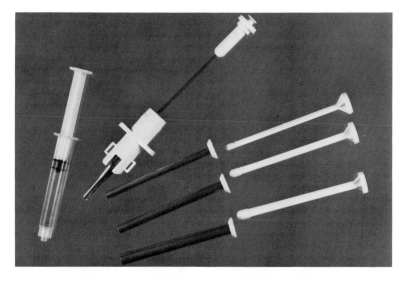

ointment can be applied with the laryngoscope blade itself. Once the lower pharynx and posterior larynx become visible, the tongue is gently lifted anteriorly, and 4% lidocaine solution is sprayed into the pharynx and toward the glottis. Spraying into the larynx is best timed to coincide with a deep inspiration. The total dosage of lidocaine should not exceed 4 mg/kg.

Other approaches to local anesthesia for awake intubation include bilateral glossopharyngeal nerve block, bilateral superior laryngeal nerve block, and transtracheal injection. These are described in detail in Chapter 2. In performing bilateral glossopharyngeal nerve block, which provides anesthesia to the posterior one third of the tongue and eliminates the gag reflex,[128] paralysis of the pharyngeal muscles may trigger airway obstruction in certain predisposed individuals. In performing superior laryngeal nerve block, there is the option of either applying anesthesia-soaked pledgets to the pyriform fossa or entering the neck percutaneously. Transtracheal injection of 4 mL of 2% lidocaine solution through the cricothyroid membrane provides satisfactory anesthesia to the region below the vocal cords. Superior laryngeal and transtracheal blocks—as well as any other methods that deliver anesthesia to the area of the vocal cords and below—are contraindicated in patients at risk of aspiration of gastric contents.

SPECIAL TECHNIQUES

FLEXIBLE FIBEROPTIC ENDOSCOPY

Since its clinical introduction almost one quarter of a century ago, the fiberoptic bronchoscope has had a wide variety of applications, including diagnosing pulmonary disease; assisting tracheal intubation; confirming proper placement of endotracheal, tracheostomy, and endobronchial tubes; and removing pulmonary secretions.

Details of techniques for fiberoptic endoscope use are available in several publications.[29–31] Briefly, the scope is advanced through the larynx and inserted into the trachea. The endotracheal tube is then introduced into the trachea, over the fiberscope, employing the fiberscope as a stylet.

Laryngoscopy and intubation are most easily accomplished through the nasal route, which seems to direct the instrument "naturally" toward the glottis. However, for cases in which orotracheal intubation is demanded or desirable, various oropharyngeal airways (Fig. 3–7) are available that hold the tongue forward and centrally position the fiberscope, guiding it toward the larynx. (These airway guides are particularly useful if the patient is under general anesthesia and muscle tone in the tongue has been markedly attenuated.) Because secretions obliterate or eliminate the view, it is extremely important to pretreat with antisialagogues and to apply suction as needed. Elevating the head, if possible, may aid in secretion management. The fiberoptic scope is perhaps most valuable when pharyngeal and laryngeal anatomy are normal, but access through conventional laryngoscopy is impaired. In patients with laryngeal distortion, recognition of landmarks may be extremely difficult. However, the endotracheal tube should not be inserted blindly in these difficult cases, because trauma with hemorrhage and edema may ensue. These events could trigger serious complications such as respiratory obstruction and laryngospasm. Most skillful endoscopists emphasize that successful use of the fiberoptic endoscope in difficult situations requires considerable previous experience using the instrument for elective, routine intubation in patients with normal anatomy. In addition, when fiberoptic equipment and expertise are available, a strong case should be made for using this technique *before* attempting blind nasal intubation, lest inadvertent epistaxis obscure or totally obliterate visualization.

Typical causes of failed fiberoptic intubation are listed in Tables 3–1 and 3–2.

Fiberoptic endoscopy also may be employed in the pediatric population.[32] The 5.8-mm bronchoscope may be used with a 6.5-mm inside diameter (ID) tube, and the 3.2-mm bronchoscope threads through an endotracheal tube with a minimum 4.5-mm ID. However, the 3.2-mm fiberoptic scope lacks suction or ventilating capabilities, so secretions may easily obscure the view. Furthermore, because in the small child the 3.2-mm bronchoscope significantly occludes the upper trachea, the tube must be quickly passed over the scope, and the scope must be rapidly removed to permit unobstructed oxygenation and ventilation.[32] In an infant or small child, the 2.7-mm outside diameter (OD) fiberoptic bronchoscope passes through endotracheal tubes with internal diameters ranging between 3.0 and 4.0 mm. The 2.7-mm scope has similar shortcomings to the 3.2-mm scope in its lack of a suction port and

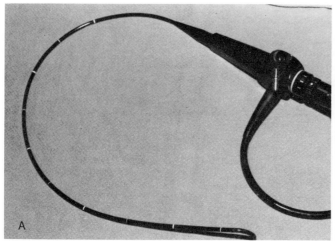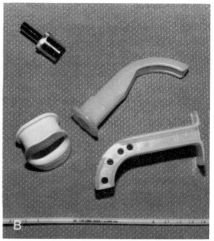

FIGURE 3–7 (A and B). *A variety of oral airways are available to facilitate endotracheal intubation with a flexible fiberoptic endoscope. (Photographs courtesy of Dorothy J. Gaal, M.D., Assistant Professor of Anesthesiology, Yale University School of Medicine.)*

the inability of patients to breathe well through an endotracheal tube, which is smaller than 3.5 mm with the 2.7-mm scope inside it. The same caveats regarding speed with instrumentation clearly apply. Moreover, 4.5 mm is the maximum size tube that should be used with the 2.7-mm instrument.[32] A larger tube is so stiff that it is difficult to use with the smallest pediatric flexible fiberoptic bronchoscope.

BLIND NASOTRACHEAL INTUBATION[21]

Not uncommonly, an individual with an anterior larynx that escapes visualization with conventional direct laryngoscopy does well with a blind nasotracheal intubation. First, the axes of the mouth, pharynx, and larynx are aligned by extending the head at the atlanto-occipital joint and flexing the neck at the cervical spine, achieving the so-called sniffing position. Intubation may be performed then under general anesthesia, with local anes-

thesia, or without anesthesia. However, for optimal results, spontaneous respiration should be preserved. Following application of a vasoconstrictor, such as cocaine, to the more patent naris, a nasotracheal tube is inserted into the chosen nostril and advanced gently into the oropharynx and then to the laryngeal entrance. Breath sounds are used to indicate the correct path through the larynx into the trachea. Skillful positioning of the head and neck may help guide the nasotracheal tube into the trachea. Head flexion tends to align the tube with the esophagus, whereas extension often aligns the axis of the tube with the trachea. In addition, tilting the head to the side on which the tube enters the naris may help align the tip of the tube with the trachea.

Clearly, blind intubation techniques should not be attempted—or even contemplated—for lesions of the tongue, pharynx, or larynx. Trauma to friable tumors or abscesses may result in airway obstruction or aspiration of pus. Hemorrhage and laryngospasm may ensue

TABLE 3–1. Causes of Failed Fiberoptic Intubation

Lack of training and experience
Presence of secretions or blood
Inadequate topical anesthesia
Decreased space between tip of epiglottis and posterior pharyngeal wall
Distorted airway anatomy
Endotracheal tube that could not be advanced
Fiberscope that could not be withdrawn

From Ovassapian A, Dykes MHM: The role of fiberoptic endoscopy in airway management. Semin Anesth 1987; 6:93–104.

TABLE 3–2. Causes of Decreased Space Between Tip of Epiglottis and Posterior Pharyngeal Wall

Large floppy epiglottis
Hypotonicity of oropharyngeal tissues or use of general anesthesia with a muscle relaxant
Elevation of floor of the mouth by edema, tumor, or hematoma
Supraglottic mass pushing epiglottis posteriorly
Severe flexion deformity of the cervical spine

From Ovassapian A, Dykes MHM: The role of fiberoptic endoscopy in airway management. Semin Anesth 1987; 6:93–104.

also. As previously mentioned, epistaxis or blood from other traumatized areas may thwart use of fiberoptic endoscopy if blind nasotracheal intubation fails.

TACTILE INTRAORAL ENDOTRACHEAL TUBE PLACEMENT

Sklar and King[33] have described a variant of blind nasotracheal intubation of a nonvisualized larynx in a child with Treacher Collins syndrome. A nasal endotracheal tube is placed into the pharynx. While it functions as a nasopharyngeal airway, inhalation anesthesia is induced and maintained with spontaneous respiration. The anesthesiologist's second and third fingers are inserted into the mouth over the anesthetized child's tongue. Following palpation of the epiglottis, the tube is directed between the two fingers into the glottis.

The same technique has been successful also in directing a nasotracheal tube in the presence of severe flexion contracture of the neck secondary to burn scarring and also in a case involving partial traumatic loss of the mandible.[32]

LIGHTED STYLET

The lighted stylet, or lightwand, is a malleable stylet equipped with a battery in its handle and a light bulb at its tip, which allows intubation without direct laryngoscopy. Prior to insertion, the lightwand is lubricated and placed in a transparent plastic endotracheal tube and angled into the typical "hockey stick" position. With the patient's head in the sniffing position, the anesthesiologist opens the patient's mouth, holds the tongue forward, and gently inserts the tube and stylet centrally over the tongue and into the glottis. Correct placement is confirmed by dimming the room lights and observing the neck. If the larynx is brightly illuminated, the position of the stylet is maintained, and the endotracheal tube is advanced through the glottic opening into the trachea. High success rates have been reported using this simple technique.[34, 35] However, the technique may prove ineffective in cases of massive obesity, neck edema, and neck neoplasia, where laryngeal illumination may be obscured. Moreover, the technique is contraindicated in patients with intraoral or laryngeal tumors, airway compromise, or laryngeal trauma. Indeed, any blind technique would be ill-advised in these situations.

RETROGRADE TRACHEAL INTUBATION

Retrograde tracheal intubation involves percutaneous introduction of a needle through the cricothyroid membrane and then threading a guidewire through the membrane and up the trachea until the wire emerges through either the mouth or a nostril. In adults, this can be accomplished with a long-arm central venous pressure (CVP) catheter or an epidural catheter passed through the accompanying needle. A J-wire technique also can be employed in adults.[36] In children, a 20-gauge IV catheter with a 0.021 extra-long flexible tip guidewire* is appropriate.[37] The endotracheal tube is then inserted over the guide into the larynx and advanced into the trachea. The tip of the tube may catch on the anterior commissure and therefore not pass. Passage may be facilitated by threading the guidewire or catheter through the distal side hole (Murphy eye) rather than through the bevel,[38] and by keeping the guide taut during insertion of the tube. Gentle rotation of the tube (usually 90 degrees counterclockwise) may prove helpful also.

The larger the outside diameter of the stylet in relation to the internal diameter of the endotracheal tube, the greater the chance the tube will enter the trachea. For nonbloody cases, Benumof[24] favors passing a 125-cm guidewire retrograde, out the mouth, and up the suction port of a fiberoptic bronchoscope. This technique enables the endoscopist to visualize the trachea; the central position of the suction port within the fiberoptic bronchoscope forces the scope to follow the guidewire faithfully into the trachea.

Retrograde intubation can be performed under either local or general anesthesia. It should not be performed, however, unless the landmarks for percutaneous puncture are easily discernible. Contraindications to use of this procedure include airway compromise; pathology of the trachea, larynx, or pharynx; and local sepsis.

UNANTICIPATED AIRWAY DIFFICULTY

Despite meticulous preoperative evaluation, difficulty with intubation is not always predictable,[2, 39] and the problem may be recognized

---

*Becton-Dickinson, 100-cm 0.021, Safeguide, Stainless Steel Guide Wire.

only after general anesthesia has been administered. After a failed intubation attempt, the anesthesiologist must *immediately* try to determine the cause of the problem. Then, with each subsequent attempt, some modification of technique should be adopted to overcome the difficulty. These modifications include using a different laryngoscope blade, using a smaller size endotracheal tube, reshaping the stylet, changing the position of the patient's head, and asking an assistant to apply or release downward laryngeal pressure.

In the majority of these patients, the larynx is anatomically normal but relatively inaccessible, and satisfactory ventilation with face mask is well maintained between attempts. One should, however, resist the temptation to persist with multiple intubation attempts with conventional equipment, because this will only cause trauma, bleeding, copious secretions, and possible deterioration of the airway. Moreover, blood and secretions interfere with the use of a flexible fiberscope if such equipment becomes necessary. Hence, after a maximum of four unsuccessful attempts, either specialized techniques should be used, e.g., flexible fiberoptic endoscopy, lighted stylet, retrograde intubation or the patient should be allowed to emerge from anesthesia; in this case, intubation should be attempted under controlled conditions at a later time.[5]

An antisialagogue should be administered as soon as the decision is made to proceed with fiberoptic endoscopy. Often, general anesthesia can be maintained with a potent inhalation agent. It may be necessary or desirable, however, to reverse a nondepolarizing muscle relaxant to allow resumption of spontaneous ventilation. (In addition to the safety that spontaneous ventilation affords, bubbling secretions in the region of the airway may assist the anesthesiologist in identifying the larynx.) If the esophagus was inadvertently intubated, or if positive-pressure ventilation produced gastric distension, a nasogastric tube should be inserted to decompress the stomach.

If the procedure is emergent and the patient's condition unstable, general anesthesia should be abandoned, and the patient should be allowed to awaken.[7] The patient whose condition is rapidly deteriorating because of hemodynamic instability or airway obstruction is almost never a candidate for fiberoptic endoscope examination, because precious time may be lost in the process. Only if equipment is immediately available in the form of a Difficult Intubation Cart, for example, and only

if a highly skilled endoscopist is in attendance, should this route even be contemplated. In general, one should proceed immediately in the fashion described.

The incidence of patients who cannot be ventilated and cannot be intubated is difficult to determine but has ranged in the literature from 0.01 to 2.0/10,000 attempts to anesthetize.[39-43] Benumof and Scheller[44] more recently reported an institutional incidence at University of California, San Diego, of approximately 1 cannot ventilate/cannot intubate situation per 10,000 attempts during the mid to late 1980s. This desperate situation has been responsible for a previously irreducible 1–28% of all deaths associated with anesthesia.[39-43]

When ventilation by face mask is ineffective and progressive hypoxemia develops, transtracheal resuscitation should be instituted immediately. Percutaneous insertion of a 14-gauge needle through the cricothyroid membrane and attachment to an oxygen source (with jet ventilation if available) will maintain oxygenation[44] until a cricothyroidotomy cannula, such as Nu-trake, is inserted or until a tracheostomy can be performed. A 3-mm endotracheal tube adapter fits the hub of a 14-gauge needle and can be employed as a connector.

Establishment of percutaneous transtracheal jet ventilation (TTJV) is much quicker and simpler than percutaneous cricothyroidotomy and tracheostomy, provided TTJV is immediately available. "Immediately available" means that present in the anesthetizing location is a high pressure oxygen source and the requisite preassembled materials to connect the high pressure source to the hub of an IV catheter. The systems of choice, in descending order of desirability, are jet injector powered by regulated wall or oxygen tank pressure (50 psi), jet injector powered by unregulated wall or tank oxygen pressure, and anesthetic machine flush valve using noncompliant tubing from the fresh gas outlet. The fresh gas outlet of the anesthesia machine is connected to noncompliant oxygen supply tubing by a standard 15-mm endotracheal tube adapter that fits a 4-mm ID endotracheal tube. Less effective transtracheal ventilation systems consist of an anesthesia machine flush valve that uses the compliant tubing of the anesthesia circle system with reservoir bag and connects a reservoir bag directly to the transtracheal catheter.[44] Regardless of the system selected, the only way the jetted inspired oxygen can be exhaled is through the natural airway. Thus, every attempt must be made to maintain the natural airway. The chest must be observed to rise and fall after each jet in an attempt to prevent barotrauma.[24] Benumof and Scheller are eloquent advocates of the immediate availability of TTJV in every anesthetizing location.[44]

Confirmation of proper endotracheal tube placement must be accomplished following every intubation. Traditional methods of confirmation, such as auscultation of breath sounds, can sometimes be misleading, as in cases of gross obesity and severe chronic obstructive lung disease, in which the breath sounds may be distant and difficult to assess. However, capnometry or capnography is especially valuable in this setting, because persistent presence of carbon dioxide in the expired gas is reliable evidence that the trachea and not the esophagus has been intubated.[45]

SUMMARY

The causes of difficult intubation as well as the techniques and special equipment helpful in accomplishing these challenging intubations are presented in this chapter. Safe practice is based on careful observation and thorough preparation, gentleness, knowledge of anatomy and physiology, common sense, and an ever-present awareness and avoidance of potential mishaps.

REFERENCES

1. Edens ET, Sia RL: Flexible fiberoptic endoscopy in difficult incubations. Ann Otol Rhinol Laryngol 1981; 90:307–309.
2. Wilson ME, Spiegelhalter D, Robertson JA, Lesser P: Predicting difficult intubation. Br J Anaesth 1988; 61:211–216.
3. Sia RL, Edens ET: How to avoid problems when using the fiberoptic bronchoscope for difficult incubations. Anaesthesia 1981; 36:74.
4. Cass NM, James NR, Lines V: Difficult direct laryngoscopy complicating intubation for anaesthesia. Br Med J (Clin Res) 1956; 1:488–489.
5. Geffin B: Anesthesia and the "problem upper airway." Int Anesthesiol Clin 1990; 28:106–114.
6. Mallampati SR, Gatt SP, Gugino LD, et al: A clinical sign to predict tracheal intubation: A prospective study. Can Anaesth Soc J 1985; 32:429–433.
7. Stehling LC: Management of the airway. In Barash PG, Cullen BF, Stoelting RK (eds): Clinical Anesthesia. Philadelphia, JB Lippincott, 1989, pp 543–561.
8. McIntyre JWR: The difficult tracheal intubation. Can J Anaesth 34:204–213, 1987.
9. Geffin B, Grillo HC, Cooper JD, Pontoppidan H: Stenosis following tracheostomy for respiratory care. JAMA 1971; 216:1984–1988.
10. Sinclair JR, Mason RA: Ankylosing spondylitis: The case for awake intubation. Anaesthesia 1984; 39:3.
11. Brechner VL: Unusual problems in the management of airways. I. Flexion-extension mobility of the cervical vertebrae. Anesth Analg 1986; 47:362.
12. Smith PH, Sharp J, Kellgren JH: Natural history of rheumatoid cervical subluxations. Ann Rheum Dis 1972; 31:222–223.
13. Audenaert SM, Schmidt TE: Peril of atlantoaxial subluxation. Soc Pediatr Anesth Newsl 1990; 3:4.
14. Hogan KJ, Rusy D, Springman SR: Difficult laryngoscopy and diabetes mellitus. Anesth Analg 1988; 67:1162–1165.
15. Warner ME, Warner MA, Narr BJ: Difficult laryngoscopy and diabetes mellitus—letter to the editor. Anesth Analg 1989; 69:550.
16. Hogan KJ, Rusy D, Springman SR: Difficult laryngoscopy and diabetes mellitus—letter to the editor. Anesth Analg 1989; 69:550–551.
17. Rogers LF: Radiology of Skeletal Trauma. New York, Churchill Livingstone, 1982, p 280.
18. Harris JH Jr: Radiology of Acute Cervical Spine Trauma. Baltimore, Williams and Wilkins, 1978, pp 31–34.
19. Templeton PA, Young JW, Mirvis SE, Buddemeyer EU: The value of retropharyngeal soft tissue measurements in trauma of the adult cervical spine. Skeletal Radiol 1987; 16:98–104.
20. Meakem TD, Meakem TJ, Rappaport W: Airway compromise from prevertebral soft tissue swelling during placement of halotraction for cervical spine injury. Anesthesiology 1990; 73:775–776.
21. McGoldrick KE: Management of the airway in anesthesia. In Pillsbury HC, Goldsmith MM (eds): Operative Challenges in Otolaryngology Head and Neck Surgery. Chicago, Year Book Medical Publishers, 1990, pp 822–831.
22. Donlon JV Jr: Anesthesia and eye, ear, nose, and throat surgery. In Miller RD (ed): Anesthesia, 3rd ed. New York, Churchill Livingstone, 1990, pp 2001–2003.
23. Meyers EF: Cocaine toxicity during dacryocystorhinostomy. Arch Ophthalmol 1980; 98:842.
24. Benumof JL: Management of the difficult/impossible airway. 1990 Annual Refresher Course Lectures. Park Ridge, Illinois, American Society of Anesthesiologists, 1990, 163 pp 1–7.
25. Benumof JL: Anesthesia for Thoracic Surgery. Philadelphia, WB Saunders, 1987, p 331.
26. Palva T, Jokinen K, Saloheimo M, Karvonen P: Ultrasonic nebulizer in local anesthesia for bronchoscopy. J Otol Rhinol Laryngol 1975; 37:306.
27. Bourke D, Katz J, Tonneson A: Nebulized anesthesia for awake endotracheal intubation. Anesthesiology 1985;63:690–692.
28. Barton S, Williams JD: Glossopharyngeal nerve block. Arch Otolaryngol 1971; 93:186–188.
29. Taylor PA, Towey RM: The broncho-fiberscope as an aide to endotracheal intubation. Br J Anaesth 1972; 44:611–612.
30. Raj PP, Forestner J, Watson TD, et al: Techniques for fiberoptic laryngoscopy in anesthesia. Anesth Analg 1974; 53:708–712.
31. Ovassapian A, Dykes MHM: The role of fiberoptic endoscopy in airway management. Semin Anesth 1987; 6:93–104.
32. France NK, Beste DJ: Anesthesia for pediatric ear, nose, and throat surgery. In Gregory GA (ed): Pediatric Anesthesia, 2nd ed. New York, Churchill Livingstone, 1989, pp 1097–1147.
33. Sklar GS, King BD: Endotracheal intubation and Treacher-Collins syndrome. Anesthesiology 1976; 44:247.

34. Holtzman RS, Nargozian CD, Barry FF: Lightwand intubation in children with abnormal upper airways. Anesthesiology 1988; 69:784–787.
35. Robelen GT, Shulman MS: Use of the lighted stylet for difficult intubations in adult patients. Anesthesiology 1989; 71:439.
36. King HK, Wang LF, Khan AK, Wooten DJ: Translaryngeal guided intubation for difficult intubation. Crit Care Med 1987; 15:869.
37. Borland LM, Swan DM, Leff S: Difficult pediatric endotracheal intubation: A new approach to the retrograde technique. Anesthesiology 1981; 55:577.
38. Bourke D, Levesque PR: Modification of retrograde guide for endotracheal intubation. Anesth Analg 1974; 53:1013.
39. Keenan RL, Boyan CP: Cardiac arrest due to anesthesia. JAMA 1985; 253:2373–2377.
40. Taylor G, Larson CP, Prestwich R: Unexpected cardiac arrest during anesthesia and surgery. An environmental study. JAMA 1976; 236:2758–2760.
41. Bolander FMF: Deaths associated with anaesthesia. Br J Anaesth 1975; 47:36–40.
42. Harrison GG: Death attributable to anaesthesia. Br J Anaesth 1978; 50:1041–1046.
43. Davis DA: An analysis of anesthetic mishaps from medical liability claims. Int Anesthesiol Clin 1984; 22:31–42.
44. Benumof JL, Scheller MS: The importance of transtracheal jet ventilation in the management of the difficult airway. Anesthesiology 1989; 71:769–778.
45. Birmingham PK, Cheney FW, Ward RJ: Esophageal intubation: A review of detection techniques. Anesth Analg 1986; 65:886–891.

4

Endoscopy Procedures and Laser Surgery of the Airway

Kathryn E. McGoldrick
Michael D. Ho

MICROLARYNGOSCOPY

Kleinsasser described the technique of using the suspension laryngoscope and operating microscope in 1961.[1] This was a watershed in the field of laryngology, affording the surgeon enhanced diagnostic accuracy and surgical precision.

Although local anesthesia, in combination with intravenous (IV) sedation, has been used for microlaryngoscopy, the consensus is that general anesthesia is vastly superior. Unfortunately, an awake patient may experience discomfort and pain resulting in sudden movement intraoperatively that could compromise the surgical outcome. In addition to immobility of the vocal cords and patient safety, surgical goals include conditions that afford an adequate view of the area under scrutiny and sufficient space for instrumentation. Anesthetic concerns focus on protecting the lower airways, minimizing secretions and reflex activity, and ensuring satisfactory oxygenation and ventilation. In addition, because microlaryngoscopy is frequently performed on an outpatient basis, rapid, smooth emergence with return of protective airway reflexes is highly desirable. The importance of blunting intraoperative reflex responses that trigger hypertension, tachycardia, and other dysrhythmias cannot be overemphasized. Especially in patients with coronary artery disease, it is important to provide sufficient anesthetic depth and to avoid hypoxia and hypercarbia. IV or topical lidocaine, small doses of fentanyl (1–2 μg/kg IV), and a β-adrenergic receptor blocking agent, such as esmolol, can obtund the sympathetic response to airway manipulation. Labetalol may also be useful. The incidence of myocardial infarction or ischemia following microlaryngoscopic surgery has been reported to range between 1.5 and 4%.[2] Clearly, monitoring must be meticulous and include pulse oximetry, electrocardiography, continuous use of a precordial stethoscope, blood pressure determinations, and, in intubated patients, capnography.

PREOPERATIVE EVALUATION AND INDUCTION

Many different anesthetic techniques have been described for microlaryngoscopy, and each has inherent advantages and disadvantages. Regardless of the method ultimately selected, some basic principles of preoperative management are vital to patient safety.

It is imperative to assess the degree, if any, of airway obstruction, the adequacy of ventilation, and the feasibility of successful intubation. This evaluation is aided by noting the quality of the patient's voice, the presence or absence of stridor (Fig. 4–1) and retractions, and the patient's physiognomy and range of motion of the head and neck. Consultation with the ear, nose, and throat (ENT) surgeon

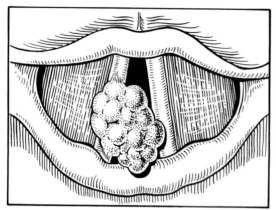

FIGURE 4–1. *A proliferative laryngeal tumor can significantly compromise the patient's airway and produce stridor.*

is invaluable in determining the findings from indirect laryngoscopy. Other diagnostic tools may include pertinent radiographs, computed tomography (CT), and magnetic resonance imaging (MRI). Moreover, pulmonary function and arterial blood gases should be documented in patients with respiratory impairment.

Patients at risk for respiratory obstruction or those with severe pulmonary disease are best brought to the operating room unpremedicated except for an antisialagogue. Those not at risk for airway obstruction may receive sedative premedication if they are anxious. However, light premedication is preferred to allow quick recovery postoperatively.

If preoperative examination suggests that the airway is unlikely to be visualized after the patient loses consciousness, the airway should be secured prior to administration of general anesthesia. In patients with significant airway obstruction, intubation is best performed over a fiberoptic endoscope rather than blindly in order to prevent tissue trauma and bleeding, which might exacerbate the obstruction or obscure the view. A tracheostomy performed under local anesthesia with the patient awake may be the optimal means of securing the airway when the degree of obstruction is severe. Once chest auscultation and capnography confirm proper tube placement, the patient may then be anesthetized.

If intubation seems feasible, anesthesia may be induced before the airway is secured. Following preoxygenation, either an IV or an inhalation induction can be performed. However, whenever anesthesia is induced in a patient with a challenging airway, a surgeon skilled in performing tracheostomy should be gowned and gloved in the operating room in case the planned method of airway management fails. Moreover, materials for performing cricothyroidotomy and rigid bronchoscopy should be immediately available in case emergency intervention is necessary.

INTRAOPERATIVE MANAGEMENT AND COMPLICATIONS

Microlaryngoscopy can be performed with or without a tracheal tube in place. When the anterior or posterior commissure area is involved, it may be advantageous to employ an anesthetic technique that does not require tracheal intubation in order to maximize the surgeon's view of the operative site. However, the overwhelming majority of these procedures can be adequately and safely performed without compromising the surgeon's view by using a narrow (5-mm), long (31-cm) endotracheal tube with a high-volume, low-pressure cuff[3] and controlling ventilation with 50% oxygen and a flow rate of 12 L/minute.[4] The use of a small endotracheal tube still allows proper oxygenation and ventilation, protects the trachea from aspiration, permits the application of positive-pressure ventilation, and gives the surgeon ample time to execute the operation. In addition, the likelihood of gastric distension and subsequent regurgitation is minimized in an intubated patient. Complete immobility of the vocal cords can be provided with IV administration of neuromuscular blocking agents.

Techniques that do not require endotracheal intubation have the advantage of maximizing surgical exposure. Ventilation can be accomplished through a metal needle attached to a Sanders-type jet-injector affixed to the operating laryngoscope.[5, 6] At the glottic opening, the surgeon directs a high velocity jet of oxygen that entrains room air as a result of the Venturi effect. The surgeon must position the jet in proper alignment with the glottis and trachea to maintain satisfactory ventilation and to avoid gastric dilatation and barotrauma. Only IV anesthetics can be given, because potent inhalational agents cannot be administered appropriately with this technique. The vocal cords must be fully relaxed to allow satisfactory inflow and free egress. Scrupulous surveillance of chest wall motion is essential at all times if the risk of barotrauma is to be minimized. Generally ventilation begins at pressures of 30–50 psi. The length of time allowed for passive exhalation should usually be at least three times the inspiratory duration. The jet Venturi technique is not appropriate for obese patients, those with bullous emphysema, or those with large tumors of the upper airway, in whom blood or tissue debris may be forced into the lungs or stomach or in whom the large size of the airway lesion makes obstruction during exhalation likely. The latter development greatly predisposes to severe barotraumatic injury.

Another anesthetic technique for microlaryngoscopy places a small catheter between the vocal cords for insufflation of potent anesthetic gases at high flows, with the patient breathing spontaneously. This technique has several disadvantages, including problems with regulation of anesthetic depth, because the inhaled anesthetic is subject to entrainment dilution and potential problems from an essentially unprotected airway. Moreover, with insufflation techniques, ambient air is contaminated with anesthetic gases. Lastly, because muscle relaxants cannot be used with spontaneous ventilation, there may be unwelcome motion of the vocal cords.

In 1980, Eng and associates[7] reported using high frequency positive-pressure ventilation (HFPPV) for laryngoscopy. Small tidal volumes at respiratory rates of 60 or more breaths per minute are delivered through a stiff 3.5- or 4.0-m catheter situated between the vocal cords. HFPPV is less apt to cause barotrauma than Venturi jet ventilation, especially in patients with obstructive airway disease. However, barotrauma may still occur. Studies have also explored the use of high frequency jet ventilation (HFJV) for laryngoscopy.[8] Indeed, the literature is replete with clinical applications of the several different modalities to provide high frequency ventilation (HFV). In addition to HFPPV and HFJV, these include high frequency flow interrupters (HFFI)[9] and high frequency oscillation (HFO).[10] The common characteristics of all forms of HFV is ventilation at small tidal volumes (less than dead-space) with high rates (60–3000 breaths per minute). These systems are said to enhance diffusive transport, minimize bulk transport, and improve intrapulmonary gas distribution. However, in addition to barotrauma, problems and complications associated with HFV include inadequate humidification, necrotizing tracheobronchitis, bronchospasm, and inadequate monitoring capabilities.[11] Although HFV appears to be effective in maintaining satisfactory pulmonary gas exchange at lower mean airway pressures, its precise role is yet to be defined. It is unclear whether HFV techniques possess any distinct advantage over traditional ventilation methods.

All of the aforementioned techniques performed without endotracheal intubation are contraindicated in patients in whom an unprotected airway is unwise.

LASERS AND AIRWAY SURGERY

Laser is an acronym for "light amplification by stimulated emission of radiation." The quantum optical theories of Albert Einstein, describing stimulated emission in 1917,[12] were the basic principles suggesting the possibility of laser action. However, it was not until 1960 that Maiman[13] described the first laser constructed in the United States. This discovery, followed shortly thereafter by the development of the carbon dioxide laser in 1964 by Patel, led to the rapid emergence and expansion of medical applications of lasers. The laser has emerged as a vital tool in ophthalmology and otolaryngology, as well as in dermatology and such subspecialties as plastic, gynecological, urological, and neurological surgery.

Laser surgery has the advantage of being precise and nontraumatic to healthy tissue, thereby producing less postoperative edema and pain. Moreover, the hemostasis associated with laser surgery is generally superb. However, lasers pose a potential risk to both patients and health care providers. These hazards include damage to eyes and skin, electric shock, fire and explosion, and the production of noxious fumes that may be mutagenic, may transmit infectious disease, and may cause acute bronchial inflammation.[14–16] When infrared lasers are used, toxic fumes must be evacuated from the operative site by suction of smoke and carbonaceous debris. Because the neodymium:yttrium-aluminum-garnet (Nd:YAG) and argon lasers can penetrate windows, any windows in the operating room should have an opaque covering. Moreover, a warning sign should be prominently displayed on the operating room door (Fig. 4–2). It is perhaps the potential for combustion, however, that most troubles the anesthesiologist when the surgical field lies near the airway.

Although communication and cooperation between anesthesiologist and surgeon are always important, they become crucial for safe laser surgery of the airway. Clearly, the choice of laser technique determines which anesthetics can be safely administered, and the selection of anesthetic techniques directly af-

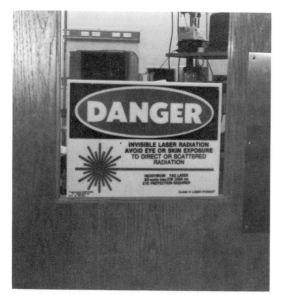

FIGURE 4-2. A conspicuous warning sign should be displayed whenever the laser is used. (Photograph courtesy of Dorothy J. Gaal, M.D., Assistant Professor of Anesthesiology, Yale University School of Medicine.)

fects the surgeon's ability to successfully execute a laser resection.

This section focuses on the types of lasers available, emphasizing their special applications in otolaryngological surgery and the important safety considerations about which all anesthesiologists should be vigilant when caring for patients having laser surgery of the airway.

PRINCIPLES OF LASER TECHNOLOGY

The physics of lasers is well described elsewhere[17] and is beyond the scope of this chapter. Suffice it to say that laser radiation has the following properties:

1. It is monochromatic. Hence, all the photons have the same wavelength, energy, and frequency.
2. It is coherent; all the photons are in phase. It is this coherence that allows the precision associated with laser surgery.
3. It is collimated, so its beam is nondivergent.
4. It has an extremely high energy density, affording great power.

The amount of radiant energy (joules) absorbed by tissues is the product of power (watts) multiplied by duration (seconds). In general, surgical lasers are employed in either a continuous or a pulsed mode.

The effect a particular laser beam may exert on tissue depends predominantly on its wavelength and power density. A particular laser's wavelength depends on its lasing medium, which also gives the laser its name. In general, the longer the wavelength, the more strongly absorbed the light. Hence, the power of the laser beam is converted to heat at a shallow depth. The converse is true: the shorter the wavelength, the more scattered the light. Because carbon dioxide (CO_2) lasers emit long wavelengths that are almost totally absorbed at the tissue surface, precise excision of lesions is possible. The much shorter wavelength of the Nd:YAG laser accounts for its ability to effectively heat large tissue masses for tumor debulking.[18] Moreover, coherent light of high power density excels in cutting or vaporizing tissue. Lower power densities are useful to coagulate and foster hemostasis. Another variable that can be manipulated to produce a given effect of optical energy on tissue is the duration of contact between laser beam and tissue.

TYPES OF LASERS

Carbon Dioxide Laser

The CO_2 laser has been used for a wide variety of surgical procedures, including general, plastic, neurological, and gynecological surgery (Table 4-1). It has had particularly extensive use in laryngology, where it has enjoyed popularity in the treatment of cysts, laryngeal carcinoma, laryngeal papillomas, and laryngeal webs. Carbon dioxide lasers have proven useful also in the resection of hemangiomas of the aerodigestive tract, and even for choanal atresia repair. Although laser excision of tonsils may perhaps result in fewer postoperative complications, it is a time-consuming, tedious process that is not considered efficient by many ENT surgeons.

The CO_2 laser beam is easily applied to lesions in the upper airway and proximal trachea. Hence, it often proves valuable for resection of stenoses or hemangiomas of the subglottic region. An innovative use of the CO_2 laser was more recently reported in two children with Hurler's syndrome who had upper tracheal obstruction secondary to progressive mucopolysaccharide deposition.[19] The upper tracheal lesions were successfully excised

TABLE 4–1. Features of Some Medical Lasers

Laser Type	Wavelength (nm)	Fiberoptic Transmission	Absorbed By	Mode	Uses in ENT or Eye Surgery
CO$_2$	10,600 (far infrared)	No	Water of all tissues	Pulsed/Continuous	Wide applications in airway surgery
Argon	488/515	Yes	Melanin/Hemoglobin	Continuous	Myringotomy, stapedectomy, and tympanoplasty; retinal work
Nd:YAG*	1064 (near infrared)	Yes	Darkly pigmented tissue	Pulsed	Lower airway tumor debulking; posterior segment work
Nd:YAG:KTP†	532	Yes	Melanin/Hemoglobin	Pulsed	Myringotomy, stapedectomy, and tympanoplasty
Ruby	695	Yes	Melanin/Cytochrome	Pulsed	Photocoagulation (ophthalmology)

*Neodymium:yttrium-aluminum-garnet
†Neodymium:yttrium-aluminum-garnet:potassium-titanyl-phosphate

with this laser. However, the Nd:YAG laser produces a greater depth of burn and can be transmitted through a fiberoptic cable, so this type of laser is used for tumor debulking and resection of lower tracheal and bronchial lesions.

Because of its infrared wavelength (10.6 μm), the radiation of the CO$_2$ laser is readily absorbed by blood, water, and all biological materials, regardless of tissue pigmentation. It literally vaporizes cells. Although CO$_2$ laser irradiation is invisible, most commercial CO$_2$ lasers incorporate a helium-neon (He-Ne) laser for aiming purposes. The low-intensity He-Ne laser emits a red light that facilitates directing the laser at the target. Although the He-Ne laser readily passes through the special goggles and glasses used for laser surgery, its low power is innocuous unless the laser is directed specifically at the eye.

Indeed, the nature of ocular damage caused by lasers depends on the wavelength as well as the intensity and duration of exposure. Exposure to a 10,600–nm wavelength produced by the CO$_2$ laser can cause corneal opacification, because the energy is largely absorbed on the surface of the eye. Hence, personnel working with or near the laser should wear protective goggles to prevent ocular damage. Because the wavelength of the CO$_2$ laser is absorbed by almost all surfaces, eyewear of any color, even clear glasses, will stop the beam. Such eyewear should have side protectors to prevent injury from reflected beams.[18] However, for other lasers, goggles must be tinted for the specific wavelength they are intended to block. Clearly, no one should look directly at the output from any laser. Moreover, for all types of lasers, the patient's

eyes should be closed during surgery and covered with moist eye patches. If the patient is having laser surgery under local anesthesia, the patient should wear goggles tinted appropriately.

The CO$_2$ laser cannot be propagated through an ordinary fiberoptic bundle, as can the Nd:YAG laser. Its output travels in a straight line from its source to the target. Of all medical lasers, the CO$_2$ laser penetrates the most superficially. Ninety percent of its energy is absorbed within the first 0.03 mm of tissue it irradiates.[20]

The precision of the CO$_2$ laser is superb, and it has good hemostatic action. The discrete, thin path of destruction and the preservation of adjacent tissue associated with the CO$_2$ laser is thought to account for the rapid healing, minimal scarring, and lack of pain seen postoperatively. The lack of postoperative edema is especially advantageous in children with small-caliber airways. Clearly, precision of tissue destruction and lack of hemorrhage and edema are especially valuable in managing juvenile laryngeal papillomatosis. Unlike the Nd:YAG laser, the CO$_2$ laser does not produce late postoperative complications.

Argon Laser

The argon laser emits blue-green light with a wavelength of approximately 0.5 μm. This laser has low maximum power and is easily transmitted by fiberoptic bundles. Because it is absorbed strongly by hemoglobin and other pigments, the argon laser has proven useful in dermatological and plastic surgery for hemangioma excision, tattoo removal, and port wine stain lightening.[21] In ophthalmology, the argon laser is useful in retinal detachment surgery and for diabetic retinopathy. In otolaryngological surgery, its usefulness has been limited primarily to myringotomy, stapedectomy, and tympanoplasty (see Table 4–1).

Because the emissions of the argon laser can penetrate the cornea and lens, severe retinal damage can ensue. Orange protective goggles should be worn by personnel in the vicinity of the argon laser.

Neodymium:Yttrium-Aluminum-Garnet Laser

The Nd:YAG laser is employed for photocoagulation and deep thermal necrosis in the destruction of obstructing bronchial carcinoma (Fig. 4–3). It has been employed also in a variety of other settings, which include the treatment of gastrointestinal (GI) bleeding owing to the Rendu-Osler-Weber syndrome[22]; during splenic and hepatic resections; and during ophthalmological surgery involving the vitreous and posterior capsule. Its radiation is usually in the infrared range (wavelength 1.06 μm). Because its radiation is invisible, an He-Ne laser is often recruited for aiming. However, the Nd:YAG laser can be adapted to emit radiation in the visible or ultraviolet portions of the spectrum by employing frequency doubling or tripling techniques.[22] A distinct advantage of Nd:YAG laser radiation is its ready transmissibility by fiberoptic bundles. However, this mode of transmission decreases collimation and increases divergence upon exiting the fiber bundle.

Nd:YAG radiation is absorbed by both hemoglobin and melanin. Indeed, it has the highest tissue penetration of all currently (1991) available medical lasers. The high power (greater than 100 W) available from this laser makes it extremely effective in the thermal necrosis of large amounts of tissue. Although this laser has superb hemostatic properties, it is less precise than the CO_2 laser. Because the Nd:YAG laser interacts with tissues by causing relatively slow coagulation of proteins and carbonization, the late effects of this laser can be extensive and difficult to predict. Tissue necrosis secondary to the Nd:YAG laser is indolent, and the resultant thermal damage frequently takes the form of delayed edema and tissue sloughing.

The Nd:YAG laser can produce severe retinal injury. Hence, personnel working in the vicinity of this laser should wear green goggles that absorb light maximally at 1064 nm. These glasses, it should be noted, make cyanosis difficult to detect. Clearly, pulse oximetry is invaluable in this milieu.

Potassium-Titanyl-Phosphate Laser

The potassium-titanyl-phosphate (KTP) laser emits green light with a wavelength of 532 nm or 0.532 μm, and it can be propagated by fiberoptic filaments. Because it is readily absorbed by blood and pigmented tissue, it is useful for neurosurgical procedures involving vascular tumors. Moreover, the KTP laser has been used in otolaryngological surgery for myringotomy, stapedectomy, and tympanoplasty.

Orange-red goggles should be worn by health care providers when the KTP laser is in use (Table 4–2).

Ruby Laser

Largely of historical interest, the ruby laser emits blue-green light with a wavelength of

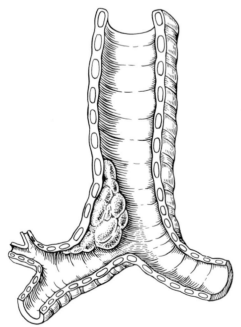

FIGURE 4–3. *The Nd:YAG laser is useful for resection of lower tracheal and endobronchial lesions.*

TABLE 4–2. Color of Protective Goggles Needed with Various Lasers

Laser Type	Goggles
CO_2	Clear
Argon	Orange
Nd:YAG	Green
Nd:YAG:KTP	Orange-red

0.695 μm. It had been useful in photocoagulating vascular and pigmented retinal lesions and for treating giant retinal tears.

ANESTHESIA MANAGEMENT

Although standard anesthetic techniques require no special modifications for laser surgery when the operative site is distant from the airway, such is not the case with ENT laser surgery. Vigilance takes on added importance with laser surgery of the airway.

A laser beam can ignite flammable materials used for general anesthesia, such as endotracheal tubes, anesthesia circuits, oil-based lubricants, ointments, sponges, and drapes.[23, 24] Incandescent debris produced by the explosive vaporization of tissue in contact with the laser beam can injure the patient's adjacent healthy tissue or operating room personnel. Nontarget tissue should be protected by layers of moist gauze. As previously mentioned, it is crucial that safety goggles of the appropriate tint be worn by all personnel in the operating room (see Table 4–2) and that the eyes of the anesthetized patient be closed and covered with saline-soaked gauze pads. The patient must be immobilized lest the laser beam strike and injure normal tissue or strike flammable material such as surgical drapes. Although the energy density of reflected beams decreases as the distance from the focal point increases, instruments used with lasers should have a dull matte finish to reduce reflections. In addition to fire hazards, other potential complications of ENT endoscopic laser surgery include dental trauma, airway obstruction, hypoventilation, hypoxemia, aspiration of resected material, hypertension, dysrhythmias, and ischemia.

The choice of anesthetics depends largely on the technique of ventilation during surgery. When the surgical field is near the airway, general anesthesia may be conducted either with an endotracheal tube or without an endotracheal tube employing special techniques, such as Venturi jet ventilation. If ventilation through an endotracheal tube is elected, prevention of a fire or explosion demands the use of special methods and appropriate tubes.

Specifics of anesthetic management for both upper and lower airway laser surgery are discussed next, including factors influencing the appropriate selection of endotracheal tubes from the potpourri of available designs.

Preoperative Considerations and Induction Techniques

Patients undergoing laser surgery frequently have some degree of respiratory compromise. A careful assessment of the individual's airway must be made prior to induction of anesthesia.

Patients not at risk for respiratory obstruction can be induced in a conventional manner and monitored as outlined in the section entitled "Microlaryngoscopy" at the beginning of this chapter.

Those at risk for obstruction or those with severe chronic obstructive or restrictive pulmonary disease should not receive premedication except for an antisialagogue. A variety of equipment, including a wide assortment of laryngoscope blades, a rigid bronchoscope, and a tracheostomy tray, should be available in the operating room for patients at risk for obstruction. In addition, the ENT surgeon should be present, gowned, and gloved in the operating suite in the event that a surgical airway needs to be established immediately. Awake tracheal intubation, often accomplished with fiberoptic endoscopy, is usually recommended for these cases.

Intraoperative Management

Upper Airway Lesions. The decision to employ a polyvinylchloride (PVC), red rubber, or silicone tube for laser surgery is controversial. Each of these three tubes can be ignited by the CO_2 laser in an environment of 100% oxygen.[24] Additional special endotracheal tubes, including the Bivona tube and the Norton metal tube, are also available; they, too, have disadvantages.

PVC tubes have the lowest ignition temperature of the currently available tubes.[25] In addition, they are most easily penetrated by the laser beam, especially at the cuff. The combustion of PVC endotracheal tubes produces hydrochloric acid, a potent respiratory irritant that can cause pulmonary toxicity.[26] Osoff and colleagues[27] studied pulmonary damage in dogs when PVC, red rubber, or silicone tubes were ignited by a CO_2 laser. The changes seen with red rubber tubes were much less extensive than those observed with the PVC tube fires, possibly because red rubber tubes char and melt before they burn and because they produce carbon monoxide rather than highly toxic hydrochloric acid. Moreover, white ash was present in the entire tracheobronchial tree following combustion of silicone tubes. The authors concluded: "This finding should put the final ban on the use of the PVC tube for carbon dioxide laser surgery."[27] They stated, furthermore, that until the morbidity associated with the inhalation of ash has been determined, silicone tubes should not be used for laser surgery.

Sosis and Heller[28] also do not recommend the Xomed Laser Shield silicone endotracheal tube (Fig. 4–4) for laser surgery; they reported a blow torch fire that was difficult to extinguish when an extremely high powered CO_2 laser was directed perpendicularly at the tube. (In fairness, it must be mentioned that the manufacturer warns that the tube should be used solely with the CO_2 laser; that no more than 25 W of CO_2 laser power in the pulse mode, with pulse durations not to exceed 0.5 seconds per pulse, should be used; and that the fractional inspired oxygen (FIO_2) should be limited to 25%. Sosis and Heller also studied the Bivona laser endotracheal tube. This latter tube has an aluminum core, a silicone covering, and a polyurethane foam cuff with a silicone envelope. These investigators concluded that they could not recommend the Bivona tube for either CO_2 or Nd:YAG[29] laser surgery because a fire ignited quickly when these lasers, operating at high power, were applied to the tube.

The Mallinckrodt Laser-Flex endotracheal tube has received a more favorable evaluation, however, than the aforementioned tubes (Fig. 4–5). The Laser-Flex—constructed exclusively from stainless steel except for two PVC cuffs

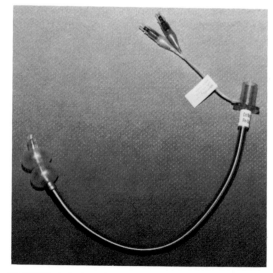

FIGURE 4–5. *The Mallinckrodt Laser-Flex endotracheal tube, complete with double cuff, is a highly recommended tube for use with the CO_2 laser. (Photograph courtesy of Dorothy J. Gaal, M.D., Assistant Professor of Anesthesiology, Yale University School of Medicine.)*

and a PVC 15-mm adaptor—is available in 4.5- and 6.0-mm inside diameter (ID) sizes. The double cuff is a valuable safety feature of this tube. Sosis and Heller recommend the Mallinckrodt Laser-Flex tube for use with the CO_2 laser,[28] but not with the Nd:YAG laser.[29]

The Norton endotracheal tube, constructed of spiral wound stainless steel, is another special tube for laser surgery. The only commercially available completely nonflammable endotracheal tube, the Norton tube has no cuff, and it has not enjoyed great popularity. Although designed to obviate the risk of tracheal tube ignition, metal tubes introduce other problems, including specular reflectance of the beam.[30] In addition, their limited flexibility has a proclivity to injure friable mucosa. Not surprisingly, the thick walls of these tubes make them unsuitable for small-sized pediatric airways. The Norton tube is available in 4.0-, 4.8-, and 6.4-mm ID. However, the 4.8-mm size has a wall thickness of 1.3 mm. Although a Norton tube may be equipped with a separate latex cuff to reduce environmental contamination with anesthetic gases and to enhance ventilation in the presence of an excessive gas leak, the addition of the cuff increases the risk of combustion.

The shafts of combustible endotracheal tubes, whether PVC or rubber, can be rendered reasonably resistant to the effects of both the CO_2 and Nd:YAG lasers by wrapping

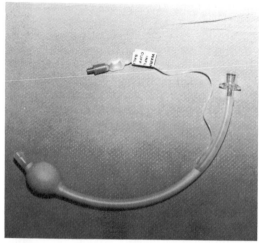

FIGURE 4–4. *The Xomed Laser Shield endotracheal tube. (Photograph courtesy of Dorothy J. Gaal, M.D., Assistant Professor of Anesthesiology, Yale University School of Medicine.)*

them properly with the correct metallic tapes.[31, 32] The most efficacious tapes are the aluminum tapes, 3M No. 425 and 433, and a copper foil tape (Venture Tape Corporation, Rockland, Massachusetts). Tubes should be wrapped in an overlapping spiral fashion, commencing just above the cuff. Foil-wrapped tubes are not a panacea, however. They may have a rough surface that could injure tissue, and the reflection of the laser beam from tape could harm the patient or operating room personnel. Moreover, if small endotracheal tubes are wrapped with metallic tape, kinking can occur,[33] causing acute airway obstruction.

Clearly, the cuff of a foil-wrapped endotracheal tube still remains vulnerable to combustion despite the presence of a protected shaft. Hence, the cuff should be filled with saline to which a small amount of methylene blue has been added. Thus, cuff perforation will be readily noted. Although saline reduces the risk of fire when the cuff is hit by a CO_2 laser, it does not totally prevent such a complication.[34] As an added precaution, wet pledgets should be placed on the cuff and moistened periodically.

Another effective method of protecting the shaft of a combustible tube is the Laser-Guard (Americal Corporation, Mystic, Connecticut). This device, consisting of a layer of embossed silver foil with adhesive on one side and a sponge-like substance on the other side, effectively protects the shafts of PVC endotracheal tubes from a CO_2 laser operating at 70 W and directed perpendicularly at the tube for 1 minute.[35] Moreover, a reflected beam from a Laser-Guard device is less apt to cause damage than with foil-wrapped endotracheal tubes.[35] (It is imperative to keep the spongy layer wet so it can function as a heat sink).

During laser endoscopic surgery, the fraction of inspired oxygen should be minimized to that which will satisfactorily oxygenate the patient, as assessed by pulse oximetry. In general, 30% oxygen should be the upper limit. The remainder of the inspired gas should not include nitrous oxide, which supports combustion to approximately the same extent as oxygen. Rather, helium or nitrogen should be used. Pashayan and Gravenstein[36] claim that helium, with its greater thermal diffusivity, is superior to nitrogen in retarding combustion. Simpson and Wolf,[37] however, report no difference in flammability between He and O_2 mixtures *versus* N_2 and O_2 mixtures (Table 4–3).

Alternatives to Endotracheal Tubes. To ob-

TABLE 4–3. Suggested Safety Precautions with Lasers

Regular testing of equipment
Laser drills for involved personnel
Warning sign on door
Eye protection for patients and health care workers
No oil-based ointments
Properly protected endotracheal tubes
Saline and methylene blue for cuff inflation
Moist gauze and towels as needed
Limit FIO_2
Avoid N_2O
Suction toxic fumes from infrared lasers
Water and CO_2 extinguishers immediately available

viate the problem of endotracheal tube combustion, an alternative is to use a Venturi ventilation technique with no endotracheal tube. However, even in this setting, an airway fire can occur. Tissue can become desiccated, can carbonize, and can ignite in the high jet flow of oxygen. Clearly, the only absolute way to prevent laser-induced combustion is to avoid using the laser.

Other disadvantages of Venturi ventilation include barotrauma, such as pneumomediastinum or pneumothorax; airway obstruction; regurgitation; and aspiration. Recently, Cozine and associates[38] retrospectively investigated whether ventilatory technique alters outcome in CO_2 laser airway surgery. The survey disclosed that the group that received Venturi jet ventilation had a significantly higher incidence of ventilatory complications, whereas the only reported death, the result of an airway fire, occurred in the standard ventilation group.

Juvenile Laryngeal Papillomas. Laryngeal papillomas, virus-induced warty lesions that tenaciously recur at the glottis and other portions of the airway, are the most common benign tumor of the pediatric larynx. Children afflicted with this disease initially present with hoarseness; later symptoms include aphonia and respiratory distress. Severe, chronic obstruction from these growths may eventually result in right ventricular hypertrophy, pulmonary hypertension, and cor pulmonale.[39] If possible, however, tracheostomy should be avoided, because it is said to seed the papillomas along the tracheobronchial tree.[39] Autogenous vaccine[39, 40] and interferon treatment have been used in attempts to control juvenile papillomas, but at this time the only effective way to maintain airway patency appears to be repeated endoscopic CO_2 laser excisions until the papillomas spontaneously regress at puberty.[41]

The anesthetic management of these children is extremely challenging. Because these children commonly have had multiple operating room experiences, they may be extremely anxious. However, preoperative sedation should be withheld if the child has significant airway obstruction. Clearly, the anesthesiologist must be especially calm, gentle, and reassuring with the child and his or her parents. In the unlikely event that the child has a preexisting tracheostomy, general anesthesia can be induced easily and safely simply by replacing the tracheostomy cannula with a metal tracheostomy tube, adapting and connecting the latter to the anesthesia circuit.[42] Unfortunately for the anesthesiologist, he or she usually does not have the luxury of such a secure airway prior to induction.

The authors' preference for most small children with laryngeal papillomas is to induce by mask with nitrous oxide, oxygen, and halothane with the usual monitors, including a precordial stethoscope, electrocardiogram (ECG), a blood pressure cuff, a pulse oximeter, a capnograph, and a nerve simulator. After IV access is secured, atropine (0.02 mg/kg) and succinylcholine (1.5 mg/kg) are administered. The child is then intubated with a red rubber endotracheal tube (of smaller than usual diameter), wrapped either with a copper foil tape or with an appropriate aluminum tape (3M No. 425, 433). All oil-based ointments used to lubricate endotracheal tubes must be avoided, because they are combustible and can be ignited by a laser beam. If the child's airway is especially difficult, the anesthesiologist should avoid using succinylcholine and instead intubate under deep halothane anesthesia, with the child breathing spontaneously. Often in this setting there is a valuable clue to the location of the glottic opening, which is obscured by a dense growth of papillomas, in the presence of a tiny air bubble generated during spontaneous ventilation.

The currently available metal endotracheal tubes with their thick walls and limited flexibility are usually too large and cumbersome for use in small children. Moreover, we avoid Venturi ventilation in these children for a variety of reasons, including fear of barotrauma if exhalation becomes obstructed by the extensive growths along the airway.

A metal adapter connects the specially modified endotracheal tube to the anesthesia circuit. Nitrogen or helium is then substituted for nitrous oxide. Once the child has recovered from succinylcholine, vecuronium (0.05 mg/kg) or atracurium (0.25 mg/kg) is administered as needed to guarantee complete vocal cord immobility. Anesthesia is maintained with halothane or isoflurane, nitrogen or helium, and oxygen. Inspired oxygen concentration is kept at 30% or less, as long as oxygen saturation is at least 96%. Saline-soaked gauze gads and towels are used to cover the patient's eyes and the portion of the endotracheal tube unprotected by foil, respectively. Dexamethasone (0.3–0.4 mg/kg) is frequently administered prophylactically, because surgical manipulation and the foil-wrapped tube may traumatize the laryngotracheal mucosa. Once the child is awake and breathing well following reversal of neuromuscular blockade, extubation is accomplished. The child is given humidified oxygen and is carefully observed in the postoperative period for any signs of bleeding, edema, or respiratory distress. If laryngeal edema develops, nebulized racemic epinephrine is administered by mask or, preferably, intermittent positive-pressure breathing (IPPB) in a dose of 1 mL of 2.25% solution diluted with 5 mL of normal saline.

Lower Airway Lesions. CO_2 and Nd:YAG lasers can be used to treat lower airway lesions. When the lesion is more distally located, the Nd:YAG laser is used because it can travel through a fiberoptic cable. Many patients selected for lower airway laser treatments have terminal cancer with inoperable obstructive lesions. Hence, they may be fragile and require, in addition to the routine monitoring described previously, more invasive methods of monitoring, including an arterial line for direct, continuous blood pressure measurements. Many of them are poorly nourished and volume depleted and thus are vulnerable to hypotension. Moreover, evaluation of left ventricular performance is particularly important in patients with airway obstruction, because obstruction in the tracheobronchial tree necessitates generation of increased negative intrathoracic pressures to ensure adequate ventilation. Buda and colleagues[43] have demonstrated that an increase in negative intrathoracic pressure increases true left ventricular afterload. Therefore, a patient with a compromised left ventricle and superimposed airway obstruction is predisposed to failure and pulmonary edema.[44]

Surgical access to the lower airway is achieved with a rigid, metal bronchoscope when the CO_2 laser is used. Ventilation may be maintained through the side arm of the bronchoscope. As long as a flammable cuff has not been used to seal the airway, the hazard of fire should be slim with a metal broncho-scope. The risk of misdirecting the beam, although not completely eliminated, can be minimized by using a specially designed bron-choscope with a matte finish to reduce specular reflectance.[18] In place of a cuff, saline-soaked gauze applied around the bronchoscope in the upper airway may be used to effect a seal during ventilation. Although the FIO_2 need not be limited if no flammable materials are used, the addition of helium to the inspired gases may improve gas flow past the obstruc-tive lesion. If an IV induction is deemed ap-propriate, it can be achieved with sodium thiopental, etomidate, ketamine, or narcot-ics—either alone or in combination. Boyce[44] finds the sequence of 0.07 mg/kg midazolam, 0.2–0.5 µg/kg sufentanil, and 1–2 mg/kg of sodium thiopental to be highly effective in providing a smooth induction, protection from cardiovascular effects of laryngoscopy, intu-bation, or placement of the bronchoscope, and prevention of intraoperative recall. Lidocaine 1.5 mg/kg is administered either IV or intra-tracheally. Potent inhalation anesthetics can be administered if standard means of convec-tion ventilation are employed. Muscle relax-ants are given as needed. To minimize pul-monary exposure to laser smoke, ventilation should be interrupted for laser firing.

Instead of conventional ventilation, jet ven-tilation may be elected. Jet adapters are avail-able to connect to the 15-mm side arm venti-lation port of metal bronchoscopes. Most clinicians manually apply 10–20 jets per minute with a duration of 0.5–1.0 second per jet while assessing adequacy of ventilation.[45] HFJV (300 breaths per minute) has also been used for laser bronchoscopy, but Vourc'h and associates[46] reported modest hypercapnia when employed in patients with bronchial stenosis.

If the Nd:YAG laser is used, either a flexi-ble or a rigid metal bronchoscope can be employed. Many bronchoscopists favor using the metal bronchoscope and having the patient under general anesthesia. They claim that this setup provides better access, suctioning, ven-tilation, and target immobility of the laser. Ventilation can be maintained by any of the several techniques previously described. Ron-tal and coworkers[47] recommend passing the fiberoptic bronchoscope through a rigid bron-choscope when peripheral lesions are to be treated. The rigid bronchoscope affords an enhanced view of airway lesions, improved ability to suction, the ability to easily remove tissue fragments, and the option of applying

epinephrine-soaked cottonoids to achieve he-mostasis.[48, 49] Although a metal bronchoscope reduces the risk of fire, nonetheless suction catheters and the fiberoptic cable carrying the Nd:YAG laser beam remain potential sources of ignition; combustion of the fiberoptic bron-choscope using this technique has been re-ported.[50] Because the Nd:YAG wavelength is well absorbed by darkly pigmented substances, the risk of fire is increased if the cable becomes soiled with charred tissue. Thus, attention must be directed toward keeping the fiberoptic tip clean throughout the resection. Power lev-els should be kept under 50 W in short pulsa-tions in order to avoid injuring underlying structures.[22] At high power, the penetration of a laser cannot be properly controlled, and perforation of a large vessel can occur.[48]

Although many favor general anesthesia for Nd:YAG treatment of central airway lesions, the use of topical anesthesia has been advo-cated if only a flexible fiberoptic bronchoscope is being used. To maximize patient comfort, a carefully titrated volume (not to exceed 1.5 mL) of 10% cocaine is applied to the nasal cavity; glossopharyngeal and superior laryn-geal nerve blocks are administered with 2% lidocaine; and 5 mL of 2% lidocaine is admin-istered intratracheally through the cricothyroid membrane. IV midazolam and sufentanil are used to enhance patient comfort and minimize recall. The anesthesiologist must be vigilant about ventilatory depression and hypoxia in this setting. Pulse oximetry is invaluable as a continuous monitor of adequacy of oxygen saturation, especially because the green gog-gles the anesthesiologist must wear during Nd:YAG laser procedures interfere with the ability to discern cyanosis. Patient cooperation is essential, because movement could cause misdirection of the laser beam, resulting in tracheal perforation. In addition, smoke inha-lation is likely in a conscious, spontaneously breathing patient. However, Rontal and colleagues[47] believe that local anesthesia is preferable to general anesthesia if a high-grade obstruction of the airway is known or sus-pected. These authors recommend local anes-thesia with spontaneous respiration whenever the middle or lower tracheal lumen is reduced in excess of 50% of its cross-sectional area.

The use of the metal bronchoscope in con-junction with the fiberoptic scope with the patient under general anesthesia has already been discussed. When general anesthesia is used, moreover, the fiberoptic scope can also either be inserted through a large-diameter tracheal tube or be placed alongside a small-diameter tube. Because wrapping with metallic tape does not protect tracheal tubes during Nd:YAG laser bronchoscope surgery, the clear plastic tracheal tubes with no markings are said to be preferable to standard PVC tubes with markings and radiopaque stripe or to red rubber tubes.[51] However, even the clear portions of PVC tubes burn with sufficient output from the Nd:YAG laser. The amount of inhaled smoke and debris can be minimized by resecting during a held inspiration and suctioning during exhalation. However, it is essential to recognize the fire hazard of both the endotracheal tube and the flexible endoscope in this milieu. Moreover, safe limits for FIO_2 and power density have not been established for this system.[18]

Perioperative complications of Nd:YAG laser treatments to the lower airway include hypoxia, hypotension, hemorrhage from penetrated pulmonary vessels, intraoperative awareness, barotrauma, and fire. Signs of barotrauma such as pneumothorax and subcutaneous emphysema are not secondary exclusively to excessively high inflation pressures or obstructed exhalation. In addition, these complications can occur following laser penetration of the airway. Moreover, delayed or late postoperative complications are not uncommon with the Nd:YAG laser and can include delayed, but clinically significant, edema and tissue sloughing.

Airway Fires. Because fire is a ubiquitous concern during laser surgery of the airway, surgeons, anesthesiologists, and all other operating room personnel should be trained in fire safety measures and be well equipped to manage such an occurrence. Both Type A (water) and Class C (carbon dioxide) extinguishers should be immediately available, as well as a bowl of saline or water to quickly flood airway flames. Type A fire extinguishers are adequate to stop a fire involving the surgical drapes, for example, but Class C extinguishers are necessary for fires involving, or extremely near to, live-circuit electrical equipment.

In the event of an airway fire, the anesthesiologist must stop ventilation immediately and interrupt the oxygen supply, either by clamping the endotracheal tube or turning off the flowmeter (Table 4–4). If this does not stop the flame, the surgical field should be doused with water immediately. If the surgical drapes are in flames, they must be doused with water and removed from the patient as well as from

TABLE 4–4. Management of Airway Fire*

Stop ventilation
Disconnect oxygen source/douse with water if needed; remove burned tracheal tube/endoscope
Mask ventilate/reintubate
Diagnose injury/provide therapy by bronchoscopy and laryngoscopy
Monitor patient for at least 24 hours
Administer short-term steroids
Administer antibiotics/ventilatory support as needed

*Measures listed in order of importance.
From Pashayan AG: Anesthesia for laser surgery. *In* Barash PG (ed): ASA Refresher Courses in Anesthesiology, Vol 17. Philadelphia, JB Lippincott, 1989, pp 215–226.

any nearby electrical equipment. The burned tracheal tube or endoscope must be removed immediately from the airway, and ventilation must be resumed either by mask or through reintubation. The extent of airway injury should be diagnosed before the patient is allowed to emerge from anesthesia. This is accomplished by careful laryngoscopy and bronchoscopy to delineate the rostral and caudad limits of thermal or chemical damage and, if necessary, to remove any particulate matter from the airways. Based on information obtained from laryngoscopy, bronchoscopy, and oximetry, a decision should be made regarding whether extubation is appropriate or, in the presence of severe damage, a tracheostomy is indicated.

Postoperatively, the patient should be monitored intensively for a minimum of 24 hours with oximetry, serial chest radiograph, and arterial blood gases, if necessary. Humidified oxygen is given, and short-term steroids may be useful to reduce airway edema. If superimposed infection is a possibility, antibiotics should be administered. In the event of severe burns, prolonged mechanical ventilation may be necessary, along with repeated laryngoscopic and bronchoscopic re-evaluations.

BRONCHOSCOPY

The first reported endoscopic examination was performed in the early 1900s by Killian, who placed a translaryngeal tube into the trachea to retrieve aspirated foreign bodies.[52] Since that time, bronchoscopy has become the most common invasive procedure in the management of intrathoracic diseases of the respiratory system. Applications of bronchoscopy are threefold: in diagnostics, in therapy, and as part of the preoperative evaluation. Diagnostically, bronchoscopy is used to evaluate persistent cough, hemoptysis, wheezing, recurrent pneumonia, or atelectasis; following inhalation injury; or to obtain cytology specimens. Therapeutic indications include removing foreign bodies or secretions, draining abscesses, and aiding in the placement of endotracheal tubes. Preoperatively, bronchoscopy is used to assess the extent of pathology, be it neoplastic or anatomical (e.g., tracheobronchial esophageal fistula.)[53] Because bronchoscopy entails sharing the airway with the surgeon during a procedure that can cause cardiac and respiratory compromise, the anesthesiologist often has to balance patient safety with optimal surgical conditions. Such a dilemma has led to the development of a variety of anesthetic techniques and means of ventilation.

RIGID BRONCHOSCOPY

Indications

Rigid bronchoscopy offers several distinct advantages over flexible bronchoscopy. For management of foreign bodies, it is the instrument of choice, because removal of the entire object can be accomplished without its fragmentation, often a necessity with fiberoptic bronchoscopy (FOB). Rigid bronchoscopy also allows better visualization, suctioning, and control of massive bleeding. Furthermore, the rigid bronchoscope may be the only instrument capable of passing through an obstructing tumor or granuloma tissue. Large biopsy specimens can be obtained also. Finally, the rigid bronchoscope permits palpation of the carina, a procedure used to assess operability and extent of disease.[53–55]

Local Anesthesia

The chances of sudden patient movement during rigid bronchoscopy are significant, given the stimulation of the scope and the extremes of neck extension required for its placement and use. Because this potentially disastrous complication can never be eliminated with exclusive use of local anesthesia, general anesthesia is usually preferred. If, however, topical anesthesia is required, the same approach described for the FOB can be used. In fact, successful rigid bronchoscopy with topical anesthesia has been reported, with supplementation with agents such as benzodiazepines.[56]

General Anesthesia

The choice of general anesthesia technique to be used for rigid bronchoscopy depends on the goals and duration of bronchoscopy, the skills and experience of the anesthesiologist and surgeon, the patient's underlying medical condition, and the mode of ventilation to be used.

As with all types of general anesthesia, ventilation during bronchoscopy can be either spontaneous or controlled. Unfortunately, spontaneous ventilation invites patient injury with bucking or coughing, especially under light anesthesia. To minimize this risk, deeper levels of anesthesia can be provided. Doing so, however, is not without its own hazards. The MAC EI_{50} and MAC EI_{95} are defined as the minimum alveolar concentrations of inhaled anesthetics required to permit laryngoscopy and endotracheal intubation without patient movement in 50% and 95% of the population, respectively.[57] For halothane, these concentrations are 1.3 MAC and 1.7 MAC, respectively; for enflurane, they are 1.4 MAC and 1.9 MAC, respectively[58]—levels that may cause significant cardiopulmonary depression during intubation as well as bronchoscopy. Clearly, the same compromise of cardiopulmonary function can occur also when using IV agents. Because of the fine line between overdose (leading to hypoventilation) and inadequate anesthesia (risking patient movement or bronchospasm), controlled as opposed to spontaneous ventilation is usually preferred.

The development of different techniques to provide general anesthesia for rigid bronchoscopy has essentially paralleled the evolution of different ventilatory modes. These have been many.[59, 60] Early rigid bronchoscopies employed intermittent ventilation with apneic oxygenation during the brief periods of bronchoscopy. Although hypercarbia and hypoxemia were constant threats, limiting the apneic episodes to 2–3 minutes offered some degree of safety. Interestingly, Frumin and associates reported a healthy subject tolerating up to 53 minutes of apneic oxygenation and a Pa_{CO_2} of 250 mmHg, apparently without harm.[61] This is, of course, by no means advocated. In fact, obese patients and those with diminished functional residual capacities may be incapable of tolerating even brief periods of apnea.[62]

Controlled ventilation through the bronchoscope became possible with the invention of the side-arm ventilating bronchoscope by Muendrich and Hoflehner in 1953.[63] After years of modification,[64] today's ventilating bronchoscope operates much like the original. Scavenging of exhaled gases is achieved through the bronchoscope or an indwelling endotracheal tube.[65] Leaks around the bronchoscope can be prevented by applying manual pressure over the larynx, fitting an inflatable cuff around the bronchoscope, or oropharyngeal packing.[55] The rigid ventilating bronchoscope allows delivery of a known amount of oxygen and reliable ventilation. Anesthesia can be given as known concentrations of volatile agents or IV agents. A major disadvantage of this bronchoscope is the interruption of ventilation and dependence on apneic oxygenation during removal of the proximal end for obtaining surgical samples. Pollution of the environment with inhaled agents can occur during such periods. These concerns, as well as the duration of the overall procedure, limit the duration of apnea to 1–2 minutes.[53] Various attempts have been made to deal with these difficulties. Simultaneous placement of either an inflation catheter[66] or a 4.0-mm cuffed endotracheal tube[67] alongside the bronchoscope has been suggested to facilitate oxygenation and ventilation. The Hopkins lens telescope best circumvented these problems with the addition of sideports for suction catheters and biopsy instruments, obviating the need to open the proximal end.[55]

An important advance in rigid bronchoscopy occurred in 1967 with the introduction of the Sanders rigid Venturi bronchoscope.[68] This adaptation consisted of directing a 16- or 18-gauge needle down the lumen of a rigid bronchoscope and injecting oxygen under high pressure through the needle through a Sanders injector, a simple reducing valve. The high velocity of the injected oxygen creates a negative pressure immediately adjacent to the open end of the needle by Bernoulli's law, entraining room air with the oxygen. This phenomena is known as the Venturi effect. Thus, large volumes of the oxygen-room air mixture can be delivered as a large tidal volume. With an 18-gauge needle and oxygen source of 50 psi, peak airway pressures of 27 cm H_2O can be produced. By using the side arm of the bronchoscope to inject oxygen, Carden was able to increase this pressure to 55 cm H_2O with only a 30 psi oxygen source.[69] At the same time, the amount of entrained room air was reduced, and ventilation was improved. Thus, the rigid Venturi bronchoscope, especially with the Carden modification, allows superior ventilation and the attainment of lower Pa_{CO_2} values compared with the ventilating bronchoscope.[70, 71] Prolonged periods of bronchoscopy can be provided also with constant uninterrupted minute ventilation, because the proximal eyepiece of the bronchos-

scope does not need to be removed. The ventilatory characteristics of different types of bronchoscopes are summarized in Table 4–5.[53]

The greatest drawback of this mode of ventilation, however, is the uncertain inspired concentration of delivered gases, notably oxygen, due to the variable amount of entrained room air. Although oxygenation can usually be maintained, hypoxemia is more likely than with the ventilating bronchoscope.[71] In addition, inadequate ventilation can occur in patients with low thoracic compliance.[78] Scrupulous attention must be paid to the adequacy of chest wall excursion in such patients. The use of muscle relaxants may be particularly helpful to achieve this goal.

More recently, the rigid Venturi bronchoscope has been used to deliver HFJV[73] and HFPPV.[74] By delivering small tidal volumes at rapid respiratory rates (HFJV at 100–400/minute, HFPPV at 60–120/minute), lower inspiratory pressures and a quiet surgical lung field can be achieved. Oxygenation is usually acceptable for both techniques, even though the inspired concentration of oxygen and delivered gases is known only for HFPPV, not for HFJV. However, carbon dioxide retention can occur at frequencies above 360/minute with HFJV.[72]

General anesthesia for rigid bronchoscopy can be provided by inhalational or IV agents. The time-honored combination of intermittent doses of thiopental and intermittent doses or continuous infusion of succinylcholine has served anesthesiologists well in the past.[75] The same success with these agents has been reported for the rigid Venturi bronchoscope.[64, 69, 71, 76] However, the relatively large doses of thiopental used have been associated with respiratory depression.[77] Today, judiciously administered barbiturates, benzodiazepines, neuroleptics, opiates, and short-acting muscle relaxants are used most commonly. Delivery of inhaled anesthetics is also a popular method of administering anesthesia, often in combination with the IV agents. It is only with the rigid ventilating bronchoscope that a known concentration of agent can be delivered. The Venturi bronchoscope, however, has been used to deliver a nitrous oxide–oxygen mixture, an application found to have less prolonged recovery times than barbiturates.[78] Others feel the problem of environmental pollution argues against its use.[55] Nitrous oxide also can cause optical distortion because of its alteration of the refractive index of the gas mixture.[72]

The hemodynamic response to bronchos-

TABLE 4–5. Ventilation Characteristics and Anesthetic Implications
of the Three Different Types of Bronchoscopes

Type of Bronchoscope	FIO$_2$	Concentration of Inhalation Anesthesia	Constancy of Minute Ventilation	Suitable Duration of Procedure	Preferred Type of Anesthesia
Flexible fiberoptic	Known	Known	Constant	Long	Local or general anesthesia
Rigid ventilating	Known	Known	Inconstant	Short (15–20 min)	Inhalational or IV general anesthesia
Rigid Venturi	Unknown	Unknown	Constant	Long	IV general anesthesia

From Benumof JL: Anesthesia for special elective diagnostic procedures. *In* Benumof JL (ed): Anesthesia for Thoracic Surgery. Philadelphia, WB Saunders, 1987, p 327.

copy can be dramatic. Deep general anesthesia could probably abolish these hyperdynamic changes as well as coughing,[57, 58] but such a level is not always compatible with rapid emergence at the end of the case, as signaled by the abrupt withdrawal of the bronchoscope. Not uncommonly, deep anesthetic levels have to be maintained up to the end of the procedure, necessitating reinsertion of the endotracheal tube pending return of airway reflexes.[79]

Numerous means of attenuating the hemodynamic response to laryngoscopy and intubation have been described. Achieving this goal also allows a reduction in the amount of volatile anesthetic that must be administered. IV or topically applied lidocaine has been recommended by several authors.[80–87] Careful scrutiny of these earlier reports, however, has revealed several methodological flaws challenging their validity.[88] More recent, better controlled investigations have failed to show any benefit of lidocaine during intubation.[88, 89] Thus, the hemodynamic efficacy of lidocaine remains open to question. Other agents reported to blunt the cardiovascular response to intubation include β blockers (practolol,[90, 91] propranolol,[92, 93] esmolol[94–101]); α blockers (phentolamine,[102] droperidol[103]); mixed α and β blockers (labetalol[91, 104–106]); vasodilators (nitroglycerine,[107, 108] nitroprusside,[109] hydralazine[110]); calcium entry blockers (diltiazem,[111] nifedipine,[112] verapamil,[113] isosorbide dinitrate[114]); and opiates (buprenorphine,[115] fentanyl,[116–123] sufentanil,[124–127] alfentanil[128, 129]). Finally, concurrent use of topical anesthesia can reduce the amount of general anesthesia required and should be considered an adjunct to all general anesthetics for bronchoscopies.

FIBEROPTIC BRONCHOSCOPY

Indications

In 1870 Tyndall first discovered that visual images could be transmitted through glass rods that had been melted and pulled into threadlike fibers. The first medical application of this finding was the flexible gastroscope in 1930. After further development of the early endoscope in the 1950s, the standards for the first FOB were described by Ikeda in 1968.[130] The flexible nature of the instrument, allowing visualization and sampling of deep endobronchial lesions, accounts for its principal advantage. Upper lobe and even fifth order bronchi become accessible.[59] Localization of distal sites of hemoptysis, obtaining localized culture and biopsy specimens, and selective bronchography are possible as well.[53] Its small size also improves patient comfort, decreases the risk of dental and other injury, and facilitates spontaneous ventilation. Indeed, because patients can assume a sitting or semisitting position, ventilatory mechanics are improved. An obvious aid to the anesthesiologist, the FOB can be indispensable in difficult intubations. Thus, additional indications for the FOB include troublesome airway anatomy, facial trauma, unstable or fused cervical spines, and vertebral artery insufficiency. Finally, use of the FOB for an intubated patient can confirm tube placement (especially for double-lumen tubes) and provide bronchial toilet.

Local Anesthesia

Unlike rigid bronchoscopy, which is usually performed under general anesthesia, FOB can be performed under either local or general anesthesia. If such a procedure were to be done through the nose, local anesthesia would involve blocking three nerves: the trigeminal, glossopharyngeal, and vagus nerves (Fig. 4–6). The trigeminal nerve provides sensory innervation to the nasal mucosa, nasopharynx, palate, and anterior two thirds of the tongue. The glossopharyngeal nerve provides sensation to the posterior one third of the tongue, most of the oropharynx, and the anterior (pharyngeal surface) epiglottis.[131, 132]

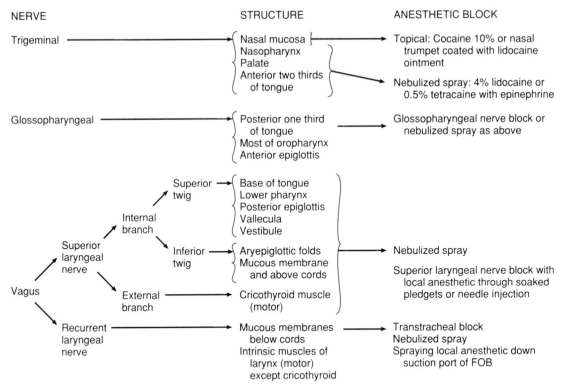

FIGURE 4–6. *Nerves to be blocked during local anesthesia for fiberoptic bronchoscopy.*

The vagus nerve has two major components relevant to bronchoscopy: the superior laryngeal and recurrent laryngeal nerves (Fig. 4–7). The superior laryngeal nerve (primarily vagal, but also containing a small branch from the superior cervical ganglion) descends along the lateral pharynx behind and medial to the internal carotid artery. At the hyoid, it divides into the internal and external branches. The internal branch enters the thyroid membrane and divides into superior and inferior twigs. The superior twig provides sensation to the base of the tongue, lower pharynx, posterior (laryngeal surface) aspect of the epiglottis, vallecula, and vestibules. The inferior twig provides sensation to the aryepiglottic folds and mucous membranes above the vocal cords. The external branch has no sensory function, but provides motor innervation to the cricothyroid muscle.[132, 133]

The other relevant branch of the vagus, the recurrent laryngeal nerve, has paths that are asymmetric. The right recurrent laryngeal nerve arises from the right vagus as it passes in front of the subclavian artery, winds below it, and ascends between the trachea and esophagus. The left recurrent laryngeal nerve arises from the left vagus at the aortic arch, loops under the arch lateral to the ligamentum arteriosum, and ascends between the articulation of the inferior thyroid cornu and the cricoid cartilage. The recurrent laryngeal nerves provide sensation to the mucous membranes below the vocal cords and motor innervation to all intrinsic muscles of the larynx, except the cricothyroid muscle.[133, 134]

Anesthesia for the nose may be performed by spraying the nasal mucosa with 0.5% tetracaine with epinephrine or 4% lidocaine with epinephrine. Alternatively, pledgets soaked in 4% cocaine (maximum of 3 to 4 mL) can be applied topically for both anesthetic and vasoconstrictive effects.[53] Spraying the nares with neosynephrine followed by progressive dilation with increasing sizes of soft nasal trumpets coated with 10% lidocaine jelly may be effective also. With all these methods, providing vasoconstriction is important to reduce bleeding into the pharynx, which can impair fiberoptic visualization.

Anesthesia for the pharynx can be achieved by simply spraying the oropharyngeal surfaces with the same lidocaine or tetracaine used for the nose, or by gargling viscous lidocaine.[53] The pharynx can be further anesthetized with a glossopharyngeal nerve block. This is accom-

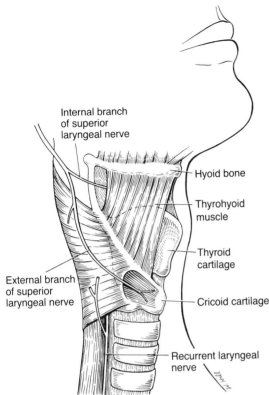

FIGURE 4–7. Anatomy of the larynx illustrating the course of the superior and recurrent laryngeal nerves.

Internal branch of superior laryngeal nerve

Hyoid bone

Thyrohyoid muscle

Thyroid cartilage

External branch of superior laryngeal nerve

Cricoid cartilage

Recurrent laryngeal nerve

plished by depressing the tongue and inserting a 26- or 27-gauge needle behind the tonsillar pillar at the base of the tongue. At this location in the lateral pharyngeal wall, the lingual branch of the glossopharyngeal nerve is relatively superficial and can be anesthetized by injecting 2 mL of 1% lidocaine, after negative aspiration is confirmed to avoid carotid injection.[135, 136]

The larynx may be anesthetized by a variety of means. An intraoral superior laryngeal nerve block can be performed by placing local anesthetic–soaked pledgets into both pyriform sinuses. More invasively, a superior laryngeal nerve block can be accomplished by directing a 25-gauge needle into the thyrohyoid membrane between the greater cornu of the hyoid bone and the superior cornu of the thyroid cartilage. The superior laryngeal nerve is blocked at its point of entry into the membrane by infiltrating 2 mL of 2% lidocaine. To anesthetize the mucous membranes below the vocal cords, the recurrent laryngeal nerve can be blocked by injecting local anesthetics down the suction port of the FOB or by a transtracheal block. For the latter technique, percu-

taneous puncture of the cricothyroid membrane is performed with a 22-gauge needle attached to a syringe. Entry into the trachea is detected by aspiration of air and is followed by injection of 4 mL of local anesthetic. The patient's ensuing cough helps disperse the anesthetic along the subglottic trachea. Rather than using a simple needle, inserting a 22-gauge IV Teflon catheter and withdrawing the needle before injecting the anesthetic reduces the chances of puncturing the posterior tracheal wall.[137]

If the bronchoscopy is to be done orally or if one needs to supplement nasal anesthesia, the simplest method of providing local anesthetic for bronchoscopy is by administering aerosolized local anesthetic to a spontaneously ventilating patient. A nebulizing device can be easily assembled by connecting an atomizer with a directed nozzle to an oxygen tank through extension tubing. Delivery of 10 seconds of mist every 10 to 20 seconds anesthetizes not only the oropharynx but also the tracheobronchial tree below the cords. To minimize the amount of agent deposited on the mouth and posterior oropharynx, the use of an ultrasonic nebulizer has been described.[138] Given sufficient time, the use of nebulized local anesthetics, perhaps supplemented with moderate amounts of IV agents for sedation, is all that is needed for FOB. For oral fiberoptic bronchoscopy, the FOB can be inserted through a Williams[139] or Ovassapian[140] intubation airway to help maintain airway patency, as well as protect both the teeth and the bronchoscope.

Attainment of adequate local anesthesia for the larynx blunts the gag reflex, predisposing the patient to aspiration. Consequently, a full stomach warrants consideration of general as opposed to local anesthesia with an appropriate method of induction. Conversely, even though superficial sensation to the mucous membranes can be abolished with topical techniques, anesthesia of the deeper pressure receptors is not provided and may require glossopharyngeal or superior laryngeal nerve blocks.[55]

Because the average adult trachea has a diameter of 18 mm, bronchoscopes with outside diameters of 5.0 mm, 5.7 mm, and 6.0 mm occupy only 6%, 10%, and 11% of the total cross-sectional area, respectively.[53] In an otherwise healthy patient, this presents little impediment to spontaneous ventilation.

Hypoxemia during fiberoptic bronchoscopy is well documented.[141–146] One suspected mechanism is atelectasis, perhaps due to overzealous suctioning through the side-port of an FOB wedged in a distal bronchus. For instance, a 2-mm suction port can remove 14.2 L/minute of gas at 760 mmHg.[147] Hypoventilation in an oversedated patient also may contribute to hypoxemia. Therefore, supplemental oxygen should be provided either by nasal cannula or, for delivery of a higher oxygen concentration, by a special Patil-Syracuse face mask with a diaphragm allowing passage of an FOB.[148, 149]

General Anesthesia

When fiberoptic bronchoscopy is performed in the intubated patient under general anesthesia, ventilation becomes a more important issue. A 5.7-mm outside diameter bronchoscope reduces the cross-sectional area of a 9.0-mm and 8.0-mm endotracheal tube by 41% and 52%, respectively (Fig. 4–8).[53] Because laminar flow is directly proportional to the fourth power of the radius by Poiseuille's law, resistance to flow would be expected to be markedly increased. Furthermore, rather than providing a perfectly tubular path for airflow, the FOB probably creates some turbulence as it courses eccentrically down the length of the endotracheal tube. Because resistance to turbulent flow is inversely proportional to the fifth power of the radius, even greater difficulty with air exchange is expected. Inadequate ventilation with CO_2 retention, gas trapping, inadvertent positive end-expiratory pressure (PEEP), and barotrauma can result, especially with smaller endotracheal tubes.

To overcome the problems of increased airway resistance with fiberoptic bronchoscopy through an endotracheal tube, ventilation should be controlled or vigorously assisted. The largest sized endotracheal tube possible should be used. For example, a PEEP of 35 cm H_2O was observed when a 5.7-mm FOB was placed into a patient's 7.0-mm endotracheal tube. No PEEP values above 20 cm H_2O were observed when the same FOB was inserted into an 8.0- or 8.5-mm endotracheal tube.[150] Thus, depending on the size of the FOB, the average adult should receive an endotracheal tube no smaller than 8.0 or 8.5 mm. Carden and Raj designed a special endotracheal tube for use with fiberoptic bronchoscopy with a wide internal diameter of 11 mm above the vocal cords and a narrow portion below the cords.[151] Because most of the airflow occurs in the portion with the wide lumen, the major resistance occurs in the infraglottic portion, which is only one fourth the total length. Resistance is only one fourth that of an endotracheal tube of similar infraglottic diameter. A special elbow connector between the endotracheal tube and circuit is used with the Carden as well as a regular endotracheal tube, allowing passage of the FOB through an airtight diaphragm.

Adequate oxygenation and CO_2 elimination can usually be achieved as long as the scope is not too large for the endotracheal tube and the patient's pulmonary mechanics are normal. Unfortunately, these conditions are not always met. In such situations, a prolonged expiratory time may be needed to allow adequate ventilation and prevent air trapping. If gas exchange is still unacceptable, the FOB may have to be

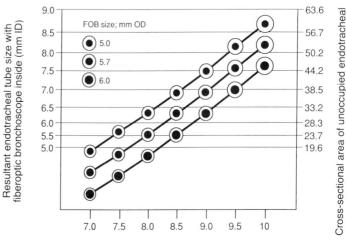

FIGURE 4–8. *Resultant cross-sectional area and equivalent endotracheal tube size following placement of 5.0-, 5.7-, or 6.0-mm fiberoptic bronchoscopes within variously sized endotracheal tubes. (Reprinted from Lindholm CE, Ollman B, Snyder JV, et al: Cardiorespiratory effect of flexible fiberoptic bronchoscopy in critically ill patients. Chest 1978; 74:362–368, with permission.)*

removed and the patient ventilated intermittently. Alternatively, jet ventilation can be supplied through the suction port of the FOB[152] or through a chest tube placed alongside the FOB.[153] If endotracheal tubes below 8.0 mm are to be employed, the use of helium-oxygen mixtures has been reported to decrease resistance to flow and enhance ventilation.[154]

The selection of general anesthetic technique for FOB depends on the same factors as with rigid bronchoscopy. Again, the task of having to provide deep levels of anesthesia and then having to wake the patient immediately is a recurrent motif. Inhalational agents, with their ability to be eliminated relatively quickly, may be helpful in this regard. However, the concentrations required to tolerate laryngoscopy may not be conducive to rapid arousal. A nitrous-narcotic technique has the advantage of allowing a smooth wake-up, but predicting the amount of narcotic can be difficult, especially in patients with limited respiratory reserve. High concentrations of nitrous oxide can predispose also to hypoxemia. Newer agents with short elimination half-lives, such as propofol, alfentanil, and even desflurane,[55] could have a new application in this setting. Airway hyper-reactivity and bronchospasm are also not uncommon in patients requiring bronchoscopy, who are often smokers with irritative lung pathology. Avoidance of agents known to release histamine (e.g., morphine, metocurine, gallamine, d-tubocurarine), cautious use of agents known to precipitate bronchospasm (e.g., β_2 antagonists, anticholinesterases), and utilization of bronchodilators (inhalational agents, ketamine, and atropine) may be prudent. These considerations are by no means exhaustive, but serve to illustrate that as long as care is individualized, a wide variety of anesthetics can be used.

Complications

The insertion of rigid or flexible fiberoptic bronchoscope in patients who are compromised by coexistent cardiopulmonary disease is fraught with potential hazard, both surgical and anesthetic.

From a respiratory standpoint, several mechanical changes are known to occur during fiberoptic bronchoscopy. A decrease in vital capacity, forced expiratory volume in 1 second, peak expiratory flow rate, and midmaximal expiratory flow rate have been observed following topical lidocaine anesthesia and immediately after fiberoptic bronchoscopy, perhaps owing to stimulation of airway reflexes or mucosal edema.[155] Increases in residual volume and functional residual capacity during fiberoptic bronchoscopy are other changes consistent with bronchospasm found to occur in patients with chronic airway obstruction.[156] Systemic administration of atropine[157, 158] or glycopyrrolate[159] can offset these adverse effects, presumably by the bronchodilating effects of vagal blockade. Anticholinergics also have the added benefit of decreasing secretions, thereby improving visualization.

Hypoxemia, seen with both rigid and flexible fiberoptic bronchoscopies, can be minimized by the techniques that allow uninterrupted ventilation. When using rigid bronchoscopy, adequate oxygenation can be provided by ventilation through the side arm of the bronchoscope.[160, 161] Oxygenation can be satisfactory with a rigid Venturi bronchoscope,[64, 65, 76, 162] but the likelihood of hypoxemia is heightened by the inability to guarantee the concentration of inspired oxygen. The arterial oxygen pressure (Pa_{O_2}) with fiberoptic bronchoscopy can drop by an average of 20 mmHg; a decrease can last for up to 4 hours after the procedure.[14]

Inadequate ventilation during bronchoscopy can lead to CO_2 retention. This condition seems to be more likely to occur with the ventilatory rigid bronchoscope than the Venturi bronchoscope,[71, 76] although in patients with normal pulmonary function, normocapnea is achievable with either bronchoscope. Indeed, several reports have observed the ability of Venturi jet ventilation to produce adequate Pa_{CO_2} levels without change from preoperative values.[64, 65, 70] It should be noted, however, that in patients with significant respiratory derangements, normalization of the Pa_{CO_2} may not be possible, no matter what mode of ventilation is used. Patients with decreased total thoracic compliance can be especially worrisome when the Venturi bronchoscope is used. Delivery of adequate tidal volumes in such patients may require higher peak airway pressures.

Bronchospasm has an increased incidence during bronchoscopy compared with its rate in patients undergoing general anesthesia for other procedures. In one study of more than 100,000 patients, the overall incidence of bronchospasm was 1.6/1000 for patients under general anesthesia for nonbronchoscopic surgery, but up to 16.4/1000 for patients undergoing bronchoscopy.[163] Other investigations, however, have reported incidences as low as 0.2/

1000 for patients having bronchoscopy.[164] This bronchospasm, occurring in both rigid and flexible bronchoscopy, can be the result of light levels of anesthesia and is especially common in patients with reactive airway disease.[165] Similarly, laryngospasm has an incidence of up to 14.0/1000 with bronchoscopy, compared with 7.9/1000 for general anesthesia[166] for non-bronchoscopic surgery. Again, lower limits of laryngospasm with bronchoscopy have been cited to be as infrequent as 1.3/1000.[164]

Other more infrequent complications involving the respiratory system during bronchoscopy exist. Pneumothorax, pneumomediastinum, and subcutaneous emphysema can occur secondary to biopsy or gas trapping from reduction of the cross-sectional area required for gas emptying with resultant barotrauma.[53, 164, 165] A post bronchoscopy chest radiograph is recommended to exclude this event. Subglottic edema can be caused by traumatic manipulation of the soft tissues, especially with rigid bronchoscopy. Bronchial and tracheal perforations are also more likely with the rigid bronchoscope, as are dental damage and hemorrhage, which can sometimes be massive.[165, 167] These possibilities reinforce the need for muscle relaxation. With the FOB, animal studies have demonstrated desquamation of tracheobronchial ciliated epithelium, but probably without significant effect on mucociliary transport.[168] Finally, the high gas velocity used with the rigid Venturi bronchoscope may propel blood or tumor particles into distal bronchioles or damage the airway.[53]

Cardiovascular complications of bronchoscopy are similar to those of laryngoscopy and intubation. The literature is replete with descriptions of tachycardia and hypertension seen with these procedures.[169–175] These hemodynamic surges are the result of the reflex sympathetic discharge from upper airway stimulation.[176] Hypertensive patients in particular seem to be prone to increases in blood pressure.[177, 178] Deleterious effects of such hyperdynamic changes include rupture of pre-existing intracranial aneurysms,[132, 179–181] dysrhythmias,[182-184] elevation of pulmonary artery pressures,[185] myocardial ischemia,[132, 186–188] and myocardial dysfunction.[189–191] In fact, myocardial ischemia is known to occur on induction in patients both with and without coronary artery disease.[192, 193] Although there is reason to believe the ischemia from induction and endotracheal tube placement is due to tachycardia[188] or hypertension,[187] brief periods of ischemia do not necessarily lead to later

myocardial necrosis.[194, 195] Brief is the key word, however. Unlike a speedy laryngoscopy and intubation, some bronchoscopies can subject patients to prolonged periods of intense stimulation. This underscores the importance of providing adequate anesthesia as described in the preceding sections, especially in high risk patients.

The dysrhythmias seen during fiberoptic bronchoscopy deserve further comment. The bradycardia occasionally seen with laryngoscopy and thought to be vagally mediated[169, 172–174] seems to be rare with FOB. In fact, the procedure is usually accompanied by sinus tachycardia.[196] Other dysrhythmias, such as premature atrial contractions, atrial fibrillation, atrial flutter, superventricular tachycardia, premature ventricular contractions, bigeminy, trigeminy, and other ventricular dysrhythmias, have been reported.[164, 197, 198] Patients with cardiopulmonary disease seem to have more rhythm disturbances during the procedure than those without such disease have.[196] Furthermore, although one investigation did find that FOB increased the incidence of ventricular and atrial ectopy over that recorded in the hour before the procedure,[199] more extensive monitoring of baseline dysrhythmias failed to corroborate such findings.[197] In either case, the majority of these dysrhythmias seem to be self-limited and require no treatment.[199] Nevertheless, because retrospective reports of deaths owing to cardiac arrest during FOB have been documented,[165] careful electrocardiographic monitoring should be performed on all patients receiving bronchoscopy. The delivery of supplemental oxygen would also be prudent, because hypoxia seems to increase the chances of producing dysrhythmias.[199] Although of unproven efficacy, the generous use of topical lidocaine has been recommended by some authors for its protective effect against dysrhythmias if systemically absorbed.[197]

Other cardiovascular complications seen during bronchoscopy are the same as those associated with anesthetic use in any procedure. An additional special consideration during bronchoscopy, however, occurs when the FOB occupies a significant cross-sectional area of the endotracheal tube or when the rigid bronchoscope fits too tightly around the larynx. If the resistance to exhalation is sufficient to cause inadvertent PEEP, venous return can be impeded, thereby reducing cardiac output. This scenario may be especially likely in young children, whose conical cricoid cartilage predisposes to a tight fit with the bronchoscope.

Toxic reactions to an overdose of local anesthetic have been reported with bronchoscopy. Central nervous system toxicity is a dose-dependent phenomenon, with low levels causing drowsiness; higher levels causing tinnitus, numbness of the lips and tongue, a metallic taste in the mouth, diplopia, and nystagmus; and still higher levels causing tremors in the face and hands, eventually leading to generalized tonic-clonic seizures.[200] Cardiovascular toxicity manifests as depression of conduction and contractility, with subsequent conduction blocks, dysrhythmias, and hypotension.[200, 201] The negative inotropic effect of local anesthetics is potentiated by hypercardia and hypoxia, two problems commonly encountered during bronchoscopy. Toxicity with tetracaine may not be heralded by early neurological warnings, as with lidocaine, but rather by syncope and cardiovascular collapse,[202] giving it a narrower margin of safety. In one large series of patients undergoing FOB, six out of seven major complications ascribed to local anesthetics, including one death, involved tetracaine.[164] This is not to say that toxic reactions due to lidocaine are not unknown. Limiting the total dose to 2–3 mg/kg,[203, 204] however, decreases the chances of exceeding the lidocaine blood levels of 5–6 $\mu g/mL$ associated with adverse symptoms.[205] Allergic reactions to esters, derivatives of allergenic para-aminobenzoic acid (PABA), are much more likely than to amides. Thus, in addition to its other disadvantages, tetracaine (or other esters) carries a higher risk of allergic reactions than lidocaine (or other amides) unless the lidocaine solution contains methylparaben, a preservative similar in structure and allergenic potential to PABA.

Intraoperative awareness, found to occur in 1–2% of patients undergoing general anesthesia,[206, 207] has an incidence of 4 to 8% with bronchoscopy.[208–210] Although the studies from which such values were obtained used a barbiturate-relaxant technique as the primary anesthetic, detection of such awareness may be underestimated, both by investigators in studies and by experienced clinicians.[208, 210]

The overall incidence of complications during bronchoscopy in the operating room has been estimated by several authors.[164, 165, 167, 198, 211] In these studies, the highest incidences of major and minor complications reported are 1.0% and 6.5%, respectively.[198] Death rates have been found to be as high as 0.7%[11] and as low as zero.[165] To be sure, some of these studies were retrospective, whereas others were prospective. The definitions of what constituted complications also varied. Despite these difficulties in comparing investigations, they emphasize the need for careful preoperative assessment and meticulous intraoperative monitoring, including use of capnometry and pulse oximetry.[55]

BRONCHOGRAPHY

Bronchography is a diagnostic radiographic procedure that involves selective application of radiopaque contrast into the bronchopulmonary tree to aid in the definition of parenchymal lung disease. Injection of the contrast into the lung region of interest is performed through either a rigid bronchoscope or flexible FOB, which is usually inserted into an endotracheal tube. Anesthesia can be provided as for any bronchoscopic procedure, with the understanding that spontaneous ventilation allows for the most even distribution of contrast into the peripheral airways. However, because spontaneous ventilation during bronchoscopy incurs its own risks, and because coughing during contrast injection leads to its unpredictable distribution, gentle controlled ventilation under general anesthesia and muscle relaxation may be the best approach.[53] Suctioning as much of the contrast material as possible is usually performed after the radiographs have been completed.

ESOPHAGOSCOPY

Like bronchoscopy, esophagoscopy has both diagnostic and therapeutic indications and can employ either flexible or rigid esophagoscopes. Diagnostically, esophagoscopy allows examination of strictures, upper GI bleeding, and mucosal abnormalities. Therapeutically, esophagoscopy is used for removal of foreign bodies, dilation of strictures, injection sclerotherapy of bleeding varices, and placement of stinting prostheses across obstructing strictures. Fiberoptic esophagoscopy permits greater patient comfort, superior visualization of the entire upper GI tract, and greater safety. Rigid esophagoscopy offers easier removal of foreign bodies and localization of massive esophageal bleeding.[53]

Both general and local anesthesia can be used with esophagoscopy, although local anesthesia alone is usually avoided with the rigid esophagoscope because of the greater chances of perforation. When topicalization is needed, lidocaine gargle and spray, used in conjunction with moderate doses of sedative, hypnotics, opiates, or propofol,[212] enable most patients to tolerate the procedure. However, patients considered to have full stomachs, significant reflux, or actively bleeding varices require rapid sequence induction and endotracheal intubation because of the risk of aspiration.

Certain aspects of airway management during esophagoscopy for foreign body removal require special attention. For instance, one would expect patients with foreign bodies trapped in the esophagus to require a rapid sequence intubation. However, if the object is sharp, cricoid pressure can cause esophageal perforation. An awake intubation is perhaps the best approach to this dilemma. A large foreign body can cause tracheal collapse also if it presses against the posterior tracheal wall, which lacks cartilaginous support. Using a reinforced endotracheal tube may help relieve this obstruction. Furthermore, selecting a smaller sized endotracheal tube may be necessary to allow insertion of the esophagoscope. Deflating the cuff of the endotracheal tube may aid in passing the esophagoscope also.

Complications of esophagoscopy are fewer than those of bronchoscopy, but no less important. Perforation is most likely to occur in the hypopharynx because of the apposition of the esophagus against the lower cervical spine during neck extension, the deficiency of muscle fibers in the posterior pharynx and upper esophagus, and the likelihood of pressure necrosis in that region, especially in aged individuals. Such perforations are known to have a 34–84% mortality.[213] Massive hemorrhage may occur from biopsies, trauma to bleeding varices, and mucosal tears at the gastroesophageal junction from retching. Dysrhythmias, usually transient, are seen occasionally as the esophagoscope brushes against the posterior border of the heart. Finally, the danger of aspiration pneumonia is augmented in patients requiring esophagoscopy, not only for the reasons mentioned earlier, but because agents used to reduce the gastric acidity, such as H_2-blockers and oral antacids, may be ineffective in patients with achalasia.[55]

REFERENCES

1. Kleinsasser O: Ein laryngomikroskop zur Fruhdiagnose und Differentialdiagnose von Krebsen in Kehlkope, Rachen und Mundhohle. Laryngol Rhinol Otol 1961; 40:276–279.
2. Strong MS, Vaughn CW, Mahler DL, et al: Cardiac complications of microsurgery of the larynx: Etiol-

ogy, incidence and prevention. Laryngoscope 1974; 84:908.
3. Keen RI, Kotak PK, Ramsden RT: Anaesthesia for microsurgery of the larynx. Ann R Coll Surg Engl 1982; 64:111–113.
4. Berenyi KJ, Harris RS, Harmel MH: General anaesthesia for endoscopy and interlaryngeal operations. A clinical study with determination of arterial blood gases and acid-base parameters. Acta Anaesthesiol Scand (Suppl) 1966; 23:529–537.
5. Weeks DB: Use of jet Venturi ventilation during microsurgery of the glottis and subglottis. Anesth Rev 1985; 12:32.
6. Crockett DM, McCabe BF, Scamman FL, et al: Venturi jet ventilaton for microlaryngoscopy: Technique, complications, pitfalls. Laryngoscope 1987; 97:1327.
7. Eng UB, Eriksson I, Sjostrand U: High frequency positive pressure ventilation (HFPPV): A review based upon its use during bronchoscopy and for laryngoscopy and microlaryngeal surgery under general anesthesia. Anesth Analg 1980; 59:594.
8. Babinski M, Smith RB, Klain M: High frequency jet ventilation for laryngoscopy. Anesthesiology 1980; 52:178–180.
9. Gettinger A, Glass DD: High frequency positive pressure ventilation use in neonatal and adult intensive care. *In* Carlon GG, Howland WJ (eds): High Frequency Ventilation in Intensive Care and During Surgery. New York, Marcel Dekker, 1985, p 63.
10. Kolton M: A review of high frequency oscillation. Can Anaesth Soc J 1984; 31:416.
11. McCullock PR, Froese AB: High frequency ventilation. *In* Shapiro BA, Cane RD (eds): Positive Airway Pressure Therapy: PPV and PEEP, Vol 5. Philadelphia, WB Saunders, 1987, p 873.
12. Einstein A: Zur Quantentheorie der stralung. Physikalische Zeitschrift 1917; 18:121–128.
13. Maiman TH: Stimulated optical radiation in ruby. Nature 1960; 187:493–494.
14. Garden JM, O'Banion MK, Shelnitz LS, et al: Papillomavirus in the vapor of carbon dioxide-treated verrucae. JAMA 1988; 259:1199–1202.
15. Tomita Y, Mihashi S, Nagita K, et al: Mutagenicity of smoke condensates induced by CO_2-laser irradiation and electrocauterization. Mutat Res 1981; 89:145–149.
16. Freitag L, Chapman GA, Sielczak M, et al: Laser smoke effect on the bronchial system. Lasers Surg Med 1987; 7:283–288.
17. Fuller TA: The physics of surgical lasers. Lasers Surg Med 1980; 1:5–14.
18. Pashayan AG: Anesthesia for laser surgery. *In* Barash PG (ed): ASA Refresher Courses in Anesthesiology, Vol 17. Philadelphia, JB Lippincott, 1989, pp 215–226.
19. Adachi K, Chole RA: Management of tracheal lesions in Hurler syndrome. Arch Otolaryngol Head Neck Surg 1990; 116:1205–1207.
20. Albert PW: The complications of CO_2 laser surgery in otolaryngology. Acta Otolaryngol (Stockh) 1981; 91:375–381.
21. Council on Scientific Affairs: Lasers in medicine and surgery. JAMA 1986; 256:900–907.
22. Sosis M: Anesthesia for laser surgery. *In* Lebowitz PW (ed): International Anesthesiology Clinics: Anesthesia for Eye, Ear and Airway Surgery, Vol 28. Boston, Little, Brown, 1990, pp 119–131.
23. Cozine K, Rosenbaum LM, Askanazi J, Rosenbaum SM: Laser-induced endotracheal tube fire. Anesthesiology 1981; 55:583.

24. Hermens JM, Bennett MJ, Hirshman CA: Anesthesia for laser surgery. Anesth Analg 1983; 62:218.
25. Keon TP: Anesthetic considerations for laser surgery. Int Anesthesiol Clin 1988; 26:50.
26. Esch VH, Dyer RF: Polyvinylchloride toxicity in fire fighters. JAMA 1976; 235:393–397.
27. Osoff RH, Duncavage JA, Eisenman TS, Karlan MS: Comparison of tracheal damage from laser-ignited endotracheal fires. Ann Otol Rhinol Laryngol 1983; 92:333–336.
28. Sosis M, Heller S: A comparison of special endotracheal tubes for use with the CO_2 laser. Anesthesiology 1988; 69:A251.
29. Sosis M, Heller S: A comparison of special endotracheal tubes for use with the Nd-YAG laser. Anesth Analg 1989; 68:S271.
30. Norton ML, DeVos P: New endotracheal tube for laser surgery of the larynx. Ann Otol Rhinol Laryngol 1978; 87:554–557.
31. Sosis MB: Evaluation of five metallic tapes for protection of endotracheal tubes during CO_2 laser surgery. Anesth Analg 1989; 68:392–393.
32. Sosis M, Dillon F, Heller S: A comparison of metallic tapes for protection of endotracheal tubes during Nd-YAG laser surgery. Anesth Analg 1989; 68:S270.
33. Kaeder CS, Hirshman CA: Acute airway obstruction: A complication of aluminum tape wrapping of tracheal tubes in laser surgery. Can Anaesth Soc J 1979; 26:138–139.
34. Sosis M, Dillon F, Heller S: Saline filled cuffs help prevent polyvinylchloride laser induced endotracheal tube fires. Can J Anaesth 1989; 36:S142.
35. Sosis M, Dillon F, Heller S: Prevention of CO_2 induced laser tracheal tube fires with the Laser-Guard. Can J Anaesth 1989; 36:S88.
36. Pashayan AG, Gravenstein JS: Helium retards endotracheal tube fires from carbon dioxide lasers. Anesthesiology 1985; 62:274–277.
37. Simpson JI, Wolf GL: Helium does not reduce endotracheal tube flammability. Anesth Analg 1989; 68:S266.
38. Cozine K, Stone JG, Shulman SM, Flaster E: Ventilatory technique alters outcome in CO_2 laser airway surgery. Anesthesiology 1989; 71:A992.
39. Hawkins DB, Udall JN: Juvenile laryngeal papillomas with cardiomegaly and polycythemia. Pediatrics 1979; 63:156.
40. Oleske JM, Kushnick T: Juvenile papilloma of the larynx. Am J Dis Child 1971; 121:417.
41. France NK, Beste DJ: Anesthesia for pediatric ear, nose, and throat surgery. In Gregory GA (ed): Pediatric Anesthesia, 2nd ed. New York, Churchill Livingstone, 1989, pp 1097–1147.
42. Motoyama EK: Anesthesia for ear, nose, and throat surgery. In Motoyama EK, Davis PJ (eds): Smith's Anesthesia for Infants and Children, 5th ed. St. Louis, CV Mosby, 1990, pp 649–674.
43. Buda AJ, Pinsky MR, Ingels NB: Effect of intrathoracic pressure on left ventricular performance. N Engl J Med 1979; 301:453.
44. Boyce JR: Laser therapy for bronchscopy. Anesthesiol Clin North Am 7:597–609.
45. McElvein RB, Zorn G: Treatment of malignant disease in trachea and mainstem bronchi by carbon dioxide laser. J Thorac Cardiovasc Surg 1983; 86:858.
46. Vourc'h G, Fischler M, Michon F, et al: Manual jet ventilation versus high frequency jet ventilation during laser resection of tracheo-bronchial stenosis. Br J Anaesth 1983; 55:969–972.
47. Rontal M, Rontal E, Wenokor ME, Elson L: Anesthetic management for tracheobronchial laser surgery. Ann Otol Rhinol Laryngol 1986; 95:556–560.
48. Brutinel WM, Cortese DA, McDougall JC: Bronchoscopic phototherapy with the neodymium-YAG laser. Chest 1984; 86:157–158.
49. Vourc'h G, Fischler M, Persome C, Colchen A: Anesthetic management during Nd-YAG laser resection for major tracheobronchial obstructing tumors. Anesthesiology 1984; 61:636–637.
50. Casey KR, Fairfax WR, Smith SJ, Dixon JA: Intratracheal fire ignited by the Nd-YAG laser during treatment of tracheal stenosis. Chest 1983; 84:295–296.
51. Geffin B, Shapshay SM, Bellack GS, et al: Flammability of endotracheal tubes during Nd-YAG laser application in the airway. Anesthesiology 1986; 65:511–515.
52. Sacker MA: Bronchofiberoscopy. Am Rev Resp Dis 1975; 111:62–88.
53. Benumof JL: Anesthesia for special elective diagnostic procedures. In Anesthesia for Thoracic Surgery. Philadelphia, WB Saunders, 1987, pp 326–342.
54. Landa JF: Indications for bronchoscopy. Chest 1978; 73:686–690.
55. Ehrenwerth J, Brull SJ: Anesthesia for thoracic diagnostic procedures. In Kaplan JA (ed): Thoracic Anesthesia. New York, Churchill Livingstone, 2nd ed (in press).
56. Kortilla K, Tarkkanen J: Comparison of diazepam and midazolam for sedation during local anesthesia for bronchoscopy. Br J Anaesth 1985; 57:581–586.
57. Yakaitis RW, Blitt CD, Angillo JE: End tidal enflurance concentration for endotracheal intubation. Anesthesiology 1979; 50:59–61.
58. Roizen MR, Horrigan RW, Frazer MB: Anesthetic doses blocking adrenergic (stress) and cardiovascular response to incision—MAC BAR. Anesthesiology 1981; 54:390–398.
59. Curling PE: Anesthesia for thoracic diagnostic procedures. In Kaplan JA (ed): Thoracic Anesthesia. New York, Churchill Livingstone, 1983, pp 319–345.
60. Carden E: Recent improvements in techniques for general anesthesia for bronchoscopy. Chest 1978; 73:697–700.
61. Frumin MJ, Epstein RM, Cohen G: Apneic oxygenation in man. Anesthesiology 1959; 20:789–798.
62. Fraioli RC, Sheffer LA, Steffenson JC: Pulmonary and cardiovascular effects of apneic oxygenation in man. Anesthesiology 1973; 39:588–596.
63. Muendrich K, Hoflehner G: Die narkose-beatmungs bronchoscopic. Anesthetist 1953; 21:121–123.
64. Duvall AJ, Johnson AF, Buckley J: Bronchoscopy under general anesthesia using the Sanders ventilating attachment. Ann Otol Rhinol Laryngol 1969; 78:490–498.
65. Carden E, Trapp WG, Oulton J: A new and simple method for ventilating patients undergoing bronchoscopy. Anesthesiology 1970; 33:454–458.
66. Grillick JS: The inflation-catheter technique for ventilation during bronchoscopy. Anesthesiology 1974; 40:503–506.
67. El-Naggar M: The use of a small endotracheal tube in bronchoscopy. Br J Anaesth 1975; 47:390–392.
68. Sanders RD: Two ventilating attachments for bronchoscopes. Del Med J 1967; 39:107–175.
69. Carden E: Positive-pressure ventilation during anesthesia for bronchoscopy: A laboratory evaluation of two recent advances. Anesth Analg 1973; 52:402–406.

70. Carden E, Burns WW, McDevitt NB, Carson T: A comparison of Venturi and side-arm ventilation in anaesthesia for bronchoscopy. Can Anaesth Soc J 1970; 20:569–574.

71. Giesecke AH, Grebershagen HU, Dortman C, Lee D: Comparison of the ventilating and injecting bronchoscopes. Anesthesiology 1973; 38:298–303.

72. Eisenkraft JB, Neustein SM: Anesthesia for special surgical problems in thoracic surgery. *In* Brodsky JB (ed): Problems in Anesthesia: Thoracic Anesthesia, Vol 4. Philadelphia, JB Lippincott, 1990, pp 326–354.

73. Schlenkhoff D, Droste H, Scieszka S, Vogt H: The use of high-frequency jet ventilation in operative bronchoscopy. Endoscopy 1986; 18:192–194.

74. Eng UB, Eriksson I, Sjostrand U: High-frequency positive-pressure ventilation (HFPPV): A review based upon its use during bronchoscopy and for laryngoscopy and microlaryngeal surgery under general anesthesia. Anesth Analg 1980; 59:594–603.

75. Safer P: Ventilating bronchoscope. Anesthesiology 1958; 19:406–408.

76. Morales GA, Epstein BS, Cinco B, et al: Ventilation during general anesthesia for bronchoscopy: Evaluation of a new technique. J Thor Cardiovasc Surg 1969; 57:873–878.

77. Reitman JS: General orotracheal anesthesia for bronchoscopy. JAMA 1957; 165:943–946.

78. Carden E, Schwesinger WB: The use of nitrous oxide during ventilation with the open bronchoscope. Anesthesiology 1973; 39:551–555.

79. Gal TJ: Anesthetic considerations for bronchoscopy. 1989 IARS Review Course Lectures. International Anesthesia Research Society, Cleveland, Ohio, 1989, pp 43–46.

80. Abou-Madi MN, Keszler H, Yacoub JM: A method for prevention of cardiovascular reactions to laryngoscopy and intubation. Can Anaesth Soc J 1975; 27:316–329.

81. Denlinger JK, Ellison N, Ominsky AJ: Effects of intratracheal lidocaine on circulatory responses to tracheal intubation. Anesthesiology 1974; 41:409–412.

82. Stoelting RK, Peterson C: Circulatory changes during anesthetic induction: Impact of d-tubocurarine pretreatment, thiamylal, succinylcholine, laryngoscopy and tracheal lidocaine. Anesth Anagl 1976; 55:77–81.

83. Stoelting RK: Circulatory changes during direct laryngoscopy with or without prior lidocaine. Anesthesiology 1977; 47:381–384.

84. Stoelting RK: Blood pressure and heart rate changes during laryngoscopy for endotracheal intubation: Influence of viscous or intravenous lidocaine. Anesth Analg 1978; 57:197–199.

85. Hamill JF, Bedford RF, Weaver DC, Colohan AR: Lidocaine before endotracheal intubation: Intravenous or endotracheal? Anesthesiology 1981; 55:578–581.

86. Youngberg JA, Graybar G, Hutchings D: Comparison of intravenous and topical lidocaine in attenuating the cardiovascular responses to intubation. South Med J 1983; 76:1122–1124.

87. Hartigan ML, Cheary JL, Gross JB, Schaffer DW: A comparison of pretreatment regimens for minimizing the haemodynamic response to blind nasotracheal intubation. Can Anaesth Soc J 1984; 31:497–502.

88. Chraemmer-Jorgensen B, Holland-Carlson RF, Marving J, Christensen V: Lack of effect of intravenous lidocaine in hemodynamic response to rapid sequence induction of general anesthesia: A double-blind controlled trial. Anesth Analg 1986; 65:1037–1041.

89. Laurito CE, Baughman VL, Polek WV, et al: Aerosolized and intravenous lidocaine are no more effective than placebo for the control of hemodynamic responses to intubation. Anesthesiology 1987; 67:A29.

90. Prys-Roberts C, Foex P, Biro GP, Roberts JG: Studies of anaesthesia in relation to hypertension V. Adrenergic beta-receptor blockade. Br J Anaesth 1973; 45:671–680.

91. Maharaj RJ, Thompson M, Brock-Utne JG, et al: Treatment of hypertension following endotracheal intubation: A study comparing the efficacy of labetalol, practolol, and placebo. S Afr Med J 1983; 63:691–694.

92. Kopriva CJ, Brown ACD, Pappas G: Hemodynamics during general anesthesia in patients receiving propranolol. Anaesthesia 1978; 48:28–33.

93. Safwat AM, Fung DC, Bilton DS: The use of propranolol in rapid sequence anesthetic induction: Optimal time interval for pretreatment. Can Anaesth Soc J 1984; 31:638–641.

94. Gold MI, Brown M, Salem JS: The effects of esmolol after ketamine induction and intubation. Anesthesiology 1984; 61:A19.

95. Merkhaus PG, Reves JG, Kissin I, et al: Cardiovascular effects of esmolol in anesthetized humans. Anesth Analg 1985; 64:327–334.

96. Lui PL, Gatt S, Gugino LD, et al: Esmolol for control of increases in heart rate and blood pressure during tracheal intubation after thiopentone and succinylcholine. Can Anaesth Soc J 1986; 33:556–562.

97. Murthy VS, Patel KD, Elangovan RG, et al: Cardiovascular and neuromuscular effects of esmolol during induction of anesthesia. J Clin Pharmacol 1986; 26:351–357.

98. Cucchiara RF, Benefiel DJ, Matteo RS, et al: Evaluation of esmolol in controlling increases in heart rate and blood pressure during endotracheal intubation in patients undergoing carotid endarterectomy. Anesthesiology 1986; 65:528–531.

99. Bernstein JS, Ebert TJ, Stowe DF, et al: Single IV bolus esmolol prior to rapid sequence induction effectively blunts the intubation response. Anesth Analg 1989; 68:S24.

100. Ebert TJ, Bernstein JS, Stowe DF, et al: Attenuation of hemodynamic response to rapid sequence induction in healthy patients with a single bolus of esmolol. J Clin Anesth 1990; 2:243–252.

101. Mallon JS, Hew E, Wald R, Kapala D: Bolus doses of esmolol for the prevention of postintubation hypertension and tachycardia. J Cardiothor Anesth 1990; 2:27–30.

102. Devalt M, Greifenstein FE, Harris LG: Circulatory responses to endotracheal intubation in light general anesthesia: The effects of atropine and phentolamine. Anesthesiology 1960; 21:360–362.

103. Curran J, Crowley M, O'Sullivan G: Droperidol and endotracheal intubation: Attenuation of pressor response to laryngoscopy and intubation. Anaesthesia 1980; 35:290–294.

104. Leslie JB, Kalaysian RW, McLoughlin TM, Plachetka JR: Attenuation of the hemodynamic responses to endotracheal intubation with intravenous labetalol. Anesthesiology 1967; 67:A30.

105. Inada E, Cullen DJ, Nemeskal R, Teplick R: Effect of labetalol on the hemodynamic response to intubation: A randomized double-blind study. Anesthesiology 1987; 67:A31.

106. Bernstein JS, Nelson MA, Ebert TJ, et al: Beat-by-beat cardiovascular response to rapid sequence induction in humans: Effects of labetalol. Anesthesiology 1987; 67:A32.

107. Corat P, Daluz M, Bousseau D, et al: Prevention of intraoperative ischemia during noncardiac surgery with nitroglycerine. Anesthesiology 1984; 61:193–196.

108. Thompson TR, Mutch WH, Culligan JD: Failure of intravenous nitroglycerine to prevent intraoperative ischemia during fentanyl pancuronium anesthesia. Anesthesiology 1984; 61:385–393.

109. Stoelting RF: Attenuation of blood pressure response to laryngoscopy with sodium nitroprusside. Anesth Analg 1979; 58:116–119.

110. Davis MJ, Cronin KD, Cowie RW: The prevention of hypertension: A controlled study of intravenous hydralazine on patients undergoing intracranial surgery. Anesthesia 1984; 36:147–152.

111. Mikawa K, Ikeaki J, Maekawa N, et al: The effect of diltiazem on the cardiovascular response to tracheal intubation. Anaesthesia 1990; 45:289–293.

112. Puri GD, Batra YK: Effect of nifedipine on cardiovascular responses to laryngoscopy and intubation. Br J Anaesth 1988; 60:579–581.

113. Nishikawa T, Namiki A: Attenuation of the pressor response to laryngoscopy and tracheal intubation with intravenous verapamil. Acta Anaesthesiol Scand 1981; 33:232–235.

114. Hatano R, Imai R, Komatsu K, Mori K: Intravenous administration of isosorbide dinitrate attenuates the pressor response to laryngoscopy and tracheal intubation. Acta Anaesthesiol Scand 1989; 33:214–218.

115. Khan FA, Kamal RS: Effect of buprenorphine on the cardiovascular response to tracheal intubation. Anaesthesia 1989; 44:394–397.

116. Bennett GM, Stanley TH: Human cardiovascular responses to endotracheal intubation during morphine-nitrous oxide and fentanyl-nitrous oxide anesthesia. Anesthesiology 1980; 52:520–522.

117. Dahlgren N, Messeter K: Treatment of stress response to laryngoscopy and intubation with fentanyl. Anaesthesia 1981; 36:1022–1026.

118. Kautto UM: Attenuation of the circulatory response to laryngoscopy and intubation by fentanyl. Acta Anaesthesiol Scand 1982; 26:217–221.

119. Parker EO, Ross AL: Low dose fentanyl: Effects on thiopental requirements and hemodynamic response during induction and intubation. Anesthesiology 1982; 57:A322.

120. Martin DE, Rosenberg H, Aukberg JS, et al: Low-dose fentanyl blunts circulatory responses to tracheal intubation. Anesth Analg 1982; 61:680–684.

121. Barash PG, Giles R, Marx P, et al: Intubation: Is low dose fentanyl really effective? Anesth Analg 1982; 61:168–169.

122. Cork RC, Weiss JL, Hameroff SR, Bentley J: Fentanyl preloading for rapid-sequence induction of anesthesia. Anesth Analg 1984; 63:60–64.

123. Ebert JP, Pearson JD, Gelma S, et al: Circulatory responses to laryngoscopy: The comparative effects of placebo, fentanyl and esmolol. Can J Anaesth 1989; 36:301–306.

124. Brizgys RU, Morales R, Cowens B: Low dose sufentanil: Effects on thiopental requirements and hemodynamic response during induction and intubation. Anesthesiology 1985; 63:A377.

125. Komatsu T, Shibutani K, Okamoto K, et al: Is sufentanil superior to fentanyl as an induction agent? Anesthesiology 1985; 63:A378.

126. Kleinman J, Marlar K, Silva DA, et al: Sufentanil attenuation of the stress response during rapid sequence induction. Anesthesiology 1985; 63:A379.

127. Marty J, Couderc E, Servin F, et al: Plasma concentrations of sufentanil required to suppress hemodynamic responses to noxious stimuli during nitrous anesthesia. Anesthesiology 1988; 64:A631.

128. Wark KJ, Lyons J, Feneck RO: The haemodynamic effects of bronchoscopy: Effect of pretreatment with fentanyl and alfentanil. Anaesthesia 1986; 41:162–167.

129. Black TE, Bay B, Healy TEJ: Reducing the haemodynamic responses to laryngoscopy and intubation: A comparison of alfentanil with fentanyl. Anaesthesia 1984; 39:833–837.

130. Ikeda S: Flexible bronchofiberscope. Keio J Med 1968; 17:1–16.

131. Berkovitz BKB, Maxham BJ: A Textbook of Head and Neck Anatomy. Barcelona, Spain, Yearbook Medical Publishers, 1988, pp 277–331.

132. Bedford RF: Circulatory responses to tracheal intubation. In Bishop MJ (ed): Problems in Anesthesia. Philadelphia, JB Lippincott, 1988 2(2), pp 201–210.

133. Katz J: Atlas of Regional Anesthesia. Norwalk, CT, Appleton-Century-Crofts, 1985, pp 56–60.

134. William PL, Warwick R, Dyson M, Bannister LH: Gray's Anatomy. New York, Churchill Livingstone, 1989, p 1117.

135. Barton S, Williams JD: Glossopharyngeal nerve block. Acta Otolaryngol 1971; 93:186–189.

136. Woods AM, Cander CJ: Abolition of gagging and hemodynamic response to awake laryngoscopy. Anesthesiology 1987; 67:A220.

137. Stiffel P, Hameroff SR: A modified technique for transtracheal anesthesia. Anesthesiology 1979; 51:274–275.

138. Christofordis AJ, Tomashefski JF, Mitchell RA: Use of an ultrasonic nebulizer for the application of oropharyngeal, laryngeal and tracheobronchial anesthesia. Chest 1971; 59:629–633.

139. Williams RT, Maltby JR: Airway intubator. Anesth Analg 1982; 61:309.

140. Ovassapian A, Dykes HM: The role of fiber-optic endoscopy in airway management. Semin Anesth 1987; 67:93–104.

141. Kreinholz EJ, Fussel J: Arterial blood gas studies during fiberoptic bronchoscopy. Am Rev Resp Dis 1973; 108:1014.

142. Dubrawsky C, Awe RJ, Jenkins DE: Effect of fiber-optic bronchoscopy on oxygenation of arterial blood. Chest 1973; 64:393.

143. Albertini RE, Harrell JH, Moser KM: Hypoxemia during fiberoptic bronchoscopy. Chest 1974; 65:117–118.

144. Albertini RE, Harrell JH, Kurihara N, Moser KM: Arterial hypoxemia induced by fiberoptic bronchoscopy. JAMA 1974; 230:1666–1667.

145. Dubrawsky C, Ames RJ, Jenkins D: The effect of bronchofiberoptic examination on oxygen status. Chest 1975; 67:137–140.

146. Albertini RE, Harrell JH, Mosner KM: Management of arterial hypoxemia induced by fiberoptic bronchoscopy. Chest 1975; 67:134–135.

147. Lampton LM: Bronchoscopy: Caution! JAMA 1975; 231:138.

148. Mallios E: A modification of the Laerdil anesthetic mask for nasotracheal intubation with the fiberoptic laryngoscope. Anesthesia 1980; 35:559–560.

149. Patil V, Stehling LC, Zavder HL: Mechanical aids for fiberoptic endoscopy. Anesthesiology 1982; 57:69–70.

150. Lindholm CE, Ollman B, Snyder JV, et al: Cardio-respiratory effects of flexible fiberoptic bronchoscopy in critically ill patients. Chest 1978; 74:362–368.

151. Carden F, Raj PP: Special new low resistance to flow tube and endotracheal tube adaptor for use during fiberoptic bronchoscopy. Ann Otol Rhinol Laryngol 1975; 84:631–634.

152. Satyanarayam T, Lapan L, Ramanathan S, et al: Bronchofiberscope jet ventilation. Anesth Analg 1980; 59:350–354.

153. Smith RB, Lindholm CE, Klain M: Jet ventilation for fiberoptic bronchoscopy under general anaesthesia. Acta Anaesthesiol Scand 1976; 20:111–116.

154. Pingleton SK, Bone CR, Ruth WC: Helium-oxygen mixtures during bronchoscopy. Crit Care Med 1980; 8:50–53.

155. Belen J, Neuhaus A, Markowitz D, Rotman HH: Modification of the effects of fiberoptic bronchoscopy on pulmonary mechanics. Chest 1981; 74:516–519.

156. Salisbury BG, Metzger CF, Altose MD, et al: Effect of fiberoptic bronchoscopy on respiratory performance in patients with chronic airway obstruction. Thorax 1975; 30:441–446.

157. Matsushima T, Jones RL, King EG, et al: Alterations in pulmonary mechanisms and gas exchange during routine fiberoptic bronchoscopy. Chest 1984; 86:184–188.

158. Neuhaus A, Markowitz MD, Weg JG: The effects of fiberoptic bronchoscopy with and without atropine premedication on pulmonary function in humans. Ann Thorac Surg 1978; 25:393–398.

159. Thorburn JR, James MF, Feldman C, et al: Comparison of the effects of atropine and glycopyrrolate on pulmonary mechanics in patients undergoing fiberoptic bronchoscopy. Anesth Analg 1986; 65:1285–1289.

160. Schoenstadt DA, Doneker TG, Arnold HA, Swisher LB: A reexamination of the ventilating bronchoscope. J Thorac Cardiovasc Surg 1965; 49:525–530.

161. Smith FR, Kundohl PE, Fouty R: The safety of general anesthesia for bronchoscopy demonstrated by a study of arterial and venous oxygen saturation levels. Dis Chest 1967; 51:53–58.

162. Smith CO, Schroff PF, Steele JD: General anesthesia for bronchoscopy: The use of the Saunders bronchoscopic attachment. Ann Thorac Surg 1969; 8:348–354.

163. Olsson GL: Bronchospasm during anaesthesia: A computer aided incidence study of 136,529 patients. Acta Anaesthesiol Scand 1987; 31:244–252.

164. Gredle WF, Smidely JE, Elliott RC: Complications of fiberoptic bronchoscopy. Am Rev Resp Dis 1972; 109:67–72.

165. Lukomsky GI, Ouchinnikov AA, Bilas A: Complications of bronchoscopy: Comparisons of rigid bronchoscopy under general anesthesia and flexible fiberoptic bronchoscopy under topical anesthesia. Chest 1981; 79:316–321.

166. Olsson GL, Hallen B: Laryngospasm during anaesthesia: A computer aided incidence study in 136,929 patients. Acta Anaesthesiol Scand 1984; 28:567–575.

167. Suratt PM, Smiddy JF, Gruber B: Deaths and complications associated with fiberoptic bronchoscopy. Chest 1970; 69:747–751.

168. Holding AC: Experimental bronchoscopy in calves: Injury and repair of tracheobronchial epithelium after passage of bronchoscope. Am Rev Resp Dis 1968; 48:646–652.

169. Reid LC, Brace DE: Irritation of the respiratory tract and its reflex effect on the heart. Surg Gynecol Obstet 1940; 70:157–162.

170. King BD, Harris LC, Greifenstein FE: Cardiovascular effects of orotracheal intubation during light anesthesia. Surg Forum 1950; 1:620–624.

171. Burnstein CL, LoPinto FJ, Newman W: Electrocardiographic studies during endotracheal intubation. Anesthesiology 1950; 11:224–237.

172. King BD, Harris LC, Greifenstein FE, et al: Reflex circulatory response to direct laryngoscopy and tracheal intubation performed during general anesthesia. Anesthesiology 1951; 12:556–566.

173. Wycoff CC: Endotracheal intubation: Effects on blood pressure and pulse rate. Anesthesiology 1959; 21:153–158.

174. Takeshima IC, Noda K, Higaki M: Cardiovascular response to rapid anesthesia induction and endotracheal intubation. Anesth Analg Curr Res 1964; 43:201–208.

175. Forbes AM, Dally FG: Acute hypertension during induction of anaesthesia and endotracheal intubation in normotensive man. Br J Anaesth 1970; 42:618–624.

176. Tomori Z, Widdacomb JG: Muscular, bronchomotor, and cardiovascular reflexes elicited by mechanical stimulation of the respiratory tract. J Physiol 1969; 200:25–49.

177. Prys-Roberts C, Green LT, Meloche R, Foex P: Studies of anaesthesia in relation to hypertension II: Haemodynamic consequences of induction and endotracheal intubation. Br J Anaesth 1971; 43:531–546.

178. Bedford RF, Feinstein B: Hospital admission blood pressures: A predictor for hypertension following endotracheal intubation. Anesth Analg 1980; 59:367–370.

179. Shapiro HM, Wyte SR, Harris AS, Galindo A: Acute intracranial hypertension in neurosurgery patients: Mechanical and pharmacologic factors. Anesthesiology 1972; 37:399–405.

180. Fox EJ, Sklar GS, Hill CH, et al: Complications related to the pressor response to tracheal intubation. Anesthesiology 1977; 47:524–525.

181. Tsementas SA, Hitchcock ER: Outcome from "rescue clipping" of ruptured intracranial aneurysms during induction anesthesia and endotracheal intubation. J Neurol Neurosurg Psychiatry 1985; 48:160–163.

182. Ganthler J, Bosomworth P, Page D: Effects of endotracheal intubation on electrocardiographic patterns during halothane anesthesia. Anesth Analg 1962; 41:466–470.

183. Katz RL, Bigger JT: Cardiac arrhythmias during anesthesia and operation. Anesthesiology 1970; 33:193–213.

184. Mackenzie RA, Gould AS, Bardsley WT: Cardiac arrhythmias with endotracheal intubation. Anesthesiology 1980; 53(Suppl):102.

185. Sorenson MB, Jacobson E: Pulmonary hemodynamics during induction of anesthesia. Anesthesiology 1977; 46:246–251.

186. Roy WL, Edelist G, Gilbert B: Myocardial ischemia during noncardiac surgical procedures in patients with coronary artery disease. Anesthesiology 1979; 51:393–397.

187. Rao TRL, Jacobs KH, El-Etr AA: Reinfarction following anesthesia in patients with myocardial infarction. Anesthesiology 1983; 59:499–505.

188. Slogoff S, Keats AL: Does perioperative myocardial ischemia lead to postoperative myocardial infarction? Anesthesiology 1985; 62:102–114.

189. Barash PG, Kopriva CJ, Giles RW, et al: Global

ventricular function and intubation: Radionuclear profiles. Anesthesiology 1980; 53:S109.

190. Giles RW, Berger HJ, Barash PG, et al: Continuous monitoring of left ventricular performance with computerized nuclear probe during laryngoscopy and intubation before coronary artery bypass surgery. Am J Cardiol 1982; 50:735–740.

191. Chraemmer-Jorgenson B, Hoilund-Carlsen BF, Marving J, Pederson JF: Left ventricular performance monitored by radionuclide cardiography during induction of anesthesia. Anesthesiology 1985; 62:278–286.

192. Coleman AJ, Jordon C: Cardiovascular response to anaesthesia: Influence of beta-adrenoreceptor receptor blockade with metoprolol. Anaesthesia 1980; 35:972–978.

193. Coriat L, Harari R, Doloz M: Clinical predictors of intraoperative myocardial ischemia in patients with coronary artery disease undergoing noncardiac surgery. Acta Anaesthesiol Scand 1982; 26:287–290.

194. Whalen DA Jr, Hamilton DY, Ganote CE, Jennings RB: I. Effect of a transient period of ischemia on myocardial cells. Am J Pathol 1974; 74:381–397.

195. Geft IL, Fishben MC, Ninomiya K, et al: Intermittent brief periods of ischemia have a cumulative effect and may cause myocardial necrosis. Circulation 1982; 66:1150–1153.

196. Luck JC, Messender OH, Rubenstein MJ, et al: Arrhythmias from fiberoptic bronchoscopy. Chest 1987; 74:139–143.

197. Elguindi AS, Harrison GN, Abdulla AM, et al: Cardiac rhythm disturbances during fiberoptic bronchoscopy: A prospective study. J Thorac Cardiovasc Surg 1979; 73:557–561.

198. Pereira W, Konvat DM, Snider GI: A prospective cooperative study of complications following flexible fiberoptic bronchoscopy. Chest 1978; 73:813–816.

199. Shrader OL, Lakshminarayan S: The effect of fiberoptic bronchoscopy on cardiac rhythm. Chest 1978; 73:821–824.

200. deJong RH: Toxic effects of local anesthetics. JAMA 1978; 239:1164–1168.

201. Strichartz GZ, Covino BJ: Local anesthetics. *In* Miller RN (ed): Anesthesia. New York, Churchill Livingstone, 1990, pp 437–470.

202. Adriani J, Campbell D: Fatalities following topical application of local anesthesia to mucous membranes. JAMA 1956; 162:1527–1530.

203. Pelton D, Daly M, Cooper PD, Conn AW: Plasma lidocaine concentrations following topical aerosol application to the trachea and bronchi. Can Anaesth Soc J 1970; 17:250–255.

204. Viegas O, Stoelting RK: Lidocaine in arterial blood after laryngotracheal administration. Anesthesiology 1975; 43:491–493.

205. Foldes FF, Malloy R, McNall PG, Koukal LR: Comparison of toxicity of intravenously given local anesthetics in man. JAMA 1960; 172:1493–1498.

206. Brickenridge JL, Atkenhead AR: Awareness during anaesthesia: A review. Ann R Coll Surg Engl 1983; 65:93–96.

207. Wilson SL, Vaughan RW, Stephen CR: Awareness, dreams and hallucinations associated with general anesthesia. Anesth Analg 1975; 54:609–617.

208. Barr DM, Wong RM: Awareness during general anaesthesia for bronchoscopy and laryngoscopy using the apnaeic oxygen technique. Br J Anaesth 1973; 45:894–900.

209. Fairlie HB: An evaluation of local and general anaesthesia for diagnostic bronchoscopy. Can Anaesth Soc J 1956; 3:366.

210. Moore JK, Seymour A: Awareness during bronchoscopy. Ann R Coll Surg Engl 1987; 69:45–47.

211. Dreisin RB, Albert RK, Talley PA, et al: Flexible fiberoptic bronchoscopy in the teaching hospital: Yield and complications. Annu Rev Resp Dis 1977; 115:102A.

212. Steegers PA, Foster PA: The use of propofol in a group of older patients undergoing oesophagoscopy. S Afr Med J 1981; 73:279–281.

213. Steyne JH, Brunner BL: Perforation of cervical oesophagus at oesophagoscopy. S Afr Med J 1962; 7:494–482.

5

Anesthesia for Major Head and Neck Surgery

Francis X. McGowan

CARCINOMAS OF THE OROPHARYNX AND LARYNX

LESIONS OF THE ORAL CAVITY AND OROPHARYNX

Epidemiology

Oral and pharyngeal carcinomas (primarily squamous cell carcinomas) account for between 3 and 5% of human cancers and can have an overall 5-year survival rate as low as 60%.[1] Males are affected more than females by approximately 2.5:1, and blacks are affected more than whites by a factor of 1.8. Of 100 deaths from cancer in the United States, 5 are from these tumors; in Asia and some parts of the Third World, nearly 50% of all cancers are composed of tumors in these locations.

Approximately 75% of patients are over age 60 years at the time of initial presentation. Despite the ready accessibility of the oral cavity to examination and biopsy, most of these tumors are at an advanced stage at the time of diagnosis.[2] Lip carcinomas account for 20–30% of all oral cavity tumors; other frequent sites include the floor of the mouth, the ventral or lateral tongue surfaces (Fig. 5–1), and the soft palate. Risk factors for the development of these lesions include tobacco consumption (either inhaled or chewed), heavy alcohol ingestion for extended periods, and betel nut chewing. Pipe smoking, sunlight exposure, and fair complexion particularly have been linked to the occurrence of lip cancer.

Prognosis is determined by several factors, including size and location of the lesion, his-tological grade, and most important, the presence of metastasis to the cervical lymph nodes.[3] For smaller oral lesions without evident spread, radiation therapy and surgical resection seem about equally effective. Clinically apparent disease in the neck is considered an indication for surgery. Radiation therapy is usually combined with resection to treat lesions of the neck and may be employed (1) preoperatively, followed by excision and neck dissection; (2) for recurrences only, following surgical extirpation of the primary lesion and cervical node disease; (3) as curative therapy to the primary lesion, followed by neck dissection and irradiation; and (4) postoperatively, to both the primary site and the neck.[1, 4] The exact sequence chosen depends on multiple factors, including the surgeon's preference and the patient's overall condition. Successful control of cervical disease is believed to be the same regardless of the timing of radiation therapy.[4] Management is more controversial for the patient without apparent neck involvement, as may occur in 25–35% of cancers of the lip and oral cavity. Neck dissection and irradiation are felt to be equally effective in treating occult cervical metastasis, with the former favored in patients believed to have a high likelihood of cervical spread based on tumor type, size, and so forth, and in patients not being considered for initial radiation to the primary neck lesion.

Oropharyngeal carcinomas (soft palate, tongue base, uvula, retromolar trigone, tonsil) have a lower survival rate because of the likelihood of advanced local disease at the time of discovery and because of an incidence of

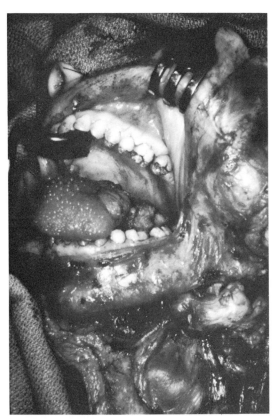

FIGURE 5–1. Hemiglossectomy for squamous cell carcinoma of the lateral tongue. (Photograph courtesy of Clarence T. Sasaki, M.D., Professor of Otolaryngology, Yale University School of Medicine.)

metastasis of 40–70%.[3] These tumors are also more frequently anaplastic or less well differentiated than their oral cavity counterparts. The risk factors of smoking and ethanol intake are similar for these lesions. Aggressive surgery, irradiation, and combinations of these have all been advocated as optimal treatment, with high-voltage radiation therapy being the mainstay. Numerous surgical approaches are used for these lesions, including intraoral excision, mandibular osteotomy, various pharyngotomies, and composite resection.

Carcinomas in the hypopharyngeal region (superior aspect of epiglottis to inferior cricoid border) are also frequently associated with alcohol and tobacco use. In females, these carcinomas may also be associated with the Plummer-Vinson syndrome, which consists mainly of achlorhydria, anemia, and mucous membrane atrophy. Primary lesions are found most frequently in the pyriform sinus. High rates of metastasis (40–70%) and the delayed onset of noticeable symptoms contribute to poor survival rates. Dysphagia and sore throat

may be symptoms. Therapy consists of pharyngolaryngectomy with neck dissection, along with postoperative irradiation. Extensive disease and specifically involvement of the postcricoid region or cervical esophagus mandate esophagectomy as well.

LARYNGEAL CARCINOMAS

Cancers of the larynx account for 2–3% of malignancies. Incidence is higher in males than females (5.5:1); 80% occur in patients 50–80 years of age.[5] Again, the most frequently cited etiological factors are heavy tobacco and alcohol use. Other factors that have been implicated in laboratory and epidemiological studies include exposure to organic compounds (hydrocarbons and amines) and their combustion products, viral infection (herpes simplex), and neck irradiation.

For purposes of classification, the larynx is divided into three anatomical regions: (1) supraglottis, which includes epiglottis, aryepiglottic folds, arytenoids, and the false vocal cords; (2) glottis, composed of the true vocal cords and the anterior and posterior commissures; and (3) subglottis, which extends from the lower margin of the glottis inferiorly to the lower border of the cricoid cartilage. Tumors in the glottis are the most common, accounting for 50–60% of laryngeal cancers.[5] Supraglottic lesions constitute 20–30%, and true subglottic tumors approximately 1%. Because of their shared boundaries and consequent therapeutic implications, pyriform fossa and inferior hypopharyngeal tumors are often considered with carcinomas of the larynx. By comparison, laryngeal lesions often have more favorable prognoses, owing to an increased degree of differentiation, confinement by local anatomical boundaries, and less frequent incidence of metastasis.

Common symptoms include weight loss, dysphagia, odynophagia, and cough. Dyspnea and stridor owing to airway obstruction may occur late in the disease. Hoarseness is the hallmark symptom in glottic carcinoma; it is delayed with supraglottic and subglottic tumors. In patients with these risk factors, hoarseness persisting for greater than 2–3 weeks is an indication for laryngeal evaluation.

Diagnostic laryngeal evaluation includes (1) physical examination of the laryngeal cartilage, tongue base, and cervical soft tissues, looking for tenderness, masses, and so forth; (2) mirror indirect or flexible nasopharyngoscopic examination; (3) direct laryngoscopy and biopsy;

and (4) xeroradiographic and computed tomographic (CT) scanning. The primary goal of these studies is to define as precisely as possible the extent of tumor involvement for both the surgical and anesthetic teams.

Supraglottic tumors tend to remain above the true vocal cords, their spread hindered by tissue planes (Fig. 5–2). As a result, some of these tumors are amenable to treatment that conserves the glottic and subglottic regions[6] (Fig. 5–3). This involves resection of the supraglottis, the pre-epiglottic space, and the associated lymphatic channels through the thyrohyoid membrane. The major advantage is potential cure without loss of speech. As for many of the lesions discussed previously, high-dose irradiation and supraglottic laryngectomy give similar results for smaller, confined lesions. If surgery is chosen, pre- or postoperative radiation therapy is usually employed also. The presence or suspicion of neck disease requires a neck dissection as well. More extensive lesions are usually treated by irradiation followed by total laryngectomy. Technical and

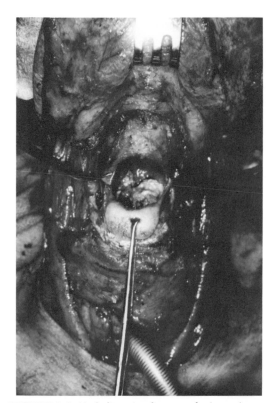

FIGURE 5–2. *Neck dissection for supraglottic carcinoma. The upper margin of fungating tumor can be seen at the center of photograph. Also note a wire-reinforced endotracheal tube emerging inferiorly. (Photograph courtesy of Clarence T. Sasaki, M.D., Professor of Otolaryngology, Yale University School of Medicine.)*

wound-healing difficulties, availability of appropriate patients, and concerns about sacrificing potential cure (i.e., if total laryngectomy is done) in an attempt to preserve function have led to some questions about the validity of this procedure.

Glottic carcinomas are usually confined to the region of the true vocal cords and are well-differentiated, slow-growing tumors. Because lymphatic drainage of the cords is limited, these more often remain localized and have a less frequent rate of cervical metastasis. Here again, the less extensive, localized lesions can be treated with irradiation, surgery, or both, with irradiation being somewhat preferred because of its ability to preserve speech. A hemilaryngectomy may be performed in cases of invasion of the subglottic, anterior commissure, or vocal processes. More extensive lesions are treated with a total laryngectomy and neck dissection, along with irradiation. A particularly lethal site of recurrence is the tracheal stoma. As with the other lesions, failure to eradicate local disease and cervical node involvement are indicative of less favorable prognosis.

Another consideration is the possibility of associated malignancies in these patients. These often occur elsewhere in the respiratory or gastrointestinal (GI) systems, with an incidence estimated to be as high as 15–20%[2, 3] These malignancies may take the form of coexistent or subsequent oral cancers, bronchogenic carcinomas, esophageal cancer, or lesions at more distant sites. It is likely that patient age, risk factors common to several tumor types (e.g., smoking), and an inherent susceptibility to cancer all play a role in this phenomenon.

PREOPERATIVE ASSESSMENT

Preoperative evaluation of these patients is complicated by their age, the likelihood of dysfunction of multiple organ systems, and the location and extent of their neoplastic process. Salient aspects of these considerations are summarized.

Airways and Pulmonary Disease

Lesions in this region have the obvious capability of obstructing the upper digestive and respiratory tracts. Oral cavity tumors may impair handling of secretions, occasionally contribute to secretion volume, and hemorrhage into the area as well. Pharyngeal sensation and

FIGURE 5–3. Example of glottic conservation following resection of supraglottic tumor. (Photograph courtesy of Clarence T. Sasaki, M.D., Professor of Otolaryngology, Yale University School of Medicine.)

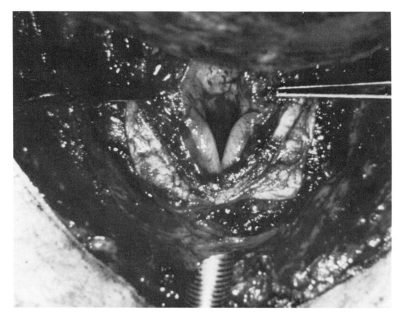

coordination may be impaired also. Prior surgery and irradiation can add to the dysfunction and the potential for aspiration, hemorrhage, anatomical distortion, and a variety of other complications.

As discussed previously, hoarseness owing to vocal cord involvement of glottic tumors is common. Impairment of cord motion may result in aspiration or severe airway obstruction. An obstructed airway may ensue with any of the laryngeal lesions as a result of mass effect, secretions, or cord fixation. A subacute degree of obstruction may be precipitously exacerbated by infection of instrumentation (e.g., laryngoscopy or biopsy). Patient symptoms and physical examination are the best indications of these difficulties. The results of indirect and direct inspection (mirror, fiberoptic, and so forth) performed by the head and neck surgeon should be obtained also. CT scanning can be helpful in documenting and quantifying the extent of airway compromise.

The link between tobacco use and the tumors raises the potential for emphysema and chronic bronchitis in these patients. Dyspnea owing to upper airway obstruction should be distinguished from dyspnea owing to chronic lung disease. Again, the history and the cited examinations are most helpful in this regard.

Overall, pulmonary complications such as respiratory failure, atelectasis, and pneumonia are more common in older patients, smokers, obese individuals, and those with underlying pulmonary dysfunction. Thoracic and upper

abdominal sites of operation are considered to be potent risk factors for postoperative pulmonary morbidity,[7] an important consideration for patients having intestinal interposition as part of their pharyngo- or laryngoesophagectomy. Although duration of anesthesia is an unclear contributor to perioperative pulmonary complications, the length of many of the more extensive of these operations may be an additional factor.

The extent and severity of symptoms such as cough, hemoptysis, sputum production, dyspnea, and bronchospasm should be ascertained. Perhaps the most important consideration in these patients is identifying and treating any reversible component(s) of their pulmonary process. Hence, therapy may include antibiotics for infection and exacerbation of chronic bronchitis as well as initiation or optimization of bronchodilator therapy for any reactive component of chronic airway disease. All but emergent procedures for airway obstruction should be delayed until treatable aspects of chronic bronchitis or emphysema are under the best possible control. Other important considerations in planning perioperative care include humidification of inspired gases, avoidance of anticholinergics (to minimize drying of secretions), and judicious use of respiratory depressants. Vigorous pulmonary toilet, incentive spirometry, and early ambulation have been shown to be valuable in the care of these patients. Discontinuation of smoking decreases carboxyhemoglobin levels within 24 hours (thereby improving tissue oxygen delivery) and dissipates the autonomic nervous system effects of nicotine. However, mucous production, mucociliary clearance, airway hyperactivity, and immune dysfunction improve only after weeks to months following cessation of smoking.[8]

In addition to studies detailing airway caliber, the chest radiograph should be examined for evidence of pneumonia, emphysema, pulmonary hypertension, cor pulmonale, and other neoplasms. Preoperative pulmonary function testing (PFT) is indicated in patients over age 70, those with significant smoking history, obese patients, those with pulmonary complaints, and those in whom an abdominal approach will be used. PFT abnormalities predictive of postoperative pulmonary morbidity include (1) a forced expiratory volume in 1 second (FEV_1) less than 1.2–2 L; (2) a forced vital capacity less than approximately 1.85 L; and (3) an arterial CO_2 tension greater than 50 mmHg.[7] Decreased preoperative Pa_{O_2} is of unclear significance in this regard.

Cardiovascular Status

Cardiovascular risk assessment has been reviewed by Mangano[9] and others.[10] Cardiac events, such as infarction, congestive heart failure (CHF), and dysrhythmias, are the most common causes of death following general anesthesia and surgery. Increasing age alone is associated with an increased prevalence of coronary artery disease (CAD). Male sex and tobacco smoking are also common to these patients. Well-substantiated predictors of perioperative cardiac events are the history of recent (<6 months) myocardial infarction and evidence of preoperative CHF by clinical or laboratory methods (specifically, an ejection fraction <0.4 is predictive of perioperative myocardial infarction and CHF). Of valvular lesions, aortic stenosis may increase morbidity and mortality. Peripheral vascular disease, and especially cerebrovascular disease (e.g., the asymptomatic carotid bruit), may be an important predictor of underlying CAD. The predictive value of asymptomatic ventricular dysryhthmias is uncertain, but they appear to be more important when they occur in the setting of acute myocardial ischemia, infarction, or underlying ventricular dysfunction. Similarly, conduction disturbances become worrisome if they are associated with CAD. Hypertension has not been consistently shown to predict untoward perioperative cardiac

events, but it may contribute to intraoperative hemodynamic lability and myocardial ischemia. Stable angina does not appear to independently predict perioperative morbidity and mortality. Because some 75% of ischemia episodes may be "silent" (i.e., pain-free), it has been suggested that the presence of symptomatic ischemia conveys little additional risk.[11] From a practical standpoint, lack of chest pain in a patient believed to be at risk for CAD who is about to undergo major surgery does not indicate low risk.

The exact role of preoperative diagnostic testing remains unclear. Cardiomegaly on chest radiograph, because it correlates fairly well with the presence of a depressed ejection fraction, is a useful sign. The significance of abnormalities detected on routine, 12-lead electrocardiograms (ECGs) is controversial, but the chance of poor outcome may be increased in patients with ST-T ischemic changes, ventricular ectopy, or intraventricular conduction disturbances. Exercise tolerance testing in at-risk patients may identify some who are more likely to experience perioperative events. Exercise- or dipyridamole-thallium scanning can be both sensitive and specific for myocardial ischemia and also can predict outcome events, especially when employed in high risk patients (those with history of angina, CHF, prior myocardial infarction, or diabetes).[12] Emergency surgery, vascular operations, and prolonged (>3 hours) upper abdominal or thoracic procedures have all been identified as independent predictors of cardiac risk. Other intraoperative risk factors include hypotension, elevated left ventricular end-diastolic pressure (as measured by a pulmonary artery catheter), tachycardia, and perhaps evidence (by ECG or transesophageal echocardiography) of myocardial ischemia.[9, 10] Patients undergoing major vascular surgery with significant underlying CAD have been shown repeatedly to be at increased risk of perioperative myocardial infarction, heart failure, and cardiac death. If, as has been suggested, the high complication rates in these patients is due to the stresses of major abdominal and aortic surgery, the author believes that this information is applicable to the head and neck cancer patient. Namely, it is well recognized that manipulation of the larynx, pharynx, and trachea can provoke near-maximal stimulation of the stress response. Gastric mobilization as performed in the pharyngolaryngectomy patient is certainly major upper abdominal surgery. Additionally, the duration of these operations, and specifically the duration of airway stimulation, is long. As a result, these patients also may represent a significantly increased risk for cardiac morbidity and mortality, because of the interplay of historical, physiological, and operative risk factors. Clinical investigations analogous to those performed in other high risk groups[9] are indicated.

Little substantive information is available about risk factors in the postoperative period. Persistent tachycardia is a common finding in postoperative patients, which may predispose to ischemia. Preliminary monitoring does show frequent postoperative ischemia, which is usually silent.

Optimal management of these patients follows directly from the considerations described earlier. If possible, surgery should be postponed so that an interval of 6 months has elapsed from a myocardial infarction (admittedly not always feasible when dealing with cancer surgery). CHF should be well controlled. The utility of dysrhythmia and hypertension control is unclear from a risk standpoint, but sound medical practice alone would suggest investigation as to cause, followed by initiation of therapy when indicated. Most cardiac medication should be continued up to the time of surgery and should be reinstituted immediately thereafter. This is certainly true of drugs with a high potential for rebound withdrawal, such as clonidine and the β blockers. There is also evidence to indicate increased likelihood of ischemia, myocardial infarction, and dysrhythmia following preoperative discontinuation of the β and calcium channel blockers. More recent evidence suggests that β blockade may be protective in at-risk patients in the perioperative period.[13] Intraoperatively, control of heart rate and maintaining blood pressure within acceptable limits are important. Patients with ventricular dysfunction or other significant risk factors may benefit from invasive monitoring, including a pulmonary artery catheter to measure left ventricular filling pressures. In the postoperative period, a high index of suspicion and continued aggressive management of hemodynamic parameters, pulmonary toilet, fluid status, and pain control are indicated.

Alcohol and Liver Disease

Although acute ethanol intoxication should be a rare finding, because the majority of these operations are elective, chronic abuse is prevalent in this population. Major systemic disturbances associated frequently with this problem are shown in Table 5–1. In its terminal stages, chronic alcoholism predisposes these patients to liver dysfunction and hepatic failure, resulting in portal hypertension and esophageal varices, coagulopathy, renal failure, ascites, hypoglycemia, and encephalopathy. Increased volume of distribution, decreased protein binding, and impaired drug metabolism may be seen also. Pulmonary function in cirrhotic patients may be altered by both diminished lung volumes and intra- and extrapulmonary shunts.

Chronic alcoholism increases tolerance and resistance to the effects of anesthetic agents, which can result in prolonged and difficult induction and in increased anesthetic requirements for both induction and maintenance. Alcohol-stimulated hepatic enzyme induction can result in enhanced drug biotransformation. This tolerant state usually persists for 50–60 days following cessation of alcohol consumption.

Delirium tremens, which results from alcohol withdrawal, may occur in up to 5–10% of chronic alcoholics. Consumption of amounts in the range of 15–20 oz/day for at least 1–2

TABLE 5–1. Systemic Disturbances Due to Chronic Alcoholism

Pulmonary (with Cirrhosis)
1. Diminished lung volumes with compensatory increase in alveolar ventilation
2. Decreased Pa_{O_2} due to arteriovenous shunting

Cardiac
1. Beriberi—due to thiamine deficiency. Congestive heart failure, paresthesias
2. Alcoholic cardiomyopathy—occasionally hypertrophic cardiomyopathy, more often congestive. Frequently manifested as atrial dysrhythmias, sometimes as congestive heart failure

Gastrointestinal
1. Gastritis
2. Esophagitis

Metabolic
1. Hypokalemia, hypocalcemia, hypomagnesemia. These may result in muscle and cardiac dysfunction, increased frequency of dysrhythmias
2. Idiopathic hypoglycemia

Hematological
1. Anemia, frequently mixed vitamin deficiencies, and idiopathic macrocytic anemia of alcoholism
2. Generalized impairment of immunity

Neurological
1. Peripheral polyneuropathy. May result in impaired circulatory reflexes
2. Wernicke-Korsakoff syndrome—ataxia and memory loss. Thiamine-responsive

weeks is required for the development of this syndrome; so-called binge drinking (periods of intense consumption separated by abstinence) does not lead to symptomatic alcohol withdrawal. Major manifestations include tremors, diaphoresis, nausea, vomiting, fevers, tachycardia, and hyperreflexia. In its fulminant form, the symptoms progress to delirium, seizures, hyperthermia, coma, and death. Peak onset is at 2–4 days following cessation of consumption; the risk is probably minimal if the patient has consumed no alcohol for longer than 7 days. Perioperative mortality can range from 8–25%, with the highest seen in patients with other major disease processes (e.g., CAD). Numerous treatment options have been suggested, but central to all is the careful titration of sedative/hypnotic medications with the patient under close observation. The aim is to control symptoms without inducing somnolence, respiratory depression, loss of airway reflexes, or other complications. This task may be especially difficult in the postoperative period, when narcotics for pain control are required as well. Chloral hydrate, 1–2 g orally every 6–8 hours, or diazepam, 10–20 mg orally every 6–8 hours, have been shown to be efficacious for milder forms of this syndrome. In more severe cases, diazepam, 5–10 mg intravenously (IV) (or its equivalent), is carefully titrated in repeated doses to gain control of symptoms while maintaining the awake state, and then continued as needed.[15] More recently, other benzodiazepines have become popular, although superiority to diazepam has not been demonstrated. Other agents, including chlordiazepoxide and paraldehyde, may be less efficacious than the benzodiazepines. IV ethanol has also fallen out of favor because of its narrow therapeutic index, difficult maintenance of blood levels, and frequent treatment failures.

Aging

Because many of these patients are middle-aged or older, a consideration of the implications of the aging process is appropriate. Overall, the organ systems can be characterized as possessing decreased reserve. Cardiac output decreases by 1% per year after age 30; although resting cardiac index and ejection fraction may remain normal with advancing age, the ability to increase these in response to exercise or stress is often diminished or absent. Beta-receptor function (but not absolute number) is decreased also. Normal resting heart rate is decreased 20% by age 80; maximal achievable heart rate falls with age and can be approximated by the equation maximal heart rate (beats/minute) $= 220 -$ age in years. In other words, a 70-year-old with a heart rate of 125/minute is effectively experiencing a near-maximal stress test. Cardiovascular responses to hypoxia, hypercarbia, catecholamines, and atropine are diminished also. Decreased baroreceptor function in combination with the above may also predispose the elderly to hypotension. Arterial degeneration and sclerosis cause decreased compliance and contribute to systolic hypertension and perhaps to an increased incidence of cerebrovascular accident.

Significant effects of aging on pulmonary mechanics include decreased thoracic compliance and respiratory muscle reserve. Total lung capacity is diminished, in part by the loss of height that accompanies osteoporosis. Residual volume is increased, mainly owing to parenchymal loss. As a result of these changes, vital capacity and the forced expiratory volume (FEV) are lowered by approximately 15–20% by age 70. Also affected is the relationship of closing volume to functional residual capacity, such that small airway closure can occur in the awake and erect state by age 65. Pa_{O_2} under normal circumstances decreases by 0.5 mmHg/year after age 20; the alveolar-arterial O_2 gradient rises from 8 to 20 mmHg by age 70. The net result of all of these changes is decreased efficiency of gas exchange and an inability to compensate in the presence of increased demand.

Renal function is characterized by a reduction in renal blood flow and concentrating ability. Glomerular filtration rate declines by approximately 1 mL/minute/year. However, the serum creatinine usually remains within the normal range because of a parallel decline in muscle mass. Therefore, an elevated serum creatinine in an elderly patient reflects significant renal dysfunction. The impaired concentrating ability mandates a greater urinary volume to achieve solute excretion. These factors make the aged patient more sensitive to both volume loading and dehydration.

Hepatic microsomal enzymes may be somewhat diminished, but decreases in cardiac output and hepatic blood flow are probably the major influences affecting hepatic drug clearance. Delayed gastric emptying and impaired glucose tolerance often accompany aging. Hypothyroidism becomes more common, and subclinical hypothyroidism may be found in 10–20% of patients aged 70.

Finally, neurological function is manifested by a decline in most parameters, including overall central nervous system (CNS) activity, numbers of cortical neurons, cerebral blood flow and oxygen consumption, and nerve conduction velocity. All of these factors make elderly patients more susceptible to anesthetic effects and toxicities.

CONSIDERATIONS FOR SPECIFIC SURGICAL PROCEDURES

Microlaryngoscopy

Microlaryngoscopy most often uses a suspension laryngoscope in conjunction with an operating microscope. Indications include diagnosis of early laryngeal lesions, biopsy, and resection (e.g., for small vocal cord tumors). Surgical requirements include patient and vocal cord immobility and obtunded airway reflexes. Specific anesthetic concerns relate to maintaining airway patency and gas exchange, avoidance of aspiration, and rapid return of airway reflexes at the conclusion of the procedure.

Numerous anesthetic techniques have been employed for this procedure, including (1) topical local anesthesia, with or without deliberate glossopharyngeal, superior laryngeal, and recurrent laryngeal nerve blockade, combined with IV sedation; (2) IV or inhalational general anesthetic induction, with maintenance through an endotracheal tube, in combination with muscle relaxation; and (3) various forms of jet ventilation. Regardless of the method chosen, assessment of the potential for airway obstruction is required. This information can usually be obtained from the history and physical, along with the results of preoperative indirect laryngoscopic evaluation performed by the surgeon. If there is any question, a direct awake laryngoscopy in the operating room following thorough topical anesthesia (usually 4% lidocaine or tetracaine aerosol) and gentle IV sedation may be required. Excellent topical anesthesia of the oropharynx and larynx may be obtained also by the use of nebulized apparatus. If the patient has evidence of airway obstruction during this inspection and intubation appears possible, it is probably advisable to do so with a small-diameter endotracheal tube; following confirmation of placement, general anesthesia can be induced rapidly with IV pentothal or etomidate. In patients not thought to be at risk of obstruction, a standard IV/inhalation induction sequence is in order,

again followed by placement of a small (5.0–6.0 internal diameter) endotracheal tube in order to allow maximal view of the operative field. If prior administration of local anesthesia was not performed, it is helpful to spray the larynx and trachea with lidocaine (2–4%, 2–3 mL) to minimize stimulation and general anesthetic requirements; this is best accomplished during direct laryngoscopy prior to intubation.

These procedures are usually fairly brief, and adequate muscle relaxation can be provided often from a single dose of succinylcholine used to facilitate intubation. More precise control may be obtained with a succinylcholine infusion, provided that neuromuscular blockade is monitored to detect inadequate blockade or the onset of phase II block. The intermediate-duration, nondepolarizing muscle relaxants vecuronium and atracurium are also useful in this setting. The short-duration narcotic alfentanil, given by infusion, is an appropriate choice as part of a "balanced" anesthetic to provide sufficient analgesia with rapid awakening, especially when postoperative pain is not a major factor. These patients are best extubated once consciousness has fully returned and the airway has been inspected for residual bleeding or other problems. Of course, gentle suctioning is also performed prior to extubation.

Topical, local anesthesia in the awake, sedated patient has largely fallen out of favor because of patient discomfort, movement, and inadequate muscular relaxation.

Many surgeons express a preference for a modification of the Saunders' jet bronchoscopic ventilation technique,[16] in which the high-pressure gas jet is delivered through a modified suspension laryngoscope. The appeal of this method is the clear view of the larynx it provides, unobstructed by an endotracheal tube. Adequate muscle relaxation is essential, as is reliance on IV agents for analgesia and amnesia. Incremental doses of thiopental and fentanyl have been used, the latter in conjunction with small amounts of a benzodiazepine or droperidol. Although gas exchange is usually adequate, it may be compromised in obese patients, in those with significant obstructive pulmonary disease or critical airway obstruction, and in the presence of large laryngeal masses that can act as ball-valve. In these instances, establishment of an endotracheal airway and controlled ventilation are more suitable alternatives. Further, barotrauma from the high-pressure jet (or the catheter that delivers it) may occur to the larynx and lungs, resulting in subcutaneous emphysema, pneumothorax, and so forth. Jet ventilation techniques are probably best reserved for selected patients and situations when it is impossible to carry out the required examination in the presence of an endotracheal tube.

Regardless of the anesthetic method, airway complications may include profuse bleeding, aspiration, vocal cord dysfunction, and edema, all of which can lead to obstruction. Preparation should be completed beforehand for emergency reintubation or tracheostomy. Cardiovascular complications include hypertension, tachycardia, and dysrhythmia resulting from the prolonged laryngeal manipulation, hypoventilation, and reflex stimulation. Minimum monitoring requirements include continuous pulse oximetry and electrocardiography, frequent blood pressure determination, and auscultation of breath sounds. End-tidal CO_2 analysis in intubated patients is also helpful. Small doses of IV fentanyl may help control the tachycardia and hypertension. Esmolol, a β blocker selective for the $β_1$ receptor (cardiac) and possessing a short half-life (approximately 9 minutes), is another attractive modality. As mentioned previously, local anesthesia of the airway may be the most useful method of providing hemodynamic stability. In one study, myocardial ischemia and infarction occurred in 1.5–4% of patients undergoing microlaryngoscopy, with the highest incidence in those with underlying cardiac disease.[17] These data underscore the risks posed by these types of procedures in the patient population most likely to require them. New computerized methods of ST segment analysis, trending, and dysrhythmia detection may improve intraoperative diagnosis and result in earlier appropriate therapeutic intervention.[18]

Laryngectomy

The extent of dissection and associated complications seen with a total laryngectomy can depend on several factors, including tumor size, location, and spread. In general, the larynx is removed in continuity from above the hyoid bone to several centimeters below the lower tumor margin. Exposure and mobilization are obtained by division of the strap muscles and the thyroid isthmus. If the tumor invades beyond local laryngeal boundaries, the thyroid lobe and parathyroid glands on the affected side are removed; the glands on the contralateral side are usually preserved. With more extensive disease, an *en-bloc* dissection may be carried out, involving unilateral or bilateral neck dissections and, occasionally, complete removal of the thyroid and parathyroid tissue. Once again, airway assessment may be critical in these patients. In those who are asymptomatic and whose preoperative evaluation is without evidence of airway compromise, standard induction and intubation techniques are employed. In this instance, the oral endotracheal tube (often a wire-reinforced one) is exchanged for one in the distal trachea by the surgeon as surgery progresses. Alternatively, direct awake laryngoscopic evaluation may be indicated, as discussed earlier. In patients known or thought to have the potential for airway obstruction, an initial tracheostomy under local anesthesia with low-dose sedation is the safest option; at this time a wire-reinforced tube is inserted and sutured to the skin on the anterior chest wall. Care must be taken not to insert this tube too far distally into the trachea. Usually insertion just beyond the proximal tube cuff margin is sufficient.

Once an adequate airway has been established, these procedures are relatively uneventful. Prior to division of the trachea and removal of the endotracheal tube, it is best to ventilate with 100% oxygen and ensure adequate anesthetic depth or muscle relaxation. At this time, the tube is removed, and a sterile tracheal tube is inserted into the stoma by the surgeon. Proper positioning of this tube within the tracheal lumen (as assessed by breath sounds or end-tidal carbon dioxide) should be confirmed. Availability of adequate anesthesia circuit length and metal or rubber gooseneck-type connections to attach between the circuit and the new tracheostomy facilitates management.

Initial monitoring considerations are as discussed previously. Operation duration, laryngeal manipulation, the potential for blood loss, and coexistent pulmonary disease are all indications for arterial cannulation to provide blood gas and hematocrit monitoring, as well as continuous arterial blood pressure determination. A central venous catheter may be indicated in selected patients to more accurately assess intravascular volume. In patients with ventricular dysfunction, with pulmonary hypertension, or at risk for myocardial ischemia, a pulmonary artery catheter may be required. Obviously, central venous access must be established by either the antecubital or femoral routes, because neck and subclavian sites are inappropriate during these operations.

Laryngectomies are relatively safe procedures, with a quoted mortality of 1–3%.[19] Blood loss may be significant, especially in those requiring *en-bloc* resections with neck dissection (see later) and in those who had prior radiation therapy. These patients should be considered at significant risk for pulmonary and myocardial complications. Hypocalcemia owing to parathyroid dysfunction may rarely occur during the final stages of surgery or within 8–24 hours following laryngectomy. This may be transient and due to partial parathyroid resection and edema or transient ischemia of the contralateral glands, or permanent in the setting of total gland removal. The patient should have close monitoring for muscle weakness and ECG changes (dysrhythmias, prolongation of the Q-T$_c$ interval); serum calcium should be monitored frequently if there is any suspicion. Hypothyroidism may also occur following a total resection, although this is usually manifested days to weeks later. Air embolism, another rare complication during laryngectomy, occurs when air enters the open large veins in the neck of a patient sitting slightly head-up. Evidence of air embolism includes hypotension, dysrhythmias, a fall in the end-tidal carbon dioxide concentration, and a rise in the apparent inspired nitrogen concentration. Treatment consists of early detection, compression of the neck veins, positive-pressure ventilation, and placing the patient in the left lateral Trendelenburg position. It may be possible to aspirate air from the central venous catheter. Inotropic support may be required.

Choice of anesthetic technique is guided by the patient's general condition and the presence of coexistent diseases. Most often, a technique using an IV narcotic such as fentanyl, in conjunction with a low inspired concentration of inhalation agent, and nitrous oxide (if pulmonary status allows) is employed. These patients are usually able to ventilate spontaneously through their tracheostomy at the conclusion of the procedure. Again, a high index of suspicion and meticulous surveillance must be maintained in the postoperative period for myocardial ischemia, infarction, dysrhythmias, congestive heart failure, and pulmonary complications.

Pharyngolaryngoesophagectomy with Gastric Interposition

In contrast to laryngeal cancer treated with laryngectomy, pharyngeal cancer requires a more extensive operation involving resection of the pharynx, larynx, and most or all of the esophagus, with resultant higher morbidity and mortality. Because of difficulties with obtaining adequate tumor-free margins and problems with postoperative wound healing and nutrition, most of these operations are performed as a one-stage operation, using two surgical teams. The larynx, pharynx, and esophagus are dissected free and removed from above while a team of general surgeons mobilizes the stomach through an abdominal approach. The stomach is then brought up through the mediastinum, and its fundus is anastomosed in the neck to the cervical pharyngeal remnant. Much of the thoracic esophageal dissection is carried out blindly in the posterior mediastinum. Esophageal rupture and pneumothorax may occur, and some authors recommend prophylactic bilateral chest tube insertion at the beginning of the procedure,[20] although this is not a routine practice. Hence, vigilance must be maintained both during the surgery and in the postoperative period. Air leak and ventilatory difficulty also may occur owing to tracheal perforation.[20] Tracheal perforation occurs most often in the posterior tracheal wall following esophageal mobilization, and adequate gas exchange may become impossible. Initial treatment includes manual ventilation with 100% oxygen, attempted advancement of a cuffed endotracheal tube past the site of rupture, and endobronchial intubation if all other maneuvers fail. Placement of the stomach into its new location in the neck may help remedy this situation by producing tamponade of the leak. Moreover, the possibilities of subcutaneous and mediastinal emphysema and subsequent pneumothorax in this setting must be kept in mind; positive-pressure ventilation should be as brief and at the lowest pressures possible if this complication ensues.

Dysrhythmias, usually supraventricular, often occur, especially during esophageal and gastric mobilization. Hypotension is seen also due to both significant hemorrhage (a blood loss of 1–2 L may be expected during this operation) and the transient impairment of venous return during mediastinal and upper abdominal manipulation. All or part of both the thyroid gland and the parathyroid gland may be removed, and thus the possibility exists for hypocalcemia, myocardial dysfunction, and delayed hypothyroidism.

Monitoring requirements and intraoperative considerations are similar to those for laryngectomy. Large-bore IV access is mandatory, and central venous pressure monitoring (through an arm or leg site) quite helpful. An arterial catheter is essential, given the considerations of blood loss and mechanical interference with venous return. Airway pressures should be closely monitored as an indication of pneumothorax. Three- (or more) lead electrocardiography with ST-segment analysis and dysrhythmia surveillance, pulse oximetry, and end-tidal CO_2 analysis are extremely useful. A urinary catheter assists in the assessment of blood and volume replacement. Temperature should be monitored, and methods to warm the operating room, fluids, blood products, and inspired gases should be employed, because the extensive visceral exposure may cause significant patient cooling.

Unlike laryngeal lesions, airway obstruction is uncommon with hypopharyngeal lesions. More often these tumors are associated with swallowing difficulties and malnutrition, anemia, and hypovolemia. Vigorous preoperative nutritional therapy prior to such major surgery would appear to be an effective adjunct, but improved outcome data to support such intervention are lacking. Anesthetic induction and maintenance are routine in most of these patients, allowing one to focus on concurrent patient disease processes, such as emphysema or coronary artery disease. Postoperative ventilation is through a permanent tracheostomy; thus, some surgeons may elect to perform this procedure at the beginning of the operation. An epidural catheter should be considered for postoperative analgesia, because this may improve ventilation and decrease pulmonary complications in these patients, who may be at increased risk because of advanced age, upper abdominal surgery, underlying lung disease, and a variety of other factors.[21]

Neck Dissection

Spread to the cervical neck lymphatics is the primary route of metastases of oropharyngeal and laryngeal tumors. Neck dissection is indicated in several circumstances, including in patients who lack clinical evidence of neck involvement but whose tumor size, location, or type is associated with a high incidence of nodal spread. These tumors include those at the tongue base, in the pyriform fossa, and in the hypopharynx, and supraglottic laryngeal cancer. Moreover, a therapeutic neck dissection is indicated in patients with palpable cervical node disease. Occasionally, this may occur in patients with neck disease and an occult

primary tumor. Hence, it is important to view neck resection as diagnostic, prognostic, and crucial to the control of the disease.[22]

The two major types of neck dissection are functional and radical. Structures removed in a radical neck dissection are (1) the lymph nodes of the anterior and posterior triangles, of the carotid sheath, and those below the sternocleidomastoid muscle; (2) the internal and external jugular veins; and (3) cranial nerve XI. The sternocleidomastoid muscle may be sacrificed also. The dissection may include the submandibular triangle with removal of the submandibular gland and nodes. In contrast, a functional neck dissection usually involves node and external jugular vein removal only; cranial nerve XI, the internal jugular vein, sternocleidomastoid muscle, and the submandibular triangle are spared. Functional neck dissections are considered in patients without evidence of metastasis and in whom such spread is felt to be unlikely. Nodal involvement found during a functional neck dissection may require conversion to a radical type of operation. These wounds are usually closed primarily. However, the creation of a large oral, pharyngeal, or skin defect often necessitates the creation of a muscle flap (usually pectoralis major) to close the wound.

Blood loss may be significant during a neck dissection; estimates typically range between 400 and 1000 mL for a radical neck operation alone, and up to 2 L or more for that combined with laryngectomy.[23] Dysrhythmias, bradycardia, and wide blood pressure fluctuations may accompany neck manipulation, especially when this manipulation involves the carotid sheath. Treatment includes cessation of the stimulation until the condition resolves, and infiltration of the sheath with 1% lidocaine.

Often, these patients are malnourished. As discussed for pharyngolaryngectomy, there is some support for forced hyperalimentation (usually through the nasogastric route) to improve wound healing and metabolic status.[22] Poorly nourished patients are thought to have a higher incidence of flap failure, wound breakdown, and carotid artery rupture, all postoperative complications of neck dissection. Preoperative radiation therapy to the neck region increases the complication rate from poor wound healing, flap necrosis, and carotid "blow out." It is generally thought also that these patients have more difficult dissections with greater blood loss intraoperatively. Finally, chyle leak from the thoracic duct may occur consequent to a neck dissection. Careful inspection of the wound prior to closure during a sustained Valsalva's maneuver may reveal its presence.

RADIATION THERAPY

Radiation therapy is the primary adjunctive treatment for most of these tumors. In fact, early carcinomas of the lip, skin, and oral cavity may be cured by irradiation alone. Use as a single agent or in combination with surgery yields high cure rates for many of the more advanced lesions in these regions and in laryngeal cancer.[23] The most significant consequence of preoperative irradiation is poor wound healing. Again, changes include erythema followed by desquamation and, rarely, necrosis. Oropharyngeal irradiation commonly results in mucositis, decreased volume and thickening of saliva, and dysphagia. These reactions are usually most prominent in the 2–6 week period following irradiation. Osteoradionecrosis of the mandible and other bony structures about the face may occur somewhat later, more commonly in alcoholics, heavy smokers, and poorly nourished individuals. Early effects of laryngeal irradiation include mucositis and vocal cord and submucosal edema, all of which may result in hoarseness as well as airway compromise. In fact, patients with laryngeal lesions having evidence of airway obstruction may require tracheostomy prior to initiating radiation therapy. Inclusion of the hypopharynx in the radiation field may produce dysphagia as well. Major later reactions include cartilage necrosis and laryngeal ulceration. In addition to hoarseness and pain, recurrent aspiration may occur. Modern radiation therapy techniques have largely eliminated effects on adjacent structures, such as the lungs, heart, eyes, and spinal cord. Occasionally, a transient myelopathy occurs, in which the patient complains of neck flexion–induced back extremity pain and paresthesias. A permanent and progressive myelopathy resulting in a Brown-Séquard or transverse myelopathic state occurs 1–2 years following radiation.

MAJOR SURGICAL OPERATIONS OF THE NECK

Major surgical procedures involving the head and neck can pose unique problems for the anesthesiologist. These difficulties include (1) the location of the surgery, with its inherent potential to affect the patient's airway both intra- and postoperatively; (2) local and systemic effects of the disease process mandating the surgery; and (3) the presence of coexisting abnormalities and underlying patient disease. Understanding the interplay of these factors is essential to the derivation of a comprehensive and optimal plan of anesthetic management.

In addition to radical and functional neck dissections, other relatively commonly performed major operations of the neck involve surgery for thyroid and parathyroid disease.

THYROID DISEASE

Thyroid Function

The thyroid gland, through its hormones thyroxin (T_4) and triiodothyronine (T_3), is the primary regulator of cellular metabolic activity. Its production of these hormones proceeds through four steps, usually described as iodide trapping, oxidation, storage/coupling, and release.[24]

Plasma iodide, absorbed from the GI tract as iodine, is transported against a 20- to 40-fold gradient into the thyroid gland, where it is concentrated. Enzymatic iodine oxidation is accomplished by peroxidase, which is followed by binding to tyrosine to form iodotyrosine (organification). Mono- and diiodotyrosine residues are coupled to form T_3 and T_4, which are stored within the gland bound to thyroglobulin. Release is accomplished through proteolysis from thyroglobulin and subsequent diffusion into the circulation.

Approximately 80–90% of the hormone is released as T_4, the remainder as T_3. Eighty percent of total T_3 is the result of peripheral tissue monodeiodination of T_4. Circulating thyroid hormones are bound primarily to thyroid-binding globulin (TBG), as well as to thyroxine-binding prealbumin. T_3 is much less protein bound than T_4, which in part accounts for its shorter half-life (24 hours versus 7 days for T_4). The increased free fraction of T_3, along with its greater potency as compared with T_4, makes it likely to be the more significant effector at the tissue level. The exact mechanism of cellular T_3 effects remains uncertain but is believed to derive from binding to cellular nuclear receptors and subsequent activation of protein synthesis.[25] Although the hallmarks of thyroid hormone effects are increased oxygen consumption and elevated basal metabolic rate, other effects include increased numbers of β-adrenergic receptors,[26] increased myocardial contractility,[27] increased protein synthesis, enhanced glucose uptake and gluconeogenesis, increased lipolysis and fatty acid oxidation, reduction in circulating cholesterol and triglyceride levels, and enhanced renal free water excretion.

Numerous regulatory and feedback loop mechanisms serve to precisely control thyroid function. Thyroid-stimulating hormone (TSH) has a positive effect on the trapping, oxidation, coupling, and release reactions. In turn, TSH release is regulated by thyrotropin-releasing hormone (TRH) elaborated from the hypothalamus. TRH production appears to be stimulated by low T_3 and T_4 levels, and conversely is suppressed by elevated TSH. TSH synthesis is regulated by a negative feedback mechanism exerted by circulating T_3 and T_4. Other important factors affecting hormone synthesis and release are shown in Table 5–2.

Interpretation of Thyroid Function Tests

Evaluation of thyroid function is primarily by measurement of thyroid hormones and binding protein levels, aided by various thyroid imaging modalities.

Total T_4. Measurement of the total T_4 level

TABLE 5–2. Substances Affecting Thyroid Hormone Synthesis and Release

Compound	Effect
Excess serum iodide (I^-)	Decreased I^- transport into gland
Decreased I^-	Increased I^- transport, increased sensitivity to TSH
Perchlorate ion	Competitive inhibition of I^- transport
Thiocyanate ion	Competitive inhibition of I^- transport; responsible for hypothyroidism occasionally seen with nitroprusside administration
Propylthiouracil, methimazole, carbimazole	Inhibit thyroid peroxidase and coupling reactions
Estrogens (pregnancy, oral contraceptives)	Increased TBG levels
Infectious hepatitis	Increased TBG levels
Hypoproteinemia (malnutrition, nephrosis, cirrhosis)	Decreased TBG levels
Testosterone, salicylates, thiobarbiturates, anabolic steroids	Decreased hormone protein binding
Active acromegaly	Decreased hormone protein binding

is currently a standard screening test of thyroid function. Approximately 90% of hyperthyroid patients have abnormally high total T_4 levels, and 80–85% of hypothyroid patients have abnormally low total T_4 levels.[28, 29] Because it is the free hormone that is responsible for both hormonal effect and activation of the feedback loops, conditions that alter TBG levels and binding (see Table 5–2) significantly affect interpretation of this test. As a common example, a euthyroid patient with a primary elevation of binding protein (e.g., pregnancy, oral contraceptives) will be found to have an elevated total T_4.

Quantitation of Free Thyroxin. To overcome these difficulties, methods to assess the amount of free T_4 have been developed. Free T_4 (as well as T_3) can be measured by equilibrium dialysis. A radioimmunoassay that measures free T_4 directly may become more widely available in the clinical setting. Normal free T_4 is $1.5–5.0 \text{ ng} \cdot dL^{-1}$. Currently, the most prevalent method of assessing the free T_4 is an indirect one, obtained by calculation of the free thyroxin index (FTI). This is expressed as the product of the total T_4 times the T_3 resin uptake (RT_3U; see later). In general, primary hormone level abnormalities result in parallel changes in the T_4 and RT_3U (both increased in hyperthyroidism, decreased in hypothyroidism), whereas alterations in protein binding are accompanied by opposite shifts in these two measurements.

T_3 Resin Uptake (RT_3U). Despite its name, this is an indirect measure of the amount of unbound plasma T_4. Radiolabeled T_3 is added to patient serum, along with a binding resin. The amount of T_3 bound to resin is inversely proportional to the availability of binding sites in the patient's serum. Thus, uptake is high in hyperthyroidism (more patient sites occupied by endogenous T_4), in association with decreased numbers of binding sites (nephrosis), or abnormal binding site occupation (salicylates). RT_3U is low in hypothyroidism (more patient sites available because of diminished T_4) and in the states that elevate TBG (Table 5–3).

Serum T_3. This test is used to detect the presence of hyperthyroidism in clinically symptomatic patients who have normal T_4 levels. Elevated T_3 levels may either precede elevations in T_4 in these patients or be the only abnormality.[28] In contrast, T_3 determinations are not a sensitive indicator of hypothyroidism, being depressed in only about 50% of hypothyroid patients. It is believed that hypothyroid of thyroid cells that are unresponsive to the normal feedback control mechanisms.

Thryoiditis, another cause of hyperthyroidism, can follow viral upper respiratory infections; a more severe form with greater hormone release can accompany subacute granulomatis thyroiditis.[33, 34] Hashimoto's thyroiditis, the result of a chronic autoimmune process that usually results in gland destruction and subsequent hypothyroidism, can sometimes present with hyperthyroidism.

Various tumors and other disease states can produce either excess thyroid hormone, as in the case of pregnancy,[35] trophoblastic tumors, and thyroid tumors, or excess TSH, as in the case of certain pituitary adenomas.

An interesting form of hyperthyroidism, known as Job-Basedow's syndrome, can occur in chronically iodine-deprived individuals suddenly exposed to high levels of iodine, most often following administration of radiographic contrast dye.[36]

Symptoms and Physical Findings. The most common symptoms of excess thyroid hormone are nervousness, irritability, tremors, palpitations, weight loss, and heat intolerance. All reflect thyroid hormone's stimulation of metabolic rate and oxygen consumption. Other changes include diaphoresis, skeletal muscle weakness and atrophy, emotional liability, pruritus, lethargy, and increased stool frequency. Of note, the severity of these signs and symptoms for a given degree of hyperthyroidism may often decrease with increasing age.

Physical findings include weight loss despite adequate caloric intake, tachycardia, atrial fibrillation, and a fine distal extremity tremor. The thyroid gland is almost invariably palpably enlarged. Eye findings of lid lag, lid retraction, and decreased blinking are most likely due to the increased sensitivity to catecholamines. Patients with Graves' disease also have an infiltrative ophthalmopathy due to edema and inflammation, as well as a mucopolysaccharide infiltration that results in conjunctival chemosis, photophobia, diplopia, and the characteristic proptosis.

Of major concern to the anesthesiologist are the cardiovascular consequences of hyperthyroidism. The relevant physical findings usually include tachycardia, elevated systolic, decreased diastolic, and widened pulse pressures, and a hyperdynamic precordium. Tachydysrhythmias, especially atrial fibrillation, may be present. Congestive heart failure (CHF) is uncommon in the absence of underlying cardiac disease. New-onset atrial fibrillation or other dysrhythmias in patients without preexisting cardiac disease should raise the question of hyperthyroidism.

Medical Management of Thyrotoxicosis and Thyroid Storm. The goals of drug therapy in the hyperthyroid patient are to control the major manifestations of the thyrotoxic state and to render the patient euthyroid.

The most commonly used agents currently to control thyroid hyperfunction are the thiourea derivatives propylthiouracil (PTU; 100–150 mg orally every 8 hours) and methimazole (10–15 mg orally every 8 hours). These agents act to inhibit synthesis of thyroid hormone (PTU may also inhibit the peripheral conversion of T_4 to T_3). Because of the large glandular storage of hormone, 4–8 weeks are usually required to render a patent euthyroid with these drugs. Treatment is usually for a 12–24 month period, after which thyroid reserve and suppressive response to thyroid hormone are reassessed. The major complication of this therapy is hypothyroidism, and daily dosage is usually adjusted to the lowest possible once a euthyroid state is achieved.[37] Other side effects seen in patients taking these antithyroid drugs include leukopenia, which may be therapy-limiting, as well as rashes, agranulocytosis, hepatitis, and drug fevers.

Iodide, in the form of potassium iodide (Lugol's solution), is often used in patients with severe thyrotoxicosis and underlying cardiac disease. This is because it much more rapidly induces thyroid suppression compared with the thiourea derivatives. It is used generally in conjunction with these antithyroid agents because of an incomplete and transient response when used as a single agent.

Adrenergic antagonists, especially propranolol, 40–120 mg/day, have been used to rapidly control the effects of catecholamine stimulation, such as tachycardia, tremor, and diaphoresis.[38, 39] It acts directly on the β receptors (which, as noted earlier, may be increased in number), and also inhibits the peripheral conversion of T_4 to T_3. Propranolol should never be used as a single agent because of its lack of antithyroid effects. Beta-blocking agents are most useful as adjuncts to the other antithyroid drugs to control cardiovascular symptoms while awaiting the onset of true antithyroid effects. They are useful also in the management of patients in the preoperative period and during thyroid storm. Major side effects are those usually referable to β blockers, and the drugs should be used with caution in those with CHF, bronchospasm, diabetes, and so forth.

TABLE 5–3. Thyroid Function Testing

	T_4	RT_3U	T_3	TSH
Normal values	5–12 µg · dL⁻¹	25–35%	80–220 ng · dL⁻¹	<8 mIU · mL
Primary hypothyroidism	↓	↓	↓ or N	↑
Secondary hypothyroidism	↓	↓		↓ or ND
Sick euthyroid	N	N	↓	N
Hyperthyroid	↑	↑	↑	N, or ND
Primary TBG elevations	↑	↓	N	N

N = normal; ↑ = elevated; ↓ = low; ND = undetectable.

patients produce a disporportionately greater amount of T_3 than T_4 as the thyroid gland fails. The real utility of T_3 measurements may be in the detection of the so-called sick euthyroid syndrome, wherein peripheral conversion of T_4 to T_3 is impaired. This is most often seen in the fetus and newborn, as well as in the very aged. Disease states associated with this tissue hypothyroidism include fasting, malnutrition, renal or hepatic failure, other severe systemic illnesses, and the postoperative state.[31] This phenomenon may also accompany the administration of propranolol.

Thyroid Stimulating Hormone. Measurement of serum TSH is currently felt to be the most sensitive test for primary hypothyroidism, wherein the value is invariably elevated. In fact, early or subclinical hypothyroidism may be manifested by TSH elevation alone, reflecting diminished glandular reserve and cellular hypothyroidism with compensatory pituitary hypersecretion of TSH. Assays for TSH in current clinical use do not possess sufficient sensitivity to distinguish between hyper- and euthyroid states. Pituitary or hypothalamic dysfunction results in a low-normal or undetectable TSH, in combination with a low T_4. Most cases of thyrotoxicosis are associated with a low or undetectable TSH.

Normal values for these indices and clinical patterns of derangement are shown in Table 5–3.

Thyroid Ultrasonography and Scintigraphy

Ultrasonography of the thyroid gland provides a useful means of evaluating thyroid nodules, differentiating between cystic, solid, and mixed lesions. Cystic nodules are rarely malignant. Solid or mixed lesions have a 10–30% malignant potential and need further evaluation by fine needle aspiration.[32] Radionuclide scanning using ¹²³iodine or ⁹⁹ᵐTc can be used to determine the degree and amount of functioning tissue in cases of thyrotoxicosis, as well as to

evaluate thyroid nodules regarding their functional status. Functioning (hot) nodules are most often benign and usually occur in groups. Nonfunctional tissue, especially in the case of the single "cold" nodule, is more often malignant, although even most cold, single lesions are benign.[32]

Hyperthyroidism

Hyperthyroidism is the result of excessive circulating thyroid hormone; usually this is manifested by elevations in the levels of both T_3 and T_4. Occasionally, only one may be increased.

Etiology. A summary of the causes of hyperthyroidism is contained in Table 5–4. Graves' disease is the most common, usually presenting as a diffuse, hyperfunctioning, multinodular goiter, most often in females 20–40 years of age. Graves' disease is on a continuum of autoimmune thyroid disease and has been linked to the presence of thyroid-stimulating immunoglobulins. These patients may have other signs of autoimmune involvement also, including myositis, an infiltrative ophthalmopathy, and occasionally myasthenia gravis. Graves' disease is also the most common cause of thyrotoxicosis in childhood.

Hyperfunctioning goiters, either single or multinodular, are thought to arise from clones

TABLE 5–4. Etiologies of Hyperthyroidism

Excess Hormone Production
1. Abnormal thyroid stimulating hormones: Graves' disease, choriocarcinoma, pituitary tumors, mesothelioma
2. Intrinsic thyroid hyperfunction: toxic nodular goiter (single or multinodular, hyperfunctioning adenoma)
3. Thyroid disruption: thyroiditis (autoimmune, viral)
4. Extrathyroidal: metastatic thyroid follicular carcinoma, struma ovarii

Exogenous Factors
1. Iatrogenic: excess thyroid hormone administration
2. Iodine-induced
3. Factitious (surreptitious ingestion of thyroid hormone)

Radioactive iodine (^{131}I) has been employed to provide rapid, effective, and nonsurgical ablation of the thyroid gland. However, it also produces progressive hypothyroidism.

Treatment of thyrotoxicosis in pregnancy remains controversial. Some believe that antithyroid therapy is preferable to surgery, especially during the first and third trimesters; however, all of the antithyroid drugs cross the placenta and can induce hypothyroidism in the fetus. Thus, therapy must be closely monitored, and the lowest doses of antithyroid drugs used.

"Thyroid storm" refers to an acute and severe exacerbation of hyperthyroidism by various and usually nonspecific stresses, such as infection, surgery, or major trauma.[39, 40] This is usually manifested by the acute onset of hyperthermia (often 105–106°C), tachycardia, dysrhythmias, shock, CHF, and extreme agitation. Increased oxygen consumption and carbon dioxide production may occur also. Obviously, thyroid storm may have severe consequences in patients with underlying cardiovascular disease, in whom CHF, pulmonary edema, and myocardial infarction may be especially likely. In the perioperative setting, similarities between this entity and malignant hyperthermia are obvious[41, 42] and can pose a difficult diagnostic dilemma. Distinguishing features that support the diagnosis of malignant hyperthermia may include positive family history, the presence of masseter muscle spasm and muscular rigidity, myoglobinuria, acute oliguria, elevated serum creatinine kinase levels, and the greater tendency toward hyperkalemia and metabolic acidosis.

Therapy of thyrotoxicosis is both supportive and aimed at controlling the underlying abnormalities. Maintenance of adequate oxygen delivery is a prime concern. Cooling is provided by surface and ambient methods, as well as cold IV fluids, and also perhaps iced gastric lavage. Propranolol, 1–2 mg IV, is used every 4–8 hours or as sufficient to reduce the heart rate to less than or equal to 100 beats per minute. The aim is to control cardiovascular symptoms and tachydysrhythmias, as well as to impair the peripheral conversion of T_4 to T_3.[43] The more recently introduced β blocker esmolol, with its short half-life (approximately 9 minutes), its limited effect on bronchial tone, and its administration by infusion, may prove useful also in this regard. Sodium iodide, 500–1000 mg IV every 8 hours, promptly blocks further release of thyroid hormone.[44] However, iodide given alone in this fashion may

stimulate the further synthesis of new thyroid hormone. For this reason, as well as to initiate definitive antithyroid therapy, most authorities also recommend giving PTU either orally or through gastric tube (large doses may be required: 200–400 mg every 4–8 hours), even though its effect to block synthesis will be delayed.

Corticosteroids are often used to prevent the adrenal insufficiency that may occur as a result of increased metabolism, as well as to inhibit hormone release and impair peripheral conversion. Digitalis may be required occasionally to control the ventricular response to atrial dysrhythmias. In general, 5–7 days are usually required to treat the events of thyroid storm completely and to begin to render the patient euthyroid, although with the described regimen the serum T_3 concentration will usually become normal within 24–48 hours. Over this time period, iodide therapy is gradually tapered, and consideration of definitive therapy begun. The precise etiology of thyroid storm remains unclear. Elevated T_4 levels cannot be the major factor, because these have been found to be normal during thyrotoxicosis.[48] Beta-receptor numbers are increased by hyperthyroidism,[26] and possibly there is a derangement in the cellular interaction of T_4/T_3 and catecholamines, or a heightened sensitivity of the sympathetic nervous system to the effects of thyroid hormone.[49] Although frequently mentioned, current evidence does not support a heightened cardiovascular sensitivity to catecholamines in hyperthyroid patients.[29]

Perioperative Management and Anesthetic Considerations. Medical control of hyperthyroid states has become the preferred initial approach. Trials of antithyroid therapy are indicated in children, adolescents and young adults, and perhaps in older patients as well. As noted earlier, the issue is not resolved in pregnant patients. In a thyrotoxic woman desirous of pregnancy, a subtotal thyroidectomy is probably the treatment of choice. Other indications for ablative or resection procedures include failures or recurrent relapses during medical therapy, unacceptable drug toxicity, large or toxic multinodular goiters, goiter-induced airway compression, progressive cardiac symptoms of thyrotoxicosis despite optimal medical management, evidence of malignancy by radionuclide scanning or fine needle aspiration, and patient noncompliance. If possible, a subtotal thyroidectomy is chosen to reduce the amount of hyperfunctioning tissue or to remove a malignant lesion, while preserving some functioning thyroid tissue. [131]Iodine ablation may be elected in the elderly or the otherwise poor surgical candidate, as well as in cases of toxic multinodular goiter (which is usually a disease of the elderly).

From the foregoing discussion, it is readily appreciated that the mainstay of preoperative management of the hyperthyroid patient is achieving metabolic control and a euthyroid state. For the hyperthyroid patient coming for elective thyroid or nonthyroid surgery, a regimen begun 4–6 weeks prior to operation consisting of an antithyroid drug plus β blockade is initiated to achieve these goals. The addition of potassium iodide for 10 days prior to surgery to cause involution of the gland and reduce circulating hormone levels is felt to provide additional safety.[44] Propranolol kinetics can demonstrate increased variability with decreased plasma levels and increased clearance in the hyperthyroid patient and during the perioperative period,[45] and some prefer the longer-acting agent nadolol for these reasons.[46] Achievement of the euthyroid state is assessed by clinical signs and symptoms, plasma hormone levels, and evidence of gland shrinkage. Control of the hyperdynamic circulation is evinced by normalization of blood pressure and a heart rate less than 85–90 beats per minute. Although surgery is felt to be safe once these criteria are met, "breakthrough" thyroid storm in the perioperative period has been reported,[47] and one should be prepared with the treatment regimen outlined earlier.

Again, adequate preoperative preparation of the hyperthyroid patient is essential, and no elective surgery should be undertaken until this is accomplished. In the case of the non-optimized hyperthyroid patient presenting for emergency surgery, the author believes that management should proceed in a manner similar to that outlined for thyroid storm: IV β blockade and potassium iodide therapy should be instituted, high-dose steroid therapy considered, and oral or nasogastric antithyroid drug therapy instituted. The necessary facilities for patient cooling and intraoperative treatment of tachydysrhythmias, CHF, and so forth should be immediately available. If the patient's surgical condition allows, even 12–24 hours of these pharmacological measures prior to operation may be exceedingly beneficial.

Large goiters can cause tracheal compression and tracheomalacia and can extend substernally (Fig. 5–4). In addition to tracheal narrowing, considerable laryngeal and tracheal deviation can occur, resulting in stridor, dysp-

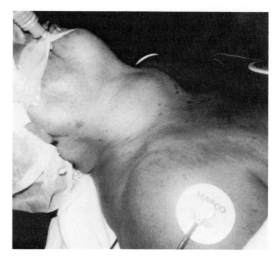

FIGURE 5–4. *Lateral view of a large goiter. (Photograph courtesy of Barbara Kinder, M.D., Associate Professor of Surgery, Yale University School of Medicine.)*

nea, and difficulties with airway management and intubation. Respiratory symptoms may be exacerbated by assuming the supine position. Analogous to other anterior mediastinal masses, a goiter with significant intrathoracic extension may result in airway obstruction, especially during supine positioning, muscle relaxation, or positive-pressure ventilation[50] (Fig. 5–5). In addition to a history of positional intolerance, flow volume loops and careful CT scanning through the neck and thorax aid in the assessment[51] (Fig. 5–6). A rigid, ventilating

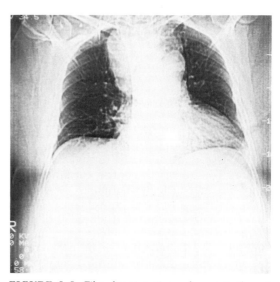

FIGURE 5–5. *Film demonstrating a large intrathoracic component of a goiter. (Photograph courtesy of Barbara Kinder, M.D., Associate Professor of Surgery, Yale University School of Medicine.)*

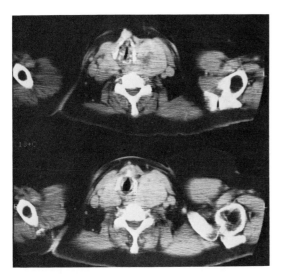

FIGURE 5–6. *CT scan showing significant tracheal compression from a goiter. (Photograph courtesy of Barbara Kinder, M.D., Associate Professor of Surgery, Yale University School of Medicine.)*

bronchoscope passed into the trachea distal to the obstruction may restore ventilation if all other maneuvers fail.[52] Intubation with spontaneous ventilation and avoidance of muscle relaxation has been advocated as a technique for such patients.[53] Patients with large neck masses or evidence of laryngeal or upper airway compromise may benefit from fiberoptic intubation or awake direct laryngoscopy and intubation following adequate sedation and topical application of local anesthetic.

No single anesthetic drug or technique has been proven superior in the management of hyperthyroid patients.[54] Rather, a rational anesthetic plan derives from the considerations outlined earlier. Preoperative medication is aimed at producing sedation, usually through a barbiturate or benzodiazepine. Anticholinergic drugs should be avoided. All medications being taken to control hyperthyroidism should be continued until surgery. Beta blockade should probably be continued intraoperatively; this can be accomplished with propranolol, labetolol, or esmolol. In the absence of mitigating factors such as underlying obesity or pulmonary or cardiac disease, noninvasive monitoring of blood pressure and electrocardiographic, oximetric, capnographic, and temperature monitoring usually suffice. Even mild increases in patient temperature or heart rate during the perioperative period should raise the question of exacerbated thyrotoxicosis.

Regional anesthesia has been described for thyroid surgery in the form of bilateral cervical plexus blockade. This may be awkward and uncomfortable for the patient, given the proximity of the surgical site to the face. In addition, the innervation of the upper pole of the thyroid is through vagal rather than cervical routes; thus, complete anesthesia may be difficult to accomplish, and the patient may be predisposed to increased stress.[55] Regional techniques for nonthyroid surgery in these patients, with their attendant interruption of both nociceptive and sympathetic pathways, are attractive options. Epinephrine should probably be omitted from local anesthetic solutions. Some recommend the use of direct-acting sympathomimetics in reduced doses to treat hypotension in these patients,[56] although experimental evidence for the invoked abnormal response to exogenous catecholamines is lacking.

Both induction and maintenance of anesthesia are directed toward ensuring adequate depth and blockade of the sympathetic responses to laryngoscopy, intubation, and surgical stimulation. Nitrous oxide/oxygen/narcotic, deep inhalational, or "balanced" techniques have all been used effectively.[54] Induction is best accomplished with a sufficient dose of barbiturate (this drug may be somewhat antithyroid as well) or, perhaps, etomitate. Ketamine should be avoided, even in the patient who has been successfully rendered euthyroid.[57] Muscle relaxation can be provided with succinylcholine or nondepolarizers; of the latter, pancuronium should probably be avoided because of its effects on sympathetic tone and heart rate. The potential for muscle weakness and myasthenia in hyperthyroid patients requires careful monitoring of neuromuscular blockade. Reversal should be undertaken with the goal of avoiding excess antimuscarinic effects. Although data are conflicting, available evidence does not support a significant increase in minimum alveolar concentration (MAC) as a consequence of hyperthyroidism.[56] However, coincident hyperthermia increases MAC approximately 5% for every degree centigrade above 37°C.[58]

Of concern is the potential for increased biotransformation and organ damage from the administration of halogenated anesthetics to hyperthyroid patients. Rats given T_3 and exposed to halothane, enflurane, or isoflurane developed centrolobular hepatic necrosis[59, 60]; the incidence was less frequent with isoflurane (28%) and enflurane (24%) than with halothane (92%). A study in humans failed to demonstrate any significant incidence of hepatic dysfunction in hyperthyroid patients receiving halothane or enflurane general anesthesia, although on postoperative day 1, lactate dehydrogenase levels were higher in the hyperthyroid patients compared with controls.[61]

As mentioned previously, some anesthesiologists think the hypotension should be treated with direct-acting sympathomimetic agents in reduced doses. The eyes of patients with exophthalmos should be protected. Surgical positioning for adequate access to the neck usually entails neck extension and shoulder support, with the arms tucked at the patient's side; a semisitting position is often used to reduce bleeding. Care must be taken to support the head without excessive extension, and also to ensure proper positioning and padding at the shoulders, arms, elbows, and wrists in order to avoid nerve injury.

Complications of Thyroid Surgery. Intraoperative complications of thyroid surgery include thyroid storm as well as venous air embolism and stimulation of the carotid baroreceptor reflex. The potential for air embolism is accentuated if the patient is in semisitting position and is breathing spontaneously. Flooding the surgical field and being prepared to treat hemodynamic complications of embolized air are the mainstays of treatment. Carotid stimulation, usually manifested by excessive bradycardia, is managed by cessation of the surgical stimulus and by use of IV atropine if needed. Lidocaine infiltration into the carotid sheath may be advisable if this problem is recurrent.

Postoperatively, thyroid storm remains a worrisome complication; its incidence is greatest within the first 24 hours postoperatively. This mandates both careful observation and continuation of β blockade and antithyroid therapy well into the postoperative period.

Trauma to, or transection of, one or both recurrent laryngeal nerves (RLN) may occur. Unilateral damage produces a single paralyzed vocal cord with resulting hoarseness. These patients are usually able to compensate well and have minimal airway difficulty. Bilateral RLN injury, which occurs rarely, most commonly follows total thyroidectomy. The RLN innervates both the abductors and adductors of the vocal cords; in the acute situation following thyroidectomy, superior laryngeal nerve innervation to the cricothyroid muscle (which when unopposed can have abductor properties) usually remains intact, and as a result the cords lie in a so-called paramedian position.[62] Interestingly, the voice is usually

fairly good in the instance of paramedian bilateral vocal cord paralysis; however, airway obstruction and stridor can be quite severe, and may even necessitate tracheostomy. Over time, atrophy of the vocal cords may ensue and render the cords in a more lateral position. Stridor is less severe, but the voice is worse and the risk of aspiration increased. Tracheal sensory innervation is lost also. For these reasons, some advocate repeat laryngoscopy with the patient asleep and breathing spontaneously at the completion of thyroidectomy in order to assess vocal cord mobility prior to extubation. In any event, extubation should be done under controlled circumstances in case reintubation is required. These patients may become obstructed immediately and require urgent reintubation or even tracheostomy. Evidence suggesting bilateral cord paralysis following surgery mandates immediate neck re-exploration in the hope of finding surgical sutures about the nerves. Attempts to reanastomose transected nerves have not been encouraging.[62] Spontaneous recovery of function can occur if nerves have been traumatized or subjected to swelling.

Postoperative respiratory embarrassment may occur with the development of an expanding neck hematoma. Prompt opening of the wound, often at the bedside, is indicated. If decompression is to be undertaken in the operating room in the extubated patient, the anesthesiologist may be confronted with many of these complications in a now emergent setting. These complications can include thyroid storm, upper airway obstruction, and tracheal deviation or compression. Tracheomalacia can be a late complication following thyroidectomy, especially in instances of removal of a large, compressing mass lesion.[63]

Hypoparathyroidism as a result of inadvertent removal of the parathyroid glands most commonly occurs after total thyroidectomy; less often, this may be the result of temporary parathyroid gland dysfunction owing to trauma and swelling.[64] Hypocalcemia and its attendant problems of tetany and cardiac dysfunction (see section on hypoparathyroidism) usually occur within 24–48 hours; however, symptoms may be manifest as early as 6 hours following gland removal. The vocal cords are sensitive to the effects of hypocalcemia, and stridor and laryngospasm may be the earliest symptoms of developing hypocalcemia. When parathyroid damage or resection is thought to have occurred, sequential physical examination and determination of serum calcium levels and the

Q-T$_c$ interval on ECG are indicated. If hypocalcemia or tetany ensue, treatment is with IV calcium chloride or gluconate.

Hypothyroidism

Hypothyroidism most often results from the decreased production of thyroid hormone and occasionally from impaired peripheral conversion of T$_4$ to T$_3$. Various causes are listed in Table 5–5.

Etiology. Chronic autoimmune thyroiditis, especially Hashimoto's, is the most common cause of primary hypothyroidism. Iatrogenic hypothyroidism, as the consequence of radioiodine therapy, thyroidectomy, or antithyroid medications, accounts for approximately one third of cases of hypothyroidism.[29] The frequency of congenital hypothyroid disease has been estimated at 1 per 4000 live births. Overall incidence in the adult population is 0.5–0.8%. The occurrence of subclinical hypothyroidism, defined as asymptomatic elevation of TSH only, may be as frequent as 5%. The incidence is increased in women in the elderly population, with perhaps as many as 20–33% of women over 65 years of age having at least mild hypothyroidism.

Although uncommon, thyroid insufficiency may be due to abnormalities in the hypothalamic-pituitary axis. This is especially true in the case of adrenocorticotropic hormone deficiency, because thyroid replacement in this setting may provoke adrenal crisis.

Symptoms and Physical Findings. Abnormalities owing to hypothyroidism usually have insidious onset and are initially nonspecific. The protean manifestations of the process have been well summarized,[65] and include lethargy, cold intolerance, weight gain (usually mild), decreased cognitive functioning, depression, headache, hoarseness, impotence, decreased libido, menorrhagia, and constipation. Physical findings can include dry skin, periorbital edema, brittle hair, goiter, bradycardia, hypothermia, distant heart sounds, and prolongation of the relaxation phase of deep tendon reflexes. Growth retardation may be prominent in children with onset after 2 years of age. In addition to poor growth, irreversible mental impairment (cretinism) may occur in infants with congenital hypothyroidism left untreated for more than 2 months.

Many of these problems result from the general slowing of metabolic activity and the lack of thyroid hormone—the so-called permissive effect of thyroid hormone on other tissues. In severely hypothyroid patients, metabolic rates may be diminished 40–50% of normal. In addition to bradycardia, impaired myocardial contractility and a compensatory elevation in systemic vascular resistance may be seen.[66] CHF is uncommon in the absence of underlying heart disease. Peripheral perfusion is usually diminished. Effects on lipid metabolism result in elevated serum triglyceride and cholesterol, pericardial effusions with diminished voltage on ECG, and perhaps accelerated atherosclerosis and coronary artery disease.

Maximal breathing capacity and the ventilatory response to both hypoxia and hypercarbia may be significantly depressed in hypothyroid individuals.[67] Renal free-water excretion is decreased; however, plasma volume may be 25% below normal.[65] Electrolyte imbalance, especially hyponatremia, can be due to hypothyroidism, as can reductions in glomerular filtration rates and tubular transport mechanisms. Capillary fragility is increased and levels of clotting factors VIII and IX reduced, as is platelet adhesiveness.[68] Adrenal function may be impaired also.

For clinical purposes, hypothyroidism can be divided into three categories:

1. Asymptomatic—patients without symptoms have subclinical disease, manifested only by an increase in serum TSH levels. All peripheral organ function and responsiveness is maintained, perhaps through stimulation of the failing gland by the elevated TSH levels. The rate of progression to overt hypothyroidism is unclear.

2. Mild to moderate hypothyroidism—patients with mild hypothyroidism have elevated

---

TABLE 5–5. Etiologies of Hypothyroidism

Primary Hypothyroidism
Acquired:
  Autoimmune–Hashimoto's thyroiditis
  Inflammatory–Riedel's thyroiditis, subacute thyroiditis
    (rare), end-stage Graves' disease (rare)
  Iatrogenic—postsurgical, radioiodine therapy,
    antithyroid drugs, external irradiation
  Dietary—iodine deficiency, food goitrogens
  Thyroid tumors (rare)
Congenital:
  Thyroid dysgenesis or dyshormonogenesis
  Maternal antithyroid therapy
  Maternal iodine deficiency

Secondary Hypothyroidism
  Pituitary disease

Tertiary Hypothyroidism
  Hypothalamic disease

TSH levels and borderline-low T_4. Mild physical signs, including lethargy and constipation, may be present. These patients are not felt to be at increased perioperative risk, because cardiac and pulmonary parameters remain fairly normal.[69]

3. Severe hypothyroidism—patients with severe hypothyroidism have significant elevations of TSH and depression of circulating thyroid hormone, along with the development of the signs and symptoms outlined earlier. Diminished myocardial contractility, impaired ventilatory performance, fluid and electrolyte imbalances, and hypothermia may increase the risk of general anesthesia in these patients. Elective surgery should probably not be performed until they are rendered euthyroid. Myxedema coma, the most critical form of severe hypothyroidism, is characterized by hypothermia, bradycardia, severely impaired myocardial contractility, hypoventilation, hypovolemia, myopathy, adrenal insufficiency, and depressed mental status that may progress to frank coma.

Medical Management of Hypothyroidism. Replacement therapy with thyroid hormones can largely reverse the systemic complications of hypothyroidism, with the major manifestations such as ventilatory drive, myocardial contractility, and CNS performance returning to normal within 4–6 months of adequate replacement therapy.[29]

The most common mode of replacement therapy is with thyroxine, 0.15–0.20 mg/day. Synthetic liothyronine (L-T_3) is occasionally used, but the more gradual onset and longer half-life of T_4 make it more attractive. Use of desiccated thyroid (Thyroid [USP]) has fallen out of favor because of the sometimes unpredictable composition and efficacy of this preparation.

The major risk of thyroid replacement therapy beyond that of iatrogenic hyperthyroidism is the precipitation or exacerbation of coronary insufficiency and myocardial infarction. Patients with stable angina should have gradual thyroid replacement instituted at reduced dosage.[70] The risk of an occult coronary artery disease in the elderly and diabetics would suggest a lower dosage protocol in these patients as well. In those requiring coronary artery bypass grafting, available evidence indicates that the surgery can and probably should be performed prior to the institution of thyroid hormone replacement.[71]

Myxedema coma is treated with the prompt administration of sodium levothyroxine, 0.3–0.5 mg IV load, followed by 0.05–0.2 mg IV daily. Some prefer to use IV T_3, 5–50 μg, because of its more rapid onset.[29] Again, given the risk of exacerbating myocardial ischemia, extreme care, comprehensive monitoring, and dosage reductions should be utilized in those with known or possible CAD.

Perioperative Anesthetic Management and Considerations. Although a reasonable goal would be to have all hypothyroid patients euthyroid prior to surgery, and despite popular beliefs to the contrary, there is no well-controlled evidence to support either an increased overall operative or anesthetic risk in mild or moderately hypothyroid patients, or an unusual sensitivity of the cardiac or nervous system to anesthetic drugs.[29, 72, 73] In the absence of severe, overt hypothyroidism, it would appear that elective surgery may be performed safely without prior thyroid replacement therapy, although the incidence of mild intraoperative hypotension and postoperative ileus and mental status changes may be somewhat higher in hypothyroid patients. As discussed previously, thyroid hormone replacement is not indicated prior to coronary artery bypass grafting. Patients with severe hypothyroidism or myxedema coma are at increased risk of perioperative hypotension, hypothermia, hypoventilation, respiratory muscle insufficiency, ileus, delayed gastric emptying, adrenal insufficiency, hyponatremia, free-water excess, and coma. If possible, these patients should be rendered euthyroid for a period of 3–4 months prior to elective surgery.[29, 66, 67]

Obviously, narcotic and sedative premedicants must be used with caution, and probably in small doses. Thiopental has been used safely[72]; the intravascular volume and myocardial considerations as discussed earlier mandate careful titration and perhaps reduced dose as well. Ketamine is a theoretically attractive drug because of its indirect sympathetic stimulating properties, but there are no controlled studies reporting its use in these patients.

Nitrous oxide and all potent inhalation agents have been used safely in hypothyroid patients. Again, the potential for hypotension and myocardial dysfunction must be kept in mind. As with hyperthyroidism, there is no evidence to support a change in MAC (in this case it would be decreased) related directly to hypothyroidism.[56, 74] Nevertheless, increased anesthetic sensitivity could be related to the underlying hemodynamic, respiratory, CNS, and plasma volume abnormalities. Awakening may be delayed. The potential for depressed ventilatory drive and respiratory muscle weakness postoperatively must be remembered. Sensitivity to narcotics may be increased, perhaps in part owing to impaired hepatic metabolism.[29] Obviously, careful attention must be paid to monitoring and maintenance of body temperature, using the standard methods. Steroid coverage should be continued (or begun) in the severely hypothyroid patient because of the possibility of adrenal crisis.

These patients need to be observed well into the postoperative period for the development of fluid overload, hyponatremia, hypothermia, ileus, and respiratory insufficiency and depression (which will be potentiated by narcotic analgesics).

Thyroid Neoplasms

Thyroid neoplasms either are of the benign, adenomatous variety or, less frequently, represent thyroid carcinoma. Adenomas fall into three histological cell types: follicular, papillary, and Hürthle cell. Unlike normal thyroid tissue, most adenomas function autonomously, independent of TSH stimulation. They usually present as a solitary, painless nodule that is "hot" on radioiodine scintiscanning, with growth being slowly progressive over many years. Eventually, they may achieve a state of hyperfunction (toxic adenomas) sufficient to cause suppression of TSH secretion that results in involution of the normal gland, along with the development of thyrotoxic symptoms. Treatment of these lesions is usually by subtotal thyroidectomy of ^{131}I ablation. Anesthetic considerations are those related to hyperthyroidism and subtotal thyroidectomy discussed earlier.

Thyroid carcinomas also occur in three histological cell types.[75] The most common is papillary carcinoma, which occurs both in elderly persons and in persons 20–40 years old. This is a slowly growing tumor that spreads through regional lymph nodes. Follicular carcinoma, in contrast, is a more uncommon lesion and undergoes early hematogenous spread, frequently resulting in bone and pulmonary metastases. The most uncommon malignant thyroid lesion is anaplastic carcinoma, which occurs principally in the aged. This tumor is usually poorly differentiated, spreads by aggressive local invasion, and is typically resistant to most forms of intervention. Solitary "cold" thyroid nodules are malignant in approximately 10–30% of patients; patients with such lesions who receive neck irradiation early in life have an approximately 33% incidence of carcinoma. Suspicion is aroused by the findings of a rapidly growing, firm, nontender nodule with reduced or absent uptake on radioiodine scanning. A solitary "cold" nodule surrounded by normal thyroid tissue is especially worrisome for tumor. Lesions that are cystic on ultrasound are less likely to be malignant than are solid ones. Evidence of laryngeal involvement such as hoarseness, tracheal deviation, and so forth should be sought out and evaluated by CT scanning of the neck. Initial diagnosis is usually established by needle aspiration or incisional biopsy.

Treatment of most thyroid carcinomas is usually by wide excision that is often a near-total, if not total, thyroidectomy, along with examination of the regional lymph nodes. Large doses of ^{131}I are often used to scan for distal functional metastases as well as to ablate any remaining thyroid tissue. Treatment is then continued by close follow-up for residual or recurrent disease, as well as with suppressive dosages of T_4.

PARATHYROID DISEASE

Parathyroid Physiology

The major role of the parathyroid gland is, in conjunction with vitamin D, to precisely control serum calcium (Ca^{2+}) concentration. The active form of calcium in plasma is ionized Ca^{2+} (approximately 50% of the total calcium), which is also the form that is crucial to myocardial and skeletal muscle function, glandular activity, neurotransmitter release, coagulation, and so forth. Forty percent of the total calcium is bound to albumin; alterations in pH (acidosis increases the free fraction of ionized calcium) and competition by other drugs bound to albumin affect the ionized calcium concentration by this mechanism.

The effects of parathyroid hormone (PTH) include stimulating osteoclastic bone resorption and distal tubular resorption of calcium, as well as promoting the synthesis of 1,25-dihydroxyvitamin D.[76] Renal effects also include magnesium reabsorption, phosphaturia, and bicarbonaturia. PTH release is stimulated primarily by depressed ionized calcium concentration, although hyperphosphatemia (perhaps through decreased calcium level), acute hypomagnesemia, and serum catecholamines also cause PTH secretion. In a normal gland, elevated serum calcium level effectively inhibits release. The mechanism of action of PTH secretion is through stimulation of the adenylate cyclase system with resultant formation of adenosine 3':5'-cyclic phosphate (cyclic AMP) and phosphorylation of the protein kinase system.

Vitamin D is produced from dietary calciferol by 25-hydroxylation in the liver, followed by the synthesis of 1-25 hydroxyvitamin D (aPTH-stimulated step) in the kidney. 1,25-hydroxyvitamin D promotes the intestinal, renal, and bone absorption of calcium and phosphate. The synthesis of vitamin D is stimulated by both hypocalcemia and hyperphosphatemia. The goal of this complex, interrelated system is to precisely maintain serum ionized calcium levels within a narrow normal range.

Hyperparathyroidism

Hyperparathyroidism is the usual indication for parathyroid surgery. Primary hyperparathyroidism most commonly is the result of a benign, functioning parathyroid adenoma, less often of glandular hyperplasia, and rarely is due to adenocarcinoma. Secondary hyperparathyroidism results from increased parathyroid function due to hypocalcemia or hyperphosphatemia. Causes include (1) renal failure, with its hyperphosphatemia and hypocalcemia, and diminished hydroxylation of vitamin D; (2) dietary vitamin D deficiency; and (3) intestinal malabsorption of calcium or vitamin D.

Hypercalcemia is responsible for the majority of signs and symptoms of primary hyperparathyroidism. These include muscle weakness and fatigue, peptic ulcers, hypertension, depression, memory loss, psychosis, and nephrolithiasis. Polyuria and polydipsia may occur also. All of these symptoms usually resolve with successful treatment.

The serum calcium is almost always significantly elevated in primary hyperparathyroidism. The diagnosis is confirmed by the presence of elevated PTH (by radioimmunoassay). Other laboratory features include elevated urinary cyclic AMP levels, anemia, and hyperchloremic acidosis. Shortening of the Q-T$_c$ interval on ECG is an uncertain indication of the degree of hypercalcemia.[77]

Hypercalcemia can result from a variety of other causes, including multiple myeloma, vitamin D intoxication, sarcoidosis, thyrotoxicosis, ingestion of large amounts of milk combined with absorbable antacids, and malignancy. Malignancy causes hypercalcemia through osteolytic metastases, production of

PTH hormone (pseudohyperparathyroidism), or the production of hormonal substances chemically distinct from PTH that possess PTH-like effects.

Anesthetic Considerations. As with symptoms, the major goals of preoperative management are directed toward treatment of hypercalcemia, the mortality of which increases significantly when total serum calcium rises above 15–16 mg · dL^{-1}.[77] Other prominent abnormalities involve hypovolemia, hyperchloremia, and the aforementioned renal, cardiac, and neuromuscular effects. Vigorous hydration accompanied by a sodium diuresis with furosemide (which also promotes calcium excretion) is the initial treatment and is usually effective. Mithramycin may be effective in malignant states and may reduce PTH-induced osteoclastic bone resorption. Calcitonin can have significant and rapid effects to lower serum calcium, but resistance to this usually develops in 1–2 days. Glucocorticoids are not effective treatment in primary hyperparathyroidism, but may be helpful in malignancies, sarcoidosis, and thyrotoxicosis. Other than specific considerations mentioned previously, no particular anesthetic technique or agent seems especially favored. Neck dissection to locate a single parathyroid adenoma can be a long, painstaking process. Careful patient positioning and padding is indicated because of the generalized bone demineralization. The potential for cardiac rhythm disturbances must be kept in mind. It is important to remember the potential for underlying renal dysfunction, as well as the need to maintain intravascular volume and urine output. Response to neuromuscular blocking drugs may be unpredictable. Hypercalcemia-mediated muscle weakness would theoretically increase sensitivity to these drugs, whereas elevated serum calcium concentrations could potentially antagonize the effects of nondepolarizing muscle relaxants. Monitoring of neuromuscular blockade is clearly indicated.

The consequences and complications of parathyroidectomy are much the same as those discussed for thyroid surgery. Air embolism is rare. More often, transient hypoparathyroidism can result owing to edema and dysfunction of the remaining (if any) glandular tissue. The serum calcium is usually at its lowest point 24–48 hours after surgery, but patients may be symptomatic (see later) as early as 6–8 hours postoperatively. Obviously, such problems will be permanent in the case of a total parathyroidectomy. Unilateral or bilateral recurrent laryngeal nerve injuries and expanding neck hematomas are also infrequent problems. Postoperative stridor and airway obstruction may result from recurrent laryngeal nerve injury, expanding neck hematoma, or hypocalcemia.

Hypoparathyroidism

The most common cause of hypoparathyroidism is glandular removal during thyroid or parathyroid surgery. Other causes are neck trauma (including laryngeal and pharyngeal cancer surgery), neck irradiation, and infiltrating malignancy or amyloidosis. Pseudohypoparathyroidism is usually an inherited disorder wherein PTH secretion is normal but the peripheral tissues are resistant to its effects. In addition to hypocalcemia and hyperphosphatemia, these patients have growth failure, obesity, mental retardation, and calcified basal ganglia.[78]

Acute hypocalcemia, such as may occur following surgery on or about the parathyroid glands, is commonly manifested as perioral paresthesias, restlessness, muscle spasms, and neuromuscular irritability. Tetany and seizures may occur. Stridor and complete airway obstruction may develop, because the laryngeal muscles are especially sensitive to the effects of hypocalcemia. The tendency toward neuromuscular irritability may be elicited as Chvostek's and Trousseau's signs. The former is facial muscle contracture induced by tapping over the facial nerve as it crosses the mandible below the parotid gland; the latter is carpopedal spasm produced by 3 minutes of tourniquet-induced ischemia. Cardiovascular complications include Q-T prolongation, congestive failure, and hypotension. Interestingly, dysrhythmias are uncommon. More chronic manifestations include lethargy, depression, and fatigue.

Severe hypocalcemia is treated with the administration of IV calcium gluconate 10–20 mg/kg slowly over several minutes. This is usually followed with an infusion at a rate of 100–250 mg/kg/day of calcium gluconate. Continuous ECG monitoring and frequent serum calcium determinations should be performed. If persistent, oral calcium and vitamin D supplementation may be required.

MULTIPLE ENDOCRINE NEOPLASIA

Rarely, lesions of the thyroid or parathyroid glands occur in the setting of multiple glandular abnormalities. Collectively these are referred to as the multiple endocrine neoplasia

disorders (MEN), each of which is inherited in an autosomal dominant fashion. MEN type 1, also known as Wermer's syndrome, is defined by hyperplasia or tumors of the parathyroids, pancreatic islet cells, pituitary, adrenal cortex, and thyroid. Lesions may appear in two or more glands simultaneously or may be individually manifest separated by a period of years. The parathyroid and pituitary lesions are often benign, but pancreatic and adrenal tumors are frequently malignant. Symptoms of hyperparathyroidism are common, and the islet cell tumor component can liberate insulin, gastrin, vasoactive inhibitory peptide, and glucagon.

MEN type 2, called the Sipple syndrome, consists of medullary thyroid carcinoma, pheochromocytoma (often bilateral), and occasional parathyroid hyperplasia. Type 2b of this disease consists of pheochromocytoma and medullary thyroid carcinoma, but these patients have multiple neuromas also involving the larynx, oral mucosa, and conjunctiva.

REFERENCES

1. Batsakis JG: Tumors of the head and neck. Clinical and pathological considerations. Baltimore, Williams and Wilkins, 1982, pp 144–76.
2. Oral cancer. A stubborn problem. Lancet 1972; 1:299.
3. Johns ME: Carcinomas of the oral cavity and pharynx. *In* Lee KJ (ed): Essential Otolaryngology. New Hyde Park, Medical Examination Publishing, 1983, pp 571–616.
4. Jesse RH: The philosophy of treatment of neck nodes. Ear Nose Throat J 1977; 56:58–66.
5. Ogura JH, Thawley SE: Cysts and tumors of the larynx. *In* Paparella MM, Shumrick DA (eds): Otolaryngology. Philadelphia, WB Saunders, 1980, pp 2504–2527.
6. Son ML: Conservative surgery for carcinoma of the supraglottis. J Laryngol Otol 1970; 84:655–670.
7. Tisi GM: Preoperative evaluation of pulmonary function. Am Rev Respir Dis 1979; 119:293–310.
8. Stoelting RG, Dierdorf SF, McCammon RL: Anesthesia and coexisting disease. New York, Churchill Livingstone, 1988; pp 207–208.
9. Mangano DT: Perioperative cardiac morbidity. Anesthesiology 1990; 72:153–184.
10. Mangano DT (ed): Preoperative Cardiac Assessment. New York, JB Lippincott, 1990.
11. Gottlieb SO, Weisfeldt ML, Ouyang P, et al: Silent ischemia as a marker for unfavorable outcomes in patients with unstable angina. N Engl J Med 1986; 314:1214–1219.
12. Eagle KA, Singer DE, Brewster DC, et al: Dipyridamole-thallium scanning in patients undergoing vascular surgery. JAMA 1987; 257:2185–2189.
13. Chung F, Houston PL, Cheng DCH, et al: Calcium channel blockade does not offer adequate protection from perioperative myocardial ischemia. Anesthesiology 1988; 69:343–347.
14. Eckhardt MJ, Harford TC, Kaelber CT: Health haz-

ards associated with alcohol consumption. Anesthesiology 1981; 56:648–666.

15. Thompson WL, Johnson AD, Muddrey WL, et al: Diazepam and paraldehyde for treatment of severe delirium tremens: A controlled trial. Ann Intern Med 1975; 82:175–180.

16. Godden DJ, Willey RF, Fergusson RJ, et al: Rigid bronchoscopy under intravenous general anesthesia with oxygen Venturi ventilation. Thorax 1982; 37:532–534.

17. Strong MS, Vaughan CW, Mahler DC, et al: Cardiac complications of microsurgery of the larynx. Laryngoscope 1974; 84:908–920.

18. Kotrly KJ, Kotter GS, Mortara D, et al: Intraoperative detection of ischemia with an ST-segment trend monitoring system. Anesth Analg 1984; 63:343–348.

19. Ogura JH, Thawley SE: Surgery of the larynx. In Paparella MM, Shumrick DA (eds): Otolaryngology. Philadelphia, WB Saunders, 1980, pp 2528–2588.

20. Plant M: Anaesthesia for pharyngolaryngectomy with extrathoracic oesophagectomy and gastric transportation. Anaesthesia 1982; 37:1211–1213.

21. Bromage PR, Camporesi E, Chestnut D: Epidural narcotics for postoperative analgesia. Anesth Analg 1980; 59:473–480.

22. Shumrick DA: Neck dissection. In Paparella MM, Shumrick DA (eds): Otolaryngology. Philadelphia, WB Saunders, 1980, pp 2966–2986.

23. Feinstein R, Owens WD: Anesthesia for ENT. In Barash PG, Cullen BF, Stoelting RK (eds): Clinical Anesthesia. Philadelphia, JB Lippincott, 1989, pp 1067–1078.

24. Brennan MD: Thyroid hormones. Mayo Clin Proc 1980; 55:33–44.

25. Eberhardt NW, Apulette JW, Baxter JB: The molecular biology of hormone action. In Litwok G (ed): Biochemical action of hormones. New York, Academic Press, 1980, pp 309–311.

26. Williams LT, Lefkowitz RJ, Watanabe AM, et al: Thyroid hormone regulation of beta-adrenergic number. J Biol Chem 1977; 252:2787–2789.

27. Buccins RA, Spann JF, Pool PE, et al: Influence of the thyroid state on the intrinsic contractile properties and energy stores of the myocardium. J Clin Invest 1967; 46:1669–1682.

28. Abuid J, Larsen PR: Triiodothyronine and thyroxine in hyperthyroidism: Comparison of the acute changes during therapy with antithyroid agents. J Clin Invest 1974; 54:201–208.

29. Murkin JM: Anesthesia and hypothyroidism: A review of thyroxine physiology, pharmacology, and anesthetic implications. Anesth Analg 1982; 61:371–383.

30. Melmed S, Geola FL, Reed AW, et al: A comparison of methods for assessing thyroid function in nonthyroidal illness. J Clin Endocrinol Metab 1982; 54:300–306.

31. Cavalieri RR, Rapoport B: Impaired peripheral conversion of thyroxine to triiodothyronine. Annu Rev Med 1978; 28:57–68.

32. Becker SP, Skolinik EM, O'Neil JV: The nodular thyroid. Otolaryngol Clin North Am 1980; 13:53–58.

33. Volpe R: Thyroiditis: Current views of pathogenesis. Med Clin North Am 1975; 59:1163–1175.

34. Cave WT: Thyroiditis. In Conn RB (ed): Current Diagnosis. Philadelphia, WB Saunders, 1985, pp 843–848.

35. Amino N, Mori H, Iwatani Y, et al: High prevalence of transient post-partum thyrotoxicosis and hypothyroidism. N Engl J Med 1982; 306:849–852.

36. Fradkin JE, Wolff J: Iodide-induced thyrotoxicosis. Medicine 1983; 62:1–20.

37. Greer MA: Antithyroid drugs in the treatment of thyrotoxicosis. Thyroid Today 1980; 3:1–18.

38. Feely J, Forrest AL, Gunn A, et al: Beta-blocking drugs and thyroid function. Br Med J 1977; 2:1352–1359.

39. Zonszein J, Santangelo RP, Mackin JF, et al: Propranolol therapy in thyrotoxicosis. A review of 84 patients undergoing surgery. Am J Med 1979; 66:411–416.

40. Mackin JF, Canary JJ, Pittman CS: Thyroid storm and its management. N Engl J Med 1974; 291:1396–1398.

41. Ingbar SH: Thyrotoxic storm. N Engl J Med 1966; 274:1252–1254.

42. Peters KR, Nance P, Wingard DW: Malignant hyperthyroidism or malignant hyperthermia? Anesth Analg 1981; 60:613–615.

43. Hamilton WFD, Forrest AL, Gunn A, et al: Beta-adrenoceptor blockade and anesthesia for thyroidectomy. Anaesthesia 1984; 39:335–342.

44. Feek CM, Sawers JSA, Irvine WJ, et al: Combination of potassium iodide and propranolol in preparation of patients with Graves' disease for thyroid surgery. N Engl J Med 1980; 302:883–885.

45. Feely J, Stevenson IH, Crooks J: Increased clearance of propranolol in thyrotoxicosis. Ann Intern Med 1981; 94:472–474.

46. Peden NR, Gunn A, Browning MCK, et al: Naldolol and potassium iodide in combination in the surgical treatment of thyrotoxicosis. Br J Surg 1982; 69:638–640.

47. Strube PJ: Thyroid storm during beta blockade. Anaesthesia 1984; 39:343–346.

48. Brooks M, Waldstein SS: Free thyroxine concentrations in thyroid storm. Ann Intern Med 1980; 93:694–697.

49. Jacobs HS, Mackie DB, Eastman CJ, et al: Total and free triiodothyronine and thyroxine levels in thyroid storm and recurrent hyperthyroidism. Lancet 1973; 2:236–238.

50. Neumann G, Weingarten AE, Abramowitz RM, et al: The anesthetic management of the patient with an anterior mediastinal mass. Anesthesiology 1984; 60:144–147.

51. Wade JSH: Respiratory obstruction in thyroid surgery. Ann R Coll Surg Engl 1980; 62:15–24.

52. De Soto H: Direct laryngoscopy as an aid to relieve airway obstruction in a patient with a mediastinal mass. Anesthesiology 1987; 67:116–117.

53. Sibert KS, Biondi JW, Hirsch NP: Spontaneous respiration during thoracotomy in a patient with a mediastinal mass. Anesth Analg 1987; 66:904–907.

54. Stheling LC: Anesthetic management of the patient with hyperthyroidism. Anesthesiology 1974; 41:585–595.

55. Benson DW: Anesthesia for thyroid surgery. Semin Anesth 1984; 111:168–180.

56. Stoelting RK, Dierdorf SF, McCammon RL: Anesthesia and Coexisting Disease, 2nd ed. New York, Churchill Livingstone, 1988, p 480.

57. Kaplan JA, Cooperman LH: Alarming reactions to ketamine in patients taking thyroid medication treated with propranolol. Anesthesiology 1971; 35:229–230.

58. Steffey EP, Eger EI: Hyperthermia and halothane MAC in the dog. Anesthesiology 1980; 41:392–396.

59. Wood M, Berman ML, Harbison RD, et al: Halothane-induced hepatic necrosis in triiodothyronine-pretreated rats. Anesthesiology 1980; 52:470–476.

60. Berman ML, Kuhnert L, Phython JM, Holaday DA: Isoflurane and enflurane-induced hepatic necrosis in

triiodothyronine-pretreated rats. Anesthesiology 1983; 58:1–5.

61. Seino H, Dohi S, Aiyoshi Y, et al: Postoperative hepatic dysfunction after halothane or enflurane anesthesia in patients with hyperthyroidism. Anesthesiology 1986; 64:122–125.
62. Howard D: Neurological affections of the pharynx and larynx. *In* Stell PM (ed): Scott-Brown's Otolaryngology, Laryngology. London, Butterworths, 1987, pp 169–185.
63. Green WER, Sheppard HWH, Stevenson HM, Wilson W: Tracheal collapse after thyroidectomy. Br J Surg 1979; 66:544–547.
64. Waldstein SS: Medical complications of thyroid surgery. Otolaryngol Clin North Am 1981; 13:99–107.
65. Ingbar SH, Worbar KA: The thyroid gland. *In* Williams RH (ed): Textbook of Endocrinology. Philadelphia, WB Saunders, 1981, pp 117–247.
66. Bough EW, Crowley WF, Ridgway C, et al: Myocardial function in hypothyroidism: Relation to disease severity and response to treatment. Arch Intern Med 1978; 138:1476–1480.
67. Zwillich CW, Pierson DJ, Hofeldt FD, et al: Ventilatory control in myxedema and hypothyroidism. N Engl J Med 1975; 292:662–665.
68. Edson JR, Fecher DR, Doe RP: Low platelet adhesiveness and other hemostatic abnormalities in hypothyroidism. Ann Intern Med 1975; 82:342–346.
69. Hellman DE: The thyroid gland. *In* Brown BR, Blitt CD, Gisecke AH (eds): Anesthesia and the patient with endocrine disease. Philadelphia, FA Davis, 1980, pp 109–144.
70. White VA, Kumagai LF: Preoperative endocrine and metabolic considerations. Med Clin North Am 1979; 63:1321–1334.
71. Becker C: Hypothyroidism and atherosclerotic heart disease: Pathogenesis, medical management, and the role of coronary bypass surgery. Endocr Rev 1985; 6:432–440.
72. Weinberg AD, Brennan MD, Gorman CA, et al: Outcome of anesthesia and surgery in hypothyroid patients. Arch Intern Med 1983; 143:893–897.
73. Ladenson PW, Levin AA, Ridgway EC, Daniels GH: Complications of surgery in hypothyroid patients. Am J Med 1984; 77:261–266.
74. Babad AA, Eger EI: The effects of hyperthyroidism and hypothyroidism on halothane and oxygen requirements in dogs. Anesthesiology 1968; 29:1087–1093.
75. James AG, Farrar WB, Cooperman M: Tumors of the thyroid and parathyroid. *In* Pilch YH (ed): Surgical oncology. New York, McGraw-Hill, 1984, pp 405–429.
76. Martin KJ, Hruska KA, Freitag JJ, et al: The peripheral metabolism of parathyroid hormone. N Engl J Med 1979; 301:1092–1098.
77. Heath DA: Emergency treatment of disorders of calcium and magnesium. Clin Endocrinol Metab 1980; 9:487–502.
78. Hebener JF, Potts JT: Biosynthesis of parathyroid hormone. N Engl J Med 1978; 299:580–585.

Anesthetic Management of Maxillofacial Trauma

Alexander W. Gotta
Colleen A. Sullivan

Maxillofacial trauma challenges the anesthesiologist to recognize the nature and severity of the injury, concurrent medical and surgical problems, and the integrity of the airway. Adequate understanding and prudent therapy of these problems requires consideration of the following:

1. the normal anatomy of the facial skeleton
2. etiology of facial fractures
3. usual lines of fractures of the facial skeleton
4. evaluation of the airway
5. preoperative evaluation of the patient with maxillofacial trauma
6. common medical problems in the traumatized patient
7. common surgical problems in the traumatized patient
8. choice of anesthetic agent and technique.

As Rene LeFort demonstrated almost 100 years ago, diagnosis of traumatic disruption of the facial skeleton is often difficult to recognize because of the lack of correlation between bone disruption and external signs of trauma.[1]

NORMAL ANATOMY

It is conventional to divide the facial skeleton into thirds. The lower third consists of the mandible, composed of the body, the ramus, the coronoid process, and the condyle and its articulation in the temporomandibular joint. The maxillae, zygomatic bones, nasal bones, and orbits constitute the middle third. The upper third consists of the frontal bone and frontozygomatic processes. The craniofacial skeleton contains a series of arches and bony buttresses that together disperse and redistribute forces applied to the face, protecting the intracranial contents from the effects of facial trauma. There is an arch created by the zygomatic process of the temporal bone, continuing by the zygoma, to the zygomaticomaxillary suture. Another arch joins the head and neck of the mandibular condyle to the coronoid process.

The bony buttresses limit displacement of the facial skeleton in its relationship to the cranium. Horizontal posterior displacement is limited by the zygomatic process of the temporal bone, oblique posterior displacement is limited by the pterygoid process of the sphenoid bone, and vertical posterior displacement is limited by the greater wing of the sphenoid bone. Upward displacement is limited by the zygomatic process of the frontal bone, the nasal part of the frontal bone, and the roof of the mandibular fossa, although the latter is thin, translucent, and easily fractured.

ETIOLOGY OF FACIAL FRACTURES

The combination of buttresses and arches protects the craniofacial skeleton from the effects of the physiological forces generated during mastication, and also creates a vector of force dispersion that redistributes and dissipates the impact of a blow directed to the mandible along this vector. Thus, although a blow to the mandible may fracture this bone, the fracture line rarely extends into the cranium, because the force follows a normal dispersion vector and is redistributed and directed away from the skull. Similarly, a blow to the skull may cause a cranial fracture, but it is unlikely that the fracture will extend into the face. A patient with a fractured mandible may, at the same time, have a fractured skull; almost invariably, however, this is the result not of one blow, but of a series of blows to both the mandible and the skull.

However, a blow to the face from the front, especially the front and above, does not follow a normal vector of force dispersion and may generate an abnormal shearing force that tends to tear the facial skeleton away from the cranium and may extend the fracture into the base of the skull (Fig. 6–1).

Because the mandible is tubular, it derives its strength from the cortex. The mandible is least vulnerable to fracture at its anterior-inferior border, where the cortex is thickest.[2] Posteriorly, the cortex thins, and the mandible becomes more susceptible to fracture.

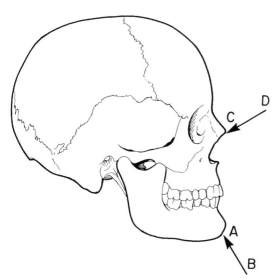

FIGURE 6–1. *A blow delivered along vector AB may fracture the mandible, but the force will be dispersed and usually will not cause a fracture of the skull. A blow along vector CD, however, will generate an abnormal shearing force tending to tear the facial skeleton away from the cranial skeleton, and thus extend a midface fracture into the base of the skull. (From Gotta AW: Maxillofacial trauma: Anesthetic considerations. ASA Refresher Courses in Anesthesiology, Vol 15. Philadelphia, JB Lippincott, 1987.)*

USUAL LINES OF FRACTURE

Most fractures of the mandible occur in the ramus and may be at or near the condyle,[3–6] possibly involving the temporomandibular joint, interfering with its operation and rendering direct visualization of the larynx difficult. The second most common site of fracture is in the body of the mandible at the level of the first or second molar.[5] Bimandibular fractures may result in posterior-inferior displacement of the anterior fracture segment, as the segment is pulled posteriorly by the muscles of the floor of the mouth, impacting the tongue and paraglottic soft tissues into the upper airway and causing acute airway closure.[7] Because of the foreshortened jaw, this type of fracture is often called an Andy Gump fracture after a misshapen cartoon character popular many years ago.

Because of the shape of the mandible, a blow delivered anywhere to the bone creates shearing forces within it and causes the forces to gather at points of vulnerability, i.e., the ramus or body at the level of the molars. Thus, a fracture may occur at the point of impact of a blow, but the same blow may cause fractures also at remote locations.[5]

In 1901, Rene LeFort of Lille, France, published the results of his series of studies on cadaver skulls.[1] He attempted to determine the relationship between external (soft tissue) signs of facial trauma and skeletal disruption, and the usual lines of midface fracture. His delineation of these fracture lines led to the LeFort classification of fractures (Fig. 6–2).

The LeFort I is a horizontal fracture of the maxilla, passing above the floor of the nose, involving the lower third of the septum and mobilizing the palate, the maxillary alveolar process, the lower third of the pterygoid plates, and part of the palatine bones. The fracture segment may be displaced posteriorly or laterally, may be rotated about a vertical axis, or may be moved in combination of these directions.

The LeFort II is a pyramidal fracture, beginning at the junction of the thick upper part of the nasal bone and the thinner portion forming the upper margin of the anterior nasal aperture. The fracture crosses the medial wall of the orbit, including the lacrimal bone, and then beneath the zygomatic-maxillary suture, crossing the lateral wall of the antrum, and then posteriorly through the pterygoid plates. The mobile segment may be displaced posteriorly or rotated about an axis.

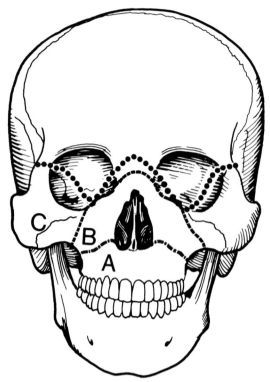

FIGURE 6–2. The LeFort classification of fractures. A identifies the line of fracture for a LeFort I; B, LeFort II; and C, LeFort III. (From Gotta AW: Maxillofacial trauma: Anesthetic considerations. ASA Refresher Courses in Anesthesiology, Vol 15. Philadelphia, JB Lippincott, 1987.)

In a LeFort III fracture, the fracture line runs parallel with the base of the skull, separating the midfacial skeleton from the cranial base. The fracture extends through the base of the nose and the ethmoid, through the orbital plates, and near the cribriform plate, which may be fractured also. The line crosses the lesser wing of the sphenoid, then moves downward to the pterygomaxillary fissure and sphenopalatine fossa. From the base of the inferior orbital fissure, the fracture line extends laterally and upward to the frontozygomatic suture, and downward and backward to the root of the pterygoid plates. The zygomatic arch of the temporal bone is fractured also. Because the cribriform plate may be fractured, a LeFort III fracture can involve basal skull fracture and access to the subarachnoid space. Cerebrospinal fluid (CSF) rhinorrhea is a definite indication of basal skull fracture. Even without this sign, LeFort III fractures demand basal skull x-ray examination (e.g., through computed tomography).

In a LeFort III fracture, the midface is mobilized and often distracted posteriorly. The normal convexity of the face may be replaced with a concavity, giving the patient a characteristic "dish-face deformity."

LeFort fractures rarely present in the classic form. They are usually incomplete fractures of one side, presenting singly or in combination with incomplete fracture of the other side. Thus, one may see, for example, a hemi LeFort I, combined with a hemi LeFort II of the other side, or any combination. Recognition of the fracture type is important because of the possibility of basal skull fracture.

EVALUATION OF THE AIRWAY

Severe maxillofacial trauma may cause disruption of the bony, cartilaginous, and soft tissue components of the airway and cause respiratory distress or even airway closure. Fresh and clotted blood can occlude the airway also. Stertorous, labored breathing with flaring of the alae nasi, cyanosis, and an anxious countenance are obvious indicators of respiratory distress. Use of the accessory muscles of respiration is a more subtle sign of breathing difficulty.

With a bimandibular (Andy Gump) fracture and posterior displacement of the fractured segment, it may be possible to pull the fractured segment forward by traction at the symphysis and lower central incisors, thus pulling the tongue and soft tissues forward in restoring the airway. This maneuver may be life-saving.

Mobility in the jaw may be limited after facial trauma. Trismus, spasm of the masseter muscles, may occur secondary to the trauma and lock the jaw shut. Trismus is overcome by anesthesia and muscle relaxant. Edema and pain may limit mobility but can be minimized by anesthetic and relaxant. A dangerous form of immobility, unresponsive to either anesthetic drugs or relaxants, can occur with a fracture through or near the temporomandibular joint, or with a fracture that involves the zygomatic process of the temporal bone (Fig. 6–3). Fractures involving the joint directly may lock the jaw closed, or the jaw may open only partly, making direct visualization of the larynx difficult or impossible.

The zygomatic process of the temporal bone is enveloped in the tough temporal fascia. If this fascia is ruptured by a blow, usually directed downward at the side of the head, and the zygomatic process is fractured, the fracture segments may be displaced and impinge di-

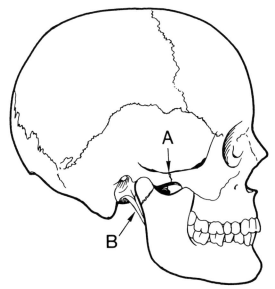

FIGURE 6–3. Mechanical impairment of the temporomandibular joint, and a jaw locked shut and unresponsive to anesthetics and muscle relaxants, may occur after fracture of the zygomatic arch of the temporal bone (A) or after a fracture of the condyle of the mandible (B). (From Gotta AW: Maxillofacial trauma: Anesthetic considerations. ASA Refresher Courses in Anesthesiology, Vol 15. Philadelphia, JB Lippincott, 1987.)

rectly on the temporomandibular joint and the condyle, locking the jaw shut.

The cause of jaw immobility must be determined prior to attempting intubation. Awake intubation or tracheostomy is mandated if one cannot determine with reasonable certainty whether a patient will be able to open the mouth sufficiently to allow visualization of the larynx.

COMMON MEDICAL PROBLEMS

In the patient with maxillofacial trauma, concurrent medical problems influencing anesthetic management may include (1) acute alcoholic intoxication, (2) chronic alcoholism, (3) drug intoxication, (4) myocardial infarct, and (5) stroke.

Acute alcoholic intoxication is a frequent concomitant of facial trauma and may render physical examination and adequate evaluation of the history extremely difficult. Chronic alcoholism must always be suspected in the acutely intoxicated patient, and the effects of chronic alcohol ingestion on hepatic function, metabolism, and blood clotting must be considered. Acute drug intoxication and chronic

drug abuse also can make the patient poorly responsive and vulnerable to a wide variety of major organ dysfunctions, e.g., hepatitis, bacterial endocarditis, renal failure. A major problem of the drug addict is the risk of withdrawal when the drugs of abuse are not available. Addicts are usually polyaddicted, and the narcotic addict is almost invariably also an alcoholic.[8]

The possible presence of myocardial infarct or stroke must be considered in elderly traumatized patients, because they predispose to trauma and may have been major causative factors.

COMMON SURGICAL PROBLEMS

Concurrent surgical problems in patients with maxillofacial trauma may include fracture of the skull, intracranial hemorrhage, subdural hematoma, fracture of the cervical spine, fat embolism, pneumothorax, flail chest, cardiac tamponade, cardiac hematoma, ruptured spleen, and ruptured liver. Repeated blows to the face and head may fracture both the mandible and the skull. Midface fractures, especially LeFort III fractures, should always arouse suspicions of possible extension of the fracture line into the base of the skull.

Blows to the head and face may be of sufficient magnitude to cause intracranial bleeding, either into the substance of the brain itself or into the subdural space. Diagnosis of intracranial bleeding depends on a strong index of suspicion.

Fracture or subluxation of the cervical spine influences the technique of endotracheal intubation and must be investigated whenever it is suspected. Radiographs of the cervical spine must be obtained if there is any possibility of spinal damage.

Fat embolism and its confusing clinical manifestations must always be considered after major trauma; it is not just a sequela of long bone fracture.

Pneumothorax may occur as a result of blows to the chest or in an automobile accident in which the thorax is thrown violently against the steering column or dashboard. Bony or cartilaginous fragments of broken ribs can penetrate the lung and be almost undetectable by radiography. Trauma may be sufficient to produce a flail chest or to compress the heart forcibly between the steering column and the vertebral column and cause extensive intramyocardial hemorrhage. A ruptured intra-abdominal organ may cause massive blood loss, often not easily recognized.

PREOPERATIVE EVALUATION

Knowledge of the mechanism of trauma, the nature of the facial fractures, and possible concurrent medical and surgical complications assists the anesthesiologist in the preoperative evaluation of the patient.

An adequate history is important. The nature of significant prior illness must be determined, if possible. The physician must assess the acute problem—not only the obvious trauma to the face, but also the possibility of trauma elsewhere. Certain questions should guide the evaluation: What was the form of the blow or force causing the injury? Were there other blows directed to other parts of the body? Was there loss of consciousness? Is there a history of drug (including alcohol) use?

Adequate physical examination demands evaluation of the face and jaw. Is there sufficient mobility to allow visualization of the larynx? Is there any possibility of concurrent skull fracture? Are there signs of CSF rhinorrhea? The patient should be able to flex and extend the head; limitation of motion suggests cervical spine injury and possible instability.[9] Bleeding within the closed fascial planes of the neck may cause pressure on the larynx or trachea and cause respiratory distress.

When possible, a neurological examination should be performed to establish a baseline and to evaluate the possibility of concurrent nervous system dysfunction. Laboratory and x-ray data should include the following:

1. hemoglobin or hematocrit as a crude index of oxygen-carrying capacity or blood volume
2. urinalysis as an indicator of trauma elsewhere
3. chest radiograph (if indicated) to detect pneumothorax if there is evidence of chest injury
4. electrocardiogram (if indicated) to detect cardiac injury.

Other useful data include liver function tests and coagulogram in patients known or suspected to be alcoholic.

ANESTHETIC AGENT AND TECHNIQUE

If there is any question about jaw mobility and the ability to visualize the larynx and effect

endotracheal intubation, the airway must be secured with the patient awake. It may be possible to use guided fiberoptic techniques for intubation. However, anatomical distortion secondary to trauma, coupled with blood or edema in the upper airway, may make these techniques impossible.

The insertion of a nasotracheal tube into the awake patient is often painful and unpleasant. However, the airway can be anesthetized to facilitate tube placement. A local anesthetic (e.g., 2–4% lidocaine) can be instilled with a few drops of vasoconstrictor (e.g., phenylephrine 0.25–0.50%).[10]

Sensory innervation of the larynx is provided by the internal branch of the superior laryngeal nerve, which can be blocked usually without great difficulty.[11, 12] The superior laryngeal nerve is a branch of the vagus and arises from the nodose ganglion. It travels with the main trunk of the nerve to the level of the larynx, where it springs forward and terminates in an internal (sensory) branch and an external (motor) branch (Fig. 6–4). The cricothyroid muscle, a tensor of the vocal cords, is innervated by the motor branch.[13]

The internal branch penetrates the thyrohyoid membrane and ramifies immediately to provide sensory innervation from the base of the tongue to the vocal cords. After penetrating the thyrohyoid membrane, the nerve rests in a closed space bounded medially by the laryngeal mucosa, laterally by the thyrohyoid membrane, superiorly by the inferior border of the hyoid, and inferiorly by the superior border of the thyroid cartilage.

Thus, for a block of the internal branch of

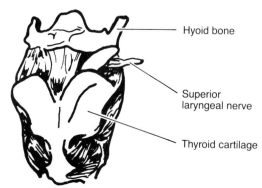

FIGURE 6–4. *The internal branch of the superior laryngeal nerve penetrates the thyrohyoid membrane and ramifies to provide sensory innervation to the interior of the larynx. (From Gotta AW: Maxillofacial trauma: Anesthetic considerations. ASA Refresher Courses in Anesthesiology, Vol 15. Philadelphia, JB Lippincott, 1987.)*

the superior laryngeal nerve, the landmarks are (1) the hyoid bone, a freely movable bone in the upper neck, articulating with no other bone; (2) the thyroid cartilage; and (3) the thyrohyoid membrane binding the two together.

As the patient lies on the table, she or he should be asked to extend the head fully. A 22-gauge needle, attached to a syringe containing 2 mL of 2% lidocaine, is directed at the hyoid, parallel to the coronal plane (perpendicular to the sagittal plane). After the needle strikes the hyoid, it is walked caudad until it just slips off the bone and is advanced through the thyrohyoid membrane. A sudden loss of resistance may be noted as the membrane is penetrated. Aspiration should yield nothing. Aspiration of air reveals penetration into the larynx, whereas aspiration of blood indicates entry into the carotid sheath or superior laryngeal artery. If there is no aspirate, the local anesthetic may be injected and the block repeated on the opposite side.

Contraindications to a superior laryngeal block include (1) a full stomach, because the block obtunds the laryngeal protective mechanisms; (2) infection at the site of block; and (3) tumor at the site of block. Complications of the block include possible intravascular injection into one of the large blood vessels of the neck, or hematoma secondary to blood vessel puncture.

The recurrent laryngeal nerve provides sensory innervation to the trachea below the vocal cords. Because it also provides motor innervation to the muscles of the larynx, block of this nerve is contraindicated because of the possibility of a laryngeal motor dysfunction and airway closure.

Sensory analgesia can be obtained by translaryngeal instillation of local anesthetic through cricothyroid puncture. Usually the cricoid is easily identified in the neck, with the cricoid membrane joining it to the thyroid cartilage, immediately superior. A 22-gauge needle attached to a syringe containing 4 mL of 2% lidocaine is thrust through the membrane in the midline, and air is aspirated. The bevel of the needle is turned caudad, toward the carina. The patient is instructed to inhale deeply, then exhale maximally. At the end of expiration, the lidocaine is rapidly injected, and the needle is quickly removed. The vigorous coughing that ensues sprays local anesthetic droplets along the tracheal walls and the inferior surface of the vocal cords.

With complete anesthetization of the airway from nose to carina, the patient is ready for intubation. The patient should extend his or her own head, thus avoiding painful manipulation of the injured face. The tube should be inserted parallel to the hard palate, through the right nostril, if possible. It should be advanced gently; if resistance is felt, it should be replaced by a smaller tube or positioned in the other nostril. Clear loud breath sounds should be heard as the tube is advanced to the glottis. If the sounds disappear, the tube should be withdrawn until they reappear. The fiberoptic bronchoscope may be inserted through the tube, the vocal cords visualized, and the bronchoscope advanced through the cords and into the trachea. With identification of the tracheal rings and carinii, the endotracheal tube may be slipped off the bronchoscope into the trachea. If blind awake intubation is elected, the tube is advanced near the larynx as indicated by clear breath sounds, and the patient is instructed to hyperventilate through the nose. At the beginning of inspiration, the tube is quickly but gently thrust forward, and the patient almost invariably aspirates it without difficulty. There are no dermatome representatives of the nerves blocked by the techniques described, and proper block technique is evidenced only by ready acceptance and tolerance of the endotracheal tube. Nasal intubation is contraindicated in the presence of known or suspected basal skull fracture.[14] Even positive-pressure ventilation runs a risk of introducing foreign matter into the subarachnoid space.[15]

After intubation, any inhalation anesthetic agent may be used. We caution against the use of halothane because of its tendency to cause dangerous ventricular dysrhythmias, often preceded by aberrant conduction.[16] The halogenated ethers are safer and allow the use of judicious amounts of epinephrine, if the surgeon prefers its use. Intravenous narcotics may be used as the primary anesthetic agent. However, the dosage may be difficult to determine in the addict. Ketamine should be used with great caution (if at all), especially if used in an attempt to avoid endotracheal intubation. Ketamine may depress respiration,[17] increase intracranial pressure, and alter cerebral metabolism,[18–20] none of which would be desirable in a patient with concurrent intracranial trauma.

REFERENCES

1. LeFort R: Etude experimentale sur les fractures de la machoire superieure. Rev Chir 1901; 23:208–227, 360–379, 479–507.

2. Haskell R: Applied surgical anatomy. Rowe NL, Williams JL (eds): Maxillo Facial Injuries. Edinburgh, Churchill Livingstone, 1985, pp 3–4.
3. Huelke DF: Mechanics in the production of mandibular fractures: A study of the "stresscoat" technique. I. Symphyseal impacts. J Dent Res 1961; 40:1042–1056.
4. Huelke DF, Patrick LM: Mechanics in the production of mandibular fractures: Strain-gauge measurements of impacts to the chin. J Dent Res 1964; 43:437–446.
5. Halazonetis JA: The "weak" regions of the mandible. Br J Oral Surg 1968; 6:37–48.
6. Nahum AM: The biomechanics of facial bone fracture. Laryngoscope 1975; 85:140–156.
7. Seshul MB, Sinn DP, Gerlock AJ: The Andy Gump fracture of the mandible: A cause of respiratory obstruction or distress. J Trauma 1978; 18:611–612.
8. Stimmel B, Vernace S, Tobias H: Hepatic dysfunction in heroin addicts; the role of alcohol. JAMA 1972; 222:811–812.
9. Dauphinee K: Orotracheal intubation. Emerg Med Clin North Am 1988; 6:699–713.
10. Gross JB, Hartigan ML: A suitable substitute for 4% cocaine before blind nasotracheal intubation: 3% lidocaine-0.25%, phenylephrine nasal spray. Anesth Anagl 1984; 63:915–918.
11. Gotta AW, Sullivan CA: Superior laryngeal nerve block: An aid to intubating the patient with fractured mandible. J Trauma 1984; 24:83–85.
12. Gotta AW, Sullivan CA: Anaesthesia of the upper airway using topical anaesthetic and superior laryngeal nerve block. Br J Anaesth 1981; 53:1055–1058.
13. Durham CF, Harrison TS: The surgical anatomy of the superior laryngeal nerve. Surg Gynecol Obstet 1964; 118:38–44.
14. Seebacher J, Rozik D, Mathieu A: Inadvertent intracranial introduction of a nasogastric tube, a complication of severe maxillofacial trauma. Anesthesiology 1975; 42:100–102.
15. Kitahata LM, Collins WF: Meningitis as a complication of anesthesia in a patient with a basal skull fracture. Anesthesiology 1970; 32:282–283.
16. Gotta AW, Sullivan CA, Pelkofski J, et al: Aberrant conduction as a precursor to cardiac arrhythmias during anesthesia for oral surgery. J Oral Surg 1976; 34:421–427.
17. Zsigmand EK, Matsuki A, Kothafy SP: Arterial hypoxemia caused by intravenous ketamine. Anesth Analg 1976; 55:311–314.
18. Gardner AE, Olson BE, Lichtiger M: Cerebrospinal-fluid pressure during dissociative anesthesia with ketamine. Anesthesiology 1971; 35:226–228.
19. Takeshita H, Okuda Y, Sari A: The effects of ketamine on cerebral circulation and metabolism in man. Anesthesiology 1972; 36:69–75.
20. Crosby G, Crane AM, Sokoloff L: Local changes in cerebral glucose utilization during ketamine anesthesia. Anesthesiology 1982; 56:437–443.

GLOMUS TUMORS[15]

In 1941, Guild[16] first reported the presence of small structures in and near the temporal bone in association with the adventitia of the jugular bulb just below the floor of the middle ear. These structures are also in the bony walls of tympanic canals that transmit the tympanic branches of the ninth and tenth cranial nerves. Guild named these structures, which are composed of epithelioid cells and are histologically similar to the carotid body, glomus bodies. In contrast to the cells in the adrenal medulla, these epithelioid cells fail to stain with chromium salts and are termed nonchromaffin.

As part of the autonomic nervous system, glomus bodies develop from the ectodermal neural tube.[17] Anatomically, glomus bodies are considered part of the chemoreceptor system, which includes the carotid, aortic, and ciliary bodies.[18] The physiological function of glomus bodies remains to be delineated. Some believe they are functionally inert,[19] whereas others think that, similar to the carotid bodies, they act as chemoreceptors.[18]

On rare occasions, glomus bodies may create an unusual tumor, variously called nonchromaffin paraganglioma, receptoma, chemodectoma, or most frequently, glomus tumor. Such tumors are usually single, but they may be multicentric. There is a notable genetic proclivity to development of glomus tumors, and, in one study,[19] one third of familial glomus tumors were multicentric. Approximately 80% occur in women.[20] The glomus tumor that originates from the tympanic plexus on the medial wall of the middle ear is designated a glomus tympanicum tumor. It is surgically removed either through the ear canal or through a more liberal mastoid exposure. Rarely, a glomus tumor may extend through the eustachian tube and become a nasopharyngeal lesion.[20] Glomus jugulare tumors are those that occur within the adventitia of the jugular bulb. The following comments focus on this type of glomus tumor, and the hazards of glomus tumors are listed in Table 7–1.

Glomus jugulare tumors are usually histologically benign but have a predilection for local invasion. Nonetheless, malignant metastases have been known to occur.[21] Extraordinarily vascular, these tumors derive their main blood supply through branches of the external carotid artery, chiefly the ascending pharyngeal branch. If the tumor is especially large, it may derive some of its blood supply through the internal carotid and vertebral arteries. Bruits may be audible over these highly vas-

TABLE 7–1. Hazards of Glomus Tumors

Highly vascular
Involvement of cranial nerves IX, X, XI, and XII, causing dysphagia, aspiration, and upper airway obstruction
May secrete catecholamines
Prophylactic embolization may trigger cerebrovascular accident
Cerebrospinal fluid leaks
Venous air embolism

cular tumors. Additional symptoms are produced by invasion of surrounding structures. Often, unilateral tinnitus is the patient's presenting complaint.[22] As the tumor grows to interfere with eardrum mobility or ossicular movement, or as it invades the cochlea, a conductive hearing loss results. The patient may have a pulsatile feeling of fullness in the ear and develop a facial nerve palsy. Other symptoms may include pain, aural discharge, and vertigo. If the glomus jugulare tumor spreads through the base of the skull, palsies of cranial nerves IX, X, XI, and XII may ensue. Not uncommonly, glomus tumors invade the lumen of the internal jugular vein, and they may even grow finger-like projections that can reach into the right atrium.[23]

Occasionally, glomus jugulare tumors and other paragangliomas secrete catecholamines and cause symptoms similar to those of a pheochromocytoma.[24] However, Brown[20] documented that when glomus tumors have secretory activity, it is norepinephrine rather than epinephrine that is elaborated.

Preoperative Evaluation

Carotid arteriography is necessary to evaluate the suspected tumor's blood supply as well as the tumor's location and extent. Retrograde venography to assess tumor growth into the internal jugular vein and preoperative computed tomography (CT) scanning for intracranial extension and bone erosion are also mandatory. If the patient has endocrinological symptoms, measurement of catecholamine levels and their metabolites in urine and blood is indicated. Indeed, Levit and associates[25] recommend routine preoperative determination of urinary levels of catecholamines and metabolites in all patients with craniocervical paraganglioma. In addition, thorough neurological examination of the cranial nerves is important. Debilitating problems include the dysphagia and aspiration that results from palsies of cranial nerves IX and X. Those patients with involvement of cranial nerves XI and XII have difficulty removing their airway secretions and are susceptible to upper airway obstruction.

Treatment

If possible, complete surgical excision is the best therapy for glomus jugulare tumor.[26] Irradiation is less effective but may be used for poor risk patients or those with extensive tumors. Although glomus jugulare tumors are generally more radiosensitive than paragangliomata at other sites, symptomatic relief results largely from involution of the mass secondary to an induced endarteritis resulting in parenchymal infarction and fibrosis.

Embolization with absorbable gelatin sponge or Teflon balls is frequently used preoperatively to reduce surgical blood loss.[27] However, embolization carries the risk of cerebrovascular accident, because active arterial-venous shunting permits the embolizing material to pass through the tumor and lodge in a cerebral artery. Embolization is contraindicated for tumors having a blood supply from the internal carotid or vertebral artery.

Tumors with significant intracranial extension are usually managed in two stages: first the neurosurgical procedure is performed through a suboccipital craniotomy, and about 6 weeks later the temporal bone component is removed. Staging of the neurosurgical and otologic-cervical procedures allows healing of the communication between the posterior fossa and the temporal bone, thus diminishing the incidence of cerebrospinal fluid leaks.

Some surgeons routinely perform cricopharyngeal myotomy at the time of removal of the glomus tumor if new injuries to cranial nerve IX, X, or XII are anticipated. This results in improvement of dysphagia and aspiration. In those with unilateral vocal cord damage, Teflon or absorbable gelatin sponge augmentation of the paretic vocal cord may result in marked improvement in deglutition and voice.

Anesthetic Implications

Because these tumors are vascular, the anesthesiologist must anticipate and be prepared to manage massive blood loss.

Detailed knowledge of the extent of intravascular extension of the tumor is mandatory before inserting a central venous or pulmonary artery catheter. The involved internal jugular vein should not be cannulated. Moreover, internal jugular vein involvement may cause fragments of the tumor to break off and embolize into the pulmonary circulation.

Because surgical resection may take over 15 hours, IV fluids should be warmed and inhaled gases humidified to prevent hypothermia and drying of secretions. Controlled hypotension may be useful in minimizing blood loss, but if the tumor extends intracranially and if intracranial pressure is increased, sodium nitroprusside is best avoided, because it produces cerebral vasodilation.

Venous air embolism is possible, particularly if the surgery is performed with the patient in the sitting position, though it may occur even if the patient is supine. Clearly, excision of tumor invading the temporal bone is likely to result in exposure of veins that cannot collapse because of bony attachments. Whereas placing the patient with the head inclined slightly facilitates venous drainage, thereby decreasing venous congestion and blood loss, zealous elevation of the head increases the risk of air embolism. If the internal jugular vein is involved and the surgeon plans to open it, venous air embolism may occur, so a right atrial catheter should be inserted preoperatively. The patient is monitored to detect this complication with measurement of end-tidal CO_2 and with a precordial Doppler ultrasound device. In cases in which venous air embolism is a distinct possibility, it is wise to control ventilation. Adornato and colleagues[28] showed that even a minimal air embolism may precipitate a gasp reflex that in turn may cause a large bolus of air to be sucked into the opened vein. This action transforms a minor air embolus into a major one. However, the gasp reflex complication can be obviated by controlling respiration.

If the surgeon must identify the facial nerve with a nerve stimulator, as is usually required, temporary, partial reversal of muscle relaxants is indicated. In patients with intracranial extension of glomus tumors, the principles of neuroanesthesia relative to any patient with a space-occupying lesion are germane, including use of drugs to decrease the intracranial pressure and use of patterns of ventilation consistent with producing a Pa_{CO_2} of approximately 30 mmHg.

Although Levit and associates[25] recommend routine preoperative determination of urinary catecholamines and their metabolites in all patients with craniocervical paragangliomas, others[15] make such measurements only when there is an associated history of hypertension or pheochromocytoma-like symptoms. If the tumor is secreting catecholamines, perioperative management is similar to that employed in patients with pheochromocytomas.[29]

SINUS SURGERY

The paranasal sinuses are air-filled cavities whose mucous membrane lining is continuous with that of the nasal cavity. The ethmoidal sinuses, situated between the upper part of the nose and the orbit, and the sphenoidal sinus, located behind the upper part of the nose, open directly into the superior meatus. The frontal sinuses, situated in the supraorbital frontal bone, drain through the frontonasal ducts into the anterior middle meatus. The maxillary sinuses open directly into the middle meatus. Of all the paranasal sinuses, the maxillary is the most frequently affected by infection and inflammation.[30]

Some salient features of intranasal anatomy and pathology should be familiar to the anesthesiologist. The thick mucous membrane, with its liberal blood supply, is especially vulnerable to congestion, infection, and significant bleeding. Congestion compromises the patency of the nasal airway and may result in total obstruction, especially with pre-existing bony aberrations in the lateral walls or septum. Although such obstruction may be relatively insignificant when the patient is able to breathe through the mouth, during induction of anesthesia the oral airway may be lost, and total respiratory obstruction can ensue. Hence, a patent oral airway should be preserved until the trachea is intubated.

The richly vascularized nasal mucosa has a propensity to bleed copiously with surgical manipulation, sometimes obscuring the view sufficiently to interfere with surgical access. Brisk bleeding may occlude the airway or, occasionally, cause serious hypotension. Therefore, the patient should be placed in a head-up 15-degree tilt to reduce bleeding and enhance visibility. In addition, a cuffed tube and a posterior pharyngeal pack should be employed to prevent aspiration of blood or infected material. Hypertension should be avoided.

Because of the impressive nasal blood supply, an appropriate topical vasoconstrictor should be used. Cocaine, in 4% solution, is used often in nasal surgery, but because cocaine interferes with catecholamine uptake, its sympathetic potentiating effect must be appreciated. Meyers[31] described two cases of cocaine toxicity during dacryocystorhinostomy, emphasizing that cocaine is contraindicated in hypertensives or in patients receiving adrenergic-modifying drugs such as guanethidine, reserpine, tricyclic antidepressants, or monoamine oxidase inhibitors (Table 7–2).

In the past, epinephrine was commonly mixed with cocaine to augment vasoconstriction. This dangerous practice failed to enhance vasoconstriction and triggered dysrhythmias.

The usual maximum dose of cocaine given clinically is 200 mg for a 70-kg adult, or 3 mg/kg. However, 1.5 mg/kg is preferable if a volatile anesthetic agent is being used, because this lower dose does not exert any clinically significant sympathomimetic effect in combination with halothane.[32] One gram is the usual lethal dose for an adult, but considerable variation occurs, and systemic reactions may transpire with as little as 20 mg.

Clearly, before applying cocaine, the physician should carefully rule out any contraindications, including the use of various concurrent medications. To avoid toxic levels, doses of dilute solutions should be meticulously calculated, measured, and administered. If serious cardiovascular effects occur, propranolol[33] or labetalol[34] may be given therapeutically. Because a lethal hypertensive exacerbation has been attributed to unopposed α stimulation,[35] labetalol may be preferable, because it offers the advantage of both α and β blockade.

Anesthesia may be maintained with halothane, but if catecholamines or cocaine is administered, isoflurane, enflurane, or any other agent less likely to trigger dysrhythmias may be substituted. Alternatively, a balanced technique with nitrous oxide, oxygen, narcotics, and muscle relaxant may be used as long as hypertension is avoided. (Although the sinuses are air-containing cavities, nitrous oxide is commonly used without difficulty during sinus surgery.)

Some surgeons inject air into the maxillary antrum after irrigating it with fluid.[36] Most investigators advise against this course and warn of the hazard of air embolism.[37, 38] Indeed, death has occurred during lavage of nasal sinuses.[37-39]

TABLE 7–2. Dangers of Cocaine

Hazardous interactions with adrenergic-modifying drugs
Dysrhythmias
Hypertension
Toxicity at relatively low dosages
Respiratory and cardiac arrest

Although venous air embolism can be produced any time air is forced into the body deliberately, the amount of air and rate of delivery are primary factors affecting the severity of an injury produced by venous air emboli.[40, 41]

The main specific sign of venous air embolism (Table 7–3) is the mill wheel murmur, a loud, churning sound audible over the precordium. Hence, a precordial or esophageal stethoscope is mandatory whenever the possibility of air embolism exists.[42] A Doppler precordial detector placed over the right heart is even more sensitive in detecting entry of air into the circulation.

Another early sign includes a fall in the fraction of end-tidal CO_2 in each breath, secondary to an increase in dead space with a resultant increase in areas of ventilation-perfusion mismatch in the lungs. Other findings, usually occurring later and with large emboli, include wheezing and systemic hypotension in conjunction with elevated right heart pressure. Electrocardiographic changes are nonspecific and tend to occur relatively late. Inversion of the T waves, followed by ST segment elevation and then a right bundle branch block pattern,[43] have been reported, as have ST segment depression and ventricular fibrillation.

Although most cases of venous air embolism involve only small amounts of air and are frequently not diagnosed, when massive air embolism occurs, treatment consists of aspirating air from a well-positioned right atrial or pulmonary artery catheter, adding 100% oxygen, turning the patient into the left lateral decubitus position[43] so that the pulmonary outflow tract assumes a position inferior to the body of the right ventricle, and applying closed chest cardiac massage (Table 7–4).

Upon completion of surgery, the pharynx is cleared before extubation by removing the posterior pharyngeal pack and gently suctioning the area. (Failure to remove pharyngeal packs has caused severe cyanosis on more than one occasion.) Moreover, an oropharyngeal airway should be inserted prior to extubation. (The oral airway is especially important in patients who have any form of nasal pack left in place.) Clearly, the packing must be secure

TABLE 7–3. Symptoms of Venous Air Embolism

Mill wheel murmur
Reduction in end-tidal carbon dioxide
Wheezing and hypotension
ECG changes often late and nonspecific

TABLE 7–4. Treatment of Massive Venous Air Embolism

Aspirate air from right atrial or pulmonary artery catheter
Administer 100% oxygen
Place patient in left lateral decubitus position and perform closed chest cardiac massage

so there is no aspiration hazard, and the patient's airway must be adequate following extubation.

Postoperative surgical complications following sinus surgery include bone infections, periorbital cellulitis, and intracranial pathology, including brain abscess, meningitis, cavernous sinus thrombosis, and sagittal sinus thrombosis. A dural abscess can occur also, with associated elevation of intracranial pressure.

NASAL SURGERY

The special problems of nasal surgery requiring anesthetic attention are essentially the same as for sinus surgery. These factors are as follows:

1. the possibility of pre-existing nasal obstruction
2. the propensity of blood and other material, such as pus, to drain into the pharynx intraoperatively with the attendant risk of pulmonary aspiration
3. the possibility of systemic, toxic effects from topically applied vasoactive agents
4. the use of nasal packing that remains in place postoperatively, with the associated hazard of airway obstruction.

Surgery on the nose includes operations such as repair of choanal atresia, nasal polypectomy, removal of juvenile nasopharyngeal angiofibroma, lateral rhinotomy for inverted papilloma, correction of deviated nasal septum, reconstructive plastic procedures, and control of epistaxis. Most cases of nasal surgery are performed on an elective basis, but procedures such as repair of choanal atresia and epistaxis must be done on a more urgent basis.

Some brief, relatively simple nasal procedures, including those of a primarily cosmetic nature, may be performed under local anesthesia. Nasal packing containing 4% cocaine or 2% lidocaine with epinephrine (1:100,000) is placed high and adjacent to the septum near the anterior ethmoid artery and also at the posterior end of the middle turbinate to produce a sphenopalatine ganglion block. The infraorbital, infratrochlear, and external nasal nerves may be infiltrated locally. However, general anesthesia is required commonly for nasal surgery for safety and comfort.

NASAL POLYPS

The management and implications of nasal polyps are often age-related. Congenital nasal lesions appearing in infancy are extremely rare and usually associated with a grave prognosis. In this age group, polypoid nasal tumors tend to be intranasal components of encephalocoeles, gliomas, or hemangiomas originating within the cranium.[44] Ill-advised attempts to "treat" these masses transnasally may result in disaster.

In older children, nasal polyps are relatively unusual; when they do occur, it is often in association with cystic fibrosis. In addition to the local problem of nasal obstruction and infection and the propensity of nasal polyps to bleed, other much more severe systemic complications interact to make anesthetic management challenging in patients with cystic fibrosis.

Cystic fibrosis, an autosomal recessive disorder, is characterized by generalized dysfunction of the exocrine glands. Pancreatic deficiency, cirrhosis, abnormally high sweat electrolyte concentrations, and chronic obstructive pulmonary disease (COPD) secondary to tenacious tracheobronchial secretions are hallmarks of the disorder. COPD with alveolar hypoxia results in the development of pulmonary hypertension and eventual cor pulmonale.[45] Pulmonary function testing of those with severe disease shows a significant consistent increase in the ratio of the residual volume to total lung capacity[45] and the presence of marked hypoxemia. Other respiratory parameters are also abnormal, but less consistently so.[45] For example, carbon dioxide tension may not begin to rise significantly until the end stage of the disease.[46] Although chemosensitivity is normal in individuals with cystic fibrosis, they are unable to respond appropriately to hypoxia or adequately to hypercapnia, because their pulmonary mechanics are impaired. Therefore, their ventilatory response to CO_2 is blunted, and their response to hypoxia is a paradoxical decrease in tidal volume and minute ventilation. The latter phenomenon is presumably a response to respiratory muscle fatigue secondary to the reduced supply of oxygen.[46]

Preoperative therapy, including chest physiotherapy, antibiotics, and hydration, ensures that the patient is in optimal condition consistent with the stage of the disease. Baseline arterial blood gases should be obtained, prothrombin and partial thromboplastin times should be checked, and parenteral vitamin K should be given the night before surgery, if indicated.[47] Respiratory depressants should be omitted perioperatively, for the reasons cited earlier. Atropine premedication is commonly omitted because of its effect on the viscosity of secretions. However, atropine may be administered intraoperatively, as needed, to treat dysrhythmias.[48] An anesthetic goal should be rapid recovery from anesthetic agents so that the patient may engage in vigorous coughing and pulmonary physiotherapy postoperatively (Table 7–5).

Ventilation-perfusion abnormalities predispose to a prolonged inhalation induction. Preoxygenation, IV induction, and oral intubation followed by administration of an appropriate inhalation agent with controlled ventilation is a suitable technique. Muscle relaxants may be employed to prevent reflex movement under the requisite light plane of anesthesia. Gases should be humidified and, throughout the operation, the endotracheal tube should be aspirated frequently, but gently, with a soft catheter to remove tenacious tracheobronchial secretions. If any apparently unexplained clinical deterioration occurs, pneumothorax must be ruled out. Profuse bleeding may occur, and transfusions may be indicated, because malabsorption of fat-soluble vitamins and decreased gastrointestinal synthesis of vitamin K may predispose the patient with cystic fibrosis to an increased risk of hemorrhage.[47] Upon completion of surgery, the patient may be extubated unless there is persisting nasal obstruction (by packing, for example) or persistent bleeding. Adequate humidification of inspired oxygen is important in the immediate recovery period. Active chest physiotherapy, postural drainage, bronchodilators, and anti-

TABLE 7–5. Perioperative Management of Cystic Fibrosis

Chest physiotherapy, postural drainage, antibiotics, and bronchodilators
Liberal hydration
Baseline arterial blood gases checked
Prothrombin and partial thromboplastin times checked
Vitamin K, if indicated
No respiratory depressants
Gases humidified
Frequent, gentle suctioning

biotics should be recommended as soon as possible in the postoperative course.

In adults, nasal polyps usually grow in the middle turbinate area and are commonly associated with allergic rhinitis, chronic sinus infection, or both. When accessible and few, the polyps can be excised sometimes under local anesthesia. Multiple or remote polyps mandate general anesthesia, though the physician must bear in mind the presence and degree of preoperative nasal obstruction. A topical vasoconstrictor is often applied to decrease bleeding. Most anesthesiologists tend to avoid halothane in this setting because of concern about dysrhythmias. As always, the airway must be protected against soiling from pus or blood by insertion of both a cuffed endotracheal tube and a posterior pharyngeal pack.

JUVENILE NASOPHARYNGEAL ANGIOFIBROMA

Although rare, juvenile nasopharyngeal angiofibroma is the most common benign pediatric tumor of the nasopharynx, with the exception of allergic polyps. The typical patient is an adolescent male, but occasionally older individuals may be afflicted. The tumor is extraordinarily vascular; intermittent, impressive episodes of epistaxis is usually the presenting history. Although benign, an aggressive local growth pattern renders it dangerous. Nasopharyngeal angiofibromas have a propensity to enlarge and erode adjacent vital structures, including the skull or orbit. CT and bilateral carotid angiography are mandatory to delineate tumor margins, discern intracranial extension, and identify the predominant arterial supply vessel (usually the internal maxillary artery).

In cases of intracranial or orbital extension, radiation therapy is the therapeutic modality selected. When surgical removal is possible, the approach is transpalatal. Life-threatening hemorrhage may occur at any moment.[50] The safety of removing this extremely vascular lesion has been improved in recent years by preoperative selective arterial embolization with absorbable gelatin sponges or silastic beads. Hypotensive anesthesia has been useful also in reducing blood loss, but the systolic blood pressure should not be allowed to drop below 60 mmHg. If sodium nitroprusside is used to maintain controlled hypotension, cyanide toxicity must be prevented, as evidenced by the development of metabolic acidosis. Sodium thiosulfate may be given as an antidote.

The anesthesiologist must be prepared to manage massive blood loss through at least two functioning large-bore IV cannulae. Appropriate monitors should include a central venous pressure catheter, a urinary catheter, and an intra-arterial catheter. Following IV induction and orotracheal intubation, a posterior pharyngeal pack is inserted and ventilation controlled with the aid of muscle relaxants. Anesthesia may be maintained with inhalation agents or narcotics, along with nitrous oxide and oxygen. (The inhalation agents offer the advantage of lowering blood pressure to a greater extent than is generally possible with a balanced technique.) In general, management of the recovery period is the same as for nasal operations, with emphasis on maintaining a patent oral airway and prevention of aspiration.

BRONCHOGRAPHY

In Chapter 4, a detailed discussion of the management of anesthesia for laryngoscopy, bronchoscopy, and laser surgery is presented. Some highlights pertinent to bronchography are repeated here.

Following bronchoscopy, diagnostic bronchography may be required to further localize and define airway pathology. This is accomplished by elective instillation of contrast media into the tracheobronchial tree under fluoroscopic guidance. Propyliodone can be a valuable contrast material for delineating lesions such as congenital abnormalities, cysts communicating with the lower airways, vascular malformations, and bronchiectasis.[51] However, bronchography is not an entirely benign procedure, because it carries the hazard of acute small airway obstruction secondary to the presence of the contrast medium. Furthermore, bronchography is associated with a temporary reduction in pulmonary function,[52] and these patients commonly have pre-existing pulmonary disease.

Following the anesthetic principles described for bronchoscopy, the patient is intubated, and an angle connector complete with a side port is incorporated into the system. A small radiopaque catheter is introduced through the side port into the endotracheal tube. Under fluoroscopic control, the catheter tip is positioned in the region of the airway to be studied. Under conditions of spontaneous or gently controlled ventilation, the contrast medium is carefully and slowly injected onto the bronchial walls. Inadvertent coughing is avoided at all costs, because rapid alveolarization of the dye could interfere with radiographic interpretation.[51] Monitoring must take into account the darkened conditions of the room and should include continuous ECG display, a precordial stethoscope, and pulse oximeter.

Propyliodone, an iodized oil contrast medium, is not water-soluble and must be eliminated by coughing, suctioning, and gravity draining. Upon completion of bronchography, as much of the dye as possible should be removed by suctioning. The endotracheal tube is removed once the patient is sufficiently awake to cough vigorously. Observation for 12–24 hours in either the recovery room or the intensive care unit is recommended. During this time, humidified oxygen is administered, and chest percussion and postural drainage are employed to remove any residual dye.

Although young children require general anesthesia for bronchography, with adolescents and adults it may be preferable to do this study while the patient is conscious and able to assume and maintain the different positions required for various radiograph views. Any of the methods of topical anesthesia employed for bronchoscopy should give satisfactory results, especially if combined with appropriate sedation.[53]

TRACHEOSTOMY

Traditionally, tracheostomy was frequently performed under dramatic and stressful conditions on moribund patients. However, tracheostomy ideally should be an unhurried procedure, performed calmly in a well-lighted operating room under sterile conditions with the patient in proper position and the airway secured with an endotracheal tube or rigid bronchoscope. An awake endotracheal intubation transforms an emergency situation into an orderly, semielective procedure and circumvents many postoperative complications.[54]

INDICATIONS

Indications for tracheostomy tend to be relative rather than absolute and vary from institution to institution depending on the philosophy regarding prolonged nasotracheal intubation. In adults, tracheostomy is favored if an artificial airway is needed beyond a week or so, although tracheal intubation has been used successfully for more extended periods.[55] Moreover, infants and children with normal airway anatomy requiring prolonged mechanical ventilation may be satisfactorily managed with nasotracheal intubation for weeks.[56] The general indications for tracheostomy are prolonged mechanical ventilation, protection against pulmonary aspiration in unconscious or other patients whose protective laryngeal reflexes are obtunded, as a planned part of major operations involving the face and neck, or to relieve upper airway obstruction (Table 7–6).

There are two main types of tracheostomy tubes: disposable plastic tubes, often with inflatable cuffs, for short-term use in patients who require mechanical ventilation or in whom the airway needs to be sealed, and nondisposable metal tubes for long-term use in individuals not requiring ventilatory support and in whom there is minimal risk of aspiration. These tubes are physiologically inert and radiopaque. They are designed so that the tip of the tube lies at least 2 cm above the adult carina, and the cuff, if inflated, will be positioned entirely within the trachea. Because the cuff is responsible for most of the tracheal damage and subsequent stenosis associated with tracheostomy, considerable attention has been devoted to cuff design and use. Hence, high volume, low pressure cuffs are popular. Pressures greater than 20 mmHg have been implicated in the development of mucosal ischemia, and high volume cuffs are much more apt to provide a satisfactory seal at lower inflation pressures. Moreover, the high volume cuff has an additional advantage in providing symmetrical inflation.[57] It is postulated that intermittent deflation of the cuff, for 5 minutes every hour, allows for local restoration of capillary perfusion in the cuff region and, hence, diminishes or retards tracheal mucosal necrosis. However, the patient may be vulnerable to aspiration during deflation periods and may be underventilated owing to an excessive airway leak during this interval.

TABLE 7–6. Indications for Tracheostomy

Relief of airway obstruction
Prolonged mechanical ventilation
Protection against aspiration
Facilitation of tracheobronchial toilet
Part of major, extensive head and neck surgery

SURGICAL TECHNIQUES

The patient is placed in the supine position on the operating table with a roll under the shoulders to partially extend the neck. A transverse skin excision is made at the level of the second or third tracheal ring. Retraction of the strap muscles and division of the pretracheal fascia reveals the thyroid. The isthmus of the thyroid is then either retracted or divided. A vertical incision extending down the second and third tracheal cartilages is made into the anterior tracheal wall. The first cartilage must be assiduously avoided, because trespass in this area may lead to eventual subglottic stenosis. The cuff in the endotracheal tube should be deflated, and the tube should be withdrawn until its lower end is at the upper limit of the tracheal incision. The tracheostomy tube is now inserted. As soon as the latter tube has been safely and properly placed, the endotracheal tube is removed. The anesthesia circuit is attached to the tracheostomy tube. Once the tracheostomy has been connected, the lung fields must be auscultated bilaterally to confirm proper tube placement and satisfactory ventilation. The skin wound is then closed, a dressing applied, and the tracheostomy tube firmly secured by sutures and by tape attached around the patient's neck.

An alternative surgical technique—aimed at facilitating reinsertion of a dislodged tube—involves making the incision in the form of an inverted U, fashioning a tracheal "trap door" and suturing the flap so formed to the skin. Regardless of which surgical technique is selected, it is essential to focus on proper fixation of the tube. Because a tracheostomy tract takes almost a week to form, if a tube is inadvertently displaced during this interval, it may be impossible to reinsert. Usually, this crisis can be resolved successfully by performing an emergency orotracheal intubation.

Tracheostomy may pose certain additional challenges in children, because the pediatric trachea is softer and often more difficult to locate accurately. The latter problem is minimized when an endotracheal tube or rigid bronchoscope is in place. Furthermore, the risk of damaging the innominate vessels is very real in children, because these vessels traverse the trachea at a higher level in the infant than in the adult. Tracheostomies are performed somewhat lower in infants and children in an attempt to prevent laryngeal or subglottic injury.

ANESTHESIA FOR TRACHEOSTOMY

Prior securing of the airway through an endotracheal tube or a rigid bronchoscope is the key to a relatively uncomplicated tracheostomy. Indeed, the majority of patients presenting for tracheostomy are already intubated, and anesthesia may be induced and maintained in any reasonable fashion. If the patient is not already intubated and has no significant degree of airway obstruction, an IV induction and muscle relaxant may be employed to accomplish endotracheal intubation. However, if significant obstruction exists or is likely to suddenly develop, an inhalation induction without muscle relaxants should be used. In this setting, it is often necessary to insert a tube much smaller than usual.

In some individuals, including those with marked stridor at rest, any form of general anesthesia may be too risky. If an awake endotracheal intubation cannot be accomplished, tracheostomy must be performed under local anesthesia in the awake patient. Simple infiltration of the skin and subcutaneous tissue in the area of the proposed incision is often adequate. If necessary, this may be supplemented by a bilateral superficial cervical plexus block.[58] Blocking the clavicular branches of the superior cervical plexus provides excellent cutaneous anesthesia of the lower half of the neck. This is easily accomplished by bilaterally injecting 5 mL of local anesthesia just beneath the midpoint of the posterior border of the sternomastoid muscle. Then, to minimize coughing when the trachea is incised, 4 mL of 2% lidocaine should be injected transtracheally.

COMPLICATIONS

The overall incidence of complications associated with tracheostomy is approximately 16–33%. The most common short-term complications are hemorrhage, pneumothorax, mucous plugs, tube displacement, cardiovascular collapse, and subcutaneous emphysema[59, 60] (Table 7–7). Pneumothorax is most likely to occur in a struggling patient or in a child, because the pleural apices are higher in youngsters. Pneumothorax may occur because of inadvertent opening of the cervical pleura or rupture of an emphysematous bulla by positive-pressure ventilation. Subcutaneous neck or mediastinal emphysema is most likely to occur when the neck dissection has been especially extensive or the incision tightly closed.

TABLE 7–7. Complications of Tracheostomy

Hemorrhage
Pneumothorax
Esophageal perforation
Cardiovascular collapse
Subcutaneous emphysema
Tracheostomy tube malposition and displacement
Tracheostomy tube obstruction
Infection
Dysrhythmias during suctioning
Tracheal stenosis
Erosion of major vessels
Esophageal erosion

Early hemorrhage usually involves superficial bleeders, but a fatal hemorrhage can transpire 1–2 weeks postoperatively owing to erosion of the innominate artery or other major vessel. Such erosion is frequently associated with a low tracheostomy, off midline, and is also commonly due to extension of pressure necrosis from the trachea. Often, the first signs of the problem are tracheal tube pulsations and hemoptysis, but occasionally massive bleeding occurs virtually *de novo* after routine deflation of the cuff. Acute treatment demands insertion of an endotracheal tube into the tracheal stoma and overinflation of the cuff to temporarily control the bleeding until definitive surgery can be performed. If cuff overinflation fails, blind digital dissection through the tracheostomy wound to compress the innominate artery against the posterior sternum should be attempted. (Pressure over the neck is usually ineffective as a means to control exsanguination.)

Although pneumonia is rare, tracheitis occurs to some degree in every patient subjected to tracheostomy. Meticulous postoperative nursing care, focusing on frequent cleansing of the wound and dressing changes, helps control infection. Bacteriological surveillance of the tracheostomy wound, the tracheal aspirates, the tracheostomy tube, and the humidification system must be vigilantly maintained, and the appropriate antibiotic must be administered when a pathogen is identified.

Tube malpositions and displacements are best circumvented by excellent surgical technique, careful and frequent checking of ventilation by chest auscultation, and meticulous fixation of the tube. Tube displacement becomes less of a problem after the first postoperative week, because the tracheostomy tract is more clearly established.

Obstruction of the tube by clot or inspissated secretions can be avoided by providing highly humidified oxygen through a tracheostomy mist collar and by removing and cleaning the inner cannula at least every 6 hours. Frequent suctioning—initially as often as every half hour—of blood or secretions is essential, and the technique employed is extremely important. Full sterile technique must be used, and prolonged suctioning must be avoided. Cardiac dysrhythmias, such as nodal tachycardia, premature ventricular contractions, and transient sinus arrest, have been noted during tracheal suctioning.[61] To prevent these dysrhythmias, the patient should receive 100% oxygen for at least 2 minutes prior to suctioning, a 10-second limit should be imposed on duration of suctioning, and the lungs should be re-expanded with several deep breaths with positive pressure. Humidification, proper suctioning, chest physiotherapy, and early ambulation also help to ward off pneumonia.

The late complications of tracheostomy are all related to the mechanical effects of the tracheostomy tube or its cuff in causing trauma and necrosis. Important predisposing factors include the duration of the tracheostomy, especially the length of time an inflated cuff was essential, and the presence of infection or hypotension. Tracheal stenosis virtually always follows tracheostomy, but most cases are asymptomatic. However, dyspnea, impaired expectoration, and inspiratory stridor occur when reduction of the tracheal lumen exceeds 50%. Diagnosis is verified by bronchoscopy and radiological studies. If severe, resection of the stenotic segment and tracheal reconstruction are necessary.

The problem of erosion of major vessels is described earlier. Esophageal erosion may occur also and has a similarly grim prognosis. Again, esophageal erosion is caused by the spread of ischemic necrosis and, hence, is usually found at cuff level. Predisposing factors include reflux esophagitis, systemic steroids, and presence of a nasogastric tube allowing the tissues to be compressed between the rigid tracheal tube anteriorly and the relatively rigid nasogastric tube posteriorly.

REFERENCES

1. Bluestone CD: The status of tonsillectomy and adenoidectomy—1977. Laryngoscopy 1977; 87:1233–1243.
2. Tate N: Deaths from tonsillectomy. Lancet 1963; 2:1090–1091.
3. Rowland TW, Nordstrom LG, Bean MS, et al: Chronic upper airway obstruction and pulmonary hy-

pertension in Down's Syndrome. Am J Dis Child 1981; 135:1050.

4. King DH, Jones RM, Barnett MB: Anesthetic considerations in the mucopolysaccharidoses. Anaesthesia 1984; 39:126–131.

5. Kravath RE, Pollack CP, Borowiecki B: Hypoventilation during sleep in children who have lymphoid airway obstruction treated by nasopharyngeal tube and tonsillectomy and adenoidectomy. Pediatrics 1977; 59:865.

6. Meyers EF, Krupin B: Anesthetic management of emergency tonsillectomy and adenoidectomy in infectious mononucleosis. Anesthesiology 1975; 42:490–491.

7. Paradise JL, Bluestone CD: Toward rational indications for tonsil and adenoid surgery. Hosp Prac 1976; 11:79.

8. Dong M-L: Arnold-Chiari malformation type I appearing after tonsillectomy. Anesthesiology 1987; 67:120–122.

9. Simpson JI, Wolf GL: Endotracheal tube fire ignited by pharyngeal electrocautery. Anesthesiology 1986; 65:76–77.

10. Sommer RM: Preventing endotracheal tube fire during pharyngeal surgery. Anesthesiology 1987; 66:439.

11. Boliston TA, Upton JJM: Infiltration with lignocaine and adrenaline in adult tonsillectomy. J Laryngol Otol 1980; 94:1257–1259.

12. Broadman LM, Spellman GF, Patel RI: Effects of peritonsillar infiltration upon the reduction of operative blood loss and postoperative pain in children having tonsillectomies. Anesth Analg 1988; 67:S22.

13. Gefke K, Anderson LW, Friesel E: Intravenous lidocaine as a suppressant of cough and laryngospasm with extubation after tonsillectomy. Acta Anaesthesiol Scand 1983; 27:112.

14. Klein JO: Middle ear disease in children. Hosp Prac 1976; 11:45.

15. Ghani GA, Sung Y-F, Per-Lee JH: Glomus jugulare tumors—origin, pathology, and anesthetic considerations. Anesth Analg 1983; 62:686–691.

16. Guild SR: A hitherto unrecognized structure, the glomus jugulare in man. Anat Rec 1941; 79 (Suppl 2):28.

17. Steinberg N, Holz WG: Glomus jugulare tumor. Arch Otolaryngol 1965; 82:387–394.

18. Fuller AM, Brown HA, Harrison EG, et al: Chemodectomas of the glomus jugulare tumor. Laryngoscope 1966; 76:218–238.

19. Lawson W: Glomus bodies and tumors. NY State J Med 1980; 80:1567–1575.

20. Brown JS: Glomus jugulare tumors. Methods and difficulties of diagnosis and surgical treatment. Laryngoscope 1967; 77:26–67.

21. Monroe J, Lore JM Jr: Metastatic glomus jugulare tumor. Ear Nose Throat J 1977; 56:7–13.

22. Gardner G, Cocke EW Jr, Robertson JT, et al: Combined approach surgery for removal of glomus jugulare tumors. Laryngoscope 1977; 87:665–688.

23. Chretien PB, Engleman K, Hoye RC, et al: Surgical management of intravascular glomus jugulare tumor. Am J Surg 1971; 122:740–743.

24. Newland MC, Hurlbert BJ: Chemodectoma diagnosed by hypertension and tachycardia during anesthesia. Anesth Analg 1980; 59:388–390.

25. Levit SA, Sheps SG, Espinosa RE, et al: Catecholamine-secreting paraganglioma of glomus jugulare region resembling pheochromocytoma. N Engl J Med 1969; 281:805–811.

26. Rosenwasser H: Glomus jugulare tumors. Proc R Soc Med 1974; 67:259–270.

27. Simpson GT, Konrad HR, Takahash M, et al: Immediate postembolization excision of glomus jugulare tumors. Arch Otolaryngol 1979; 105:639–643.

28. Adornato DC, Glidenberg PL, Ferrario CM, et al: Pathophysiology of intravenous air embolism in dogs. Anesthesiology 1978; 49:120–127.

29. Pratilas V, Pratile MG: Anesthetic management of pheochromocytoma. Can Anaesth Soc J 1979; 26:253–259.

30. Axelsson A, Chidekel N, Grebelius N, et al: Treatment of acute maxillary sinusitis. Ann Otol Rhinol Laryngol 1973; 82:186–191.

31. Meyers EF: Cocaine toxicity during dacryocystorhinostomy. Arch Ophthalmol 1980; 98:842.

32. Barash PG, Kopriva CJ, Langon R, et al: Is cocaine a sympathetic stimulant during general anesthesia? JAMA 1980; 243:1437.

33. Rappolt RT, Gay GR, Inaba DS: Propranolol: A specific antagonist to cocaine. Clin Toxicol 1977; 10:265.

34. Gay GR, Loper KA: Control of cocaine-induced hypertension with labetalol. Anesth Analg 1988; 67:91–94.

35. Ramoska E, Sacchetti AD: Propranolol-induced hypertension in treatment of cocaine intoxication. Ann Emerg Med 1985; 14:1112–1113.

36. Boyle S, Ockerman R, Barton CR, et al: Venous air embolism during anesthesia for maxillary sinus irrigation: A case study. J Assoc Nurse Anesthetists 1986; 54:126–129.

37. Honolulu TH, Pang LQ: Air embolism during lavage of the maxillary sinus. A report of two cases. Laryngoscope 1952; 62:1205–1224.

38. Thompson KFM: Air embolism following antral lavage: A fatal case. Laryngoscope 1955; 69:829–832.

39. Bacher JA: Fatal air embolism after puncture of maxillary antrum—autopsy. Calif St J of Med 1923; 21:433.

40. O'Quin RJ, Lakshminaraya S: Venous air embolism. Arch Int Med 1982; 142:2173–2176.

41. Hybels R, Boston MA: Venous air embolism in head and neck surgery. Laryngoscope 1980; 90:946–954.

42. Gottlieb JD, Ericsson J, Sweet R: Venous air embolism: A review. Anesth Analg 1965; 44:773–779.

43. Durant T, Long J, Oppenheimer M: Venous air embolism. Am Heart J 1947; 33:269–282.

44. Bradley PG, Singh SD: Congenital nasal masses: Diagnosis and management. Clin Otolaryngol 1982; 7:87–97.

45. Stern RC, Borkat G, Hirschfeld SS, et al: Heart failure in cystic fibrosis. Am J Dis Child 1980; 134:267.

46. Bureau MA, Lupien L, Begin R: Neural drive and ventilatory strategy of breathing in normal children and in patients with cystic fibrosis and asthma. Pediatrics 1981; 68:187.

47. Brown BR, Walson PD, Taussig LM: Congenital metabolic diseases of pediatric patients: Anesthetic implications. Anesthesiology 1975; 43:197.

48. Smith RM: Anesthetic management of patients with cystic fibrosis. Anesth Analg 1965; 44:143.

49. Zakzouk SM, Elgarem A, Hafiz HA: An unusual case of nasopharyngeal angiofibroma. Ear Nose Throat J 1979; 58:351.

50. Sessions RB, Zarin DP, Bryan RN: Juvenile nasopharyngeal angiofibroma. Am J Dis Child 1981; 135:535.

51. Rita L: Anesthesia for bronchography in infants and children. Anesth Rev 1979; 6:40.

52. Surprenant E, Wilson A, Bennett L, et al: Changes in regional pulmonary function following bronchography. Radiology 1968; 91:736.

53. Stevenson HM, Pandit SK, Dundee JW: Experience with a technique of neuroleptanalgesia for bronchography. Thorax 1972; 27:334–337.
54. Greenway RE: Tracheostomy: Surgical problems and complications. Int Anesthesiol Clin 1972; 10:151.
55. Lewis FR, Schlobohm RM, Thomas RN: Prevention of complications from prolonged tracheal intubation. Am J Surg 1978; 135:452–457.
56. Battersby EF, Hatch DJ, Towey RM: Effects of prolonged nasotracheal intubation in children. Anaesthesia 1977; 32:154–157.
57. Tonnesen AS, Vereen L, Arens L: Endotracheal tube cuff residual volume and lateral wall pressure in a model trachea. Anesthesiology 1981; 55:680–683.
58. Murphy T: Somatic blockade for head and neck. *In* Cousins MJ, Bridenbaugh PO (eds): Neural Blockade. Philadelphia, JB Lippincott, 1980, pp 420–432.
59. Mead JW: Tracheotomy—its complications and their management. N Engl J Med 1961; 265:519.
60. Chew JY, Cantrell RW: Tracheostomy complications and their management. Arch Otolaryngol 1972; 95:538.
61. Shim C, Fine N, Fernandez R, et al: Cardiac arrhythmias resulting from tracheal suctioning. Ann Intern Med 1969; 7:1149.

Pediatric Airway Emergencies: Foreign Body Aspiration, Epiglottitis, Laryngotracheobronchitis, and Bacterial Tracheitis

Kathryn E. McGoldrick

There are few acute situations more challenging to the anesthesiologist than such potentially life-threatening pediatric airway emergencies as epiglottitis or foreign body removal. For a variety of reasons, affected children are vulnerable to disaster.

Even under unobstructed conditions, the pediatric airway may be difficult to manage properly. The infant's tongue, for example, is relatively large and easily obstructs the airway. The infant's larynx is higher (C_{3-4}) than the adult's (C_{4-5}) and is more anterior (Table 8–1). This higher, more anterior larynx enables the neonate to swallow and breathe simultaneously, but the position of the infant's larynx makes intubation difficult, especially in the hands of a neophyte. The infant's epiglottis is omega-shaped and angled away from the axis of the trachea. By contrast, the adult epiglottis is flat, thin, and parallel to the tracheal axis. Whereas the infant's vocal cords are angled, the adult's are perpendicular to the axis of the trachea. Moreover, in the adult the narrowest part of the airway is the glottic opening, but in the infant the narrowest part is in the subglottic region, where the cricoid cartilage completely encircles the airway. Hence, an endotracheal tube that passes through the infant's laryngeal opening easily may encounter considerable subglottic resistance, necessitating the substitution of a smaller endotracheal tube.

In the presence of airway edema, there are greater proportional changes in cross-sectional area and airway resistance with equivalent circumferential edema in the infant than in the adult. For example, 1 mm of edema in an infant's airway with an internal tracheal diameter of 4 mm causes a 16-fold increase in resistance and a 75% reduction in cross-sectional area. However, in an 8-mm adult airway, the same 1 mm of edema results in only a threefold increase in resistance and a 44% reduction in cross-sectional area. (These changes are computed assuming laminar flow. However, in the presence of obstruction, flow frequently becomes turbulent, and the deleterious effects of 1 mm of edema are even more dramatic.)

The detrimental impact of critical narrowing is compounded by the elasticity of the child's airway. Because of tracheal "softness," children with laryngeal obstruction may demonstrate collapse of the extrathoracic trachea distal to the obstruction during inspiration. The rigid upper airway of an adult requires -90 cm H_2O pressure to collapse, whereas the neonate's airway collapses at -2 to -10 cm

TABLE 8–1. Distinguishing Features of Infant and Adult Airways

Feature	Infant	Adult
Mandible	Relatively small	
Tongue	Relatively large, tending to obstruct airway	
Epiglottis	Omega-shaped; angled away from axis of trachea; relatively large and stiff	Thin, flat, and parallel to axis of trachea; relatively shorter and more malleable
Larynx	Higher (C_{3-4}) and more anterior; vocal cords angled; narrowest at cricoid cartilage	Opposite C_{4-5}; vocal cords perpendicular to axis of trachea; narrowest at glottic opening
Trachea	Soft	Relatively rigid

H_2O pressure. Moreover, dynamic collapse increases when children with obstruction become agitated because of increased negative intratracheal pressure. Crying exacerbates airway obstruction by increasing dynamic airway collapse. Crying also exacerbates the impact of obstruction by increasing oxygen consumption. Unfortunately, although avoiding crying is important, the use of sedatives or narcotics in the setting of airway compromise is contraindicated.

Signs of upper airway obstruction include stridor, retractions, cyanosis, tachypnea, tachycardia, and decreased level of consciousness (Table 8–2). Agitation, anxiety, or lethargy implies hypoxemia and hypercapnia until proven otherwise and should not be dismissed as a sign of misbehavior. Children demonstrating a preferred posture or aphonia may be on the verge of respiratory arrest.

Stridor is secondary to an increase in airflow or turbulence through a narrowed passage. The timing of stridor in the respiratory cycle may be a clue to diagnosing the site of obstruction. Inspiratory stridor and retractions suggest obstruction of the upper airway, as occurs with epiglottitis. Primarily expiratory stridor suggests obstruction of the intrathoracic trachea and bronchi, such as may occur with an endobronchial foreign body.

Causes of acute airway obstruction may be grouped into three main categories: (1) obstruction from structures of the airway; (2) obstruction from external compression; and (3) obstruction from exogenous materials. Examples of airway structures causing obstruction include angioneurotic edema, an obstructive tongue,[1] uvular edema, epiglottitis, laryngotracheobronchitis, and postextubation croup. Obstruction from external compression may occur with airway trauma, goiter, retropharyngeal abscess, peritonsillar abscess, and Ludwig's angina. Obstruction from exogenous materials may occur in the setting of foreign body aspiration or diphtheria.

For both convenience and differential diagnosis, we have chosen to group foreign body aspiration, epiglottitis, laryngotracheobronchitis, and bacterial tracheitis in this chapter on pediatric airway emergencies, although certainly these problems are not exclusively pediatric. Clearly, these entities have similarities as well as important differences. In Chapter 9, additional pediatric airway emergencies such as choanal atresia are discussed, as are other ear, nose, and throat emergencies encountered in children and adults.

POSTOBSTRUCTIVE PULMONARY EDEMA

Once airway obstruction is relieved, postobstructive pulmonary edema may follow.

Although noncardiogenic pulmonary edema is uncommon, it may arise from a variety of causes, including drugs, sepsis, head trauma, and high altitude (Table 8–3). Although airway obstruction as a rare cause of acute pulmonary edema was recognized clinically in the 1960s, no case reports[2,3] appeared until 1977. Because several of the early case reports described pediatric patients with croup or epiglottitis, there was an initial perception that postob-

TABLE 8–2. Features of Airway Obstruction

Stridor, retractions, cyanosis, decreased level of consciousness, tachypnea, and tachycardia may occur.

Agitation, anxiety, or lethargy implies hypoxemia and hypercapnia.

Children demonstrating a preferred posture or aphonia may be on the verge of respiratory arrest.

TABLE 8–3. Etiologies of Noncardiogenic Pulmonary Edema

Drugs
Sepsis
Head trauma
High altitude
Postobstruction
Miscellaneous[3]

structive pulmonary edema occurs mainly, if not exclusively, in children. However, in adults a vast spectrum of conditions resulting in airway obstruction also may be linked with fulminating pulmonary edema, including laryngospasm,[4] epiglottitis,[5] sleep apnea,[6] goiter,[7] malignancy, and strangulation.[3]

The mechanisms underlying postobstructive pulmonary edema are obscure and probably multifactorial. However, forced inspiration against a closed glottis (modified Müller's maneuver), inducing large negative intrapleural and transpulmonary pressure gradients favoring the transudation of pulmonary edema fluid from the pulmonary capillaries into the interstitium, appears to be the predominant one. (Chest wall compliance strongly influences the amount of respiratory muscle force transformed to negative intrathoracic pressure. Because children have more compliant chest walls than adults, this may explain the greater incidence of postobstructive pulmonary edema in children.) Nonetheless, the possibility that prolonged hypoxia or severe acidosis can initiate pulmonary edema, either by direct pulmonary effects or through cardiac depression, cannot be dismissed.

Certain patients, such as those with a *forme fruste* of sleep apnea or nasopharyngeal abnormalities, may be at increased risk for the development of postobstructive pulmonary edema.[8] This form of postobstructive pulmonary edema is characterized by rapid onset and, commonly, by resolution without the need for aggressive therapy or invasive monitoring, especially in children.

Those who need more aggressive therapy for this condition usually respond well to reintubation, ventilation with either continuous positive airway pressure or positive end-expiratory pressure, judicious use of diuretics and, some believe, steroids.

Because of the potentially serious consequences, patients recovering from an acute episode of upper airway obstruction should be observed closely for at least 12 hours for the appearance of postobstructive pulmonary edema. If pulmonary edema develops, untoward sequelae can be averted by judicious management.

FOREIGN BODY ASPIRATION

Bronchoscopy for foreign body removal is extremely challenging. Many potential problems arise when the anesthesiologist must share the airway with the endoscopist while simultaneously providing adequate ventilation. Furthermore, most patients in this setting have some degree of compromise of the upper or lower airway. Without question, the removal of foreign bodies from the respiratory tract is one of the most exacting procedures known, and a successful outcome requires expertise, communication, and teamwork of the endoscopist and anesthesiologist.

Foreign bodies have a predilection for the pediatric airway. Young children—commonly, those 1–3 years old—lack the teeth, the muscular coordination, and the requisite table manners to chew their food properly. The nature of objects aspirated by children encompasses a wide spectrum, but most commonly one encounters food, such as peanuts, beans, seeds, or popcorn kernels. Plastic or metal pieces of toys also are aspirated with distressing frequency. Unfortunately, approximately 90% of aspirated objects are radiolucent. The peanut is especially perfidious if retained for any period of time, because it causes serious mucosal irritation, edema, and a greater incidence of pneumonitis distal to the bronchial obstruction than most other foreign bodies. Moreover, a single aspirated peanut or bean softens and expands from liquid absorption while it is lodged. This characteristic renders the peanut or bean especially vulnerable to fragmentation when grasped in the airway by the endoscopist's instrument. Fragmentation is notorious for causing death during the course of attempted removal if the divided pieces occlude both mainstem bronchi and totally prevent ventilation. (Not all aspirated foreign bodies exist prior to induction. Iatrogenically induced foreign body aspiration may include materials such as blood, teeth, vomitus, adenoidal tissue, parts of the laryngoscope or the endotracheal tube, and soda lime dust.)

Clinical findings in patients with aspirated foreign bodies are most commonly those of partial bronchial obstruction. Hence, although air can enter around the foreign body on inspiration when the bronchus dilates, exhala-

TABLE 8–4. X-rays and Aspirated Foreign Bodies

90% of aspirated objects radiolucent

85% of inspiratory chest films normal

Majority of forced expiratory films showing the
   following:
    1. unilateral air trapping (ball-valve effect)
    2. contralateral mediastinal shift

tion is impeded because the foreign body acts as a unidirectional valve. Although 85% of inspiratory chest films are said to be normal, expiratory films often prove useful (Table 8–4). On expiration, one commonly sees unilateral hyperaeration, a lowered and flattened diaphragm, and mediastinal shift away from the affected side (Figs. 8–1 and 8–2). However, chest films may be negative, especially during the first 24 hours. Stridor, dyspnea, coughing, and wheezing are common. If the episode of foreign body aspiration was unwitnessed, the child may initially appear to be essentially asymptomatic. The diagnosis of foreign body

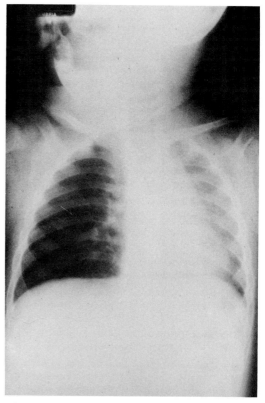

FIGURE 8–2. Expiratory film of the patient in Figure 8–1. (Photograph courtesy of Margaret A. Kenna, M.D., Department of Otolaryngology, Children's Hospital of Pittsburgh, University of Pittsburgh School of Medicine.)

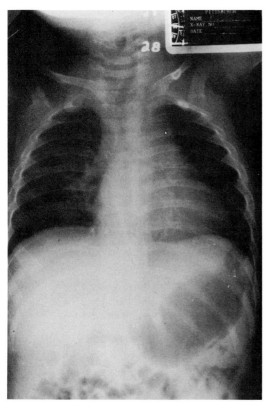

FIGURE 8–1. Inspiratory film of a child who aspirated a carrot into the right mainstem bronchus. (Photograph courtesy of Margaret A. Kenna, M.D., Department of Otolaryngology, Children's Hospital of Pittsburgh, University of Pittsburgh School of Medicine.)

aspiration might be made only after recurrent episodes of localized pneumonia or unexplained wheezing. In cases of complete laryngeal obstruction, aphonia and cyanosis occur, and death ensues within minutes unless the Heimlich maneuver or back slapping is successful. Certainly, objects retained in the larynx or trachea cause much more distress and have a higher mortality than objects positioned more peripherally.

Objects that are retained in the upper airway requiring urgent removal are relatively uncommon, compared with foreign bodies that are located more distally. Approximately 5% of aspirated objects require urgent removal; 95% lodge in a bronchus. However, most otolaryngologists maintain that, ideally, the aspirated object should be removed within the first 24 hours to minimize the incidence of secondary pneumonia or other complications.

If urgent removal is mandated by the presence of cyanosis, 100% oxygen should be administered while the child is taken immediately to the operating room under the care of an anesthesiologist and endoscopist. Awake laryngoscopy, rapid insertion of an endotracheal tube or bronchoscope, and positive-pressure ventilation may dislodge a tracheal foreign body and push it more peripherally into a mainstream bronchus with relief of the immediate crisis. Intravenous (IV) atropine is necessary to minimize secretions and reduce the incidence of bradycardia and other dysrhythmias so common with hypoxia and airway manipulation. Nitrous oxide should be withheld because of its propensity to expand the volume of trapped gas and increase pressure in the affected lung.

When bronchoscopy can be performed on a less urgent basis, atropine should be given IV, and preoperative sedation should be omitted. Following administration of IV thiopental or a mask induction, deep inhalation anesthesia with halothane and oxygen plus topical anesthetization of the larynx and trachea using 4% lidocaine, up to 4 mg/kg, allows vocal cord movement, appropriate jaw relaxation, and satisfactory anesthesia for airway endoscopy. The physician must allow for the greatly increased time required for an inhalation induction in the presence of an obstructed mainstem bronchus (Table 8–5). Extremely skillful airway management is critical, because many of these patients have full stomachs, and the appropriate precautions to prevent aspiration should be taken.

As anesthesia is deepened with halothane or another appropriate volatile agent and with oxygen, spontaneous ventilation should be preserved, at least until the location and nature of the foreign body have been ascertained by bronchoscopic examination. If the object is vegetable matter, with the potential for fragmentation during extraction, placing the patient in the lateral position with the affected

side down is strongly advised. It is desirable to have thoracotomy instruments and a thoracic surgeon immediately available, because thoracotomy and bronchotomy may be instantly indicated if a fragmented object acutely occludes both mainstem bronchi. If the object occludes the trachea, it is often possible to succeed with less invasive steps by pushing the object into a mainstem bronchus. Also, a Fogarty 3 embolectomy balloon catheter may be helpful in dislodging impacted foreign bodies.

Sometimes, the size of the foreign body may exceed the internal diameter of the bronchoscope, necessitating the simultaneous removal of the aspirated object, the scope, and the forceps as a single unit through the vocal cords. This maneuver usually requires that the cords be rendered immediately but briefly immobile, which can be accomplished by giving succinylcholine, 0.25–0.5 mg/kg IV. If the object is lost during attempted extraction, the pharynx should be inspected first. If the object is not retrieved there, the bronchoscope should be reinserted and the foreign body sought in the larynx or trachea. The value of spontaneous respiration is readily apparent if tracheal occlusion is present, because breath sounds will be minimal or absent. (A precordial stethoscope is essential and a pulse oximeter invaluable during bronchoscopy.) As mentioned previously, if the trachea is obstructed, the object must be pushed back to its initial position so that the patient can be ventilated. The foreign body must be returned to the originally affected side and not to the side of the only functioning lung, because then ventilation would be impossible in either lung. With the increased resistance inherent during bronchoscopy with the optical telescope in place, manual positive-pressure ventilation is impaired, necessitating a higher inspiratory pressure and faster rate. Sporadically, the endoscopist should remove the telescope, occlude the orifice, and allow the anesthesiologist a brief interlude of unobstructed manual ventilation.

Following extraction of the foreign body, the endoscopist needs to check for additional pieces and to suction distal secretions. Because multiple bronchoscopic reinsertions may be necessary, mucosal edema with respiratory distress is not unusual after bronchoscopy. Measures to prevent or attenuate postoperative stridor and respiratory compromise include administration of humidified oxygen, nebulized racemic epinephrine, and, arguably, steroids. Occasionally, intubation for 1–2 days may be required until the edema resolves.

TABLE 8–5. Anesthetic Management of Aspirated Foreign Bodies

Careful organization with contingency planning
No preoperative sedation
IV atropine
No nitrous oxide
Prolonged inhalation induction with topical anesthetization of larynx and trachea
Careful monitoring, including pulse oximetry
Observation for fragmentation—importance of ipsilateral return
Hypoventilation a constant hazard—excessive leak, high resistance with telescope in place, deep endobronchial placement
Postoperative care—close observation for airway edema or postobstructive pulmonary edema

Decadron is initially given in doses of 0.5–1.5 mg/kg, with smaller doses repeated as needed at intervals determined by the individual situation. With electrocardiographic monitoring, racemic epinephrine (2.25%) is administered for 10–15 minutes through a nebulizer and face mask or intermittent positive-pressure breathing (IPPB) device in a 1:6 dilution. This may be repeated every 2 hours. Indeed, if the clinical situation warrants such therapy, racemic epinephrine may be repeated as often as every 30 minutes.

Some aspirated objects may cause serious pneumonitis or other problems, including postobstructive purulent asphyxiation. Vegetable matter is likely to stimulate the proliferation of granulation tissue and attendant complications. The peanut, especially, is infamous for the variety of damage it can cause, including purulent asphyxiation. The peanut's rich content of arachidonic acid is especially likely to trigger inflammatory reactions; eventually, copious purulence may ensue. It is possible for the purulence to block the airways and cause death. However, bronchoscopic suctioning is often helpful in ameliorating this rare complication.

EPIGLOTTITIS

Acute epiglottitis is rare but one of the most feared infectious diseases in children. It can progress with extreme rapidity from a sore throat to respiratory obstruction and sudden death. Although epiglottitis most commonly occurs in youngsters under 6 years of age,[9] it can occur in adolescents and adults. Often, adult patients have a milder course,[10, 11] but fatalities owing to respiratory obstruction have been reported in adults[12] as well as children. Epiglottitis should not be mistaken for laryngotracheobronchitis or other less dangerous conditions. Delay in diagnosis may result in death, because misdiagnosis of epiglottitis can be fatal in less than 1 hour.[13]

Indeed, a more accurate designation would be "supraglottitis," because most of the supraglottic laryngeal and contiguous tissues, from the vallecula to the arytenoids, are usually involved by the infection in epiglottitis.[14] Because *Haemophilus influenzae* type B is the most common offending organism in children, *H. influenzae* type B polysaccharide vaccine is offered to children at 2 years of age; as most supraglottitis commonly occurs between the ages of 2 and 6 years, within a few years

supraglottitis in children might become obsolete.[15] Ironically, then, most cases would be in adults. Providers of care to adults may have to become as skilled in the management of this entity as their pediatric colleagues have been for years.[16]

Characteristic signs and symptoms of acute epiglottitis include sudden onset of fever; anorexia or dysphagia; drooling; a thick, muffled voice; and a preference for the sitting position, leaning slightly forward. The child may show signs of respiratory obstruction (retractions, labored breathing, cyanosis) but, early on, the child may merely appear pale and toxic without obvious signs of impending obstruction. As mentioned, the patient is commonly between the ages of 2 and 6, but infants as young as 8 days old[17] to adults over 70 years of age[18] have been afflicted. The causative organism in children is usually, as stated previously, *H. influenzae,* but occasionally *Staphylococcus aureus* or β hemolytic streptococci may be responsible. Occasionally, the clinical condition of the patient may allow time for diagnostic lateral soft tissue radiographs of the neck that would demonstrate thickening of the aryepiglottic folds and swelling of the epiglottis (Fig. 8–3). However, radiographs are generally ill-advised, because they cause delay and may involve a dangerous lapse of properly supervised observation of the patient.

Occasionally, the patient arrives in the emergency room with collapse and cyanosis. In this case, rapid oral intubation without anesthesia can be life-saving. Some prefer to use a rigid bronchoscope rather than an endotracheal tube to establish the airway. Attempting nasal intubation in this emergency setting is dangerous, because it may precipitate bleeding that further complicates an already difficult intubation. If respiratory arrest occurs before expert assistance and suitable equipment are mobilized, it may be possible to resuscitate these children using mouth-to-mouth ventilation[19] until intubation, cricothyrotomy, or tracheostomy is accomplished. (However, Holinger[20] maintains that cricothyrotomy is not possible in the infant, because the cricothyroid membrane is a mere 3 mm long, and insertion of an airway can cause glottic or cricoid cartilage injury.)

In less extreme situations when the airway is compromised but the child is not moribund, the child should be taken directly to the operating room for laryngoscopy and intubation under anesthesia. Attempts to visualize the epiglottis with the child awake and radiographs

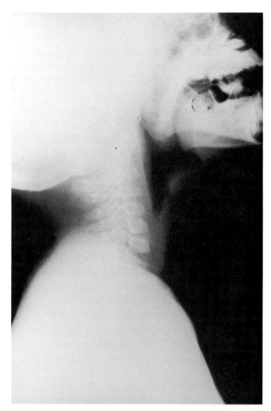

FIGURE 8–3. Lateral neck film of a child with epiglottitis. (Photograph courtesy of Margaret A. Kenna, M.D., Department of Otolaryngology, Children's Hospital of Pittsburgh, University of Pittsburgh School of Medicine.)

of the neck should not be performed to confirm the diagnosis. Any manipulation done at this time may trigger complete obstruction. Although the child must be carefully and continuously observed during transport from the emergency room to the operating room, he or she should not be disturbed. Because crying may exacerbate the degree of airway obstruction, venipuncture and arterial puncture are contraindicated, as is examination of the supraglottic region. Oxygen is given through a face mask while the child is transported to the operating room accompanied by the parents and at least one physician skilled in airway management. In addition to a mask and oxygen source, a resuscitation bag, laryngoscopes, endotracheal tubes with stylets, resuscitative drugs and syringes, and a 14-gauge needle for cricothyrotomy should accompany the patient. Racemic epinephrine is contraindicated if the presumed diagnosis is epiglottitis, as is any sedative premedication.

The operating room must be notified immediately of the urgent need for a suite where laryngoscopy, intubation, bronchoscopy, and tracheostomy may be performed. When the child arrives in the operating room, the anesthesiologist assumes control and delegates specific instructions to other colleagues and personnel (Table 8–6). The child is moved to the operating table and allowed to remain in the sitting position. A precordial stethoscope, electrocardiograph, and pulse oximeter are applied, and 100% oxygen is administered. Halothane is then gently introduced and the concentration gradually increased. When the child loses muscle tone, he or she is placed in the supine position. This may aggravate airway obstruction, but the gentle application of continuous positive airway pressure is often helpful; spontaneous ventilation may be continued, or ventilation may be gently assisted. Vigorous positive-pressure or controlled ventilation in this setting is ill-advised.

While induction is being accomplished, an assistant should apply a blood pressure cuff, start an IV infusion, and administer IV atropine 0.02 mg/kg. IV fluids are given liberally, because these children are usually dehydrated and may develop hypotension when high concentrations of halothane are employed.

(Prior to induction of anesthesia, a bronchoscope with functioning light source and a tracheostomy kit with appropriately sized tracheal tubes should be ready in the room. Furthermore, although most children with epiglottitis have been too ill to eat, a Yankauer suction tip should be attached to the suction apparatus for use in the event of vomiting.)

TABLE 8–6. Management of Epiglottitis

1. Prepare for respiratory arrest and mobilize operating room team.
2. Avoid disturbing the child.
3. Appreciate that preoperative sedatives, tranquilizers, and narcotics are contraindicated.
4. Safely transport the child in the sitting position to the operating room.
5. Perform an inhalation induction and direct laryngoscopy with ENT back-up. (Start an IV infusion and give atropine after the child is asleep.)
6. Initially secure airway control with a small, oral endotracheal tube placed in midtrachea. Change to nasotracheal tube or tracheostomy as circumstances dictate.
7. Meticulously secure tube with benzoin and tape. Apply arm and leg restraints to child.
8. Obtain cultures and start IV ampicillin and chloramphenicol.
9. Carefully monitor child postoperatively. Be prepared for postobstructive pulmonary edema.
10. Extubate after resolution of supraglottic edema.

The inhalation induction should be continued until the child is adequately anesthetized. With an obstructed airway, 15 or 20 minutes or longer may be the necessary induction duration to afford sufficient anesthetic depth for intubation. The endotracheal tube selected should be at least two sizes smaller than what would ordinarily be used, and a stylet may be useful. Muscle relaxants are assiduously avoided. If the vocal cords cannot be visualized, it may be possible to identify the glottis by gently squeezing the chest and watching for the appearance of air bubbles. If intubation is unsuccessful, the mask should be reapplied and the child ventilated and allowed to achieve an appropriately deep plane of anesthesia before intubation is again attempted. Prolonged attempts at intubation result in laryngospasm as the child becomes "light."

After the airway is secured with an orotracheal tube and the otolaryngologist has confirmed the diagnosis, the anesthesiologist usually replaces the orotracheal tube with a nasotracheal tube, which is less likely to become dislodged and is generally more comfortable for the patient. The tube should be meticulously secured and taped. Restraints should be placed on the child's arms prior to awakening, because dislodgement of the tube could precipitate catastrophe.

Once the child's larynx has been intubated and after blood and throat cultures have been obtained, IV antibiotic therapy is initiated. A starting ampicillin dose of 100 mg/kg is advised, then 150 mg/kg/day and chloramphenicol 75 mg/kg/day, because 20% of *H. influenzae* infections are resistant to ampicillin. A chest radiograph should be obtained to confirm midtracheal placement of the endotracheal tube and to rule out pneumonia or postobstructive pulmonary edema.[2]

In the past, tracheostomy for epiglottitis was popular; more recently, because of the high rate of complications associated with pediatric tracheostomy as well as the relatively short duration of airway obstruction, nasotracheal intubation for a period ranging from 12 to 72 hours has been advocated.[13, 19, 21]

The child is taken postoperatively to the intensive care unit, where nurses continuously monitor the patient to ascertain that the tube is both secure and patent. (In institutions where nurses are not comfortable caring for intubated children, and no individual skilled in intubation is available in the hospital at all times should reintubation become necessary, tracheostomy should be elected.) In addition

to restraints, sedation is usually necessary. The inspired oxygen-enriched atmosphere should be warmed and humidified, and 2 or 3 cm of continuous positive airway pressure (CPAP) should be maintained. Endotracheal tube suctioning should be performed at least once every hour using aseptic technique.

Timing of extubation depends on the child's clinical course, including increase in audible leak around the tube and diminished supraglottic swelling. Some physicians empirically extubate patients after 36–48 hours, but most recommend visual inspection of the larynx prior to extubation.[22] Equipment must be immediately available for reintubation should it become necessary.

Davis and colleagues[23] stress that the major errors in initial management of the child with a compromised airway are failure to appreciate the severity of respiratory distress, overly aggressive examination, and performance of unnecessary laboratory studies that waste valuable time and unnecessarily distress the child.

LARYNGOTRACHEOBRONCHITIS

Laryngotracheobronchitis (LTB), or croup, typically occurs in children under age 3. It is more common than epiglottitis and differs from that condition in its history, physical findings, and clinical course. The majority of children with LTB can be managed with close observation and administration of racemic epinephrine and steroids. Laryngoscopy and endotracheal intubation are necessary only when significant respiratory distress occurs or when the diagnosis is ambiguous.

Although LTB may be confused with epiglottitis, there are several distinguishing features (Table 8–7). The onset of croup is usually more gradual, often commencing with an upper respiratory tract infection followed by a stridulous or "barking" cough and inspiratory and expiratory stridor. As the disease progresses, restlessness, tachypnea, tachycardia, and chest wall retractions may ensue. LTB is primarily a viral infection, but secondary bacterial infection may follow. Parainfluenzae is the most common viral culprit. However, adenovirus, enterovirus, respiratory syncytial virus, and measles are other offending agents.

The diagnosis of LTB is primarily one of exclusion, usually arrived at when lateral neck X-ray discloses normal supraglottic structures and subglottic narrowing and haziness. The anteroposterior chest film demonstrates the

TABLE 8–7. Features of Laryngotracheobronchitis and Epiglottitis

Category	LTB	Epiglottitis
Etiology	Viral	Bacterial (in children)
Onset	Gradual	Fulminant
Age	Under 3 years	Any age; most 2–6 years
Appearance	Ill with barking cough	Toxic but not coughing
Postural preference	None	Sitting
Stridor	Inspiratory and expiratory	Inspiratory (occurs late)
Drooling	None	Common because of inability to swallow
Voice quality	Hoarse	Muffled
Antibiotics	Ineffective	Therapeutic
Racemic epinephrine	Effective	Contraindicated
Intubation	Rarely needed	Indicated in children
Recurrence	Not uncommon	Rare

"steeple" sign of tapering of the subglottic larynx. Only about 5% of children with LTB require hospitalization. Indications include stridor at rest or inability to exclude epiglottitis, foreign body aspiration, or other serious conditions.

Subglottic edema may lead rapidly to severe respiratory distress. The subglottic larynx, normally the narrowest segment of the pediatric airway above the carina, has loose areolar submucosal tissue, which permits substantial swelling at the expense of the subglottic space. Because there is no ciliated epithelium at the level of the glottis, secretions and debris arriving in the subglottic larynx through mucociliary transport accumulate as coughing becomes less effective with more severe obstruction. The formation of thick, tenacious bronchial secretions compound the more cephalad airway problems. The primary goal of therapy is to do whatever is necessary to protect the child without being unnecessarily or detrimentally invasive. Initial treatment is directed toward liquefaction of viscid secretions. Hence, all hospitalized children should receive meticulous visual surveillance, the comfort of their parent(s), humidification of supplemental oxygen provided within a mist tent, and IV hydration. High dose steroids may be helpful and are probably not harmful.[24] Dexamethasone 0.5 mg/kg (up to 30 mg) every 6 hours is commonly given in infants in danger of requiring an artificial airway.

Racemic epinephrine is used to combat edema. It usually has a dramatic, albeit ephemeral, effect as a local vasoconstrictor. Although nebulized racemic epinephrine may be given through a mask to young patients, it is more effective if delivered by IPPB.[25] One milliliter of 2.25% racemic epinephrine solution is diluted with 5 mL of normal saline and administered over 15 minutes. Because it is composed of equal parts of the dextro- and levoisomers of epinephrine, it has the same effect as half the amount of epinephrine, the active levoisomer. Hence, tachycardia and hypertension are not commonly problems, but ECG monitoring is advised nonetheless. Improvement should be evident by the time therapy is completed. Treatments are usually given every 1–2 hours but may be given as often as every 30 minutes, if necessary. Because racemic epinephrine has a short duration of action and potential for rebound hyperemia, the child must be kept in the hospital at least several hours after treatment and carefully observed for recrudescence of symptoms. As mentioned previously, racemic epinephrine is contraindicated in children with epiglottitis, because it has been reported to precipitate complete upper airway obstruction.

Transfer to the intensive care unit (ICU) is indicated if the child shows increasing agitation, heart rate, and respiratory rate. If the child is on the verge of respiratory failure despite steroids and maximal (every 30 minutes) racemic epinephrine therapy, monitoring should consist of pulse oximetry and checking arterial blood gases frequently from a percutaneous radial arterial catheter. Mask oxygen and CPAP should stent the airway, increase functional residual capacity, and hence decrease the work of breathing. The child may get some rest and then generate sufficient force to mobilize secretions that have played a significant role in her or his distress.

Some epinephrine-resistant infants, often those with underlying subglottic stenosis, fail to respond to all of the aforementioned measures and require an artificial airway. Anticipating rapidly impending respiratory arrest, the anesthesiologist may have to perform an awake intubation in the ICU. Success depends on the ability of an assistant to hold the child's shoulders down with his wrist and maintain the skull in neutral position with his hands. With suction available, after ventilating with 100% oxygen by bag and mask, atropine 0.02 mg/kg is given IV, and laryngoscopy is performed. An endotracheal tube at least 1.0 mm smaller than usual for the patient's age is inserted to avoid secondary trauma to the subglottic area.

Fortunately, in most instances there is sufficient time to move the child to the operating room, with an otolaryngologist standing by, for an inhalation induction, confirmation of the diagnosis, and intubation. Although a small tube is necessary, a 2.5-mm tube does not permit adequate suctioning and should not be used for a long period. Occasionally, only a rigid bronchoscope will pass through.

Next, a decision is made whether to convert to a nasal tube or proceed with an elective tracheostomy. Proponents of tracheostomy argue that a translaryngeal airway big enough to permit proper suctioning will be too tight-fitting, causing ischemia, necrosis, and mucosal and cartilaginous erosion. The result will be subglottic stenosis and the eventual need for a long-term tracheostomy. However, others claim a surprisingly and impressively low incidence of permanent laryngeal complications after 3–7 days of nasal intubation for LTB, even in the absence of an audible leak around the tube.

We commonly use the smallest nasotracheal tube that allows suctioning and positive-pressure ventilation as long as there is an audible air leak below 35 cm of H_2O pressure. The leak is assessed at least six times every 24 hours. When no leak is heard, a tracheostomy is performed. Details of tracheostomy are provided later in this chapter.

ICU management is similar to that for epiglottitis. For youngsters with nasotracheal tubes, liberal sedation minimizes further injury to the subglottic region that may occur secondary to head and neck motion, and humidified gases are delivered. Commonly, the subglottic edema starts to resolve within 2–4 days, as signaled by the appearance of an air leak at lower inflation pressures. With tracheostomy, inadvertent decannulation is less apt to occur with the use of a double swivel attachment to the CPAP system. The ICU staff and nurses should be instructed to manage an accidental decannulation by initially ventilating with bag and mask and then reintubating orally. Oth-erwise, attempted reinsertion of a fresh tracheostomy is likely to be unsuccessful or extremely traumatic.

BACTERIAL TRACHEITIS

Although bacterial tracheitis occurs less frequently than LTB and epiglottitis, this condition can cause acute airway obstruction and death in the pediatric population. This condition, also called membranous LTB or pseudomembranous croup,[26] is usually due to *Staphylococcus aureus*, although *Haemophilus influenzae*, pneumococci, and streptococci have been implicated also.[27] The disease produces exudative membranes that adhere to the laryngeal and tracheal wall. Severe tracheitis ensues, and the majority of children also have pulmonary infiltrates.

Most patients with this entity are between 2 and 6 years of age, and almost always less than age 10. The onset tends to be insidious, with a few days of upper respiratory infection and a barking cough followed by hoarseness and stridor. Respiratory distress with tachypnea, tachycardia, retractions, and cyanosis usually develops over the course of days but in some patients may escalate to toxicity and airway obstruction within a few hours. In the latter scenario, respiratory distress mimics epiglottitis.

The condition does not improve with racemic epinephrine, and the disease does not resolve as quickly with antibiotic therapy as does epiglottitis. Anesthetic management is similar to that of children with epiglottitis. However, laryngoscopy discloses normal supraglottic anatomy but subglottic narrowing and copious, purulent, viscid tracheobronchial secretions. This subglottic narrowing mandates the use of a smaller endotracheal tube than that usually appropriate for the youngster's age. However, repetitive obstruction of the tube by copious, tenacious secretions often necessitates tracheostomy.

TRACHEOSTOMY

It is preferable to perform a tracheostomy over an endotracheal tube or bronchoscope. However, particularly in the infant in whom cricothyrotomy is not feasible and intubation proves impossible, emergency tracheostomy may be necessary to provide airway control.

In the adult, tracheostomy is classically performed between the second and third tracheal rings. However, because of anatomical factors in infants and children, the incision must be made relatively low in the trachea. The pediatric level ranges from the fourth to the seventh tracheal rings.[28] Purportedly, certain complications associated with a high tracheostomy are eliminated. For example, tracheal stenosis can develop from the inflammatory and edematous reaction of the subglottic larynx or from drainage to the cricoid cartilage. In children, a vertical midline incision is made through the fourth and fifth tracheal rings without removing cartilage. Traction sutures inserted in the lateral margins of the tracheal incision emerge through the skin incision and expedite initial tracheostomy tube insertion. However, they cannot be relied on for facilitating reinsertion if the tube becomes displaced within the first 3 postoperative days. Hence, the necessity of meticulously securing the tracheal tube is obvious.

Advantages of tracheostomy include a reduction in pulmonary physiological dead-space and avoidance of the laryngeal stenosis that may follow prolonged orotracheal or nasotracheal intubation with attendant mucosal ulceration. Moreover, tracheostomy permits easier removal of airway secretions and allows for more comfortable swallowing, permits speech, and causes less stimulation of the cough reflex.[29-31] However, Battersby and associates[32] showed that in infants and children in whom airway anatomy is normal but who require ventilator support for other reasons, nasotracheal intubation has proven satisfactory for periods measured in weeks rather than days.

The majority of complications associated with tracheostomy relate to surgical technique, especially when tracheostomy is performed on an emergency basis. In children, tracheostomy is technically more difficult and carries a high complication rate. The comprehensive review by Holinger[20] of 4000 pediatric tracheostomies disclosed an overall complication rate of 14% and a mortality rate of 1.5%. Others[33, 34] have reported mortality directly attributable to tracheostomy from 3 to 10%. Complications included pneumothorax, mediastinal emphysema, bleeding, tracheal granuloma, obstructed tracheostomy tube, misplaced incision, inadvertent extubation, and cardiac arrest.

Postoperative care must be vigilant and include careful follow-up examinations and meticulous nursing care. Appropriate monitoring, chest radiographs, adequate humidification, and suctioning are essential to the maintenance of any artificial airway, not just in the tracheostomy patient. In addition, the patient with a tracheostomy needs fastidious local care of the incision to prevent infection.

SUMMARY

Infants and children with airway obstruction are among the most challenging patients. When difficulty with intubation is anticipated, the surgeon and anesthesiologist must decide preoperatively what strategy to follow if attempts at intubation are unsuccessful. An experienced otolaryngologist, gowned and gloved, must be in the operating room for induction of anesthesia. A tracheostomy set, rigid bronchoscopes with functioning light sources, and a varied assortment of endotracheal tubes, stylets, and laryngoscope blades and handles must be available. A fiberoptic endoscope may be of some use also. The physicians should have a plan that they disclose to the operating room personnel. The critical ingredients for a successful outcome are rapid and accurate evaluation of the patient's condition by experienced physicians and excellent organization, cooperation, and teamwork.

Children with airway obstruction, if not already hypoxic, may rapidly become so. Disturbing them may trigger complete obstruction, yet sedatives, tranquilizers, and narcotics are contraindicated until the airway is secured. Even after the obstruction is relieved, the child is still in danger, either from postobstructive pulmonary edema or from the myriad complications that may befall a patient with an artificial airway.

REFERENCES

1. Bell C, Oh TH, Loeffler JR: Massive macroglossia and airway obstruction after cleft palate repair. Anesth Analg 1988; 67:71–74.
2. Travis KW, Todres ID, Shannon DC: Pulmonary edema associated with croup and epiglottitis. Pediatrics 1977; 59:695–698.
3. Oswalt CE, Gates GE, Holmstrom FM: Pulmonary edema as a complication of acute airway obstruction. Rev Surg 1977; 34:346–347.
4. Melnick BM: Post laryngospasm pulmonary edema in adults. Anesthesiology 1984; 60:516–517.
5. Rivera M, Hadlock FP, O'Meara ME: Pulmonary edema secondary to acute epiglottitis. AJR 1979; 132:991–992.
6. Goldhill DR, Dalgleish JG, Lake RH: Respiratory problems and acromegaly. An acromegalic with hypersomia, acute upper airway obstruction, and pulmonary oedema. Anaesthesia 1982; 37:1200–1203.
7. Stradling JR, Bolton P: Upper airway obstruction as

a cause of pulmonary oedema. Lancet 1982; 1:1353–1354.

8. Lohr DG, Sahn SA: Postextubation pulmonary edema following anesthesia induced by upper airway obstruction: Are certain patients at increased risk? Chest 1986; 90:802–805.

9. Blanc VF, Weber ML, Leduc C, et al: Acute epiglottitis in children: Management of 27 consecutive cases with nasotracheal intubation with special emphasis on anaesthetic considerations. Can Anaesth Soc J 1977; 24:1–11.

10. Mayo Smith MF, Hirsch PJ, Wodzinski SF, et al: Acute epiglottitis in adults: An eight-year experience in the state of Rhode Island. N Engl J Med 1986; 314:1133–1139.

11. Shapiro J, Eavey RD, Baker AS: Adult supraglottitis: A prospective analysis. JAMA 1988; 259:563–567.

12. Gorfinkel HJ, Brown R, Kalins SA: Acute infectious epiglottitis in adults. Ann Intern Med 1969; 70:289–294.

13. Battaglia JD, Lockhart CH: Management of acute epiglottitis by nasotracheal intubation. Am J Dis Child 1975; 129:334–336.

14. Miller AH: Acute epiglottitis: Acute obstructive supraglottic laryngitis in small children caused by Hemophilus influenza, type B. Trans Am Acad Ophthalmol Otolaryngol 1949; 53:519–526.

15. Cochi SL, Broome CV: Vaccine prevention of Haemophilus influenzae type b disease: Past, present, and future. Pediatr Infect Dis 1986; 5:12–19.

16. Baker AS, Eavey RD: Adult supraglottitis (epiglottitis). N Engl J Med 1986; 314:1185–1186.

17. Baxter JD, Pashley NRT: Acute epiglottitis—25 years experience in management—The Montreal Children's Hospital. J Otolaryngol 1977; 6:473–476.

18. Barney WH, Stoll EJ, Hansbarger EA: Acute epiglottitis in adults. Va Med 1971; 98:252–257.

19. Adair JC, Ring WH: Management of epiglottitis in children. Anesth Analg 1975; 54:622–625.

20. Holinger PH: Foreign bodies in the air and food passages. XVII Wherry Memorial Lecture. Trans Am Acad Ophthal Otolaryngol 1962; 66:193–210.

21. Breivik H, Klaastad O: Acute epiglottitis in children. Br J Anaesth 1978; 50:505–510.

22. Rothstein P, Lister G: Epiglottitis—duration of intubation and fever. Anesth Analg 1983; 62:785–787.

23. Davis HW, Gartner JC, Galvis AG: Acute upper airway obstruction: Croup and epiglottitis. Pediatr Clin North Am 1981; 28:859–880.

24. Tunnessen WW, Feinstein AR: The steroid-croup controversy: An analytic review of methodologic problems. J Pediatr 1980; 96:751–756.

25. Bass JW, Bruhn FW, Merritt WT: Corticosteroids and racemic epinephrine with IPPB in the treatment of croup. Am J Pediatr 1980; 96:173–174.

26. Henry RL, Mellis CM, Benjamin B: Pseudomembranous croup. Arch Dis Child 1983; 58:180–183.

27. Weinberg S, Najajo M, Rao M: Airway management in children with bacterial tracheitis. Anesth Analg 1985; 63:860.

28. Fearon B: Laryngeal surgery in the pediatric patient. Ann Otol Rhinol Laryngol (Suppl 74) 1980; 89:146–149.

29. Spector GJ, Faw KD: Respiratory insufficiency and tracheostomy. *In* Ballenger JJ (ed): Diseases of the Nose, Throat, Ear, Head and Neck. Philadelphia, Lea & Febiger, 1985.

30. Coppel DL, Assac RAE: Tracheostomy. *In* Morrow W, Morrison J (eds): Anesthesia for Eye, Ear, Nose and Throat Surgery. Edinburgh, Churchill Livingstone, 1975.

31. Pracy R: Intubation of the larynx, laryngostomy, and tracheostomy. *In* Ballantyne J, Graves J (eds): Diseases of the Ear, Nose and Throat, Vol 4. London, Butterworth, 1975.

32. Battersby EF, Hatch DJ, Towey RM: Effects of prolonged nasotracheal intubation in children. Anaesthesia 1977; 32:154–157.

33. Filston HC, Johnson DG, Crumrine RS: Infant tracheostomy, a new look with a solution to the difficult cannulation problem. Am J Dis Child 1978; 132:1172.

34. Friedberg J, Morrison MD: Paediatric tracheotomy. Can J Otolaryngol 1974; 3:147.

CHAPTER 9

Anesthesia for Ear, Nose, and Throat Emergencies

Kathryn E. McGoldrick

BLEEDING FOLLOWING TONSILLECTOMY

Although bleeding from the tonsillar fossa or adenoidal site can occur at any time from the immediate postoperative period up to 10 days following surgery, it most commonly occurs during the first day, often within the first 4 hours. Secondary bleeding, frequently associated with infection, typically occurs between the fifth and tenth days. Anesthesia for postsurgical bleeding must be approached carefully and methodically, because affected patients have an increased incidence of morbidity and mortality.[1] Hypovolemia, hypotension, and a potential for airway obstruction and aspiration must be anticipated. It must be presumed that these patients have a full stomach.

The patient should be evaluated and volume resuscitation should be completed prior to induction of anesthesia. The anesthesiologist should not give in to the surgeon's demand to give "a little anesthesia" immediately, in a rushed fashion. Rather, the anesthesiologist should take time to carefully review the patient's chart and previous anesthetic record for details of intubation and drug dosage and should ascertain that cross-matched blood is available. (Obviously, in cases of life-threatening hemorrhage there may not be sufficient time to accomplish all of these objectives.)

The patient's volume status and the rate of ongoing bleeding should be estimated carefully. This assessment is difficult, because the patient may have swallowed large amounts of blood. However, blood pressure and pulse rate determinations in supine and upright positions often provide valuable clues. In most instances of hemorrhage, volume resuscitation should occur before anesthesia induction unless the patient is in danger of exsanguinating. A reliable, large-bore intravenous (IV) cannula for the infusion of crystalloid or the transfusion of blood is mandatory.

Monitoring should be as previously described for elective tonsillectomy. Two tonsil suction devices, forceps for removing clots, an extra laryngoscope, and a variety of blades and endotracheal tubes of various sizes with stylets must be immediately available, and expert assistance is mandatory.

Following generous preoxygenation and administration of atropine, 0.02 mg/kg, a rapid-sequence thiopental-succinylcholine induction of anesthesia with cricoid pressure is employed. (Awake intubation is performed only on patients who appear moribund.) To avoid hypotension, the dose of thiopental is reduced to 2 mg/kg, or etomidate 0.3 mg/kg may be used. Orotracheal intubation with an appropriate-size tube and stylet is performed. Before cricoid pressure is released, the presence of equal, bilateral breath sounds is confirmed. A nasogastric sump tube or large-bore suction catheter is then passed orally to empty the stomach of blood, air, clots, and gastric secretions. The gastric tube can then be removed. The cardiovascular response to the various agents is noted during the maintenance of anesthesia. If the patient becomes hypotensive when given an appropriate concentration of inhalation agents, small doses of narcotics, etomidate, or ketamine can be used.

During active, brisk bleeding, many experts preserve spontaneous ventilation until intubation can be accomplished. Their preferred technique in these circumstances is to induce anesthesia with halothane and oxygen, with the patient in the left lateral decubitus, head down position. Cricoid pressure should be applied by an expert assistant once the patient has lost consciousness. When sufficient anesthetic depth is attained, the laryngoscope is gently introduced, and the glottis is exposed. If the glottis is clearly visible, the assistant can administer succinylcholine while the anesthesiologist maintains glottic exposure with the laryngoscope. Alternatively, anesthesia can be deepened further and intubation can be performed without the administration of a muscle relaxant. When the vocal cords relax, intubation is accomplished, and the patient is turned supine. Anesthesia is then continued in any appropriate fashion.

Once bleeding is controlled and surgery is completed, the patient is turned to the lateral position and is not extubated until fully awake. The patient is then re-evaluated for airway patency, placed in the "tonsil position," and transported to the recovery room for vigilant postoperative observation.

Although bleeding from the tonsillar fossae can usually be controlled by suture, ligation, or cautery, when the bleeding has been from the adenoidal bed, frequently a posterior nasal pack is inserted and maintained for 24 hours. This pack is secured by ligatures brought out through the nares and tied securely together, while an additional ligature (for later removal of the pack) is brought through the mouth and fixed to the cheek by adhesive tape. By this procedure, the patient's nasal airway is occluded; also, the pack might become dislodged, causing complete respiratory obstruction. Clearly, in patients with posterior nasal packs, the oral airway must be perfectly adequate after extubation. These patients must be under constant surveillance until the pack is successfully removed.

PHARYNGEAL INFECTIONS

With the exception of tonsillitis, pharyngeal infections that eventually require surgical attention are infrequent and limited primarily to cases such as peritonsillar abscess, retropharyngeal abscess, and Ludwig's angina. Because these infections usually respond to appropriate antibiotic therapy, abscess formation and hence the subsequent need for surgical drainage is uncommon. This is fortuitous, because in these cases surgery creates a significant potential for airway obstruction and aspiration of infected material. Since the advent of effective antibiotics, the incidence of deep neck abscesses has dramatically decreased, and mortality has been reduced from approximately 50% to less than 5%.[2]

Inflammation is a relatively common cause of upper airway obstruction, and various mechanisms may be operative, depending on the site of inflammation. For example, external pressure distinct from the airway proper may compress the lumen of the airway, as happens with some neck abscesses or cellulitis and with retropharyngeal abscesses. Furthermore, infections of the tongue or the floor of the mouth (e.g., Ludwig's angina) may trigger obstruction secondary to posterior displacement of an edematous tongue. Other pharyngeal infections, including peritonsillar abscesses, may occlude the airway simply because of their size. In addition, nasal and nasopharyngeal infections, especially in the infant, may cause airway obstruction, because infants younger than 9 months of age are obligate nose breathers.

These problems can complicate intubation and mask ventilation. Because structures of the oral cavity, oropharynx, hypopharynx, and supraglottic larynx have tremendous potential for rapid expansion, the need for effective emergency intervention is always possible. General anesthesia in these situations is hazardous and challenging.

PERITONSILLAR ABSCESS (QUINSY)

Quinsy occurs outside the tonsillar capsule, usually in the soft palate, and is commonly unilateral. The abscess is excruciatingly painful and causes severe trismus. If swelling is significant, respiratory obstruction may ensue. This infection usually responds to appropriate antibiotic therapy, but if not, incision and drainage into the pharynx are required. General anesthesia should not be used, if possible, to avoid the risk of aspiration.[3]

In addition to aspiration of infected material, other hazards of general anesthesia include the likelihood of exacerbating any preexisting respiratory obstruction as consciousness is lost and the distinct possibility that laryngoscopy and intubation will be difficult or impossible if the trismus does not resolve following the administration of muscle relaxant.

If general anesthesia cannot be avoided, and if the anesthesiologist feels reasonably confident about the likelihood of successful intubation, the general methods for induction of anesthesia in post-tonsillectomy bleeding should be followed. Any intraoral instruments, such as an oral airway, laryngoscope, or suction catheter, must be used carefully and gently to avoid rupturing the abscess. If, however, induction of general anesthesia is considered too risky, a preliminary tracheostomy under local anesthesia to secure the airway must be performed. Once the airway is secure, the surgeon may devote his or her attention to control of bleeding, because the already rich vascularity of this area will be augmented by hyperemia in the region of the abscess.

RETROPHARYNGEAL ABSCESS

There are basically two types of retropharyngeal abscesses, differing in site of infection, chronicity, and age of the patient. In the pediatric population, acute abscesses tend to form in the lymphatic tissue located between the pharyngeal wall and the prevertebral fascia. They are usually associated with metastatic infection from nose, middle ear, or tonsil. These infections cause severe pharyngitis and marked systemic malaise. Respiratory obstruction may occur secondary to anterior displacement of the posterior pharyngeal wall (Fig. 9–1). Surgical therapy is the same as for peritonsillar abscess, with drainage into the pharynx.

The second type of retropharyngeal abscess

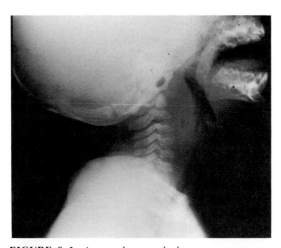

FIGURE 9–1. *A retropharyngeal abscess can compress airway structures that are positioned anterior to the abscess. (Photograph courtesy of Margaret A. Kenna, M.D., Department of Otolaryngology, Children's Hospital of Pittsburgh, University of Pittsburgh School of Medicine.)*

occurs in older patients and is usually chronic. It occurs behind the prevertebral fascia and is usually associated with osteomyelitis involving a vertebral body. With these cases, the infection is drained to the exterior through a skin incision behind the sternomastoid muscle. This type of abscess is usually less risky from an anesthetic viewpoint, because the intact prevertebral fascia should prevent spontaneous drainage into the pharynx.

LUDWIG'S ANGINA

Ludwig's angina is a life-threatening cellulitis of the floor of the mouth caused by bacterial infection of the sublingual and submandibular spaces. Of reported cases, 60 to 80% are of dental origin, with or without the trauma of tooth extraction.[4–6] Other local orodental causes include compound fractures of the mandible, traumatic laceration of the floor of the mouth, and peritonsillar abscess.[6] Furthermore, several systemic diseases, such as neutropenia, combined immunodeficiency disease, aplastic anemia, systemic lupus erythematosus, diabetes mellitus, glomerulonephritis, and hypersensitivity states, have been complicated by Ludwig's angina.[6, 7]

The syndrome was first described in 1836 by Frederick von Ludwig in a presentation before the Stuttgart Medical Society.[8] A paper entitled "Concerning a Variety of Neck Inflammations" was subsequently published. The symptomatology and the autopsy findings were accurately described by von Ludwig, and he correctly noted that the inflammatory process did not involve the lymphatics or the salivary glands. However, Ludwig failed to understand that deaths were caused by asphyxia from airway obstruction. Moreover, a distinction should be made between true Ludwig's angina and other cervical inflammatory processes.[4] If the inflammation involves the lymphatics, salivary glands, peritonsillar spaces, or other parts of the neck, the term *pseudo-Ludwig's angina* should be used.

Symptoms of Ludwig's angina include progressive trismus, drooling of secretions, and dysphonia, resulting in the aptly described "hot potato" voice. Fever is common and often marked. The progressive soft-tissue swelling of the suprahyoid area; the elevation, edema, and posterior displacement of the tongue; and the frequently associated laryngeal edema all result in increasing tachypnea, dyspnea, stridor, cyanosis and, eventually, death if appropriate intervention is not successful.[9]

Usually, the infection is mixed, and a multiplicity of organisms, including pneumococci, hemolytic and nonhemolytic streptococci, *Escherichia coli,* and assorted anaerobic bacteria, are cultured from the purulent material.[4, 6] Hence, several antimicrobial agents are needed to control the infection. Occasionally, organisms may be resistant to all common antibiotics, and surgery becomes necessary.

Proper airway management is essential, because deaths from asphyxia may occur even before surgery is attempted.[5] The presence of respiratory obstruction contraindicates general anesthesia until the airway has been safely secured either with an awake nasal intubation or by a tracheostomy under local anesthesia.[10]

Owing to the presence of infection, local anesthesia, other than for pretracheostomy infiltration, is ineffective. Local anesthesia does not open channels adequately for proper drainage. Local anesthesia should not be injected into infected tissues, because infection may spread and exacerbate the patient's condition.

If the patient's airway is apparently uncompromised—a rare and dubious situation when dealing with this life-threatening disease—general anesthesia may be administered with great caution, employing an inhalation induction and preserving spontaneous respiration until direct laryngoscopy demonstrates that intubation can be performed. This practice is extremely risky, and the surgeon must be ready to perform an emergency tracheostomy at all times. An elective tracheostomy under local anesthesia with the patient awake is the more prudent course.

ATLANTOAXIAL SUBLUXATION[11]

Atlantoaxial subluxation (AAS) is a condition that can be asymptomatic one minute and cause quadriplegia the next.

Children are at risk for AAS, particularly following trauma, because of the laxity of the transverse ligament of the young cervical spine, combined with immaturity of the odontoid process. C_1-C_2 subluxation is the most common type of cervical spine injury in children, at least until the odontoid fuses to the atlas at about age 4.

In addition, an epidemiological factor is operative. Young children have a relatively high frequency of upper respiratory infections and surgeries. Because of the close proximity of the posterior pharyngeal mucosa and the transverse ligament, pharyngeal infections may

cause serious complications in the cervical spine. Moreover, pharyngeal tumors and surgeries have been implicated in the pathogenesis of AAS. Prolonged, unusual positioning, which is necessary for many ear, nose, and throat procedures, may contribute to rotatory, transverse, or anterior-posterior subluxation. Finally, a variety of disease processes and congenital conditions predispose to AAS. In addition to pharyngeal tumors and infections, such diseases include rheumatoid arthritis and ankylosing spondylitis. Congenital conditions with the propensity for AAS include syndromes such as Down's, Klippel-Feil, Kniest, and Larsen's, as well as diseases such as chondrodystrophia calcificans congenita, chondrodysplasia punta, spondyloepiphyseal dysplasia, and mucopolysaccharidosis. Meticulous care during intubation and surgical positioning of these patients must be maintained.

Although AAS can be asymptomatic, early warning signs may include neck pain or stiffness or torticollis. Indeed, any neurological change should be sought and investigated. Complete cervical spine films, including odontoid and nonforced flexion views, should be obtained if there are postoperative symptoms. (Furthermore, these radiological studies are well advised *preoperatively* in patients with the aforementioned conditions who are at high risk for AAS.) Cervical traction or other intervention may be mandatory.

CHOANAL ATRESIA

In choanal atresia, a congenital condition said to occur once in every 8000 births, an aberrant growth of bone or soft tissue obstructs the posterior nares. Complete bilateral choanal atresia is a significant cause of neonatal mortality.[12] Hence, every immediate postdelivery physical examination of the newborn should include routine passage of a number 8 catheter through each nostril into the nasopharynx. Choanal atresia may be unrelated to other lesions but frequently is associated with conditions of craniofacial synostosis, such as Apert's syndrome and Crouzon's disease.

If a prompt diagnosis is made, inserting an oral airway may be life-saving, because neonates are obligate nasal breathers. This is an essential temporizing measure until definitive surgical removal of the obstruction can be accomplished. In a few infants the obstruction is caused by the presence of a membrane or a delicate bony plate. These cases respond to intranasal surgical perforation. However, when solid bone is the culprit, a transpalatal approach is usually necessary. The oropharyngeal airway must remain strapped in place until the time of orotracheal intubation for surgery.

Challenges in anesthetic management include the problems common to neonatal anesthesia in general—fluid balance, temperature control, and immaturity of the cardiorespiratory, renal, and hepatic systems—and the specific problems of intra-airway surgery, limited intraoperative patient access, and the potential for significant blood loss. Premedication is limited to atropine. Orotracheal intubation should be accomplished either with the patient awake or following an inhalation induction, depending on the status of the infant. A small, deep hypopharyngeal pack should be inserted to absorb blood that might otherwise leak down the trachea, past the uncuffed endotracheal tube. The orotracheal tube must be firmly and meticulously secured, because inadvertent intraoperative extubation is undesirable. A reliable IV cannula is mandatory because of the potential for major blood loss. Monitoring should include a temperature probe, a device to determine the fractional inspired oxygen (FIO_2), accurate blood pressure determination (a Doppler detector is useful), accurate measurement of sponge weight and suction volume to assess blood loss, continuous electrocardiographic and ventilatory monitoring with a precordial stethoscope, and measurement of pulse oximetry and, ideally, end-tidal carbon dioxide. The baby, placed on a heating blanket, should be in an operating room with a warm ambient temperature. At the completion of surgery, stents or nasal packs may be left in place, and the hypopharyngeal pack is removed. Extubation is performed only when the baby is awake and able to maintain airway patency.

Unilateral choanal atresia often remains undiagnosed for years. (Only about 10% of cases of choanal atresia are unilateral.) Older children present with a history of mouth breathing, copious nasal discharge, and epiphora. Indeed, unrecognized partial nasal obstruction from choanal stenosis may be one etiology involved in the enigmatic pathogenesis of sudden infant death syndrome.[13]

A special situation exists in infants with CHARGE. The acronym CHARGE, coined by Pagon and colleagues[14] in 1982, refers to a complex of malformations that includes coloboma, heart disease, atresia choanae, retarded growth or development, genital hypoplasia, and ear anomalies or deafness. The pathogenesis of the anatomical malformations is thought to be secondary to the abnormal development of the neural crest during embryogenesis. Successful repair of choanal atresia in the infant with CHARGE is more difficult than in an otherwise normal baby. Coniglio and associates[15] reported that the vast majority of their patients with CHARGE required revision surgery, and Asher and colleagues[16] reported similar findings. Because early repair of bilateral choanal atresia in these infants is rarely successful, probably owing to their abnormal nasopharyngeal anatomy that predisposes to restenosis, Asher and coworkers recommended early tracheostomy rather than early choanal repair.[16] They suggest delaying the choanal surgery until the child is at least 2 years old, when the operation is more likely to be successful.

EPISTAXIS

Surgical management of epistaxis involves ligation of the internal maxillary artery, the anterior ethmoid artery, and occasionally, the external carotid artery. The anterior ethmoid artery is approached through the orbit, and the external carotid is ligated in the neck. Hence, the operative site in these cases is outside the nasal and pharyngeal cavities and poses no threat to the patient's airway. Until an endotracheal tube has been safely placed, however, there is significant risk to the patient's airway from the continuing intranasal blood loss.

A careful preoperative evaluation is indicated, because chronic epistaxis may be associated with a spectrum of entities, including hypertension, nasal trauma, leukemia or other hematological dyscrasias, and use of medications, such as coumadin or aspirin. Furthermore, many of the conditions that require coumadin or aspirin therapy are formidable and anesthetically challenging. In addition, during the 2 or 3 days immediately prior to surgery, the majority of epistaxis patients have been subjected to unsuccessful attempts at controlling bleeding with nasal packing. These patients are often anxious, hypertensive, tachycardic, and hypovolemic. It is difficult to accurately estimate the amount of blood loss, but such patients should be assumed to have a full stomach from swallowing blood and to be hypovolemic. Blood pressures and heart rates should be compared with the patient in both the sitting and supine positions. Evaluation should include questions concerning a family history of bleeding disorders, liver function tests, and screening tests to determine coagulation parameters and bleeding time.

These patients should be kept sitting at 45 degrees before surgery. As mentioned, they almost always have a posterior pack in place. In addition to causing discomfort, anxiety, and hypertension in elderly patients with cardiopulmonary diseases, a posterior nasal pack can produce many other problems. These complications include hypercarbia, hypoxia, and dysrhythmias resulting in myocardial infarction. Moreover, extreme hypertension may precipitate a cerebrovascular accident. Cautious doses of analgesics or sedatives may be required in an attempt to avert some of these potential complications.

Before anesthesia is induced, at least 2 units of packed erythrocytes should be available. A large, functional IV line must be established to volume resuscitate the patient adequately. After preoxygenation, a rapid sequence induction of anesthesia with cricoid pressure is performed. Because the nose is still packed, an oral airway should be maintained with care as soon as the patient loses consciousness. Anesthesia is maintained with whatever agents the patient is able to tolerate hemodynamically. Extubation should be accomplished with the patient awake, responsive, and able to maintain a patent airway.

DIPHTHERIA[17]

Since the adoption of active immunization, diphtheria has largely disappeared from the developed nations,[18] although in more recent years the disease has usually occurred in patients who were either debilitated[19] or immunologically compromised.[20]

Because of transplacental transfer of maternal antibody, the disease is extremely unlikely to occur before 6 months of age. Diphtheria is most common in children 5–7 years of age and then becomes comparatively unusual after the age of 10.[17] The infecting organism, *Corynebacterium diphtheriae,* is usually spread by droplet infection. Although the bacteria remain localized primarily at the site of infection, life-threatening systemic effects may be produced by the potent exotoxin associated with the disease. Manifestations of diphtheria depend on the site of infection; the major varieties are nasal, cutaneous, and laryngeal.

Those with laryngeal diphtheria are at risk for respiratory obstruction. The incubation period is brief, usually from 2 to 5 days. The initial symptoms are nonspecific (e.g., malaise, sore throat), but within a day whitish spots appear on the tonsils. These spots rapidly enlarge and become confluent so that by the second day a leathery pseudomembrane is visible. This typical pseudomembrane, composed of necrotic tissue, exudate, and blood, has clearly defined margins and varies in color from ivory to near black. Following its characteristically rather difficult removal, a raw, bleeding surface remains. Aside from the local consequences of the membrane, devastating systemic effects may transpire also. The heart and the peripheral nervous system, particularly the cranial nerves, are especially vulnerable to the exotoxin. Approximately 50% of individuals with diphtheria have myocardial involvement, usually with impaired conduction and contractility. About 20% have neurological complications. Death is most commonly the result of either respiratory obstruction or myocardial decompensation. However, in patients who survive, neurological sequelae and cardiac perturbations are not usually permanent.

Treatment consists of relief of respiratory obstruction, specific antitoxin, antibiotics, bed rest, isolation, and public health measures to curb the spread of the disease. Although antitoxin neutralizes circulating toxin, it has no effect on toxin already in the tissues. Therefore, antitoxin should be administered early and with full precautions against sensitivity to horse serum. Elective tracheostomy is best performed early in any patient with membranous pharyngitis. If tracheostomy is delayed until evidence of respiratory obstruction becomes obvious, it may be too late.[21, 22] Because of the high incidence of toxic myocarditis, general anesthesia should be avoided, and tracheostomy should be performed under local infiltration anesthesia. Both penicillin and erythromycin suppress the growth of *C. diphtheriae* and should be administered also.

LARYNGEAL TRAUMA[17]

Injuries to the neck may be either open or closed, involving the larynx, the cervical trachea, or both. Open injuries are commonly the result of motor vehicle accidents involving broken glass, but other causes include gunshot wounds and stab wounds. Closed laryngeal injuries may be caused by forceful blows on the anterior neck, which may occur when an individual falls against the steering wheel of a car, the edge of a table, or the handlebar of a bicycle. Laryngeal fractures also may be caused by running against a taut wire or rope. In these settings, laryngeal injury can include complex damage with dislocation of the arytenoid cartilages and extensive disruption of the cricoarytenoid joint, in which the arytenoid itself may obstruct the glottis. This obstruction is exacerbated by the associated edema formation and bleeding. Tracheal damage tends to be less complicated than laryngeal; tracheal lesions usually present as relatively simple longitudinal tears.

A change in voice after a blow on the neck should alert the physician to the probability of laryngeal injury. Other signs include coughing, dyspnea, hemoptysis, and subcutaneous emphysema. Subcutaneous emphysema triggers a vicious cycle in which increased respiratory effort further exacerbates the air leak, in turn augmenting the emphysema. Although there is no direct, quantitative correlation between the degree of injury and the extent of emphysema, struggling, coughing, and positive-pressure ventilation increase the degree of subcutaneous emphysema.

Associated injuries may further complicate management. Indeed, the potential problems of cervical spine injury, hemorrhage, aspiration, hemopneumothorax, and air embolism through lacerated cervical veins are formidable (Table 9–1).

If treated properly and early, an excellent prognosis may be associated with even extremely complex laryngeal fractures. A tracheostomy is performed below the level of the injury, and the air leak is closed with laryngeal wiring and reconstruction of the airway. Tracheal injuries commonly require nothing more than suturing. However, associated damage to blood vessels, the pharynx, and the esophagus should be suspected and treated appropriately. An initially undetected esophageal tear may be a major cause of morbidity and mortality.[23]

TABLE 9–1. Potential Problems with Laryngeal Trauma

Respiratory obstruction
Cervical spine injury
Aspiration
Hemorrhage
Hemopneumothorax
Air embolism through lacerated cervical veins
Occult esophageal tear

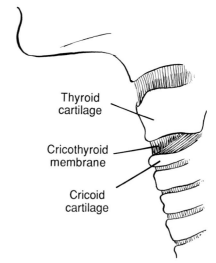

FIGURE 9–2. *The cricothyroid membrane may be punctured or incised in order to establish an emergency airway.*

Thyroid cartilage

Cricothyroid membrane

Cricoid cartilage

Initial airway management is critical because of its potential to exacerbate the degree of injury and respiratory distress,[24] and to trigger aspiration in these patients, who must be presumed to have full stomachs. In extremely rare cases, a transected cervical trachea may be visible in the wound, allowing for direct intubation of the distal segment. More commonly, attempts at glottic intubation with closed injuries may result in further anatomical disruption, or the endotracheal tube, *apparently* inserted through the glottis, may in fact exit the airway through a tear, resulting in a false passage and total respiratory obstruction. For these reasons, the airway should be initially secured either through rigid bronchoscopy or awake tracheostomy under local infiltration anesthesia.

Once the airway is secure, anesthesia can be administered in any appropriate way, but positive-pressure ventilation should not be administered if there is uncertainty about the extent of the laryngotracheal injury. Nitrous oxide is contraindicated also in the presence of surgical emphysema, as is the application of cricoid pressure over a damaged larynx.

CRICOTHYROIDOTOMY

In a life-threatening emergency, cricothyroidotomy is an alternative to a tracheostomy. Cricothyroidotomy is simple and establishes an airway in less than 2 minutes by puncturing the cricothyroid membrane[25, 26] (Fig. 9–2).

However, in infants cricothyroidotomy is not advisable, because the cricothyroid membrane is only 3 mm in length, and insertion of an airway can cause glottic or cricoid cartilage damage.[27]

Cricothyroidotomy has a complication rate of approximately 9%, which is considerably less than that associated with *emergency* tracheostomies. Although a properly performed cricothyroidotomy may be the technique of choice in an acute airway emergency when endotracheal intubation is impossible, under *elective* circumstances a formal tracheostomy is preferable and should have fewer long-term complications. Disadvantages of cricothyroidotomy include potential damage to the cricoid cartilage, resulting in laryngeal collapse or stenosis; bleeding in the neck; the requirement of a small-diameter artificial airway; and the fact that subglottic or tracheal obstruction is not remedied by this method, because tracheal entry is just immediately below the vocal cords.

At the least, a cricothyroid membrane puncture may be performed with a 12- or 14-gauge needle to provide temporary transtracheal oxygenation until a proper airway can be established. (Clearly, an incision in the cricothyroid membrane, rather than a mere puncture, provides a more generous opening through which a small tracheostomy tube can be inserted.) Properly used, transtracheal oxygenation can remedy hypoxia. Neff and colleagues[28] maintain that to serve as an adequate airway, a 15-gauge transtracheal needle must be connected to intermittent jet oxygen at 50 psi for an oxygen flow rate of 15 L/minute. The intermittent rate is kept slow (6–8 per minute) with a 1:4 inspiratory:expiratory cycle[29] to allow sufficient time for passive expiration, especially in the presence of expiratory obstruction. Otherwise, high airway pressures quickly build up, impeding venous return and precipitating cardiovascular collapse and pneumothorax. Jet ventilation is adequate only if egress of gases is satisfactory. An alternative setup following percutaneous cricothyrotomy involves the administration of 100% O_2 by positive pressure through a 14-gauge catheter using a 3.0 endotracheal tube adapter or the barrel of a 3-mL syringe and a 7.5-mm endotracheal tube adapter.

EMERGENCY TRACHEOSTOMY

As previously mentioned, tracheostomy ideally should be an unhurried procedure, performed with either an endotracheal tube or a rigid bronchoscope in place. The complication rate may exceed 30% even with so-called elective tracheostomy, and it is much higher for tracheostomy performed as an emergency, lifesaving measure. Pneumothorax, for example, is more common in struggling patients as well as in children because of their higher pleural apices. Additionally, inadvertent esophageal perforation is a more frequent complication in tracheostomies performed on an emergency basis.

Emergency tracheostomy may be indicated for upper airway obstruction secondary to infections, exudate, edema, burns, impacted foreign bodies, trauma, and large airway tumors. Although the normal adult trachea can be compromised by as much as 50% before respiratory distress becomes apparent, stridor at rest occurs when the tracheal diameter is reduced to 4 mm.[30]

For emergency tracheostomy, local infiltration with 1% lidocaine is used. This may be supplemented with a bilateral superficial cervical plexus block, as described in Chapter 2. When intubation is not possible, the anesthesiologist must continue to focus on the airway and try to preserve whatever marginal airway remains. Hence, 100% oxygen is administered by mask, and the patient is carefully monitored with an electrocardiogram, pulse oximeter, blood pressure determinations, and precordial stethoscope. Considerable effort should be devoted to calming and reassuring the patient. The preservation of spontaneous respiration is a major goal until the tracheostomy tube is inserted. Cardiovascular collapse may occur suddenly during tracheostomy upon establishing a patent airway.[31] It is postulated that rapid correction of hypoxia, reduction in carbon dioxide levels, reversal of respiratory acidosis, and alterations in electrolytes may be contributing factors to such dramatic hemodynamic instability. Regardless of pathogenesis, the anesthesiologist must be prepared to treat this situation should it occur.

Once the tracheostomy tube is inserted, its position should be verified by bilateral auscultation of the lung fields and end-tidal carbon dioxide measurement. Postoperative tracheostomy care should be as previously described, and a postoperative chest radiograph should be obtained.

REFERENCES
1. Alexander DW, Graff TW, Kelley E: Factors in tonsillectomy mortality. Arch Otolaryngol 1965; 82: 409.

L133

132 ANESTHESIA FOR EAR, NOSE, AND THROAT EMERGENCIES

2. Heindel DJ: Deep neck abscesses in adults: Management of a difficult airway. Anesth Analg 1987; 66:774–776.

3. Tucker A: Peritonsillar abscess—a retrospective study of medical treatment. J Laryngol Otol 1982; 96:639–643.

4. Ashhurst Astely PC: Ludwig's angina. Arch Surg 1929; 18:2047–2078.

5. Garland Boyd JM: A memo about Ludwig's angina. Anaesthesia 1963; 18:29–31.

6. Meyer BR, Lawson W, Hirshman SZ: Ludwig's angina: Case report with review of bacteriology and current therapy. Am J Med 1972; 53:257–260.

7. Barkin KG, Bovis SL, Elghammer RM, et al: Ludwig's angina in children. J Pediatr 1975; 87:563–565.

8. von Ludwig WF: Ueber eire neue artz von halsentzundung. Mediz Korr Blatt des Wuremberg arztl Vereins 1836; 6:21–23.

9. Finch RG, Snider GE, Sprinkle PM: Ludwig's angina. JAMA 1980; 243:1171–1173.

10. Dalili H, Adriani J: Ludwig's angina: Anesthetic management. Anesth Rev 1983; 10:11–15.

11. Audenaert SM, Schmidt TE: Perils of atlanto-axial subluxation. Soc Pediatr Anesth Newsletter 1990; 3:4.

12. Ferguson CF: Congenital choanal atresia. In Ferguson CF, Kendig EL (eds): Pediatric Otolaryngology. Philadelphia, WB Saunders, 1972.

13. France NK: Anesthesia for pediatric ENT. In Gregory GA (ed): Pediatric Anesthesia. New York, Churchill Livingstone, 1983, p 812.

14. Pagon RA, Graham JM, Zonana J: Coloboma, congenital heart disease, and choanal atresia with multiple anomalies: CHARGE association. J Pediatr 1981; 99:223–227.

15. Coniglio JU, Manzione JV, Hengerer AS: Anatomic findings and management of choanal atresia and the CHARGE association. Ann Otol Rhinol Laryngol 1988; 97:448–453.

16. Asher BF, McGill TJ, Kaplan L, et al: Airway complications in CHARGE association. Arch Otolaryngol Head Neck Surg 1990; 116:594–595.

17. Morrison JD: Otolaryngological diseases. In Katz J, Steward DJ (eds): Anesthesia and Uncommon Pediatric Diseases. Philadelphia, WB Saunders, 1987, pp 297–299, 306–308.

18. Hodes HL: Diphtheria. Pediatr Clin North Am 1979; 26:445.

19. Heath CW, Zusman J: An outbreak of diphtheria among skid row men. N Engl J Med 1962; 267:809.

20. Brooks GF, Bennett JV, Feldman RA: Diphtheria in the United States 1959–1970. J Infect Dis 1974; 129:172.

21. Dobie RA, Tobey TN: Clinical features of diphtheria in the respiratory tract. JAMA 1979; 242:2197.

22. Naiditch MJ, Bower AG: Diphtheria: A study of 1433 cases observed during a ten year period at the Los Angeles County Hospital. Am J Med 1954; 17:229.

23. Defore WW, Mattox KL, Hansen HA, et al: Surgical management of penetrating injuries of the esophagus. Am J Surg 1977; 134:734.

24. Schaefer SD: Primary management of laryngeal trauma. Ann Otol Rhinol Laryngol 1982; 81:399.

25. Boyd AD, Romita MC, Conlan AA, et al: Clinical evaluation of cricothyroidotomy. Surg Gynecol Obstet 1979; 149:365.

26. Schecter WP, Wilson RS: Management of upper airway obstruction in the intensive care unit. Crit Care Med 1981; 9:577.

27. Holinger PH: Foreign bodies in the air and food passages. XVII Wherry Memorial Lecture. Trans Am Acad Ophthal Otolaryngol 1962; 66:193–210.

28. Neff CC, Pister RC, Sonnenberg E: Percutaneous transtracheal ventilation: Experimental and practical aspects. J Trauma 1983; 23:84.

29. McSwain NE: Percutaneous transtracheal ventilation (editorial). J Trauma 1983; 23:1076.

30. Pearson FG, Goldberg M, deSilva AJ: Tracheal stenosis complicating tracheostomy with cuffed tubes. Arch Surg 1968; 97:380.

31. Greenway RE: Tracheostomy: Surgical problems and complications. Int Anesthesiol Clin 1972; 10:151.

10

Anesthesia for Otologic Surgery

Kathryn E. McGoldrick
John G. Muller

ANATOMY[1,2] AND PHYSIOLOGY OF THE EAR, INCLUDING PATHOPHYSIOLOGY[3]

The external ear consists of the auricle (pinna), the external auditory meatus, and the tympanic membrane (eardrum). The tympanic membrane separates the medial end of the external auditory meatus from the middle ear cavity. The handle of the malleus is embedded in the relatively thin tympanic membrane. The sensory nerve supply of the external ear and the middle ear includes the auriculotemporal nerve, the great auricular nerve, the tympanic nerve, and the auricular branch of the vagus.

The middle ear is a biconcave air-filled cavity in the temporal bone that communicates, through the eustachian tube, with the nasopharynx. Although the eustachian tube is usually closed, it opens during swallowing to swallow equalization of pressure between the middle ear cavity and the nasopharynx. The middle ear houses three mobile bones—the malleus, incus, and stapes—that connect the lateral wall to the medial wall and transmit the vibrations of the tympanic membrane to the inner ear. In addition, the middle ear communicates with the mastoid air cells through the mastoid antrum. The head of the malleus articulates with the incus, which articulates with the head of the tiny, delicate stapes. The footplate of the stapes is positioned in the oval window by the annular ligament (Fig. 10–1).

The lateral wall of the inner ear is characterized by a promontory resulting from the basal turn of the cochlea. This wall behind the promontory has two small openings: the oval window, located superiorly, and the round window, located inferiorly. While a membrane closes the round window, the footplate of the stapes closes the oval window and leads into the vestibule of the inner ear. The horizontal portion of the facial nerve canal lies immediately superior to the oval window. Because the facial nerve is intimately associated with the structures of the ear, its preservation is crucial during ear surgery.

The majority of major otologic operations are for middle ear disorders, including mastoid disease, or for reconstruction and remobilization of the tympanic membrane or ossicular chain. Many different problems interfere with sound conduction through the middle ear. For example, chronic infection produces scarring of the drum, resulting in restricted movement of the tympanic membrane. In addition, impaired patency of the eustachian tube reduces air pressure in the middle ear and limits drum movement. Moreover, chronic infection in the middle ear cleft may ultimately extend to the labyrinth, triggering nystagmus, vertigo, and in cases of severe involvement, nausea and vomiting. Otalgia and otorrhea usually indicate middle ear disease. When the discharge is chronic and offensive, and particularly when the patient is a child, cholesteatoma formation should be suspected.

The labyrinth, or internal ear, is located in the petrous part of the temporal bone and consists of a series of bony canals. The interior

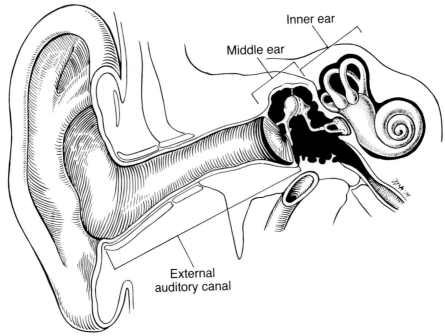

FIGURE 10–1. Anatomy of the ear.

of these bony canals is filled with perilymph and surrounds the membranous labyrinth, which is filled with endolymph. At the anterior end of the labyrinth is the cochlea, a coiled, hollow tube that is divided into three chambers: the scala vestibuli and the scala tympani, containing perilymph, and a middle chamber, containing endolymph. The cochlea can be visualized as a column of fluid within a bony tube; one end (the scala tympani) is at the oval window, and the other end (the scala vestibuli) is at the round window. The cochlea's middle chamber contains the organ of Corti with its auditory sense organs, the hair cells. Movement of cochlear fluid produces movement of the basilar membrane, where the organ of Corti is located. This mechanical excitation of the hair cells ultimately transforms mechanical movements into electrical nerve impulses.

When sound waves arrive at the tympanic membrane, it moves in and out, as does the attached handle of the malleus. The malleus and incus are one functional unit, and the long process of the incus moves the stapes in a piston-like fashion so that its footplate moves in and out of the oval window. This action of the stapes triggers reciprocal movement of the perilymph. Unimpeded movement of the cochlea's fluid column can occur in response to pressure from the footplate only if the membrane over the round window at its other end can protrude away from that pressure.

Posterior to the cochlea, in the middle ear, is a vestibule located between the middle ear and the internal auditory meatus. This vestibule communicates anteriorly with the cochlea and posteriorly with the five openings of the three semicircular canals (the posterior, superior, and lateral canals). Membranous canals suspended in perilymph are located inside the bony semicircular canals. Each membranous canal contains a sensory crista ampullaris that responds to rotational acceleration and produces the conscious perception of motion and spatial orientation. Excessive stimulation can trigger nausea, palpitations, diaphoresis, vomiting, dizziness, and fluctuations in blood pressure. The lateral semicircular canal, by virtue of proximity, may be disturbed during middle ear surgery, causing severe postoperative nausea, vomiting, and dizziness.

Imbalance and vertigo can result not only from inner ear disturbances, but also from eighth nerve and brain stem disorders. A careful neurotological evaluation is essential to differentiate among the myriad possible etiologies.

Congenital sensorineural hearing loss may result from partial or almost complete absence of the membranous cochlear duct, with or without loss of the afferent auditory neurons.

Occasionally, these aberrations are combined with other abnormalities to produce syndromes such as Usher's syndrome with retinitis pigmentosa; Alport's syndrome with hereditary nephritis; Pendred's syndrome with sporadic goiter; and Waardenburg's syndrome with a white forelock, heterochromia iridium, and broad nasal bridge. A vast array of other syndromes are associated with sensorineural hearing loss, including the Jervell and Lange-Nielson syndrome characterized by episodic fainting and electrocardiogram (ECG) abnormalities in addition to deafness (Table 10–1).

Infections such as rubella and medications taken during pregnancy may produce deafness in the infant. In addition, birth trauma and prematurity together with hypoxia and kernicterus may result in profound hearing loss.

The labyrinth may become infected by direct extension from chronic suppurative otitis media or secondarily from meningitis. Viral infections, such as mumps, influenza, and herpes zoster, similarly affect the labyrinth.

Certain ototoxic drugs can damage both the cochlea and the vestibular labyrinths. Drugs in this category include aminoglycoside antibiotics; diuretics, such as ethacrynic acid and furosemide; quinine; chloroquine; and salicylates.

Sensorineural deafness also can result from vascular insufficiency caused by thrombosis or vasospasm of the internal auditory artery. Indeed, even the hemodynamic and hormonal changes that accompany pregnancy may produce a high tone sensorineural loss and tinnitus.

Lastly, activity such as heavy lifting or straining that produces a marked increase in cerebrospinal fluid pressure can result in dramatically elevated perilymph pressure, whereby perilymph is forced from the labyrinth through a membrane or ligament rupture into the middle ear. This serious condition constitutes one of the few emergencies involving ear surgery, because sensorineural loss can be prevented if the leak is sealed quickly with a free-fat graph.

SURGICAL PROCEDURES INVOLVING THE EAR

MYRINGOTOMY AND INSERTION OF TYMPANOTOMY TUBES

Otitis media is one of the most prevalent infectious diseases of infants and young children and has a propensity to recur. Frequent recurrences can lead to irreversible middle ear damage and hearing impairment. Data suggest that certain children are predisposed to middle ear disease, and that those babies whose initial episode of otitis occurs during the first 3 months of life are frequently susceptible to multiple recurrences.[4] It is commonly acknowledged that infants with unrepaired cleft palates have recurring otitis, and a large percentage of older children with a history of cleft palate have hearing loss.[5] Likewise, a high prevalence of both hearing loss and otitis media has been reported in individuals with Turner's syndrome.[6]

Pathogenesis appears to involve abnormal eustachian tube function. Hypertrophied nasopharyngeal lymphoid tissue causes extraluminal eustachian tube obstruction. A study by Gates and colleagues[7] concluded that adenoidectomy should be considered when surgical therapy is indicated in children 4–8 years old who are severely affected by chronic otitis media with effusion. Intraluminal obstruction may be the result of mucosal edema, an abnormal opening mechanism of the tube, or excessive tubal wall compliance rendering the tube vulnerable to collapse. The crucial feature of otitis is the middle ear effusion causing diminished mobility of the tympanic membrane.

The placement of tympanotomy tubes is the most commonly performed minor surgical procedure in children in the United States today. Bilateral myringotomy, evacuation of the middle ear effusion, and insertion of a tympanotomy or myringotomy tube typically requires

TABLE 10–1. Some Etiologies of Sensorineural Hearing Loss

Genetic	*Drugs*
Usher's syndrome	Aminoglycoside antibiotics
Alport's syndrome	Diuretics
Pendred's syndrome	Quinine
Waardenburg's syndrome	Chloroquine
Jervell and Lange-Nielson	Salicylates
syndrome	
	Vascular insufficiency
Birth trauma	
	Ménière's disease
Infectious	
Bacterial	*Traumatic perilymphatic*
Direct extension from	*rupture*
chronic suppurative	
otitis media	
Secondary to meningitis	
Viral	
Congenital rubella	
Mumps	
Influenza	
Herpes zoster	

only 5–10 minutes in expert hands, although the procedure may take almost 30 minutes when performed by a neophyte. This surgery is done almost exclusively on an outpatient basis. Administration of nitrous oxide, oxygen, and halothane by mask affords a rapid and smooth induction, as well as prompt recovery. Monitoring typically includes a precordial stethoscope, ECG, blood pressure cuff, and pulse oximetry. If the surgery is anticipated to last only a few minutes, some anesthesiologists, depending on a variety of factors, may elect not to start an intravenous (IV) infusion intraoperatively. However, physicians should not minimize the potential risks when obtaining informed consent from parents just because of the brevity of the procedure. A prospective study[8] of 510 children undergoing tympanotomy tube placement documented that transient upper airway obstruction is not uncommon in this setting. (Enlarged adenoidal tissue causing obstruction in the eustachian tubes also partially obstructs the upper airway.) Therefore, it is helpful to keep the child's mouth open until he or she is anesthetized sufficiently to accept an oropharyngeal airway without gagging or without undergoing laryngospasm. Argon and potassium-titanyl-phosphate (KTP) lasers have been employed for myringotomy.

MIDDLE EAR SURGERY

Use of the operating microscope has greatly enhanced and advanced ear surgery. Anesthetic considerations for middle ear surgery include elevation of middle ear pressure using nitrous oxide (N_2O) (Fig. 10–2), techniques to ensure a bloodless surgical field, and monitoring of facial nerve integrity.

Mastoidectomy and Tympanoplasty

Chronic suppurative otitis media is treated by either myringoplasty to close perforations in the tympanic membrane, or tympanoplasty with additional ossicular reconstruction and tympanic membrane grafting. With improved medical and surgical management of otitis media, the incidence of mastoidectomy has declined considerably over the past 2 decades. However, in the setting of extremely extensive middle ear disease, a modified radical mastoidectomy may be necessary. With the latter procedure, the attic and mastoid antrum are cleared, but as much of the ossicular chain is preserved as possible. Both the external auditory meatus and the mastoid air system are converted into a single accessible bony cavity, freely communicating with the external meatal orifice. Classical radical mastoidectomy, in which all middle ear structures are removed, is seldom necessary.

Because nitrous oxide is approximately 34 times more soluble than nitrogen, it can pose problems in closed spaces within the body. Because nitrous oxide enters the closed space at a faster rate than nitrogen can be removed, the volume of any gas contained within a closed space can significantly expand (Fig. 10–2). Many reports[9–14] have documented the increase in middle ear pressure that occurs with nitrous oxide administration and the deleterious results attributed to its use. Rupture of the tympanic membrane[15] and dislodgement of tympanic membrane grafts have been described. Another concern is that when the nitrous oxide is discontinued, this withdrawal of the gas produces a negative pressure.[16] Such negative pressure could displace a fresh graft,

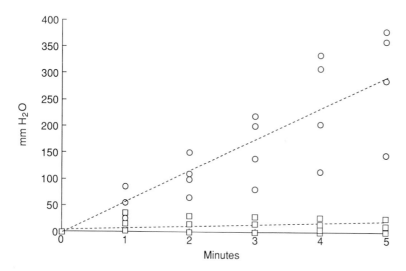

FIGURE 10–2. *Rate of increase of middle ear pressure in children during assisted ventilation with halothane and nitrous oxide in oxygen (circles), compared with the rate of increase in pressure in children breathing halothane in oxygen (squares). (From Casey WF, Drake-Lee AB: Nitrous oxide and middle ear pressure. Anaesthesia 1982; 37:896.)*

cause severe pain or transient hearing impairment, or stimulate vomiting.

During middle ear surgery, until the surgeon begins to close the middle ear, there is no closed space. It has been proposed that nitrous oxide be discontinued approximately 30 minutes before the tympanic membrane graft is positioned.[17] However, others have suggested that if nitrous oxide is discontinued for 5 minutes before the graft is placed, the gas usually does not create a problem for the surgeon.[18] Moreover, packing the middle ear with absorbable gelatin sponges usually prevents deleterious retraction of the graft postoperatively. Because surgeons have their own biases with regard to the intraoperative use of nitrous oxide, the issue should be discussed at the start of the case.

Microsurgery of the middle ear demands a nearly bloodless operative field, because even tiny amounts of blood can obfuscate anatomical landmarks (Table 10–2). During stapedectomy, for example, a blood loss in excess of 1.5 mL may be considered unsatisfactory.[19] Generally, vasoconstriction and minimal blood loss are accomplished by administering epinephrine 1:200,000, either by infiltration or by topical application. The suggested maximal doses of epinephrine with halothane, enflurane, or isoflurane are 2 μg/kg, 4 μg/kg, or 6 μg/kg, respectively.[20] Controlled hypotension is another method that has been advocated by some investigators and clinicians to minimize bleeding. A 15-degree head-up tilt in combination with moderate reductions in blood pressure (85 mmHg systolic) secondary to inhalation anesthetic agents may offer favorable operating conditions. Other methods of inducing hypotension include IV therapy with ganglionic blockers, α- and β-receptor blockers, or direct vasodilators such as sodium nitroprusside. However, these techniques are controversial, and the anesthesiologist must decide for each case if the purported benefits outweigh the potential risks. The topic of drug-induced hypotension is discussed in greater detail at the end of this chapter. Blood loss can also be minimized by using either an argon or a KTP laser for tympanoplasty.

Middle ear surgery often encompasses dissection in the region of the facial nerve. Therefore, periodic checks of facial nerve integrity may be necessary. Although neuromuscular blocking agents can provide skeletal muscle relaxation without complete paralysis (thereby enabling identification of the facial nerve from direct nerve stimulation), many surgeons request that long-acting muscle relaxants (especially if given in a fashion that would produce total paralysis) be avoided during certain otologic procedures.

The superiority of an appropriate volatile inhalation anesthetic for microsurgery of the ear seems obvious. Clearly, volatile anesthetics provide excellent analgesia and akinesia, do not require nitrous oxide or muscle relaxant for their effective use, and if indicated, can induce hypotension.

Stapedectomy

Otosclerosis, characterized by fixation of the footplate of the stapes, is one of the most common causes of conductive hearing loss or deafness in adults. It is inherited as an autosomal dominant with variable penetrance. The stapes footplate becomes increasingly fixed because of encroachment from the abnormal formation of soft, spongy bone. The limited range of motion of the footplate results in delivery of less sound energy to the inner ear; hence, a progressive conductive hearing deficit ensues. Removal of the stapes superstructure, along with partial or complete removal of the footplate, and replacement with a stainless steel or Teflon piston can result in dramatic improvement. Because the utricle and saccule of the membranous labyrinth are less than 1 mm from the footplate, surgical damage to these structures may produce permanent deafness. Some surgeons capitalize on the precision of laser surgery by using either the argon or KTP laser for stapedectomy.

In the United States, stapedectomy is commonly performed under local anesthesia, with the anesthesiologist monitoring the patient appropriately and giving sedation as needed. Having the patient awake allows the surgeon to assess the patient's hearing intraoperatively.

MÉNIÈRE'S DISEASE

Ménière's disease secondary to endolymphatic engorgement is characterized by episodic rotational vertigo, sensorineural hearing loss, and tinnitus. Additional vagal symptoms may accompany the attacks. The condition may

TABLE 10–2. Major Potential Problems During Middle Ear Surgery

Nitrous oxide-induced changes in middle ear pressure
Bleeding
Facial nerve injury

become bilateral in about 50% of patients, and the disease gradually remits as hearing acuity decreases. Most cases can be managed medically with a combination of vestibular sedatives, vasodilators, and diuretics.

Occasionally, nondestructive surgery may be indicated, either to decompress the endolymphatic sac or to divide the vestibular nerve. Ultrasonic therapy may be efficacious also. For patients with severe cases in whom little hearing remains, total labyrinthectomy may be necessary to afford relief from attacks that are perceived as inexorable by the patient.

General anesthesia with a volatile anesthetic agent is commonly administered for labyrinthectomy. Antiemetics are liberally administered perioperatively, and in cases of severe and protracted nausea, the addition of a benzodiazepine to the antiemetic therapy may prove beneficial.

COCHLEAR IMPLANTATION[21, 22]

The clinical use of implantable electronic devices to stimulate the auditory systems of profoundly deaf individuals has been a relatively recent advance. Only a decade ago, a predominant opinion among otolaryngologists was that long-term electrical stimulation of the auditory system was unworkable.

In general terms, the Food and Drug Administration (FDA) has determined that reasonable candidates for cochlear implantation without restriction include (1) those who are healthy, postlinguistically deafened adults; (2) those who are profoundly or totally bilaterally deaf; (3) those who do not benefit from high-power hearing aids; (4) those who have suffered from profound to total sensorineural deafness for a minimum of 12 months (this restriction allows time for spontaneous recovery of hearing); and (5) those who are medically, psychologically, and emotionally stable.

Under specific FDA protocols, both prelinguistically deafened adults and prelinguistically or postlinguistically deafened children may be considered candidates (investigational device exemption stage). More than 30 centers nationwide are performing clinical trials in these groups.

Following initial screening, suitable candidates are evaluated more thoroughly through a multispecialty team approach. Such evaluation includes otologic, audiologic, psychological, speech and language, and radiological assessment. Medical evaluation is essential to rule out ongoing or acute processes as well as to establish the suitability of the temporal bone for electrode implantation.

A variety of implants—single channel or multichannel devices—are available for intracochlear as well as extracochlear use. A popular implant is the Nucleus Mini-22 device. A variety of processing and transmission strategies are available with cochlear implants as well. The Symbion cochlear implant is a percutaneous device in which a biocompatible pedestal is anchored to the skull and extends through the postauricular skin for a hard wire connection. The other internal devices are powered and provided with information through transcutaneous radiofrequency stimulation or magnetic induction. Obviously, techniques of implantation differ in detail from prosthesis to prosthesis.

In addition to electrode failure, the risks of the implant procedure are much the same as those for ear surgery in general: infection, facial paralysis, cerebrospinal fluid drainage, meningitis, and the usual risks of anesthesia. Failure of incisional healing and associated minor infections appear to be the most frequent problems encountered with implant surgery. Anesthesia is generally managed as for middle ear surgery.

Results of cochlear implant stimulation are encouraging. Although an implant does not as yet restore normal hearing, it gives adults an awareness of environmental sounds, improves lipreading, and enables many patients to partially understand speech without the aid of visual cues. Children also acquire improved auditory skills, and many of them expand their speech and language skills. The patient, adult or child, likely to benefit from a cochlear implant is one who became deaf after developing verbal language skills and receives the implant within a few years of the onset of deafness.

GLOMUS TUMORS

The glomus tumor that originates from the tympanic plexus on the medial wall of the middle ear is called a glomus tympanicum tumor and is surgically removed either through the ear canal or through a mastoid exposure. These nonchromaffin-staining epithelioid tumors are histologically similar to the carotid body "glomus bodies."

Glomus jugulare tumors are discussed in detail in Chapter 7.

ACOUSTIC NEUROMA

Acoustic neuroma, a benign neurofibroma of the eighth cranial nerve, originates within the internal auditory meatus, where it can produce erosion and expansion of the auditory canal. Patients typically present with gradual unilateral sensorineural hearing loss. Eventually, ataxia occurs when the tumor has spread to the cerebellopontine angle and when the brain stem is compressed. Acoustic neuromas usually do not cause vertigo.

Combined neurotological surgical management of these cases has resulted in considerably improved morbidity, particularly with respect to facial nerve preservation.[3] Indeed, the widest application of intraoperative electromyography (EMG) has been monitoring and preserving facial nerve function during acoustic neuroma resection.[23, 24] Indwelling fine-wire electrodes are placed preoperatively into the facial muscles (orbicularis oculi, orbicularis oris, mentalis, frontalis, masseter, or temporalis), and preanesthetic recording is used to verify their location. Spontaneous muscle action potentials are recorded continuously intraoperatively, and neurotonic discharges that indicate nerve irritation signal that surgical maneuvers are affecting the facial nerve. These maneuvers may be modified to minimize potential nerve damage. Additionally, to assist localization of the facial nerve during the resection, compound muscle action potentials may be recorded from the fine-wire electrodes in response to direct electrical stimulation of the facial nerve by the surgeon through a hand-held stimulating electrode. These techniques of measuring spontaneous EMG and elicited muscle action potentials are efficacious in preserving facial nerve function, especially with larger acoustic neuromas.

To allow effective assessment of intraoperative EMG, muscle relaxants must be avoided following their initial use to facilitate tracheal intubation. Anesthetic maintenance using a combination of a potent inhalation agent, nitrous oxide, and supplemental doses of IV narcotic are generally preferred. The anesthesiologist must be skilled at assessing anesthetic depth, because immobility without the aid of muscle relaxants must be assured when the surgeon is dissecting delicate structures under the operating microscope.

The prognosis of patients with acoustic neuroma is favorable following successful surgical excision.

CONTROLLED HYPOTENSION

Controlled hypotension is a deliberate attempt by the anesthesiologist to lower a patient's arterial blood pressure during surgery in order to provide improved operating conditions for the surgeon and to reduce the amount of blood loss. In the 1940s, Endeeby[25] showed that 26 of 35 patients studied had significantly less blood loss with a controlled hypotensive technique. However, he also suggested that positioning was more important than the absolute reduction in systolic blood pressure.[25] Although elevating the head 15–30 degrees enhances venous drainage and reduces cerebral venous pressure, elevating the operative field above the level of the heart also increases the risk of venous air embolism.

In controlled hypotension techniques, mean arterial pressures of 50–65 mmHg are usually sought.[26] However, there are two contraindications to controlled hypotension, both involving situations in which lowering the mean arterial pressure to these levels may compromise end-organ function: ischemic heart disease and cerebrovascular disease. Clearly, the "ideal" candidate for this procedure is a young, healthy patient.

Techniques employed to lower blood pressure intraoperatively include deep inhalation anesthesia and IV methods. Halothane had been a popular agent for this purpose because of its ability to effectively decrease arterial pressure. However, this reduction in blood pressure is accompanied by a reduction in stroke volume and cardiac output. In recent years, halothane not surprisingly has lost favor, because isoflurane can lower mean arterial pressure through a reduction in systemic vascular resistance, with little or no change in cardiac index. When using isoflurane, the patient's volume status must be adequate, because reductions in systemic vascular resistance may be pronounced. Furthermore, isoflurane may trigger reflex tachycardia with an attendant increase in myocardial oxygen consumption.

IV agents are currently the most popular means of inducing controlled hypotension. They offer the advantages of easy titration with rapid initiation and termination of effect.

Sodium nitroprusside (SNP) is the most widely used IV agent for controlled hypotension. A smooth muscle dilator, SNP decreases peripheral and pulmonary vascular resistance and can cause a reflex increase in heart rate. Stroke volume is usually increased also. Potential problems with SNP include cyanide toxicity as well as activation of the sympathetic nervous system and renin-angiotensin system. Recent evidence suggests that pretreatment with an angiotensin-converting enzyme inhibitor both decreases the dose of SNP necessary to achieve a given mean arterial pressure and attenuates the rebound hypertensive response that can be seen with discontinuation of the drug.[27]

Nitroglycerin also is used for inducing controlled hypotension. It has no known toxic effects and acts by directly dilating all vascular smooth muscle, with capacitance vessels preferentially dilated. This may lead to a decrease in cardiac output if preload is low.[27] Diastolic and mean arterial pressures generally are higher with nitroglycerin than with SNP.[28] Although SNP decreases the blood pressure more reliably and more rapidly than nitroglycerin, SNP also has a greater tendency to produce rebound hypertension.

Trimethaphan decreases blood pressure through ganglionic blockade, which decreases both arteriolar and venous tone. Moreover, this ganglionic blocker may decrease cardiac output as it attenuates autonomic reflexes.[29] Heart rate increases secondary to parasympathetic ganglionic blockade. The pupillary dilatation that results from blockade of the ciliary ganglion can confuse postoperative neurological evaluation. Trimethaphan decreases cerebral blood flow, yet causes no change in cerebral metabolic rate or oxygen consumption. Hence, it may reduce the availability of oxygen to the brain.[30]

In order to obviate some of the complications of SNP and trimethaphan, some investigators advocate the use of a mixture of 10:1 trimethaphan:SNP.[31, 32] Comparison of the mixture against SNP alone reveals similarly rapid onset, as well as rapid recovery (sometimes difficult to achieve with trimethaphan alone) but with significantly greater reduction in cardiac output than SNP alone.[32] Moreover, because the total dose of SNP is significantly reduced,[31] cyanide toxicity is less likely. It is important, however, to avoid hyperventilation when using combined therapy, because hyperventilation may predispose to deleterious hemodynamic consequences.

Although hydralazine is effective in decreasing mean arterial pressure, it has a slower onset and longer recovery time than SNP. Hence, hydralazine is seldom used intraoperatively.[33]

Adenosine and adenosine triphosphate are naturally occurring substances that act principally on resistance vessels, cause an increase in cardiac output, and do not activate the sympathetic nervous system. They have both rapid onset and rapid termination. Disadvantages include the need for central administration (to avoid peripheral breakdown) and the potential for complete heart block.[34]

Certain subgroups of the prostaglandin family, especially PGE_1, have been suggested as hypotensive agents. PGE_1 appears to be a mild hypotensive agent with minimal systemic side effects, but it may not produce sufficient hypotension in all patients to become clinically useful.[27]

The combined α and β blocker labetalol has been employed for controlled hypotension, usually in combination with an inhalation technique. Its use is limited, however, because of the clinically significant decrease in cardiac output associated with β blockade.[27]

Calcium channel blockers have been used to provide controlled hypotension, but their use is limited because of associated reductions in cardiac output. Calcium channel blockers also cause cerebral vasodilatation and resultant increased intracranial pressure, which may be detrimental.[27] Indeed, some researchers recommend spontaneous ventilation during controlled hypotension to decrease cerebral venous pressure.[27]

The generally accepted safe lower limit for controlled hypotension is a mean arterial pressure of 50–55 mmHg, based on the observation that this reflects the lower limit of cerebral blood flow autoregulation.[27] In addition, end-organ perfusion is compromised in most healthy adults when blood pressure drops below this range. Of course, in patients with long-standing hypertension, coronary artery disease, peripheral vascular disease, or many other abnormalities that compromise end-organ blood supply, the "safe" level of mean arterial pressure is presumably significantly higher.

The actual incidence of complications arising from the use of controlled hypotension is difficult to determine, ranging from 0.24% to 13.3% in various studies. Complicating events range from minor central nervous system changes, including prolonged emergence and dizziness, to cerebral and retinal thromboses, and death.[27]

In summary, controlled hypotension may be instituted by a variety of inhalation or IV methods, but patients must be carefully screened for any evidence of end-organ dysfunction, and their blood pressure must be carefully monitored throughout the procedure.[27] It is unknown whether profound hypotension in addition to the use of potent vasoconstrictors is either necessary or desirable in microsurgical procedures of the ear.[18] Indeed, Eltringham and colleagues[35] found no correlation with the degree of hypotension deliberately induced and the surgeon's assessment of the adequacy of surgical conditions.

LOCAL ANESTHESIA

Local anesthesia is an attractive option for surgical procedures involving the ear because of the superficial nature of many of the procedures, and because it allows the surgeon to assess auditory acuity intraoperatively. Ear surgery under local anesthesia can be vexing for the patient, however, especially if manipulation near the labyrinth triggers dizziness, nausea, or vomiting. In this setting, dizziness or nausea can have a particularly protracted course, lasting several hours.

ANATOMICAL CONSIDERATIONS

The success of local anesthesia depends on a knowledge of the innervation of the ear and of the anatomical relationships involved. Four major nerves and their branches supply sensory innervation to the ear: the great auricular (C_2 and C_3), the mandibular (a branch of cranial nerve V), the vagus (cranial X), and the glossopharyngeal (cranial nerve IX).

The auricle is primarily innervated by the great auricular nerve, which supplies the medial aspect of the auricle by a posterior branch and supplies the lower and peripheral part of the lateral aspect of the auricle by an anterior branch. The upper anterior part of the lateral aspect is supplied by the auriculotemporal nerve, a branch of the mandibular nerve. The concha is supplied by the auricular branch of the vagus nerve, emerging through the tympanomastoid fissure, anterior to the mastoid process and posterior to the external auditory meatus.

The external auditory meatus is supplied by the auriculotemporal nerve and by the auricular branches of the vagus nerve. The tympanic cavity is innervated by the tympanic nerve, a branch of the glossopharyngeal nerve.

LOCAL ANESTHETIC TECHNIQUES FOR SPECIFIC PROCEDURES

Myringotomy and Insertion of Tympanotomy Tubes

Lidocaine 1% with 1:200,000 epinephrine is injected into the posterior portion of the meatus, lateral to the bony-cartilaginous juncture. The usual volume administered is 0.5 mL. An additional 0.25 mL of the lidocaine-epinephrine solution is injected into each of three areas of the meatus: superiorly, inferiorly, and anteriorly. An additional 0.2 mL of lidocaine injected superiorly and 0.2 mL injected inferiorly at points 5 mm lateral to the margin of the tympanic membrane can enhance the local anesthesia block (Fig. 10–3).

Simple paracentesis can be performed after two or three metered spray doses of 10% lidocaine are allowed to spread over the tympanic membrane. Usually, adequate analgesia results within 3–5 minutes. If possible, the spray initially should be directed superiorly and allowed to run down over the eardrum, in order to obviate the discomfort produced when cold spray is placed directly on the eardrum.

Middle Ear Surgery: Mastoidectomy, Stapedectomy, and Tympanoplasty

For middle ear surgery, the great auricular nerve must be anesthetized. This is accomplished by injecting 1–2 mL of lidocaine (0.5–1.0% with 1:200,000 epinephrine) into multiple sites over the mastoid process (Fig. 10–4). The auricular branch is blocked by injection of 2–3 mL of lidocaine, partly into the skin along the floor of the auditory canal and partly into the periosteum on the anterior mastoid process.

The auriculotemporal nerve must be anesthetized also, especially for radical mastoidectomy procedures (Fig. 10–5). Two milliliters of 0.5–1% lidocaine with 1:200,000 epinephrine are injected into the bony-cartilaginous junction of the anterior auditory canal, and the skin and periosteum of the incisura terminalis auris over the auditory canal in the anterior portion of the ear is infiltrated. Surface analgesia may be produced by placing a few drops of 10% cocaine solution directly into the external auditory canal. The tympanic membrane is usually destroyed in patients requiring middle ear surgery, and the solution enters the tympanic canal and anesthetizes the mucous membrane lining this cavity.

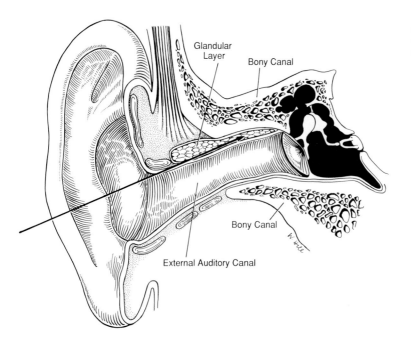

FIGURE 10–3. Injection for analgesia of the tympanic membrane and cavity.

POSTOPERATIVE MANAGEMENT

Nausea and dizziness are troublesome postoperative problems in patients undergoing middle or inner ear surgery. Avoidance of opioids as well as prophylactic administration of antiemetics, such as droperidol or promethazine, are said to be helpful.[36, 37] Antiemetics probably should be prescribed routinely for the first 24 hours after stapedectomy. Operations on the labyrinth commonly require an antiemetic for even longer periods. If the patient has associated agitation, supplementation of antiemetic therapy with a benzodiazepine is helpful in sedating the patient and minimizing

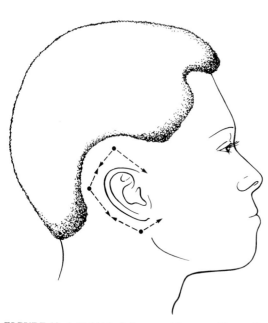

FIGURE 10–4. Field block for mastoidectomy. The needle is introduced via wheals through the dots and then is advanced subcutaneously in the direction of the arrows.

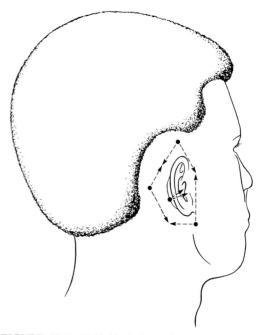

FIGURE 10–5. Field block for radical mastoidectomy. The needle is introduced via wheals through the dots and then is advanced subcutaneously in the direction of the arrows. Then the external auditory canal is injected.

superfluous movement that can exacerbate dizziness and nausea. In addition to causing nausea and dizziness, disturbances of the labyrinth may produce hypotension also.

REFERENCES

1. Morrison JD, Mirakhur RK, Craig HJL: Anesthesia for Eye, Ear, Nose and Throat Surgery, 2nd ed. London, Churchill Livingstone, 1985, pp 121–141.
2. Ellis H, McLarty M: Anatomy for Anaesthetists, 2nd ed. Philadelphia, F. A. Davis, 1968, pp 278–286.
3. Maw AR, O'Higgins JW: Diseases of the ear. In Zorab JSM (ed): Surgery for Anaesthetists. Oxford, Blackwell Scientific Publications, 1988, pp 475–483.
4. Klein JO: Middle ear disease in children. Hosp Pract 1976; 11:45.
5. Paradise JL: Otitis media in infants and children. Pediatrics 1980; 65:917.
6. Sculerati N, Ledesma-Medina J, Finegold DN, Stool SE: Otitis media and hearing loss in Turner syndrome. Arch Otolaryngol Head Neck Surg 1990; 116:704–707.
7. Gates GA, Avery CA, Prihoda TJ, Cooper JC: Effectiveness of adenoidectomy and tympanostomy tubes in the treatment of chronic otitis media with effusion. N Engl J Med 1987; 317:1444–1451.
8. Markowitz-Spence L, Brodsky L, Syed N, et al: Anesthetic complications of tympanotomy tube placement in children. Arch Otolaryngol Head Neck Surg 1990; 116:809–812.
9. Patterson ME, Bartlett PC: Hearing impairment caused by intratympanic pressure changes during general anesthesia. Laryngoscope 1976; 86:399–404.
10. Matz GL, Rattenborg CG, Holaday DA: Effects of nitrous oxide on middle ear pressure. Anesthesiology 1967; 28:948–950.
11. Casey WF, Drake-Lee AB: Nitrous oxide and middle ear pressure. Anaesthesia 1982; 37:896–900.
12. Davis I, Moore JRM, Lahiri SK: Nitrous oxide and the middle ear. Anaesthesia 1979; 34:147–151.
13. O'Neill G: Middle ear pressure measurements during nitrous oxide anaesthesia. Clin Otolaryngol 1980; 5:355.
14. Shaw JO, Stark EW, Gannaway SD: The influence of nitrous oxide anaesthesia on middle ear fluid. J Laryngol Otol 1978; 92:131–135.
15. Owens WD, Gustave F, Sclaroff A: Tympanic membrane rupture with nitrous oxide anesthesia. Anesth Analg 1978; 57:283–286.
16. Perreault L, Normandin N, Plamondon L, et al: Tympanic membrane rupture after anesthesia with nitrous oxide. Anesthesiology 1982; 57:325–326.
17. Jahrsdoerfer RA: Anesthesia in otologic surgery. Otolaryngol Clin North Am 1981; 14:699–704.
18. Feinstein R, Owens WD: Anesthesia for ENT. In Barash PG, Cullen BF, Stoelting RK (eds): Clinical Anesthesia. Philadelphia, J. B. Lippincott, 1989, pp 1067–1078.
19. Deacock AR: Aspects of anaesthesia for middle ear

surgery and blood loss during stapedectomy. Proc R Soc Med 1971; 64:44.
20. Johnston RR, Eger EI, Wilson C: A comparative interaction of epinephrine with enflurane, isoflurane, and halothane in man. Anesth Analg 1976; 55:709.
21. Balkany T: Cochlear implants. In Pillsbury HC, Goldsmith MM (eds): Operative Challenges in Otolaryngology Head and Neck Surgery. Chicago, Year Book Medical Publishers, 1990, pp 136–138.
22. Luxford WM, House WF: Cochlear implants. In Pillsbury HC, Goldsmith MM (eds): Operative Challenges in Otolaryngology Head and Neck Surgery. Chicago, Year Book Medical Publishers, 1990, pp 139–145.
23. Prass RL, Luders H: Acoustic (loudspeaker) facial electromyographic monitoring: Part 1. Neurosurgery 1986; 19:392.
24. Harner SG, Daube JR, Ebersold MJ, et al: Improved preservation of facial nerve function with use of electrical monitoring during removal of acoustic neuromas. Mayo Clin Proc 1987; 62:92.
25. Endeeby GEN: Controlled circulation with hypotension and posture to reduce bleeding in surgery: Preliminary results with pentamethonium iodide. Lancet 1950; 1:1145.
26. Gardner WJ: The control of bleeding during operation by induced hypotension. JAMA 1946; 132:572.
27. Miller ED Jr: Deliberate hypotension. In Miller RD (ed). Anesthesia, 3rd ed. New York, Churchill Livingstone, 1990, pp 1347–1367.
28. Lagerkronser M: Cardiovascular effects of nitroglycerin as a hypotensive agent in cerebral aneurysm surgery. Acta Anaesth Scand 1982; 26:453.
29. Fahmy NR: Nitroglycerin as a hypotensive drug during general anesthesia. Anesthesiology 1978; 49:17.
30. Knight PR, Lane GA, Hensinger RN, et al: Catecholamine and renin-angiotensin response during hypotensive anesthesia induced by sodium nitroprusside or trimethaphan camsylate. Anesthesiology 1983; 59:248.
31. Wildsmith JAQ, Sinclair CJ, Thorn J, et al: Hemodynamic effects of induced hypotension with a nitroprusside-trimethaphan mixture. Br J Anaesth 1983; 55:381.
32. Miller R, Toth C, Silva DA, et al: Nitroprusside versus a nitroprusside-trimethaphan mixture: A comparison of dosage requirements and hemodynamic effects during induced hypotension for neurosurgery. Mt Sinai J Med 1987; 54:308.
33. James J, Bedford RF: Hydralazine for controlled hypotension during neurosurgical operations. Anesth Analg 1982; 61:1016.
34. Belardinelli L, Belloni FL, Rubio R, et al: Atrioventricular conduction disturbances during hypoxia: Possible role of adenosine in rabbit and guinea pig heart. Circ Res 1980; 47:684.
35. Eltringham RJ, Young PN, Fairbairn MD, et al: Hypotensive anaesthesia for microsurgery of the middle ear. A comparison between enflurane and halothane. Anaesthesia 1982; 37:1028.
36. Palazzo MGA, Strunin L: Anaesthesia and emesis. I. Etiology. Can Anaesth Soc J 1984; 31:178.
37. Palazzo MGA, Strunin L: Anaesthesia and emesis. II. Prevention and management. Can Anaesth Soc J 1984; 31:407.

Anesthesia for Outpatient Ear, Nose, and Throat Procedures

_____ **Mary M. Stenger** _____

Over the past several years there has been a dramatic increase in the demand for outpatient surgery. Its many advantages for the appropriately selected patient include decreased costs, less risk of infection, avoidance of the often impersonal atmosphere associated with overnight hospitalization, and less time away from work.[1] For children undergoing outpatient surgery, there are additional benefits. Parents are actively involved with their child's care, and the child's separation from parents and home is minimized, so behavioral disturbances associated with separation and hospitalization are reduced.[2] For the anesthesiologist, however, there are disadvantages to outpatient surgery, including less time for establishing rapport with the patient, less certainty about the patient's NPO (nothing per os) status, and probably most importantly, less time for observation of postoperative complications.

There are many ear, nose, and throat (ENT) procedures particularly well suited to an outpatient setting. In determining the appropriateness of a given surgical procedure to be performed in such a setting, the type of procedure should be considered, as well as the medical condition of the patient, the reliability of the patient, and the quality and proximity of postoperative care.

APPROPRIATE SURGICAL PROCEDURES

The types of ENT procedures that are well suited to outpatient surgery include most oto-

logic, nasal, and sinus procedures; some superficial procedures of the neck; many oral and laryngeal operations; bronchoscopy; and several plastic surgical procedures. There should be no expectation of surgical complications, no need for special postoperative nursing care, and no major blood loss or anticipated need for blood transfusions. The patient should not have such severe postoperative pain that oral pain medications are inadequate. There has been no clearly defined limit of the duration of surgery for the outpatient, because the length of anesthesia has not been shown to affect the length of the recovery period.[3] From an anesthetic viewpoint, almost any procedure not requiring admission for surgical reasons can be performed as an outpatient procedure.[4]

Intrinsic to outpatient ENT surgery are several special concerns.[5] Because of the extensive vascularity of the head and neck, postoperative bleeding is always a possibility. Manipulation or obstruction of venous drainage around the airway may lead to edema and airway obstruction. Dysphagia after an oral or esophageal procedure may cause the patient to become dehydrated. Finally, nausea and vomiting may follow ENT procedures associated with blood accumulation in the stomach or with manipulation of the inner ear.

A study by Natof reviewed the complications following ambulatory surgery in 13,433 patients.[6] In general, the low complication rate confirmed the safety of outpatient surgery. However, postoperative hemorrhage that required special treatment and care was the most frequent of the serious complications (74 cases of hemorrhage out of 106 total complications), and ENT procedures constituted a majority of the cases of hemorrhage (47 out of 74 total cases of hemorrhage).

PATIENT SELECTION

The patient population appropriate for outpatient surgery consists of American Society of Anesthesiologists (ASA) class I and II and, in some cases, class III patients. To be acceptable, class III patients must be medically stable. Often, there is some other consideration, such as risk for hospital-acquired infection in the immunosuppressed patient, that favors outpatient surgery. Natof's study[6] showed no statistical difference in the complication rate of ASA III patients compared with ASA I and II patients.

Outpatients must have the same preoperative assessment as inpatients with a similar medical profile and undergoing the same procedure. This includes a complete history and physical examination and appropriate laboratory studies. There are no absolute standards for obtaining preoperative laboratory data, and decisions to obtain laboratory tests should be based on individual considerations. Levin[7] proposes the following guidelines:

Infants and children—no laboratory tests necessary for elective surgery if the patient is healthy and without risk factors (prematurity, heart disease, blood disease).

Adults—hemoglobin for all females and all males over 40, electrocardiogram (ECG) for all patients over 40, and chest radiograph for all patients older than 60.

Any finding on history or clinical examination of underlying disease would necessitate further work-up.

Because bleeding is one of the major complications in ENT surgery and because 80% of unexpected bleeding complications during surgery are caused by the use of aspirin, a bleeding time should probably be obtained in any patient who has ingested aspirin within 5 days.[8] Moreover, physicians should counsel their patients to avoid taking aspirin for 1 week prior to elective surgery.

There is some controversy regarding the age limit of children for outpatient procedures. Some anesthesiologists accept any healthy infant for outpatient procedures, whereas others accept only infants older than 6 months. An infant born prematurely has special problems and should not be operated on in an outpatient setting[2] until it has reached a postconceptual age of 60 weeks. Premature infants have a 25% incidence of apnea within the first 12 hours postoperatively. Such apnea is probably secondary to immature brain stem function with abnormal responses to hypercapnia and hypoxia.[9] Residual anesthetic drugs may further depress ventilatory responses. The premature infant has significant impairment of respiratory function until at least 1 year of age,[10] and the incidence of aspiration may be higher because of immature airway reflexes. Other problems of prematurity include bronchopulmonary dysplasia, hypothermia, hypoglycemia, retrolental fibroplasia, and problems with oxygen transport associated with anemia and hemoglobin F.

OTHER CONSIDERATIONS

SOCIOLOGICAL CONCERNS

The patient must have a responsible person accompany him or her home, and distances involved should not be excessive. An appropriate facility for transfer of the patient should be available in the event of an intraoperative or postoperative complication. Reliability is also important in patient selection. The patient must be able to understand and comply with instructions. A study by Malins demonstrated that patients often fail to remember or comply with instructions given.[11] When only verbal instructions were given regarding driving, alcohol consumption, or the necessity of having a person accompany them after the operation, 77–95% of patients failed to remember the instruction. Recall dramatically improved when both written and verbal instructions were given. However, up to 20% of patients still failed to comply with instructions given both verbally and in writing.

MINIMIZING POSTOPERATIVE COMPLICATIONS

The incidence of minor postoperative problems can be minimized to assure the patient's readiness to return home after an outpatient surgical procedure. Some outpatients expect to feel completely well after their surgical procedures, and thus a headache, dizziness, or a sore throat might concern them.[12] If the patient understands that these symptoms are short-lived, the perceived severity may be decreased. Nausea and vomiting may be minimized by avoiding inflation of the stomach with air, by avoiding postoperative narcotics, by carefully suctioning blood from the stomach and posterior pharynx, and by administering small doses of an antiemetic, such as droperidol. Considering the nature of the surgery, a sore throat after ENT procedures may be unavoidable. Gentle laryngoscopy, careful suctioning, and minimal manipulation of the head and neck while a patient is intubated may decrease the incidence of a sore throat. Muscle pain can be minimized by careful intraoperative positioning, use of nondepolarizing muscle relaxants, or prevention of succinylcholine-induced skeletal muscle fasciculations with d-tubocurarine pretreatment.[13] However, no single method of prophylaxis can reliably prevent postoperative myalgias.

Strict discharge criteria must be followed to minimize postoperative problems. The patient's vital signs must be stable, and there must be no evidence of bleeding or breathing problems. Pain should be controlled by oral medications, and there should be no significant nausea or vomiting. The patient should be able to tolerate clear liquids and should be able to sit and stand. The patient's condition should be evaluated prior to discharge by an anesthesiologist. The patient should be given lucid, written instructions for postoperative care, including how to contact the anesthesiologist or surgeon if problems arise. Up to 1 week may be required for full mental recovery following general anesthesia. Therefore, the patient also should be instructed to avoid making major decisions, performing complicated tasks, or taking drugs that may potentiate the effects of anesthetics given.[14]

INDICATIONS FOR CANCELLATION

Overall, the cancellation rate for outpatient surgery is approximately 0.7%. Usual reasons for cancellation include an upper respiratory infection, recent food ingestion, or a decision that the surgery is no longer indicated.[15] In pediatric patients, cancellation rates are usually higher because of childhood fevers, diarrhea, and anemia, as well as upper respiratory infections and inappropriate NPO status. As with any elective case, surgery should be postponed or cancelled if the patient ate recently. Because overnight fasting in children can cause asymptomatic hypoglycemia in up to 30% of

pediatric patients, young children should be allowed to drink clear liquids up to 4 hours preoperatively.[2, 16] The child's NPO status is often difficult to ascertain, and the anesthesiologist must emphasize to the parents the importance of NPO orders, as well as the necessity of keeping a watchful eye on the hungry child the morning of surgery.

Cancellation of surgery because of an upper respiratory infection remains a subject of controversy. Viral respiratory infections have been shown to increase airflow obstruction for up to 5 weeks, decrease diffusing capacity of carbon monoxide, and decrease respiratory mechanisms for clearing bacteria.[17–19] Clinically, however, it has never been shown convincingly that postponement of surgery decreases the likelihood of complications in otherwise normal patients. A retrospective study by Tait showed no increase in perioperative complications associated with an uncomplicated upper respiratory infection.[20] His data suggested that there may be increased airway reactivity in the postinfection stage, however, because there was a small increase in perioperative complications in patients who had an upper respiratory infection within 2 weeks of surgery. McGill and colleagues[21] believe that surgery should be postponed if a child has a specific history of upper respiratory infection symptoms in the previous weeks; if doubt exists on the basis of history or physical examination regarding the resolution of an upper respiratory infection, they suggest that posteroanterior and lateral chest films should be obtained. However, a more recent study from Children's Hospital of Philadelphia concluded that the presence of an active or recent (within 6 weeks) upper respiratory infection in a healthy child undergoing elective superficial surgery has little effect on the occurrence of perioperative anesthetic desaturation, laryngospasm, bronchospasm, and croup.[22]

The decision to proceed with surgery must be individualized. The urgency of the surgery, as well as the likelihood that the patient will continue to have upper respiratory infection-like symptoms until surgery is accomplished (e.g., in a patient to undergo tympanostomy, adenoidectomy, or tonsillectomy) must be considered. The severity of the symptoms and their likelihood of compromising surgical results may influence the anesthesiologist's thinking. Certainly, if a patient has any underlying pulmonary disease or is a smoker, surgery should be postponed if he or she has an upper respiratory infection to avoid compounding any respiratory problems. If surgery does proceed, instrumentation of the airway should be avoided, or a smaller endotracheal tube than usual should be used. Adequate IV hydration should be provided to loosen upper respiratory secretions and to humidify inspired gases. Because an upper respiratory infection increases the work of breathing, controlled ventilation may be necessary in children.[23] If surgery is postponed, the little data available suggest that it should be postponed 5–6 weeks.

ANESTHETIC MANAGEMENT

PREMEDICATION

In general, most outpatients do not require premedication. The concern with premedication is that it will prolong the patient's outpatient stay. However, many combinations of drugs have been used successfully, and it has been shown that premedication with meperidine and atropine does not prolong recovery to street fitness after outpatient surgery.[24]

Premedication is usually not necessary in children for outpatient surgery. In the pediatric population, delayed recovery may follow the use of narcotics, hypnotics, and other sedative drugs.[25] Children may find the route of administration of a premedication unacceptable. Pills or liquids may be hard to swallow, and an intramuscular (IM) injection may seem like an assault to the child. Rectal methohexital may be difficult to administer in the uncooperative child and may prolong recovery times slightly.[26]

However, premedication may be useful in the anxious, uncooperative child, the child who undergoes multiple surgical procedures, or the mentally retarded child. Fentanyl lollipops[27] and intranasal ketamine[28] or midazolam have been used successfully as premedications in children.

Desjardins and associates,[29] studying premedication in children undergoing day-care surgery, compared groups receiving hydroxyzine 0.5 mg/kg, promethazine 0.5 mg/kg, diazepam 0.1 mg/kg, and a placebo. Observations included the patient's emotional state on arrival, quality of induction, complications, time for emergence, and requirements for analgesia. There was no significant difference in any of the factors studied. The authors concluded that children undergoing operations on an outpatient basis should not receive pharmacological premedication, not because of

overwhelming risk from its use, but because of the absence of benefit.

Premedication with an anticholinergic agent may be indicated but usually can be given intravenously (IV) or IM after induction. Atropine or glycopyrrolate can be used to block vagal reflexes. Atropine causes more tachycardia than glycopyrrolate and also crosses the blood-brain barrier, which may cause undesirable central nervous system effects in the outpatient. Glycopyrrolate has the advantages of causing less tachycardia, not crossing the blood-brain barrier, and also providing a more intense and prolonged antisialagogic effect.

Despite NPO status, the outpatient undergoing surgery has been shown to have a higher gastric volume then the inpatient.[30] One may consider premedication to decrease gastric volume and acidity and, thus, decrease the likelihood of aspiration pneumonitis. Cimetidine is a competitive H_2 receptor antagonist that blocks secretion of hydrogen ions by gastric parietal cells. Metoclopramide is a dopamine antagonist and increases lower esophageal sphincter tone and accelerates gastric emptying by increasing gastrointestinal motility. Solanki and coworkers[31] showed that this combination of drugs when given IV 30 minutes preoperatively provides greater protection against aspiration pneumonitis than either drug does alone. Ranitidine, which has the same clinical uses as cimetidine but is five to eight times more potent in antagonizing hydrogen-ion secretion by gastric parietal cells, may be chosen instead of cimetidine, because side effects may be less likely with ranitidine.[32, 33] Alternatively, a nonparticulate antacid, such as sodium citrate, can be given to neutralize acidity,[34] although it may slightly increase gastric volume, and some patients complain that it causes nausea and vomiting. Although not indicated in every patient, premedication with an H_2 receptor antagonist and metoclopramide or a nonparticulate antacid should be strongly considered in the patient at risk for aspiration, including the patient undergoing general anesthesia by mask.[35]

MONITORING

The fact that the procedure is being performed on an outpatient basis is no reason to compromise the monitoring of the ENT patient. All of the risks inherent to anesthesia are present, and certain monitoring procedures should be provided,[36] including a blood pressure cuff, ECG, oxygen analyzer, and temperature probe. Because often in ENT surgery the surgeon and the anesthesiologist share the airway or it is difficult to obtain access to the airway, continuous monitoring of ventilation must be maintained using an esophageal or precordial stethoscope. Monitoring of end-tidal carbon dioxide, if available, is also highly desirable. In addition, continuous determination of oxygen saturation by a noninvasive pulse oximeter should be used for all operations.

ANESTHETIC TECHNIQUES

Anesthetic techniques appropriate for outpatient ENT procedures include general anesthesia (inhalation agents, nitrous/narcotic and dissociative techniques), regional anesthesia, and local anesthesia with sedation. The choice of anesthesia is based on the type and extent of surgery, the patient's characteristics and ability to cooperate, and the preferences of the surgeon. Some surgeons prefer to provide anesthesia themselves, mostly during simple procedures performed under local anesthesia in which the surgeon or assistant is able to monitor the patient adequately. However, deaths have occurred in outpatient surgical settings when patients were not adequately monitored or the airway was not properly managed. Obviously, the heavy-handed, "cookbook" approaches to "anesthesia without an anesthesiologist" that occasionally appear in journals[37, 38] should be assiduously avoided.

Selected surgical procedures can be performed safely in an office surgical setting only if personnel trained in the maintenance and monitoring of the airway are available. This point is reinforced by reviewing data from arbitration panels and insurance companies regarding the types of situations involving significant liability awards.[39] The majority of involved patients were healthy preoperatively and were undergoing relatively minor procedures. The most common injuries were brain damage or death, and the most common cause of injury was inability to secure an airway or to maintain adequate ventilation.

Local Anesthesia

Local anesthetic infiltration supplemented by IV sedation is often sufficient for many ENT and plastic surgery procedures in the cooperative patient. Many different techniques have been used successfully, and the best combination of local anesthetic and sedative agents

depends on the extent and duration of the surgery, the patient's level of anxiety and pain threshold, and the interactions of the agents used.

Local anesthetic infiltration should be performed carefully, because surgical dissection can often be facilitated by injection in the proper planes. The minimum amount of local anesthesia sufficient to produce adequate surgical anesthesia should be used, with careful attention given to maximum doses. The addition of epinephrine to the local anesthetic solution causes vasoconstriction and a less bloody surgical field and also slows uptake of the local anesthetic, decreasing the likelihood of systemic toxicity and prolonging the duration of the effect. Local anesthetic solutions combined with epinephrine 1:200,000 provide maximally effective vasoconstriction with the fewest systemic effects.

Often cocaine is used topically on the mucosa as an anesthetic and vasoconstrictor. Cocaine is used in concentrations between 4% and 10% with the maximum safe dose of 200 mg to be used at one time in an adult. Cocaine sensitizes various organs to the effects of directly acting catecholamines. It prevents reuptake of released norepinephrine at the peripheral nerve endings and also prevents uptake of exogenously administered epinephrine. Thus, the possibility exists for drug interactions when cocaine is used with other drugs that affect the adrenergic receptor.[40] Methyldopa, for example, interferes with the synthesis of catecholamines, leading to a depletion of norepinephrine. This causes increased sensitivity of the adrenergic receptor to catecholamines. Tricyclic antidepressants, such as imipramine and amitriptyline, block norepinephrine uptake. Reserpine interferes with interneuronal storage of catecholamines, and monoamine oxidase inhibitors lead to the accumulation of norepinephrine. The use of cocaine should be avoided in patients taking these drugs. The mixing of cocaine and epinephrine to provide anesthesia and enhanced vasoconstriction had been advocated in the past. However, there is no evidence that the addition of epinephrine to cocaine leads to less bleeding at the surgical site,[40] and this practice is potentially dangerous, resulting in hypertension and cardiac dysrhythmias.

Regional Anesthesia

Regional anesthesia can be an excellent alternative to general anesthesia for certain ENT procedures in the appropriately selected patient. Bridenbaugh outlines the following potential advantages especially pertinent in the outpatient[41]:

1. The nausea and vomiting seen with general anesthesia are infrequent following nerve block anesthesia.
2. Nerve block minimizes the danger of aspiration in patients who may have a full stomach.
3. Postanesthesia hospital recovery time is less than with general anesthesia.
4. Certain regional block techniques provide prolonged local anesthesia and thus delay the need for analgesics until the patient has returned home.

Regional techniques are certainly not appropriate for every patient and every procedure. The patient must be amenable to the technique. An overly anxious patient may require so much sedation that the benefits of a regional block are negated. The surgeon, too, must be willing to work with the anesthesiologist, allowing a few minutes for the block to take effect. Moreover, the surgeon should apply gentle surgical techniques, realizing the patient does perceive pressure.

The spectrum of ENT procedures performed under regional anesthesia is somewhat more limited than in other specialties, because the airway must be secured in many ENT procedures. Nevertheless, some procedures are well suited to regional block. Among the most frequently used blocks for outpatient ENT surgery are superficial and deep cervical blocks; mental, mandibular, and scalp blocks; and superior laryngeal nerve blocks. (Various nerve blocks for ENT surgery are discussed in Chapter 2.)

General Anesthesia

In many situations, general anesthesia may be appropriate for outpatient ENT procedures. No single technique of anesthesia has been shown to be superior. All inhalation techniques and IV drugs appropriate for inpatients can be used successfully in outpatients.[42] The challenge to the anesthesiologist is in combining the advantages of techniques and drugs to provide a safe, smooth induction; maintenance of light but sufficient anesthesia; and prompt recovery for discharge.[43]

General anesthesia can be performed either by mask or with an endotracheal tube in place. Some ENT procedures may require an endotracheal tube; concern about postintubation croup in the child should not preclude the use of an endotracheal tube. Smith[44] reported a 5% incidence of postintubation croup in pediatric patients, although most responded well to treatment, and only one fourth of those patients required an overnight admission. With careful laryngoscopy, minimal movement of the head, and an air leak around the endotracheal tube during the application of 20 cm H_2O positive pressure, traumatic croup should be avoided. If it does occur, it should appear within 1–2 hours after extubation at the latest, and usually within 30 minutes. This is early enough to allow for identification and treatment before discharge from an outpatient surgery setting.

The properties of nitrous oxide (N_2O) make it an attractive agent for outpatient surgery. N_2O has a slightly sweet odor and is relatively nonthreatening to the child during an inhalation induction. Speed of induction can be enhanced by the poor solubility of N_2O as well as the principles of concentration effect and the second gas effect. Its use can significantly decrease maintenance requirements for other inhalation agents. Some have suggested that N_2O may be associated with an increased incidence of nausea and vomiting, and this may delay discharge. However, Kortilla and colleagues[45] showed that omission of N_2O did not decrease the incidence or severity of emetic symptoms.

Halothane is often used in pediatric anesthesia to facilitate a smooth, relatively well-tolerated mask induction. It has an intermediate blood-gas solubility but a high potency. Therefore, induction is rapid, especially when used with N_2O. Rapid induction of anesthesia can also be achieved with both isoflurane and enflurane, although they elicit a higher incidence of breathholding and coughing than halothane. These agents provide muscle relaxation and potentiate the effects of nondepolarizing muscle relaxants, thus allowing the use of smaller amounts intraoperatively.

Different inhalation anesthetics involve different recovery times; recovery time is faster with enflurane than with halothane.[46] In short procedures there is no difference in recovery time between enflurane and isoflurane. However, in procedures longer than 90 minutes, recovery time is significantly longer for enflurane.[47, 48] Agents such as I653, now under development, may provide more rapid recovery than agents currently used and thus be especially useful in the outpatient setting.[43]

ENT surgeons often utilize the vasoconstrictive properties of epinephrine in lidocaine during general anesthesia. The anesthesiologist must be aware of the interaction of epinephrine with inhaled anesthetics and the propensity to produce premature ventricular extrasystoles. Johnston and associates[49] calculated the epinephrine dose producing ventricular irritability in 50% of patients anesthetized with halogenated agents (ED_{50}). An ED_{50} of 2.1 μg/kg for halothane, 6.7 μg/kg for isoflurane, and 10.9 μg/kg for enflurane was demonstrated, with a slight protective effect provided by the lidocaine injected with the epinephrine. The surgeon and the anesthesiologist must communicate about the maximal acceptable dose of epinephrine to avoid ventricular irritability.

Use of a balanced technique of anesthesia with N_2O, narcotics, and a muscle relaxant versus an inhalation technique for the outpatient has been a subject of debate. The main concerns are those of rapidity of recovery and incidence of postoperative nausea and vomiting. Data regarding recovery times are inconsistent, and differences between the techniques are probably negligible. However, studies have shown a significant increase in nausea and vomiting in the group receiving narcotic versus isoflurane for anesthesia.[50, 51] Also, narcotic-based anesthetics are less controllable when given as an IV bolus than are inhalation agents. A solution to this problem is the use of continuous infusion of narcotic agents. This technique may significantly decrease the drug dosage requirement and shorten the recovery time.[52] Fentanyl, sufentanil, and alfentanil have been used extensively and successfully in the outpatient setting. Recently, the sedative-hypnotic propofol, administered as a continuous infusion, has been used to advantage in ambulatory surgery.

A variety of IV induction agents can be employed in an outpatient setting. The use of an IV induction agent may delay recovery compared to recovery with a volatile anesthetic alone. However, IV induction is still preferred by most patients and anesthesiologists.[45] Sodium thiopental remains the most widely used IV induction agent, partly because of its lack of side effects. Its hypnotic effect is terminated by rapid redistribution. However, its long elimination half-life may lead to prolonged recovery if it is given in large or repeated doses. Methohexital can be used as an alternative to thiopental. It has as rapid a redistribution and recovery time as thiopental but a slower elim-

ination half-life. Disadvantages include occasional pain on injection and myoclonic muscle movements.

Midazolam, etomidate, ketamine, and propofol have been used successfully for induction in an outpatient setting.[53] Each has its unique advantages and disadvantages, but each can be used for the appropriately selected patient.

Muscle relaxants are frequently required in ENT surgery, primarily to assure an absolutely motionless field (e.g., in laser surgery or other delicate microscopic surgery). Generally, the short-acting nondepolarizing agents (e.g., vecuronium, atracurium) are used, although for a short procedure a succinylcholine drip may be preferable. If succinylcholine is to be used to facilitate intubation of the trachea, many advocate pretreatment with a nondepolarizing agent in an attempt to decrease the likelihood of postoperative myalgias from succinylcholine-induced fasciculations.[13]

In most cases, prophylactic administration of an antiemetic is unjustified, because the incidence of vomiting is generally low, and a large percentage of postoperative vomiting occurs once at emergence and does not recur. Antiemetics are not innocuous, and their use should be reserved for those patients needing specific therapy; prophylactically in the case of a patient likely to become nauseated; or when nausea and vomiting could interfere with delicate surgical work or endanger the patient. IV droperidol is an effective and long-lasting antiemetic.[54] Some investigators have shown no increase in postoperative sedation with doses less than 1.25 mg of droperidol, although others have shown prolonged sleepiness with similar or larger doses.[55] Despite reports claiming a longer recovery time, in the course of an ENT procedure many situations that warrant the use of an antiemetic may arise, and droperidol in small doses should be the drug of choice.

SPECIFIC SURGICAL PROCEDURES

TYMPANOSTOMY AND MIDDLE EAR OPERATIONS

The outpatient surgical center is ideal for the placement of tympanostomy tubes. Most often, the procedure lasts less than 15 minutes. In children, anesthesia can be induced with halothane and N_2O and spontaneous ventilation occur. No IV drugs are needed for the routine case, and atropine is given IM if needed. In the cooperative adult, the external auditory canal can be injected in four quadrants with lidocaine with epinephrine, which provides adequate anesthesia.

Tympanoplasty for the closure of a chronic perforation can be performed through a transcanal procedure or posterior auricular approach. A transcanal procedure with local anesthetic infiltration is sufficient for a small perforation. A small piece of temporalis fascia is harvested from the posterior auricular area, placed over the perforation, and held in place with absorbable gelatin sponges. A large perforation requires more extensive surgery and a postauricular approach. General anesthesia is usually required, because the surgery tends to be longer; involves periosteum, which may be difficult to anesthetize; and requires a microscope and an absolutely motionless surgical field.

The use of N_2O for middle ear surgery is controversial. Tympanic membrane rupture has occurred in patients having N_2O anesthesia.[56] Because of the high blood-gas partition coefficient of N_2O compared to nitrogen, N_2O diffuses into the middle ear cavity much faster than nitrogen diffuses out. In the presence of a blocked or narrowed eustachian tube, this produces an increase in pressure in the middle ear. When N_2O is discontinued at the end of the case, the N_2O rapidly diffuses out, and negative pressure suddenly develops in the middle ear. The concern is that the freshly applied tympanic membrane graft will become dislodged under these pressure changes. The surgeon's preference regarding the use of N_2O should be discussed preoperatively.

One of the major problems in performing middle ear surgery on an outpatient basis is the frequent occurrence of vertigo, nausea, and vomiting, which may be severe enough to prevent discharge of a patient. Small doses of droperidol should be given to these patients intraoperatively and continued as needed in the postoperative period. If the nausea and vomiting are not controlled, these patients must be admitted to the hospital overnight.

THE ORAL CAVITY

Many lesions of the oral cavity can be surgically excised in the outpatient setting; such lesions occur on the tongue, the floor of the mouth, the buccal mucosa, and the mandibular duct or gland. Either general or local anesthesia can be used. Before the patient is dis-

charged, there must be no airway compromise from hemorrhage or edema, and the patient should be able to swallow adequate amounts of fluid.

There is widespread controversy concerning the practice of outpatient tonsillectomies. The major complication of a tonsillectomy is hemorrhage, which usually occurs in the immediate postoperative period or about 1 week after surgery. Natof's study[6] of one ambulatory patient population reported an incidence of hemorrhage of 4.3% after tonsillectomy and 2.3% after tonsillectomy and adenoidectomy. Blood loss can be difficult to estimate in the tonsillectomy patient, because large amounts of blood may be swallowed. Even though complications following tonsillectomies may be relatively unusual, the potential for blood loss and airway obstruction is life-threatening.

Another consideration is postoperative pain after tonsillectomy. Patients may experience fairly severe pain and prefer to remain hospitalized overnight. The decision should be based on the needs of the patient and the preferences of the surgeon and anesthesiologist. However, at Yale, tonsillectomy was not performed as an outpatient procedure until 1990. Moreover, the procedure is scheduled early in the morning to allow an 8–12 hour inhospital observation period. Because a small percentage of children may still manifest their hemorrhage after 12 hours, careful selection of patients for outpatient tonsillectomy is mandatory. Consideration should be given to preexisting disease, adequacy of parental support, and the distance between the home and the hospital. Clearly, patients with sleep apnea are unacceptable candidates for tonsillectomy on an outpatient basis.

Natof's study showed a much lower incidence of postoperative hemorrhage after adenoidectomy alone (less than 0.5%).[6] Thus, adenoidectomy has been considered appropriate for the outpatient setting. General anesthesia is utilized with an endotracheal tube in place. The endotracheal tube should be secured with care, so kinking and dislocation are avoided when the mouth gag is placed to expose the oropharynx. Bleeding must be meticulously controlled with electrocautery and pressure packs. Gastric contents should be carefully suctioned to avoid postoperative nausea and vomiting triggered by the presence of blood in the stomach. The oropharynx should also be gently suctioned. On extubation, excessive retching should be avoided to prevent more bleeding. IV lidocaine (1 mg/kg) given just prior to extubation decreases the incidence and magnitude of laryngospasm and upper airway obstruction following tonsillectomy in children.[57] This may be especially advantageous in the outpatient, where one desires to avoid the prolongation of anesthesia caused by deepening anesthesia or utilizing muscle relaxants to treat laryngospasm.

SINUS SURGERY

Outpatient surgery of the paranasal sinuses should be limited to the maxillary and ethmoid sinuses. The potential intracranial complications from frontoethmoid or sphenoid surgery require careful postoperative monitoring in an inpatient setting.[5]

Often, antral puncture for nasal antral irrigation or intranasal antrostomy is performed for the treatment of maxillary sinusitis. Adequate anesthesia can be obtained using topical cocaine. The radical antrostomy or Caldwell-Luc operation may be performed for chronic maxillary sinusitis, diagnostic exploration of suspected tumors, or treatment of an oral antral fistula. Although this has been done under local anesthesia, general anesthesia is preferred. Local infiltration with lidocaine and epinephrine is used with general anesthesia for vasoconstrictive effects and to define tissue planes; local anesthetic toxicity and reactions to epinephrine must be avoided.

NASAL SURGERY

Nasal septoplasty is often performed as an outpatient procedure using local anesthesia with IV sedation. The nose is packed with pledgets soaked in a cocaine solution, which is carefully measured to avoid toxic doses. Lidocaine is then injected along the septum, producing elevation of the mucoperichondrium and an easier dissection. It is important to wait for the full vasoconstrictive and anesthetic effects of the local anesthesia before the surgical procedure is started, usually 5–10 minutes. IV sedative agents must be titrated conservatively, because assisting ventilation by mask under these surgical conditions is nearly impossible. During painful parts of the procedure, small amounts of narcotic may be given IV.

Often, nasal polypectomy is performed as an outpatient procedure under local anesthesia. Most often this is routine in an otherwise healthy patient. However, patients with cystic fibrosis often develop nasal polyps and present for polypectomy. These patients have multiple system disease, including severe pulmonary, pancreatic, hepatic, and gastrointestinal involvement.[58] Pulmonary complications consist of airway obstruction with viscous mucus, persistent bronchial infection, and diffuse fibrotic changes. Surgical procedures should be performed only when optimal pulmonary function is maintained by controlling infection and facilitating removal of secretions. If the patient is in optimal condition and local anesthesia is planned, nasal polypectomy in the patient with cystic fibrosis can be performed as an outpatient procedure. Sedation should be avoided if possible, because ventilatory depression can occur. Anticholinergics may increase the viscosity of already thick secretions and should be avoided also. If general anesthesia is planned, because of the severity of the patient's pulmonary disease and the possibility of postoperative problems, an inpatient procedure should be performed.

LARYNGEAL SURGERY AND ENDOSCOPY

Because of the potential for airway obstruction from edema, hemorrhage, or laryngospasm in the patient undergoing laryngeal surgery, the extent of surgery done on an outpatient basis is somewhat limited. Certain endoscopic techniques are ideally suited to the outpatient setting. These may include direct laryngoscopy, bronchoscopy, and esophagoscopy. The goals of anesthesia are a secure airway; relaxation of the jaw; protection of the teeth; elimination of coughing and gagging; and return of coughing and gagging reflexes at the end of the procedure.

Local anesthesia with IV sedation is often adequate for endoscopic procedures. Kortilla and Tarkkanen[59] studied the effects of diazepam and midazolam for sedation during local anesthesia for bronchoscopy. Use of midazolam (0.1 mg/kg) resulted in slightly greater amnesia for bronchoscopy than valium (0.2 mg/kg). However, recovery from sedation as measured by having the patient stand steadily and walk a straight line took somewhat longer with midazolam than with valium. In practice, it probably makes no difference which agent is used, because they both provide excellent amnesia, fairly rapid recovery, and a high degree of patient satisfaction (85–88% of patients would like their next bronchoscopy performed similarly). If the endoscopic procedure is prolonged or if there is any likelihood of bleeding or other airway compromise, general anesthesia with endotracheal intubation is indicated.

Suspension microlaryngoscopy is preferentially performed with the patient under local anesthesia, allowing the surgeon to evaluate neuromuscular function of the larynx during voluntary phonation and thus provide more accurate treatment.[60] Adequate anesthesia for this procedure consists of bilateral superior laryngeal nerve blocks[61] and intraoral blockade of the glossopharyngeal nerve either topically or by injection in the tonsillar pillar. Only small amounts of IV sedation are given, because the patient must be responsive and able to comply with the surgeon's instructions. Because of the anesthesia obtained, replete with potential for aspiration, patients are observed carefully and not allowed to eat or drink for 4 hours postoperatively.

Bronchoscopy can be performed under local anesthesia as described for suspension microlaryngoscopy, with the addition of a transtracheal injection of a local anesthetic. General anesthesia may be used also, which offers the advantage of controlled ventilation and oxygenation, protection of the airway, and less stress for the anxious or uncooperative patient. Topical application of local anesthetic to the oropharynx, larynx, and trachea lowers the requirement for general anesthesia. Either an inhalational technique or a balanced technique using N_2O, oxygen, a narcotic, and a short-acting nondepolarizing muscle relaxant or succinylcholine infusion may be employed.

Vocal cord papillomas can be treated as an outpatient procedure using laser surgical techniques. Laser surgery causes a minimal amount of trauma to the surrounding tissue and, thus, less edema. Because of the possibility of airway obstruction secondary to papillomas, the airway must be carefully evaluated preoperatively. The presence of hoarseness or stridor may suggest the advisability of obtaining xerographs of the airway.[62] General anesthesia with endotracheal intubation is utilized. As small a tube as is adequate for ventilation should be used to facilitate laser excision of the lesions. After the airway is secured, a short-acting muscle relaxant, such as vecuronium, atracurium, or succinylcholine drip, is used to assure a motionless target for the laser. The tube should be protected from ignition by the laser by use of a metal tube, or by foil wrapping a rubber tube. The surrounding areas should be packed with gauze-soaked sponges to absorb the scattered beam, and low (30%) fractional inspired oxygen should be employed to decrease the likelihood of combustion. Suitable goggles must be worn by all personnel, and the patient's eyes should be protected with wet gauze sponges.[63]

NECK SURGERY

Because of the problems of bleeding, edema, and airway obstruction, outpatient surgical procedures in the neck are limited to superficial lesions. Often, however, the extent of surgery is unknown, because superficial lesions may extend into the deep neck. Open biopsy of superficial lymph nodes as part of a diagnostic work-up can be performed in the outpatient setting. A cystic mass could be a congenital lesion, such as a branchial cleft cyst or thyroglossal duct cyst, and thus should not be excised in an outpatient procedure, because the surgery may be extensive.

FACIAL PLASTIC PROCEDURES

Many plastic surgery procedures can be performed in an outpatient setting. The scope of surgery of the external ear includes otoplasty, removal of small lesions, drainage of hematoma, and resection of preauricular lesions. Rhinoplasty and reduction of nasal fractures often are performed on the outpatient using the techniques already outlined for septoplasty.

Zygomatic fractures can be reduced in a closed fashion on outpatients. However, if a more extensive open reduction and interosseous wiring is necessary, it probably should be done on an inpatient basis. Reduction and fixation of mandibular fractures has been advocated in the outpatient setting.[5] However, because the use of archbars on the teeth and the wiring of the mandible to the maxilla is usually required, and because of the dangers of vomiting and aspiration with the jaw wired, we recommend that the patient be admitted to the hospital and observed overnight.

REFERENCES

1. Hatch LR: Day care surgery: Do we and our patients need it? Can Anaesth Soc J 1983; 30:542–543.
2. Johnson GG: Day care surgery for infants and children. Can Anaesth Soc J 1983; 30:553–557.
3. Meridy HW: Criteria for selection of ambulatory surgical patients and guidelines for management. Anesth Analg 1982; 61:921–926.
4. McTaggart RA: Selection of patients for day care surgery. Can Anaesth Soc J 1983; 30:543–545.
5. Gussack GS, Hudson WR: Major ambulatory surgery

of the otolaryngologic patient. Surg Clin North Am 1987; 67:819–840.

6. Natof HE: Complications associated with ambulatory surgery. JAMA 1980; 244:1116–1118.

7. Levin KJ: Laboratory evaluation: What tests and why? *In* Wetchler BV (ed): Problems in Anesthesia: Outpatient Anesthesia. Philadelphia, JB Lippincott, 1988, pp 18–22.

8. Elliot DL, Tolle SW, et al: Medical considerations in ambulatory surgery. Clin Plast Surg 1983; 10:295–309.

9. Liu LM, Cote CJ, et al: Life threatening apnea in infants recovering from anaesthesia. Anesthesiology 1983; 59:506–510.

10. Steward DJ: Preterm infants are more prone to complications following minor surgery than are term infants. Anesthesiology 1982; 56:304–306.

11. Malins AF: Do they do as instructed? A review of outpatient anesthesia. Anaesthesia 1978; 33:832–835.

12. Edelist G: Prophylaxis and management of postoperative problems. Can Anaesth Soc J 1983; 30:558–560.

13. Stoelting RK, Peterson C: Adverse effects of increased succinylcholine dose following d-tubocurarine pretreatment. Anesth Analg 1975; 54:282–288.

14. Brindle GF, Soliman MG: Anesthesia complications in surgical outpatients. Can Anaesth Soc J 1975; 22:613–619.

15. Dawson B, Reed WA: Anaesthesia for DCS (Day Care Surgery) adult surgical outpatients. Can Anaesth Soc J 1980; 27:409–411.

16. Bevan JC, Burn MC: Acid-base and blood glucose levels of pediatric cases at induction of anaesthesia. The effects of preop starvation and feeding. Br J Anaesth 1973; 45:115.

17. Hall WJ, Douglas RG, et al: Pulmonary mechanics after uncomplicated influenza A infection. Am Rev Respir Dis 1976; 113:141–147.

18. Green GM, Jakab GJ, Low RB, Davis GS: Defense mechanisms of the respiratory membrane. Am Rev Respir Dis 1977; 115:479.

19. Cate TR, Roberts JS, Russ MA, Pierce JA: Effects of common colds on pulmonary function. Am Rev Respir Dis 1973; 108:858–865.

20. Tait AR, Ketcham TR, Klein MJ, et al: Perioperative respiratory complications in patients with upper respiratory tract infection. Anesthesiology 1983; 59:A433.

21. McGill WA, Coveler LA, Epstein BS: Subacute upper respiratory infections in small children. Anesth Analg 1979; 58:331–333.

22. Miller BE, Betts EK, Jorgenson JJ, et al: URI and perioperative desaturation in children. Anesthesiology 1989; 71:A1170.

23. Pease W: Upper respiratory infection. *In* Bready LL, Smith RB (eds): Decision Making in Anesthesiology. Philadelphia, BC Decker, 1987, pp 190–191.

24. Clark AJM, Hurtig JB: Premedication with meperidine and atropine does not prolong recovery to street fitness after outpatient surgery. Can Anaesth Soc J 1981; 28:390–392.

25. Booker PD, Chapman DH: Premedication in children undergoing day care surgery. Br J Anaesth 1979; 51:1083–1087.

26. Steward DJ: Anaesthesia for paediatric outpatients. Can Anaesth Soc J 1980; 27:412–416.

27. Mock DL, Streisand JB, et al: Transmucosal narcotic delivery: An evaluation of fentanyl (lollipop) premedication in man. Anesth Analg 1986; 65:S102.

28. Aldrete JA, Roman-de Jesus, et al: Intranasal ketamine as induction adjunct in children: Preliminary report. Anesthesiology 1987; 67:3A.

29. Desjardins R, Ansara S, Charest J: A preanaesthetic medication in pediatric day care patients. Can Anaesth Soc J 1981; 28:141–148.

30. Garland TA: Outpatient surgery. *In* Bready LL, Smith RB (eds): Decision Making in Anesthesia. Philadelphia, BC Decker, 1987, pp 142–143.

31. Solanki RD, Suresh M, Ethridge HC: The effects of intravenous cimetidine and metoclopramide on gastric volume and pH. Anesth Analg 1984; 63:599–602.

32. Stoelting RK: Histamine and histamine receptor antagonists. *In* Stoelting RK: Physiology and Pharmacology in Anesthetic Practice. Philadelphia, JB Lippincott, 1987, pp 381.

33. Zeldis JB, Friedman LS, Isselbacher KJ: Ranitidine, a new H_2 receptor antagonist. N Engl J Med 1983; 309:1368–1373.

34. Eyler SW, Cullen BF, Welch WD, Murphy ME: Antacid aspiration in rabbits. Anesth Analg 1982; 61:183–184.

35. Coombs DW: Aspiration pneumonitis prophylaxis. Anesth Analg 1983; 62:1055–1058.

36. Eichhorn JH, Cooper JB, Cullen DJ: Standards for patient monitoring during anesthesia at Harvard Medical School. JAMA 1986; 256:1017–1020.

37. Silver H, Codesmith AO: Anesthesia for outpatient head and neck aesthetic surgery. Ann Plast Surg 1980; 5:483–485.

38. Vinnik CA: An intravenous dissociation technique for outpatient plastic surgery: Tranquility in the office surgical facility. Plast Reconstr Surg 1981; 67:799–805.

39. Porterfield HW, Franklin LT: The use of general anesthesia in the office surgical facility. Clin Plast Surg 1983; 10:289–294.

40. Smith RB: Cocaine and catecholamine interaction. Arch Otolaryngol 1973; 98:139–141.

41. Bridenbaugh LD: Regional anaesthesia for outpatient surgery—A summary of 12 year's experience. Can Anaesth Soc J 1983; 30:548–552.

42. Forbes RB: General anaesthesia for day care surgery patients. Can Anaesth Soc J 1983; 30:545–547.

43. Apfelbaum JL: Inhalation agents in anesthesia for ambulatory surgery. *In* Wetchler BV (ed): Problems in Anesthesia: Outpatient Anesthesia. Philadelphia, JB Lippincott, 1988, pp 55–68.

44. Smith FK, Deputy BS, Berry FA: Outpatient anesthesia for children undergoing extensive dental treatment. J Dis Child 1978; 45:142.

45. Kortilla K, Hovorka J, Erkola O: Omission of N_2O does not decrease the incidence or severity of emetic symptoms after isoflurane anesthesia. Anesth Analg 1987; 66:S98.

46. Padfield A: Recovery comparison between enflurane and halothane technique. A study of outpatients undergoing cystoscopy. Anaesthesia 1980; 35:508–510.

47. Kortilla K, Valanne J: Recovery after outpatient isoflurane and enflurane anesthesia. Anesth Analg 1985; 64:239.

48. Azar I, Karambelkar DJ, Lear E: Neurologic state and psychomotor function following anesthesia for ambulatory surgery. Anesthesiology 1984: 60:347–349.

49. Johnston RR, Eger EI II, Wilson C: A comparative interaction of epinephrine with enflurane, isoflurane and halothane in man. Anesth Analg 1976; 55:709–712.

50. Enright AC, Pace-Floridia A: Recovery from anesthesia in outpatients: A comparison of narcotics and inhalational techniques. Can Anaesth Soc J 1977; 24:5.

51. Zuurmond WWA, vanLeeuwen L: Recovery from sufentanil anaesthesia for outpatient arthroscopy: A comparison with isoflurane. Acta Anaesthiol Scand 1987; 31:154–156.

52. White PF: Outpatient anesthesia techniques: Continuous intravenous infusion of anesthesia agents. West J Med 1984; 140:437.

53. White PF, Schafer A: Clinical pharmacology and uses of injectable anesthesia and analgesic drugs. *In* Wetchler BV (ed): Problems in Anesthesia: Outpatient Anesthesia. Philadelphia, JB Lippincott, 1988, pp 37–54.

54. Patton CM, Moon MR, Dannemiller FJ: The prophylactic antiemetic effect of droperidol. Anesth Analg 1974; 53:361–364.

55. Cohen SE, Woods WA, Wyner J: Antiemetic efficacy of droperidol and metoclopramide. Anesthesiology 1984; 60:67–69.

56. Owens WD, Gustave F, Sclaroff A: Tympanic membrane rupture with nitrous oxide anesthesia. Anesth Analg 1978; 57:283–286.

57. Bidwai AV, Rogers C, Stanley TH: Prevention of post extubation laryngospasm after tonsillectomy. Anesthesiology 1979; 51:3.

58. LaSasso AM, Gibbs PS, Moorthy SS: Obstructive pulmonary disease. *In* Stoelting RK, Dierdorf SF (eds): Anesthesia and Co-Existing Disease. New York, Churchill Livingstone, 1983, p 189.

59. Kortilla K, Tarkkanen J: Comparison of diazepam and midazolam for sedation during LA for bronchoscopy. Br J Anaesth 1985; 57:581–586.

60. Calcaterra TC, House J: Local anesthesia for suspension microlaryngoscopy. Ann Otol Rhinol Laryngol 1976; 85:71–73.

61. Gotta AW, Sullivan CA: Anaesthesia of the upper airway using topical anesthetic and superior laryngeal nerve blocks. Br J Anaesth 1981; 53:1055–1058.

62. Babinski MF: Vocal cord papillomas. *In* Bready LL, Smith RB (eds): Decision Making in Anesthesiology. Philadelphia, BC Decker, 1987, pp 130–131.

63. Birch AA: Anesthetic considerations during laser surgery. Anesth Analg 1973; 52:53–58.

Complications Associated with Otorhinolaryngologic Anesthesia and Surgery

_____ Kathryn E. McGoldrick _____

Although much otorhinolaryngologic surgery seems simple and routine, it has a disproportionately significant potential for serious anesthetic and surgical complications. Few acute situations are more challenging to the anesthesiologist or more dangerous for the patient than such life-threatening airway emergencies as epiglottitis, foreign body aspiration, or posttonsillectomy hemorrhage. For instance, Holinger's comprehensive review of 4000 pediatric tracheostomies disclosed a complication rate of 14% and a mortality rate of 1.5%. Moreover, in pediatric patients, laser microsurgery of the airway has an increased risk of anesthetic complications (approximately 15%), especially in patients under 3 years of age with extensive disease who did not have their airway secured through tracheostomy.[2]

The major acute complications of ear, nose, and throat (ENT) surgery and anesthesia include airway obstruction, hemorrhage, hypotension, and dysrhythmias. Occasionally, these events may result in death. The patient's airway may be precarious because of pre-existing obstruction or because the anesthesiologist and surgeon must share the airway. Even if the patient's pre-existing airway is relatively normal and the operation does not require significant sharing of the airway (e.g., ear surgery), in most ENT surgery the patient's airway is hidden under drapes and difficult to reach. Each of these risks and potential complications underscores the necessity for meticulous attention to all facets of the patient's perioperative care.

In this chapter, some of the many complications that may be associated with ENT surgery are outlined. The complications are grouped according to a somewhat arbitrary time frame, i.e., (1) complications that occur in association with intubation; (2) complications that occur intraoperatively; (3) periextubation complications; and (4) postoperative, or delayed, morbidity and mortality. Within this framework, when applicable, assorted ENT complications that may follow general surgical procedures are mentioned.

INTUBATION-RELATED COMPLICATIONS

TECHNICALLY DIFFICULT INTUBATIONS

The incidence of difficult intubations has been estimated to be approximately 1:750,[3] although the range cited in the literature is rather wide (see Chapter 3). Considering the nature of the cases involved, an even higher incidence of challenging intubations when caring for ENT patients could be expected. Cass and colleagues[4] described prognostic signs of a potentially difficult intubation. These included a short, muscular neck with a full set of teeth; micrognathia with obtuse mandibular angles;

long, high-arched palate associated with a long, narrow mouth; increased alveolomental distance; protruding upper incisors owing to relative overgrowth of the premaxilla; and poor mobility of the mandible owing to temporomandibular arthritis or trismus. Others have mentioned the difficulties encountered with limited extension of the lower cervical vertebrae, increased posterior mandibular depth, and decreased (less than 3 fingerbreadths) distance from the symphysis of the mandible to the thyroid notch with the head fully extended. In addition, Mallampati's signs[5] describing the correlation between visibility of intraoral structures and ease of laryngoscopic exposure of the glottis may be helpful in predicting the difficult intubation. For example, if the soft palate, fauces, uvula, and pillars are visible when the sitting patient is asked to open the mouth and maximally protrude the tongue, an easy intubation should be anticipated. However, if the soft palate is not visualized, extreme difficulty with intubation may be encountered. Moreover, the presence of stridor at rest can signal a challenging intubation.

Upper airway problems may be conveniently divided into three categories:

1. patients with an unobstructed airway in whom the mask airway may be easily manageable. However, intubation is made difficult by physiognomic anomalies. Patients with a so-called anterior larynx clearly fall into this category. Certainly, all larynxes are anterior in the sense that they are anterior to the esophagus. Nonetheless, some conditions are characteristically associated with larynxes that are extremely anterior and difficult to visualize; these conditions include micrognathia, a hypoplastic mandible, or a very short neck. (A mask airway is not always easily manageable with these conditions.) A partial list of conditions associated with these problems includes arthrochalasis multiplex congenita and arthrogryposis, and the following syndromes: Cornelia de Lange's cri du chat, DiGeorge's, Goldenhar's, Klippel-Feil, Noonan's, Pierre Robin, Treacher Collins, and Turner's.

2. patients with an obviously obstructed airway.

3. patients in whom impending obstruction of the airway is compensated or concealed on presentation but occurs upon induction of anesthesia, administration of muscle relaxants, or extubation. Such situations may occur with certain supraglottic neoplasms, pedunculated intralaryngeal lesions, extremely large tonsils and adenoids, or various congenital deformities for which the patient ordinarily compensates by muscular effort.

The management of difficult airways is presented in detail in Chapter 3. However, in summary, the key to successfully accomplishing a challenging intubation lies in thorough preparation, which begins with careful preoperative examination of the mouth, pharynx, and neck, including assessment of range of motion. A variety of laryngoscope blades, including the curved Bijarri-Griffrida and Siker blades, Huffman prism clips attached to the number 3 MacIntosh blade, different-sized endotracheal tubes, stylets, and other equipment such as fiberoptic endoscopes, rigid bronchoscopes, devices for transtracheal ventilation, and tracheotomy kits should be readily available; an assistant should be available to manipulate the head and neck to apply posterior laryngeal pressure as needed.

Alternatives to routine intubation techniques are awake intubation, either oral or nasal, with topical anesthesia and direct visualization; blind nasotracheal intubation with the patient either awake or asleep, breathing spontaneously; visualized oral or nasal intubation under deep inhalation anesthesia; use of a fiberoptic laryngoscope or small-caliber fiberoptic bronchoscope; passage of a guidewire or catheter either anterograde or retrograde; and cricothyroidotomy or tracheostomy.

Nasal intubations are unwise if the patient has a coagulation or bleeding problem. Furthermore, superior laryngeal nerve blocks and transtracheal injection of local anesthesia to facilitate awake intubation are contraindicated if the patient has a full stomach. Nasotracheal intubation is contraindicated if the patient has a cribriform plate fracture or a basilar skull fracture because of the potential for passage of the tracheal tube into the cranial vault. Clinical signs such as cerebrospinal fluid rhinorrhea or otorrhea and periorbital or mastoid ecchymosis, as well as radiographs, may confirm the presence of a basilar skull fracture. However, it may be difficult or impossible to definitively rule out a basilar skull fracture; therefore, one must have a high index of suspicion when confronted with a patient with a facial fracture. Indeed, 20% of LeFort III and some LeFort II facial fractures have associated basilar skull fractures.[6]

METHEMOGLOBINEMIA SECONDARY TO TOPICAL LOCAL ANESTHETICS

Methemoglobinemia may be congenital or induced by a variety of drugs (Table 12–1), including local anesthetics, nitrites or nitrates, phenacetin, phenazopyridine hydrochloride, primaquine, and sulfonamides.[7] There are many case reports of potentially serious methemoglobin levels (greater than 30%) induced by topical anesthetics used in the airway.[8–13] Topical anesthetics known to induce methemoglobinemia include prilocaine, benzocaine, lidocaine, and procaine.

CETACAINE spray is a highly effective topical anesthetic commonly used by gastroenterologists, bronchoscopists, and anesthesiologists. CETACAINE contains 14% benzocaine, 2% butyl aminobenzoate, 2% tetracaine hydrochloride, cetyl dimethyl ethyl ammonium bromide 0.005%, and benzalkonium chloride 0.5%. The large amount of benzocaine in CETACAINE spray has the capability of triggering methemoglobinemia if more than 1 second of spray from the Jetco cannula is administered. Although benzocaine is usually poorly absorbed after topical application, the manufacturer warns against its use on inflamed or denuded tissue. Moreover, a patient can inhale CETACAINE spray into the trachea when it is used to facilitate awake intubation.

The diagnosis of acute methemoglobinemia should be suspected in any patient who has received topical anesthesia and has become suddenly cyanotic. An arterial blood gas that is chocolate brown with a normal arterial oxygen pressure suggests this diagnosis.[14] Moreover, pulse oximetry data should be used with

TABLE 12–1. Methemoglobinemia

May be congenital
May be induced by:
  local anesthetics
    benzocaine
    lidocaine
    prilocaine
    procaine
  nitrates
  nitrites
  phenacetin
  pyridium
  primaquine
  sulfonamides
Symptoms generally occur once MetHb levels exceed 20%
Levels above 70% can be fatal
Associated with spurious oxygen saturation readings
Methylene blue, 2 mg/kg IV, is effective treatment

caution in patients with methemoglobinemia.[7] Because methemoglobin (MetHb) has a high absorbency at both the red and the infrared wavelengths range, this tends to drive the ratio of absorbences (R) toward one. An R value of 1 corresponds to an oxygen saturation of 85% by pulse oximetry. Hence, high MetHb levels drive oxygen saturation (SpO_2) toward 85%, regardless of oxygen tension. Clearly, any substance with a high absorption coefficient in either of the two wavelengths used in pulse oximetry is likely to cause spurious oxygen saturation readings. In addition to methylene blue, these substances include indocyanine green and indigo carmine.[15, 16]

Although cyanosis may appear with levels as low as 15%, acquired methemoglobinemia is only rarely symptomatic when levels are below 20%. Lethargy, dizziness, and headache may occur with levels between 30 and 40%, and levels above 70% can be fatal, because MetHb increases the affinity of normal hemoglobin (Hb) for oxygen, thereby hindering oxygen release in the tissues.[17, 18] Treatment consists of administration of methylene blue, 2 mg/kg, given intravenously (IV) over 5 minutes.

Methemoglobinemia is formed normally in the body because small amounts of the ferrous iron in Hb are continuously oxidized to the ferric form, which is incapable of carrying oxygen or carbon dioxide. The red cells' defense against accumulated MetHb is primarily MetHb reduced nicotinamide adenine dinucleotide (NADH) reductase, which is responsible for 95% of in vivo reduction of the ferric iron MetHb to form normal Hb. This system normally keeps the MetHb level at less than 1%. (Hence, congenital methemoglobinemia is caused either by insufficient production of the enzyme MetHb NADH reductase or by abnormal Hb (Hb M) variants that are stable with the iron in the ferric form, and thus cannot be reduced.)

Methylene blue acts as a cofactor in the transfer of an electron from reduced nicotinamide adenine dinucleotide phosphate (NADPH) to ferric iron in a reaction catalyzed by MetHb NADPH reductase. In this reaction, methylene blue is initially reduced to leukomethylene blue, which then reduces MetHb to normal Hb. However, the total dose should not exceed 7 mg/kg, because high levels may directly oxidize normal Hb to cause methemoglobinemia.[15, 16] Moreover, methylene blue is ineffective in the presence of Hb M variants, and the drug should not be given to patients with glucose-6-phosphate dehydrogenase deficiency, because the hexose monophosphate shunt regenerates NADPH. With deficient NADPH regeneration, methylene blue may cause hemolytic anemia.

In summary, although CETACAINE is an excellent topical anesthetic for accessible mucous membranes to control pain or gagging during awake endoscopy, the spray should be used for only 1 second or less. (The average expulsion rate of residue from the spray, at normal temperatures, is 200 mg per second.) Spray duration in excess of 2 seconds is contraindicated. To avoid excessive systemic absorption, CETACAINE should not be applied to large areas of denuded or inflamed tissue.

LARYNGOSPASM

The precise definition and mechanism of laryngospasm are still debated. In clinical practice, laryngospasm usually means that either the true vocal cords or both the true and false vocal cords have become apposed in the midline to close the glottis. The sensory portion of the superior laryngeal nerve carries the afferent limb of the reflex to the cervical vagal nuclei. Efferent potentials then travel along the vagus. Depending on the mechanism one chooses to believe is at work, the intrinsic laryngeal muscles, extrinsic laryngeal muscles, or both are stimulated, resulting in glottic closure.

Stimuli that may produce laryngospasm include the presence of blood, secretions, or vomitus in the airway; visceral pain; chemical irritation of laryngeal or pharyngeal mucosa; and tracheal intubation with insufficient anesthesia. Prevention of laryngospasm includes adequate anesthesia before instrumentation, use of muscle relaxants, and the use of a full topical laryngeal block prior to intubation.

Treatment of a fully developed laryngospasm involves removing the stimulus, lifting the mandible up and out with the head in a "sniffing position," and using a rapidly acting muscle relaxant, such as succinylcholine 1 mg/kg IV, to relax and open the vocal cords. It is often advisable to give atropine, 0.01–0.02 mg/kg IV, prior to succinylcholine to avoid succinylcholine-associated or hypoxia-associated bradycardia. Gentle positive pressure with 100% oxygen by mask is often attempted prior to using succinylcholine. However, some believe that positive pressure causes the pyriform fossae to bulge and occasionally can exacerbate the laryngospasm by stimulating sensory areas supplied by the superior laryngeal nerve.

In the absence of IV access, succinylcholine can be administered intramuscularly in a 4 mg/kg dose to terminate laryngospasm. Furthermore, laryngospasm can occur intraoperatively in a nonintubated patient and can also occur postextubation.

FOREIGN BODY ASPIRATION

It is not unusual for an ENT patient to need endoscopic surgery to remove an aspirated foreign body (see Chapter 8). However, not all aspirated foreign bodies exist prior to anesthetic induction. Iatrogenically induced foreign body aspiration may include materials such as teeth, blood, vomitus, adenoidal tissue, parts of the laryngoscope or the endotracheal tube, and even soda lime dust.

Aspiration of vomitus during induction or emergence from anesthesia is one of the more common causes of anesthetic morbidity and mortality. Moreover, patients at risk of aspiration are not confined to those who have recently eaten. Well-established risk factors include hiatus hernia, pregnancy, collagen vascular diseases, obesity, anxiety, old age, diabetes, and conditions requiring upper abdominal surgery. The most common factors that precipitate active vomiting during anesthesia are partial respiratory obstruction and insufficient anesthetic depth. Other causes include strong autonomic stimulation, such as peritoneal traction or hypoxia and hypotension; administration of narcotics; and insertion of an oropharyngeal airway during light anesthesia. The passive phenomenon of regurgitation may be encouraged by the Trendelenburg position, the prone position, palpation of the abdomen during light anesthesia, and conditions associated with delayed gastric emptying and increased intragastric pressure. These conditions include pain, excessive anxiety, metabolic disturbances, elevated intracranial pressure, pyloric or intestinal obstruction, obstetrical labor, and administration of narcotics and parasympathomimetic drugs. Delaying induction of anesthesia is a common tactic to prevent aspiration, but during life-threatening hemorrhage, for example, it is not an option. Moreover, in less emergent cases, the decision of how long to wait is difficult and arbitrary. Because food may remain undigested for over 18 hours when the patient is tense and in pain, it must be assumed that these individuals have a full stomach.

Reports concerning the incidence of aspiration under anesthesia vary considerably, but a study by Olsson and colleagues[19] in 1986 cited an incidence of anesthesia-induced aspiration pneumonitis confirmed by x-ray of 2.2/10,000 cases of anesthesia, with a mortality of 0.2/10,000.

Morbidity and mortality depend on the volume, acidity, and type of material aspirated. The worst prognosis is associated with a pH below 2.5 and a volume in excess of 25 mL (0.4 mL/kg). If solid particulate material is aspirated, the tracheobronchial tree may be occluded, resulting in lung collapse distal to the blockage. Indeed, death may ensue with great rapidity when the tracheal lumen is blocked.

If a relatively large volume of highly acidic liquid is aspirated, wheezing, rales, and expiratory rhonchi may be noted rather quickly, although occasionally these signs can be delayed. Likewise, the extent of the pneumonitis may not be discernible radiologically for several hours. However, tachycardia, dyspnea, cyanosis, pulmonary edema, and hypotension may develop quickly.

Aspirated solid matter demands prompt removal by bronchoscopy. When liquid is aspirated, suctioning should be performed immediately to minimize pulmonary injury. Tracheal intubation and mechanical ventilation with positive end-expiratory pressure (PEEP) are often necessary for satisfactory oxygenation. Aminophylline may be needed to combat bronchospasm, and antibiotics are administered only if indicated (i.e., if the patient aspirated pus from a pharyngeal abscess).

Aspiration may occur during local or regional anesthesia, as well as during general anesthesia, and also may occur in any patient who is obtunded secondary to drugs or systemic illness.

Proper airway management (either an awake or rapid-sequence intubation) is the most important factor in preventing aspiration, but pharmacological prophylaxis with nonparticulate antacids, H_2 blockers, and drugs stimulating gastric motility may be helpful. Moreover, a nasogastric tube should be passed and suction applied to empty gastric contents as much as possible prior to extubation. Lastly, the high risk patient should not be extubated until he or she is awake, with reflexes intact.

LARYNGEAL AND PHARYNGOESOPHAGEAL INJURY

The trauma of a difficult intubation frequently occurs not at the vocal cord level, but some- what higher in the airway. Even apparently uneventful intubations can be followed by significant postoperative morbidity. Minor complications following endotracheal intubation are fairly frequent. The incidence of pharyngitis, for example, may be as high as 58%.[20]

Oral intubation can cause tissue trauma; damage to teeth, including dislodgement; mucosal lacerations; perforation of anatomical structures such as the esophagus or trachea; and bleeding with the risk of aspiration. Kambic and Radsel[21] performed indirect laryngoscopy on 1000 patients following intubation for anesthesia and found that the most frequent lesion was hematoma, which occurred in 52 patients; 45 of the hematomas were located on a vocal cord. Other additional potential complications of nasal intubation include damage to the septum and turbinates, nasal necrosis, epistaxis, sinusitis, and otitis media. Furthermore, a forced nasal intubation may take a false passage through the posterior pharyngeal wall from a retropharyngeal laceration. In cases of cribriform plate and basilar skull fractures, nasotracheal intubation should not be attempted because of risk of intracranial penetration.

Laceration of the larynx is extremely rare. One of the most serious complications is pseudomembranous laryngotracheitis, which may cause sudden death if not treated immediately. Pseudomembranous laryngotracheitis is not exclusively a result of trauma. The condition may occur after a completely uneventful anesthetic procedure and in the absence of a history of upper respiratory infection.[22]

Fortunately, vocal cord paralysis following intubation is uncommon and more likely to occur secondary to surgical factors such as trauma to the recurrent laryngeal nerve. However, occasionally the condition may be attributed to neuropraxia from pressure on the recurrent laryngeal nerve by the cuff of the tracheal tube. Prevention of this complication includes (1) intubating gently, followed by careful inflation of the high volume–low pressure cuff with a volume that permits a small, audible leak during inspiration; (2) abandoning the use of endotracheal tubes with cuffs that, on testing, inflate unevenly; (3) eliminating the practice of placing the cuff within the larynx in a misguided attempt to avoid inadvertent endobronchial intubation (the cuff should be placed about 2 cm below the larynx); and (4) filling the cuff with a sample of the inspired mixture of gases, regularly deflating the cuff, or using a simple pressure relief valve.[23]

obstruction and occurs secondary to postoperative hemorrhage. Indeed, the reported mortality rate in patients needing reoperation to control postoperative bleeding was approximately 1/500 patients.[42, 43]

The two most likely periods for post-tonsillectomy bleeding are 4–6 hours immediately postoperatively and then again 5–10 days postoperatively, when hemorrhage is frequently attributable to infection. A more recent study reported that 76% of postoperative bleeding occurred within the first 6 hours following tonsillectomy.[44] Only 0.06% of the patients in this 1986 study by Crysdale bled postoperatively, and of these, only 3% required reoperation to achieve hemostasis. However, other investigators have cited reoperation rates as high as 0.9%.

Another study conducted by otolaryngologists at the Portsmouth and Oakland Naval Hospitals sought to determine the risk factors for bleeding following tonsillectomy.[45] In their experience, from 1980 to 1985, 2.7% of patients experienced bleeding within 24 hours of the procedure. Age, gender, season, preoperative platelet count, surgical indication(s), simultaneous adenoidectomy, method used for hemostasis, intraoperative estimated blood loss, operative time, and anesthetic technique (local versus general) were not associated with postoperative bleeding. Interestingly, children under 10 years of age constituted 24% of patients but accounted for only 10% of bleeders. Although no patients had a history of bleeding diatheses, bleeders tended to have minimally elevated prothrombin time (PT) and partial thromboplastin time (PTT) values preoperatively, contradicting a growing literature that indicates a history of bleeding is present before these coagulation studies become abnormal. Mean operative time and intraoperative bleeding were somewhat greater when general anesthesia was used. Postoperative systolic and diastolic blood pressure tended to be higher among bleeders. The researchers concluded that local anesthesia is a safe technique, that preoperative PT and PTT studies help identify patients at risk, and that measures for controlling pain and more judicious use of epinephrine-containing local anesthetics may decrease the incidence of post-tonsillectomy bleeding. Indeed, Broadman and associates[46] demonstrated that, in children, the operative blood loss associated with tonsillectomy can be decreased by infiltrating with epinephrine 1:200,000 combined with bupivacaine 0.25% as a vehicle. Because peritonsillar injections of saline were also helpful, Broadman speculated that solutions injected into the plane of dissection between the tonsillar capsule and pillar compressed vascular structures and thus reduced bleeding.

Furthermore, as mentioned, procedures such as glossectomy, pharyngectomy, laryngectomy, radical neck dissection, and resection of glomus jugulare tumors may be associated with profuse bleeding. Glomus jugulare tumors, for example, are extraordinarily vascular, usually deriving their main blood supply from branches of the external carotid artery, although occasionally the internal carotid and vertebral arteries may be involved. In these procedures, blood loss is difficult to estimate, because much of it is hidden from view, saturating surgical sheets, pooling under the patient's head, and dripping onto the floor. (In addition, with post-tonsillectomy bleeding, a significant amount of blood may occultly enter the gastrointestinal tract.)

When caring for these ENT patients, the anesthesiologist must anticipate and be prepared for massive blood loss. Adequate numbers of wide-bore IV cannulae must be inserted and, when indicated, central venous pressure and pulmonary artery wedge pressure should be monitored, along with intra-arterial blood pressure. Gentle surgical technique with meticulous attention to hemostasis is important. Infiltration with epinephrine-containing solution may be helpful in minimizing blood loss, and in selected cases, intraoperative controlled hypotension may be useful if there are no contraindications. The technique of keeping the patient's head slightly elevated may reduce blood loss but also may increase the risk of venous air embolism. Preoperative embolization of glomus jugulare tumors may decrease surgical bleeding, but this maneuver is contraindicated if the tumor's blood supply is from the internal carotid or vertebral arteries.

MECHANICAL TRAUMA AND BAROTRAUMA

Facial, cervical, and thoracic subcutaneous emphysema can occur during surgical and dental procedures, upper airway trauma, and facial bone fractures and after equipment failure.[47–49] Subcutaneous emphysema of the face, neck, and mediastinum often occurs unexpectedly and inexplicably. Although subcutaneous emphysema does not necessarily produce serious pathophysiological consequences, it may be progressive and produce circulatory and respiratory compromises. Respiratory impairment may be secondary to airway obstruction from massive subcutaneous emphysema of the head and neck. Furthermore, tension pneumothorax results in decreased pulmonary compliance. Increasing tension within the mediastinum can dramatically decrease cardiac output and hence blood pressure owing to a tamponade effect.

Airway perforation may be the result of mechanical trauma or airway pressure.[50] During orotracheal intubation, the airway may be perforated by pressure from the laryngoscope blade, the stylet, or even the endotracheal tube. Elevated airway pressure can cause rupture anywhere between the point of its application and the alveolus. Airway perforation from any cause may introduce air to unusual locations and trigger subcutaneous and mediastinal emphysema and pneumothorax.

Pneumothorax can occur through three mechanisms: type I, intrapulmonary alveolar rupture, with retrograde perivascular dissection of air, producing mediastinal emphysema; type II, injury to the visceral pleura, with escape of air into the pleural space; and type III, injury to the parietal pleura, with entry of air from adjoining structures such as the thoracic wall or mediastinum. Type I may be associated with malfunctioning expiratory valve mechanisms on the anesthesia machine.[51, 52] Type II may be produced by subclavian or internal jugular venipuncture, tracheostomy, and mediastinoscopy. When visceral pleural discontinuity, regardless of etiology, is present, airway pressures that ordinarily would be well tolerated can produce tension pneumothorax. Type III pneumothorax may be a complication of thyroidectomy, tracheostomy, or radical neck dissection, when exposure of the deep cervical fascia offers a route through which air may enter the mediastinum, because the deep cervical fascia surrounds the trachea and extends directly into the mediastinum.[53] Usually, paratracheal air dissection is associated with excessive negative airway pressure generated during labored or obstructed ventilation.

Therefore, careful consideration of the risk-benefit ratio should precede certain procedures, such as subclavian or internal jugular venipuncture, especially prior to induction of anesthesia. Positive airway pressure and the use of high concentrations of nitrous oxide (N_2O) may escalate a small pneumothorax into a rapidly expanding tension pneumothorax. Tension pneumothorax should be included in the differential diagnosis of circulatory or respiratory instability following intubation, especially in the setting of thoracic or upper abdominal trauma, inadvertent overinflation of the lungs, or obstructive airway disease with emphysema, or when PEEP is being applied. N_2O should be immediately discontinued if surgical emphysema or pneumothorax is suspected, because this gas diffuses into the trapped air and dramatically expands its volume in a concentration-related fashion.

Signs of pneumothorax include hypotension, tachycardia, tachypnea, decreased pulmonary compliance, wheezing or distant breath sounds, and increased venous pressure. Treatment consists of insertion of a large-bore needle through the second intercostal space anteriorly, usually followed by tube thoracostomy.

To prevent barotrauma-related complications, excessive airway pressure should be avoided during anesthesia. Intubation should be accomplished gently, and anesthesia equipment should be meticulously checked for valve integrity. Poorly compliant breathing bags should be discarded because of the potential for high peak pressure to be produced during inadvertent overdistention. Furthermore, avoidance of airway obstruction or excessive negative airway pressure during neck surgery prevents most cases of pneumothorax associated with air dissection along deep cervical fascia into the mediastinum.

During the perioperative period of head and neck surgery, anesthesiologists should be alert for alterations in pulmonary compliance, circulatory decompensation, or sudden edema of the tissues of the facial, cervical, or thoracic region that may indicate undesirable air entry into the subcutaneous spaces.

VENOUS AIR EMBOLISM

Venous air embolism is possible during many types of ENT operations, including resection of glomus tumors, sinus surgery, and laryngeal trauma when cervical vein laceration is present (Table 12–4). Open neck veins in any surgical procedures on the neck can entrain air into the venous system and result in significant venous air embolism. Although an embolism may occur in supine patients, its likelihood is increased if surgery is performed with the patient in the sitting position, i.e., when the operative field is above the level of the heart. Excision of tumor invading the temporal bone, for example, is likely to produce exposure of

TABLE 12–4. Features of Venous Air Embolism

Likelihood increased by sitting position, presence of open neck veins, and irrigating sinuses with air
Incidence and severity decreased by slight head-down position and controlled ventilation

In patients at risk:
  insert right atrial catheter
  control ventilation
  listen with Doppler or stethoscope for mill-wheel murmur
  monitor end-tidal CO_2

Treatment:
  use 100% oxygen
  aspirate air from right atrial catheter
  turn patient into left lateral decubitus position
  use closed chest cardiac massage

veins that cannot collapse because of bony attachments. Venous air embolism can be reduced, if not totally eliminated, by keeping the patient slightly head down. Moreover, in cases in which venous air embolism is a distinct possibility, insertion of a right atrial catheter and controlled ventilation are advised. Adornato and colleagues[54] showed that even minimal air embolism may precipitate a "gasp reflex" that in turn may cause a large bolus of air to be sucked into the open vein. This phenomenon transforms a minor air embolus into a major one, but it can be obviated by controlling respiration.

Some surgeons inject air into the maxillary antrum following fluid irrigation. This practice is controversial, because deaths have been reported following lavage of nasal sinuses.[55–57] Most otolaryngologists advise against this maneuver to avoid air embolism.[55, 56]

Although venous air embolism can be produced whenever air is deliberately forced into the body, the amount of air and rate of delivery are key factors determining the severity of injury.[58, 59]

The main, specific sign of venous air embolism is the loud, churning mill-wheel murmur heard over the precordium. Thus, a precordial or esophageal stethoscope is mandatory whenever the possibility of an embolism exists.[60] A Doppler precordial detector placed over the right side of the heart is even more sensitive in detecting air entry into the circulation. Another early sign is a drop in end-tidal carbon dioxide (CO_2). Other findings, usually occurring later and with large emboli, include wheezing, systemic hypotension, and elevated right heart pressure. Electrocardiographic changes are nonspecific and tend to occur relatively late. Inversion of the T waves, followed by ST-segment elevation, and then a right bundle branch block pattern[61] have been reported, as have ST-segment depression and ventricular fibrillation.

Although the vast majority of cases involve only small amounts of air and frequently are not diagnosed, treatment of massive air embolism includes aspirating air from a well-positioned right atrial or pulmonary artery catheter, discontinuing N_2O if it is being administered, giving 100% oxygen, turning the patient into the left lateral decubitus position[61] so that the pulmonary outflow tract assumes a position inferior to the body of the right ventricle, and applying closed chest cardiac massage.

FIRES IN THE AIRWAY

Much has been written about tracheal fires during laser surgery, and this important topic is discussed here. However, airway fires may occur in the absence of lasers and in the absence of flammable or explosive agents such as ether and cyclopropane.

The requirements for a fire include an ignition source, oxidizing agent(s), and combustible material. These are provided, respectively, by electrocautery, N_2O and oxygen, and an endotracheal tube. In a publication by Simpson and Wolf[62] the hazard of using "spray" electrocautery during tonsillectomy and adenoidectomy in a 4-year-old boy is reported. Many measures reduce the risk of pharyngeal fire, such as reducing the concentration of oxidizing agent(s) in the oral cavity by using a moist, occlusive pharyngeal pack, especially if an uncuffed endotracheal tube is in place; by eliminating the use of N_2O; and by minimizing the inspired oxygen concentration. Also, the risk of igniting the endotracheal tube with stray electrical current could be reduced by using bipolar rather than unipolar cautery, because current density in the tissue surrounding the active electrode is much less with bipolar electrocautery.

The laser is an exciting technological advance, but its use can be hazardous. All operating room personnel should wear goggles that absorb the radiation frequency of the laser. The patient's eyes should be closed and protected with moistened eye pads. If feasible, viable tissue within the surgical field should be protected with moistened sponges, so that any accidental diversion of the laser beam is absorbed.

Endotracheal tube materials vary greatly in their ignitability and flammability. Research data are difficult to compare without standardization of ambient atmosphere both outside and inside the tube, laser type, power, pulse durations and repetitions, or maximum continuous application of the laser to the tube. The wavelength of the laser used must be safe for the tube planned.

The laser is an intense heat source capable of igniting many materials. The ease with which this occurs depends on the material, the gas environment surrounding the material, and the focus of the laser beam. Fried[63] showed in a survey that endotracheal tube explosion was the most common serious complication of CO_2 laser laryngoscopic surgery. The incidence rate of endotracheal tube fire has been reported to be as high as 1.5% in patients undergoing laryngeal surgery with the CO_2 laser.[64] Nonetheless, various precautions may be implemented to reduce the incidence of this potential catastrophe. A popular method of producing a "laser-proof" endotracheal tube is to wrap a red rubber tube with reflective metallic tape. Selection of the proper tape is critical, because some tapes have an aluminized surface on the back layer of the tape, so that the laser beam actually passes through a clear layer of a probably flammable plastic compound before encountering the reflective surface. Sosis recommends copper foil tape or 3M tape number 425.[65] The 3M number 425 tape offered the best protection against Nd:YAG laser, followed by 1 mm thick copper foil. Both tapes also protected against the CO_2 laser at high outputs.[65]

Proper technique in wrapping is essential. Otherwise, gaps occur, exposing portions of unprotected endotracheal tube to the laser, and rough edges can damage laryngeal structures. (The malleable copper foil affords smoother contour than many other tapes.) A cuffed tube manufactured by Xomed, made from silicone and metallic particles, is available. However, fires have occurred even with the silicone tube,[66] although the Xomed tube requires significantly more energy for ignition than either the red rubber tubes or polyvinylchloride tubes. The rubber tubes are substantially more resistant to ignition at both higher energy exposures and greater durations of exposure than properly wrapped plastic Portex tubes.[67] In addition, an all-metal endotracheal tube, called the Norton tube, is available but has no cuff. The Mallinckrodt Laser-Flex endotracheal tube, complete with a double cuff, is highly recommended during CO_2 laser surgery of the airway (see Chapter 4).

Although N_2O is nonflammable, it supports combustion. Therefore, N_2O is best avoided during laser surgery in the airway; rather, the minimum clinically acceptable concentration of oxygen should be used along with nitrogen or helium. The latter increases the time required for ignition of some tubes by as much as 100% because of the increased thermal diffusivity of the gas mixture.[65] Also, the cuff of the endotracheal tube should be inflated with normal saline instead of air to minimize the chance of ignition. Some anesthesiologists have recommended adding methylene blue to the saline so that if the cuff is pierced by the laser beam, a visible blue stream will be detected by the surgeon.

If a fire or explosion occurs, the anesthesiologist should extinguish the fire immediately by turning off the oxygen, stopping ventilation, occluding the tube with a clamp, quickly disconnecting it from the breathing circuit, and then removing it from the patient. The fire should be extinguished with sterile water or saline. (The saline is for the endotracheal tube, not the patient, unless flaming remnants of the tube remain in the patient's airway.) An ample supply of saline should be kept in the sterile field during laser procedures on the airway. Another small endotracheal tube and a bronchoscope should be readily available for reestablishing and examining the airway and performing pulmonary toilet. If damage is extensive, a tracheostomy may be performed, preferably below the third tracheal ring. A chest radiograph should be taken, and the patient should be admitted to the intensive care unit for observation. Any inhaled gases administered to the patient should be well humidified, and some advocate the use of steroids.

NERVE INJURY

In addition to the usual attention paid to proper patient positioning and padding on the operating table, the anesthesiologist must be aware of additional concerns about nerve integrity during ENT surgery. For example, use of muscle relaxants may be limited by the surgeon's need to evaluate intactness of nerves during neck dissection and during middle ear or parotid surgery. Even though different muscle groups have different sensitivities to muscle relaxants[68] and it is possible to provide skeletal muscle relaxation without complete paralysis, which enables the surgeon to elicit a response by direct nerve stimulation, many anesthesiologists are reluctant to use long-acting muscle relaxants in this setting. If postoperative facial or other nerve dysfunction occurs for any reason, an awkward situation exists for the anesthesiologist who used large dosages of long-acting muscle relaxants intraoperatively.

TYMPANIC MEMBRANE RUPTURE AND GRAFT DISLODGEMENT

The tremendous solubility of N_2O compared with nitrogen can present a problem in closed spaces. In the presence of N_2O, the volume of any gas contained within a closed space, such as the middle ear, can significantly expand. Numerous reports have documented the rise in middle ear pressure that occurs with N_2O and the damage produced.[69-71] Tympanic membrane rupture[72] and dislodgement of tympanic membrane grafts have been attributed to the use of N_2O. Another factor is that when the N_2O is discontinued and a previously open space is closed, a negative pressure is produced by the withdrawal of N_2O.

In middle ear surgery there is no closed space until the surgeon begins to close the middle ear. It has been suggested that N_2O be discontinued about 30 minutes prior to graft placement.[73] In actual practice, however, discontinuing N_2O approximately 5 minutes before the graft is placed seems satisfactory. Furthermore, packing the middle ear with absorbable gelatin sponge is helpful in preventing postoperative graft retraction. Surgeons have their own preferences, or biases, concerning the use of N_2O during middle ear surgery. At the start of the case, the preferences should be discussed and the anesthetic plan formulated accordingly.

MISCELLANEOUS COMPLICATIONS

Malignant hyperthermia is discussed in detail in Chapter 15.

Patients with certain ENT conditions may have hormonal and electrolyte imbalances that can complicate anesthetic management. For example, individuals with medullary carcinoma of the thyroid may have elevated levels of adrenocorticotropic hormone, producing a Cushing's syndrome-like picture, as well as increased secretion of thyrocalcitonin. Some patients with glomus jugulare tumors may secrete excessive amounts of catecholamines and should be managed the same as a patient with pheochromocytoma.

Individuals with major cancer of the head and neck may suffer from concomitant chronic obstructive pulmonary disease associated with heavy smoking and liver impairment secondary to excessive alcohol consumption. In addition, their nutritional status may be poor, and these patients may have received prior radiation therapy or chemotherapy. Therefore, awareness of potential side effects is crucial. Preoperative hemocrit, platelet count, white blood cell count, serum electrolytes, glucose, renal and liver function tests, pulmonary function tests, serum amylase, and coagulation profiles are important. Preoperative correction of fluid and electrolyte balance may be required as well as blood component therapy to prevent perioperative coagulopathy.

The three major chemotherapeutic agents sometimes used for major head and neck cancers are 5-fluorouracil (5FU), methotrexate, and cisplatin. The use of 5FU has been associated with bone marrow suppression, stomatitis, and CNS toxicity. In addition to stomatitis and bone marrow suppression, methotrexate has been linked with renal and, occasionally, pulmonary and hepatic toxicity. Cisplatin is known to produce bone marrow suppression, renal toxicity, neurotoxicity, hypercalcemia, and, rarely, cardiotoxicity.

Furthermore, aseptic technique is extremely important with all these cancer patients, because immunosuppression is to be expected.

INADVERTENT EXTUBATION

During many ENT procedures, the anesthesiologist does not have direct visual and tactile access to the patient's airway. Fixation techniques appropriate for the surgery are essential to prevent accidental dislodgement. Adhesive tape, benzoin, and even stainless steel wire can be applied to secure the tube to the teeth. Dislodgement is always a possibility; thus, appropriate continuous monitoring with either a precordial or esophageal stethoscope, as well as end-tidal CO_2 monitoring to immediately detect tube displacement, is critical, as is a plan if dislodgement occurs. Meticulous attention to detail, careful and continuous observation, rapid diagnosis, and prompt institution of remedial measures are essential. Reintubation is not always easy in the middle of a bloody, complex dissection. Prevention is the best treatment.

PERIEXTUBATION COMPLICATIONS

LARYNGOSPASM

To diminish the likelihood of postextubation laryngospasm, the anesthesiologist should extubate patients either while they are asleep but breathing adequately, or when they are wide awake. "Awake" means that the patient opens the eyes spontaneously, moves extremities well on command, and resumes a normal breathing pattern after a cough. When patients are extubated in the intermediate zone—somewhere between being asleep and being fully awake—they are much more likely to develop postextubation laryngospasm. The presence of blood in the airway as may occur following adenoidectomy, tonsillectomy, and nasal surgery is an especially potent stimulus for laryngospasm. (Furthermore, in unintubated patients who are inhaling anesthesia through a mask, upper airway secretions should be removed while the patient remains fully anesthetized to avoid laryngospasm.)

Applying positive airway pressure by mask may be briefly attempted to eradicate the laryngospasm, although some experts believe this maneuver actually exacerbates the condition. Laryngospasm that does not respond within 30 seconds to positive airway pressure and relief of soft tissue obstruction should be treated with IV succinylcholine, 1 mg/kg, to relax and open the vocal cords. Often it is advisable to give atropine, 0.01–0.02 mg/kg IV, prior to succinylcholine in order to avoid succinylcholine-induced, or hypoxia-associated, bradycardia.

ASPIRATION

To reduce the incidence of aspiration at the end of surgery, a nasogastric tube should be passed and suction applied prior to extubation. Moreover, patients at risk should be extubated only when they are fully awake; depression of the glottic reflex lasts at least 2 hours and perhaps as long as 8 hours after extubation, even in patients who seem alert.[74] This depression has implications for postoperative liquid or solid ingestion.

In conclusion, to reduce the incidence of aspiration pneumonitis, careful preoperative instructions should be given regarding the necessity for adults to fast from solid food for 8 hours prior to elective surgery; patients should be questioned thoroughly about ingestion of food and liquids when they arrive for anesthetic induction. High risk patients should be identified and treated accordingly in terms of anesthetic induction technique. Skillful airway management is essential, and pharmacological prophylaxis in high risk patients seems reasonable. Extubation should not be performed until the high risk patient is wide awake, with reflexes intact.

POSTOBSTRUCTION PULMONARY EDEMA

Noncardiogenic pulmonary edema is uncommon and may arise from a variety of causes, including drugs, sepsis, head trauma, and high altitude (Table 12–5). Although airway obstruction as a rare cause of acute pulmonary edema was recognized clinically in the 1960s, no case reports[75, 76] appeared until 1977.

Many of the early case reports described pediatric patients with croup or epiglottitis; therefore, there was an initial perception that postobstructive pulmonary edema occurs mainly, if not exclusively, in children. However, in adults, a variety of conditions producing airway obstruction may also be linked with fulminating pulmonary edema. A partial list of these entities includes laryngospasm,[77] epiglottitis,[78] sleep apnea,[79] goiter,[80] malignancy, and strangulation.[76]

The mechanisms underlying postobstructive pulmonary edema are obscure and probably multifactorial. However, forced inspiration against a closed glottis (modified Müller's maneuver), inducing large negative intrapleural and transpulmonary pressure gradients favoring the transudation of pulmonary edema fluid from the pulmonary capillaries into the interstitium, appears to be the predominant one. (The amount of respiratory muscle force transformed to negative intrathoracic pressure is affected by chest wall compliance. Because children have more compliant chest walls than adults, this may explain the increased incidence of postobstructive pulmonary edema in children.) Nonetheless, the possibility that pro-

TABLE 12–5. Features of Postobstructive Pulmonary Edema

Etiology multifactorial
May occur in adults as well as children
Sleep apnea and nasopharyngeal anomalies may predispose
Indicated therapy may be conservative or involve intubation, mechanical ventilation, and PEEP

longed hypoxia or severe acidosis will trigger pulmonary edema, either by direct pulmonary effects or through myocardial depression, cannot be ruled out.

Perhaps patients with a *forme fruste* of sleep apnea or those with nasopharyngeal anomalies may be at increased risk to develop the complication.[81] This variety of postobstructive pulmonary edema is characterized by rapid onset and, not uncommonly, resolution without the need for aggressive therapy or invasive monitoring, especially in children.

Those who require more aggressive therapy for this condition usually respond well to reintubation, ventilation with either continuous positive airway pressure or PEEP, judicious use of diuretics, and, some believe, steroids.

Because of the potentially serious consequences, patients recovering from an acute episode of upper airway obstruction should be observed closely for at least 12 hours. If pulmonary edema develops, untoward sequelae can be averted by timely management.

POSTEXTUBATION CROUP

An inflammatory response with mucosal edema in the larynx or trachea is produced by a variety of irritants (Table 12–6). Such stimuli include a traumatic intubation characterized by several attempts, the use of an endotracheal tube that is too large, a lengthy period of intubation, and surgery involving the head and neck with considerable turning of the neck. Moreover, movement of the tube in the airway occurs with each breath. Although the tube is secured externally, the tracheobronchial tree moves with ventilation, especially with swallowing, coughing, and head movement.[82]

Certain components of plastic tubes, for example, antioxidants and plasticizers, are tissue irritants. Furthermore, when tubes are reused, the residual cleaning agent may cause tissue injury. If inadequately aerated, gas-sterilized tubes may contain ethylene oxide that is liberated and then damages airway mucosa; ethylene oxide and water react to form ethylene glycol, a well-known irritant. In the past,

high-pressure, low-volume endotracheal tube cuffs caused much damage to tracheal walls. Modern cuffs use large inflation volumes requiring lower pressure that is more evenly distributed over a greater surface area. The net result is less mucosal and submucosal injury.

Children are most frequently afflicted with glottic edema or postintubation croup. The edema may occur in the supraglottic, retroarytenoid, or subglottic region. The complication of subglottic edema is most serious and requires immediate attention. Because edema encroaches on the airway lumen, resistance is greatly increased. This is especially true in infants, in whom there is a disproportionate increase in resistance with a reduction in lumen radius, because we know from Poiseiulle's law that flow in tubes varies as the fourth power of the radius. Expansion of edema outward is limited by the cricoid cartilage encircling the subglottic region, and in the infant, the narrowest part of the airway is the subglottic region. Moreover, the subglottic region has fragile respiratory epithelium with loose submucosal connective tissue that is easily traumatized and prone to edema.

The peak incidence of croup occurs between 1 and 4 years of age.[83] Croup presents with a barking cough and varying degrees of respiratory obstruction that may initially be noted minutes to hours following extubation. There is associated dyspnea, stridor, suprasternal retraction, tachypnea, and tachycardia. The persistence of glottic or subglottic edema beyond 24 hours is often associated with more serious, permanent lesions. If resolution of the insult is followed by scar formation, subglottic stenosis may develop several weeks or months later.

Preventive measures include performing intubation as gently as possible and avoiding irritating stimuli, especially an oversized endotracheal tube. A leak should be present around the endotracheal tube, especially in pediatric patients, and this leak should be audible with 20–25 cm H_2O pressure applied. If appropriate, the use of a face mask, rather than an endotracheal tube, for pediatric patients should be encouraged. If postintubation subglottic edema occurs, humidification of inspired oxygen, cool mist, and racemic epinephrine, 0.5 mL of 2.25% solution diluted with 2.5 cc of saline, nebulized with intermittent positive-pressure apparatus, are helpful therapeutic interventions.[83] In some cases, steroids have been useful.

TABLE 12–6. Croup-Inducing Stimuli

Traumatic intubation
Improper endotracheal tube size
Prolonged intubation
Excessive movement around endotracheal tube
Tissue irritants from tube
High-pressure, low-volume cuffs

POSTOPERATIVE OR DELAYED COMPLICATIONS

VOCAL CORD GRANULOMAS

The incidence of intubation-associated granuloma is estimated to be approximately one case per 1000 endotracheal anesthesias,[84] but reports range from 1:800[85] to 1:20,000 tracheal intubations.[86]

Long-term or delayed laryngeal complications are commonly a function of the size, shape, and stiffness of the endotracheal tube; the pressure characteristics of the endotracheal tube cuff; the duration of intubation; the amount of movement of the head and neck about the tube; and, to a certain extent, the gentleness of the anesthesiologist. However, granuloma of the vocal cord region is frequently unrelated to intubation. Moreover, even following intubation, the presence of granuloma is not *per se* evidence of inferior anesthetic technique. Many granulomas are caused by vocal fold trauma, ascribed to misuse of the voice.

Postintubation granulomas are thought to develop from tiny abrasions of the delicate mucosa covering the vocal process of the arytenoid cartilage. The exposed surface becomes infected, an ulcer forms, and eventually a sessile granuloma develops. Through central proliferation, the lesion becomes an inflammatory polyp or pyrogenic granuloma. Laryngoscopy typically shows unilateral or bilateral involvement of the vocal fold at the vocal process of the arytenoid cartilage, near the junction of the middle and posterior thirds of the fold. Women are afflicted five times as often as men, presumably because of their small larynx and thin mucoperichondrium.

Symptoms commonly depend on the size of the granuloma and range from slight hoarseness and a foreign body sensation, to persistent cough and pain, to dysphonia and respiratory obstruction. The initial signs may occur as early as 4 days or as late as 7 months following intubation.

Factors associated with intubation granulomas include use of a large endotracheal tube, traumatic insertion of the tube, and intubation lasting longer than 2½ hours. Furthermore, friction of the tube against the larynx is probably related to development of granuloma. Significant friction is more likely to develop during neck surgery, especially thyroidectomy, and when lubricant for the tube is omitted. Overextension of the neck presses the tube against the arytenoid and increases the risk of contact pressure during surgery. Some cite contusion of the vocal folds produced by post-extubation coughing as another contributory factor.

Prevention of intubation granuloma is predicated on etiological considerations. A sterile, well-lubricated smooth tube of appropriate diameter should be inserted as unobtrusively as possible. Extension of the head after intubation should be discouraged, and surgical manipulation of the trachea should be gentle. Extubation should be timed to avoid vigorous coughing. If persistent hoarseness develops, early otolaryngological evaluation is essential.

Treatment, depending on the severity of the lesion, ranges from voice rest to surgical excision of the granuloma.

VOCAL CORD PARALYSIS

Fortunately, vocal cord paralysis secondary to intubation is uncommon. Rather, it tends to be a complication associated with head and neck surgery, especially thyroidectomy, when direct or indirect injury to the recurrent laryngeal nerve(s) has transpired. As previously mentioned, however, the condition may occasionally be attributed to neuropraxia from pressure on the recurrent laryngeal nerve by the cuff of the tracheal tube. Its incidence may be reduced by placing the cuff sufficiently below the larynx and by eliminating the use of endotracheal tubes with cuffs that inflate unevenly.

Unilateral vocal cord paralysis is typically rather benign, with symptoms generally limited to hoarseness that appears immediately post-operatively or soon thereafter. Recovery is usually within a few weeks, although some slight degree of partial paralysis may persist.

Bilateral cord paralysis is much more serious and causes signs of increasing upper airway obstruction, which may follow immediately after extubation or be delayed for hours. The patient has difficulty vocalizing the letter "E," and auscultation over the larynx discloses inspiratory and expiratory vibrations. As respiratory obstruction worsens, stridor and paradoxical respiration develop, followed by complete obstruction. The usual methods of ameliorating obstruction, such as neck extension or oral airway insertion, do not help. Positive-pressure ventilation through a face mask should be applied, followed by reintubation. Most patients with bilateral vocal cord paralysis recover after a month or longer, but tracheostomy often is needed as a temporizing measure.

SUBGLOTTIC STENOSIS AND TRACHEAL INJURIES

Subglottic stenosis may be a congenital condition but is usually associated with prolonged intubation. This major complication becomes apparent several months after intubation and is more common in adults than in children. The stenotic lesion is usually situated where the cuff was positioned; less commonly, the site of damage coincides with the tip of the endotracheal tube. Prevention includes using appropriately sized endotracheal tubes with large volume, low pressure cuffs and not allowing the tube to remain in place for weeks before resorting to tracheostomy. Symptoms include coughing, dyspnea, and signs of respiratory obstruction. Treatment includes dilatation in the less serious cases or resection of the stenotic segment in more advanced cases.

The short-term complications of tracheostomy include hemorrhage, pneumothorax, obstruction of the tracheostomy tube by clot or inspissated secretions, tube displacement, cardiovascular collapse, and subcutaneous emphysema.[87, 88] Although tracheostomy protects the larynx from additional injury, trauma may still occur at the site of the inflated cuff and at the tip of the tracheostomy tube. In an attempt to prevent these injuries, standard tracheal tube cuffs have been replaced with large volume, low pressure cuffs, and many experts have advocated periodic deflation or inflation only during inspiration and various pressure-regulating devices. Moreover, tracheostomy may result in tracheal erosion, especially into the innominate artery or esophagus, much more often than laryngotracheal intubation, because tracheostomy tubes usually sit lower in the trachea and have a rigid, built-in curve that may exert significant pressure on tissues at the tube tip. In addition to tracheal stenosis and erosion of major vessels or the esophagus, other long-term complications of tracheostomy include tracheitis and, occasionally, pneumonia.

It is claimed that, in adults, the inverted U-flap incision in the anterior tracheal wall through the second and third tracheal rings circumvents damage to the first tracheal ring and may avoid the problem of tracheal stenosis following decannulation. It is common to deliberately place the tracheostomy site lower in children than in adults, usually at a level ranging from the fourth to seventh tracheal rings. Selection of this lower site generally avoids many of the complications associated with a high tracheostomy, because tracheal stenosis can develop from an edematous and inflammatory reaction in the subglottic larynx or the cricoid cartilage.

CEREBROSPINAL FLUID LEAKS AND MENINGITIS

Cerebrospinal fluid leaks and meningitis may follow surgery for conditions such as glomus resection, LeFort II and III fractures, and sinusitis.

TRANSIENT HEARING LOSS

Transient hearing loss following spinal anesthesia has been reported[89] and has been attributed to low intracranial cerebrospinal fluid pressure. Hughson[90] demonstrated that a decrease in cerebrospinal fluid pressure is associated with a decrease in intralabyrinthine pressure followed by a functional inability of the ear to transmit sound. More recently, Fog and associates[91] suggested that hearing loss after spinal anesthesia is related to needle size. Not surprisingly, larger needles appeared to be more apt to trigger postspinal hearing loss. Fortunately, the documented decrease in low frequency hearing acuity is usually completely reversed, as determined by repeat audiometry at 1 and 7 months following spinal anesthesia.

PROGRESSIVE SENSORINEURAL DEAFNESS

As previously mentioned, progressive sensorineural deafness has been reported when chlorhexidine gluconate accidentally enters the middle ear because of the presence of a perforated tympanic membrane.[28, 29] Care should be taken during preoperative skin preparation to keep this solution out of the eyes and ears.

REFERENCES

1. Holinger PH: Foreign bodies in the air and food passages. XVII Wherry Memorial Lecture. Trans Am Acad Ophthal Otolaryngol 1962; 66:193–210.
2. Leon DA, Hirshman CA: Pediatric laser airway microsurgery: Some problems and solutions. Anesthesiology 1980; S53:344.
3. Edens ET, Sia RL: Flexible fiberoptic endoscopy in difficult intubations. Ann Otol Rhinol Laryngol 1981; 90:307–309.
4. Cass NM, James NR, Lines V: Difficult direct laryn-

goscopy complicating intubation for anesthesia. Br Med J 1956; 1:488–489.

5. Mallampati SR: Clinical signs to predict difficult tracheal intubation. Can Anaesth Soc J 1983; 30:316–317.

6. Gotta AW: Maxillofacial trauma: Anesthetic considerations. ASA Refresher Course Lectures, 1986, Park Ridge, Illinois, American Society of Anesthesiologists, 246.

7. Barker SJ, Tremper KK, Hyatt J: Effects of methemoglobinemia on pulse oximetry and mixed venous oximetry. Anesthesiology 1989; 70:112–117.

8. Sandza JG Jr, Roberts RW, Shaw RC, Connors JP: Symptomatic methemoglobinemia with a commonly used topical anesthetic, Cetacaine. Ann Thorac Surg 1980; 30:187–190.

9. McGuigan MA: Benzocaine-induced methemoglobinemia. Can Med Assoc J 1981; 125:816.

10. Seibert RW, Seibert JJ: Infantile methemoglobinemia induced by a topical anesthetic, Cetacaine. Laryngoscope 1984; 94:816–817.

11. Kellet PB, Copeland CS: Methemoglobinemia associated with benzocaine-containing lubricant. Anesthesiology 1983; 59:463–464.

12. Deas TC: Severe methemoglobinemia following dental extractions under lidocaine anesthesia. Anesthesiology 1956; 17:204.

13. Burne D: Methaemoglobinemia following lignocaine (letter). Lancet 1964; 2:971.

14. Anderson ST, Hajduczek J, Barker SJ: Benzocaine-induced methemoglobinemia in an adult: Accuracy of pulse oximetry with methemoglobinemia. Anesth Analg 1988; 67:1099–1101.

15. Scheller MS, Unger RJ: The influence of intravenously administered dyes on pulse oximetry readings. Anesthesiology 1980; 65:A161.

16. Sidi A, Rush WR, Paulus DA, et al: Effect of fluorescein, indocyanine green, and methylene blue on the measurement of oxygen saturation by pulse oximetry. Anesthesiology 1986; 65:A132.

17. Curry S: Methemoglobinemia. Ann Emerg Med 1982; 11:214–221.

18. Wintrobe MM (ed): Methemoglobinemia and other disorders usually accompanied by cyanosis. In Clinical Hematology, 8th ed. Philadelphia, Lea & Febiger, 1981, pp 1011–1018.

19. Olsson GL, Haller B, Hambraeus Jonzon K: Aspiration during anesthesia: A computer aided study of 185,358 anaesthetics. Acta Anaesthesiol Scand 1986; 30:84.

20. Loeser EA, Kaminsky A, Diaz A, et al: The influence of endotracheal tube cuff design and cuff lubrication on postoperative sore throat. Anesthesiology 1983; 58:376–379.

21. Kambic V, Radsel L: Intubation lesions of the larynx. Br J Anaesth 1978; 50:587–590.

22. Komorn RM, Smith CP, Erwin JR: Acute laryngeal injury with short term endotracheal anesthesia. Laryngoscope 1973; 83:683.

23. Stanley HT, Foote JL, Liu W: A simple pressure-relief valve to prevent increases in endotracheal tube cuff pressure and volume in intubated patients. Anesthesiology 1975; 43:478–481.

24. Prasertwanitch Y, Schwarz JJH, Vandam LD: Arytenoid cartilage dislocation following prolonged endotracheal intubation. Anesthesiology 1974; 41:516–518.

25. Quick CA, Merwin GE: Arytenoid dislocation. Arch Otolaryngol 1978; 104:267–270.

26. Frink EJ, Pattison BD: Posterior arytenoid dislocation following uneventful endotracheal intubation and anesthesia. Anesthesiology 1989; 70:358–360.

27. Smith PH, Sharp J, Kellgren JH: Natural history of rheumatoid cervical subluxations. Ann Rheum Dis 1972; 31:222–223.

28. Bicknell PG: Sensorineural deafness following myringoplasty operations. J Laryngol Otol 1971; 85:957–961.

29. Igarashi Y, Suzuki J: Cochlear ototoxicity of chlorhexidine gluconate in cats. Arch Otorhinolaryngol 1985; 242:167–176.

30. Tabor E, Bostwick DC, Evans CC: Corneal damage due to eye contact with chlorhexidine gluconate. JAMA 1989; 261:557–558.

31. Uejima T, Birmingham PK: Refractory bradycardia during aspiration of a tracheal cyst in a young infant. Anesthesiology 1988; 69:776–778.

32. Reynod AK: On the mechanism of myocardial sensitization to catecholamines by hydrocarbon anesthetics. Can J Physiol Pharmacol 1984; 62:183.

33. Katz RL, Katz GJ: Surgical infiltration of pressor drugs and their interaction with volatile anaesthetics. Br J Anaesth 1966; 38:712.

34. Karl HW, Swedlow DB, Lee KW, Downes JJ: Epinephrine-halothane interactions in children. Anesthesiology 1983; 58:142.

35. Tucker WK, Packstein AD, Munson ES: Comparison of arrhythmogenic doses of adrenaline, metaraminol, ephedrine and phenylephrine during isoflurane and halothane anesthesia in dogs. Br J Anaesth 1974; 46:392.

36. Johnston RR, Eger EI, Wilson C: Comparative interaction of epinephrine with enflurane, isoflurane, and halothane in man. Anesth Analg 1976; 55:709.

37. Meyers EF: Cocaine toxicity during dacryocystorhinostomy. Arch Ophthalmol 1980; 98:842.

38. Gay GR, Loper KA: Control of cocaine-induced hypertension with labetalol. Anesth Analg 1988; 67:92.

39. Rappolt RT, Gay GR, Inaba DS: Propranolol in the treatment of cardiopressor effects of cocaine. N Engl J Med 1976; 295:448–449.

40. Ramoska E, Sacchetti AD: Propranolol-induced hypertension in treatment of cocaine intoxication. Ann Emerg Med 1985; 14:1112–1113.

41. Tate N: Deaths from tonsillectomy. Lancet 1963; 2:1090.

42. Keenan RL, Boyan CP: Cardiac arrest due to anesthesia. JAMA 1985; 253:2373.

43. Davies DD: Re-anaesthetizing cases of tonsillectomy and adenoidectomy because of persistent postoperative haemorrhage. Br J Anaesth 1964; 36:244.

44. Crysdale WS: Complications of tonsillectomy and adenoidectomy in 9409 children observed overnight. Can Med Assoc J 1986; 135:1139.

45. Tami TA, Parker GS, Taylor RE: Post-tonsillectomy bleeding: An evaluation of risk factors. Laryngoscope 1987; 97:1307–1311.

46. Broadman LM, Spellman GF, Patel RI: Effects of peritonsillar infiltration upon the reduction of operative blood loss and postoperative pain in children having tonsillectomies. Anesth Analg 1988; 67:S22.

47. Kirchner JA: Cervical mediastinal emphysema. Arch Otolaryngol 1980; 106:368–375.

48. Rosenberg MB, Wunderlich BK, Reynolds RN: Iatrogenic subcutaneous emphysema during dental anesthesia. Anesthesiology 1979; 51:80–81.

49. Jumper A, Sukumar D, Liu P, et al: Pulmonary barotrauma resulting from a faulty Hope II resuscitation bag. Anesthesiology 1983; 58:572–577.

50. Hawkins DB, House JW: Postoperative pneumothorax secondary to hypopharyngeal perforation during anesthetic intubation. Ann Otol Rhinol Laryngol 1974; 85:556.

51. Martin JT, Patrick RT: Pneumothorax: Its significance to the anesthesiologist. Anesth Analg 1960; 39:420.

52. Dean HN, Parsons DE, Raphaely RC: Bilateral tension pneumothorax from mechanical failure of anesthesia machine due to misplaced expiratory valve. Anesth Analg 1971; 50:195.

53. Schweizer O: Complications of anesthesia during radical surgery about the head and neck. Anesthesiology 1955; 16:927.

54. Adornato DC, Glidenburg PL, Ferrario CM, et al: Pathophysiology of intravenous air embolism in dogs. Anesthesiology 1978; 49:120–127.

55. Honolulu TH, Pang LQ: Air embolism during lavage of the maxillary sinus. A report of two cases. Laryngoscope 1952; 62:1205–1224.

56. Thompson KFM: Air embolism following antral lavage: A fatal case. Laryngoscope 1955, 69:829–832.

57. Bacher JA: Fatal air embolism after puncture of maxillary antrum—autopsy. Calif St J Med 1923; 21:433.

58. O'Quin RJ, Lakshminaraya S: Venous air embolism. Arch Intern Med 1982; 142:2173–2176.

59. Hybels R, Boston MA: Venous air embolism in head and neck surgery. Laryngoscope 1980; 90:946–954.

60. Gottlieb JD, Ericsson J, Sweet R: Venous air embolism: A review. Anesth Analg 1965; 44:773–779.

61. Durant T, Long J, Oppenheimer M: Venous air embolism. Am Heart J 1947; 33:269–282.

62. Simpson JI, Wolf GL: Endotracheal tube fire ignited by pharyngeal electrocautery. Anesthesiology 1986; 65:76–77.

63. Fried MP: A survey of the complications of laser laryngoscopy. Arch Otolaryngol 1984; 110:31–34.

64. Hermens JM, Bennett MJ, Hirshman CA: Anesthesia for laser surgery. Anesth Analg 1983; 62:218.

65. Sosis MB: Evaluation of five metallic tapes for protection of endotracheal tubes during CO_2 laser surgery. Anesth Analg 1989; 68:392–393.

66. Giffin B, Shapshay SM, Bellack GS, et al: Flammability of endotracheal tubes during Nd-YAG laser application in the airway. Anesthesiology 1986; 65:54.

67. Patel KF, Hicks JN: Prevention of fire hazards associated with use of carbon dioxide lasers. Anesth Analg 1981; 60:885–888.

68. Caffrey RR, Warren ML, Becker KE: Neuromuscular blockade monitoring comparing the orbicularis oculi and adductor pollicis muscles. Anesthesiology 1986; 65:95.

69. Matz GJ, Rattenborg CG, Holaday DA: Effects of nitrous oxide on middle ear pressure. Anesthesiology 1967; 28:948.

70. Marshall FPF, Cable HR: The effect of nitrous oxide on middle-ear effusions. J Laryngol Otol 1982; 96:893.

71. Casey WF, Drake-Lee AB: Nitrous oxide and middle ear pressure. Anaesthesia 1982; 37:896.

72. Owens QD, Gustave F, Sclaroff A: Tympanic membrane rupture with nitrous oxide anesthesia. Anesth Analg 1978; 57:283.

73. Jahrsdoerfer RA: Anesthesia in otologic surgery. Otolaryngol Clin North Am 1981; 14:699.

74. Tomlin PJ, Howarth FH, Robinson JS: Postoperative atelectasis and laryngeal incompetence. Lancet 1968; 1:1402.

75. Travis KW, Todres ID, Shannon DC: Pulmonary edema associated with croup and epiglottitis. Pediatrics 1977; 59:695–698.

76. Ostwalt CE, Gates GE, Holmstrom FM: Pulmonary edema as a complication of acute airway obstruction. Rev Surg 1977; 34:346–347.

77. Melnick BM: Postlaryngospasm pulmonary edema in adults. Anesthesiology 1984; 60:516–517.

78. Rivera M, Hadlock FP, O'Meara ME: Pulmonary edema secondary to acute epiglottitis. AJR 1979; 132:991–992.

79. Goldhill DR, Dalgleish JB, Lake RH: Respiratory problems and acromegaly. An acromegalic with hypersomia, acute upper airway obstruction, and pulmonary edema. Anaesthesia 1982; 37:1200–1203.

80. Stradling JR, Bolton P: Upper airway obstruction as a cause of pulmonary oedema. Lancet 1982; i:1353–1354.

81. Lorh DG, Sahn SA: Postextubation pulmonary edema following anesthesia induced by upper airway obstruction: Are certain patients at increased risk? Chest 1986; 90:802–805.

82. Blane VF, Tremblay NAG: Complications of tracheal intubation: A new classification with a review of the literature. Anesth Analg 1974; 53:202.

83. Jordan WS, Graves CL, Elwyn RA: New therapy for postintubation laryngeal edema and tracheitis in children. JAMA 1970; 212:585.

84. Hefter E: Das intubations granulom. Anesthetist 1959; 8:194.

85. Howland WS, Lewis JS: Mechanisms in the development of postintubation granulomas of the larynx. Ann Otol Rhinol Laryngol 1956; 65:1006.

86. Snow JC, Harano M, Balough K: Postintubation granuloma of the larynx. Anesth Analg 1966; 45:425.

87. Mead JW: Tracheotomy—its complications and their management. N Engl J Med 1961; 265:519.

88. Chew JY, Cantrell RW: Tracheostomy complications and their management. Arch Otolaryngol 1972; 95:538.

89. Wang LP, Fog J, Bove M: Transient hearing loss following spinal anaesthesia. Anaesthesia 1987; 42:1258–1263.

90. Hughson W: A note on the relationship of cerebrospinal and intralabyrinthine pressure. Am J Physiol 1932; 101:396–407.

91. Fog J, Wang LP, Sunberg A, Mucchiano C: Hearing loss after spinal anesthesia is related to needle size. Anesth Analg 1990; 70:517–522.

Anatomy and Physiology
of the Eye

Kathryn E. McGoldrick

OCULAR ANATOMY[1–6]

Knowledge of ocular anatomy enhances the anesthesiologist's understanding of surgical procedures and is mandatory for the performance of regional blocks of the eye and its associated structures. Salient subdivisions of ocular anatomy include the orbit, the globe, the extraocular muscles, the eyelids, and the lacrimal system. The eyeball, in part an extension of the central nervous system, is well cushioned by fat and suspended in the orbit by ligaments, fasciae, and muscles. The globe is protected by the bony orbit, soft tissues, and eyelids. During head and orbital trauma, these structures absorb and attenuate external forces and reduce potential ocular damage.

ORBIT

The orbit is a bony box, or pyramidal cavity, housing the eyeball as well as the extraocular muscles, blood vessels, nerves, and parts of the lacrimal apparatus. The orbit is approximately 40 mm in height, width, and depth, with a volume of approximately 29 mL.[1] The following bones compose the walls of the orbit: frontal, zygomatic, greater wing of sphenoid, maxilla, palatine, lacrimal, and ethmoid. Because the ethmoid bone is extremely thin (lamina papyracea), this sinus may rupture into the orbit when inflamed, or the bone may fracture, thereby permitting air to enter the orbit. The infraorbital fissure (sphenomaxillary) is the weakest area of the orbit[1] and is the region involved in so-called blowout fractures when the application of blunt force to the eye pro-

duces fragmentation of the orbital floor. Because the bone forming the roof of the maxillary antrum is extremely thin and fragile, the orbital contents herniate downward into the maxillary sinus, and incarceration of extraocular muscles and soft tissues ensues. This condition demands prompt surgical correction.

In addition to fractures, other orbital lesions include hemangiomas, meningiomas, dermoid cysts, neurofibromas, sarcomas, and gliomas. Graves' disease produces significant ophthalmopathy that may require orbital decompression. Typical signs and symptoms of these lesions include exophthalmos, impaired ocular motility, visual compromise, and displacement of the globe.

Comprehensive knowledge of surface relationships of the orbital rim facilitates skillful performance of regional blocks (see Chapter 18). The optic foramen, situated at the apex of the orbit, transmits the optic nerve, artery, and vein as well as sympathetic nerves from the carotid plexus. The superior orbital fissure transmits the superior and inferior branches of the oculomotor nerve, the lacrimal, frontal, and nasociliary branches of the trigeminal nerve, the trochlear and abducens nerves, and the superior and inferior ophthalmic veins. The inferior orbital or sphenomaxillary fissure contains the infraorbital and zygomatic nerves and a communication between the inferior ophthalmic vein and the pterygoid plexus. The infraorbital foramen, located about 4 mm below the orbital rim in the maxilla, transmits the infraorbital nerve, artery, and vein. The lacrimal fossa, housing the lacrimal gland, is situated in the superior temporal orbit. The supraorbital notch, located at the junction of the medial one third and temporal two thirds of the superior orbital rim, transmits the supraorbital nerve, artery, and vein. The supraorbital notch, the infraorbital foramen, and the lacrimal fossa are clinically palpable, major landmarks for administration of regional anesthesia.

GLOBE

The eye is one large sphere with part of a smaller sphere incorporated in the anterior surface, constituting a structure with two different radii of curvature. The wall of the globe has three layers: sclera, uveal tract, and retina (Fig. 13–1). The dense, opaque fibrous outer layer, or sclera, is protective, providing rigidity to maintain the shape of the eye. It is covered anteriorly by episclera, Tenon's capsule, and bulbar conjunctiva, which is reflected on to the inner surface of the eyelids as tarsal conjunctiva. The anterior portion of the sclera, the cornea, is transparent, permitting light to pass into the internal ocular structures. The scleral spur at the corneoscleral junction denotes the posterior boundary of the trabecular meshwork, the elaborate filter through which aqueous humor drains into Schlemm's canal and the episcleral veins.

Although the sclera is traversed by the optic nerve, the central retinal artery and vein, the anterior and posterior ciliary nerves and vessels, and the vena vorticosae from the choroid, the cornea is avascular except at the limbus, where a scant few vascular loops may be noted. However, the cornea is generously innervated with fibers from the ophthalmic division of the trigeminal nerve. The double spherical shape

of the eye exists because the corneal arc of curvature is steeper than the scleral arc of curvature. The focusing of light rays to form a retinal image begins at the transparent cornea. The cornea is protected and lubricated by the conjunctiva, eyelids, and lacrimal apparatus.

The highly vascular uveal tract, or middle layer of the globe, is in direct apposition to the sclera. A potential space, known as the suprachoroidal space, separates the sclera from the uveal tract. This potential space may become engorged with blood when an expulsive or suprachoroidal hemorrhage occurs during surgery. Such a complication may lead to a disastrous surgical result. The uveal tract is composed of the iris, ciliary body, and choroid. The iris includes the pupil, a structure composed of stroma-containing pigment cells and blood vessels, which, by contractions of three sets of muscles, controls the amount of light entering the eye. The iris sphincter and the ciliary muscle have parasympathetic innervation (oculomotor nerve), whereas the dilator pupillae fibers are supplied by the cervical sympathetic system. Sensory innervation is derived from the trigeminal nerve. Blood supply is through branches of the long posterior and anterior ciliary arteries.

Posterior to the iris lies the ciliary body, the site of production of aqueous humor. The internal surface of the ciliary body is divided into an anterior part containing the ciliary processes (pars plicata) and a posterior part, the pars plana. The ciliary muscles, situated in the ciliary body, adjust the shape of the lens to accommodate focusing at assorted distances. Sensory innervation is through the trigeminal nerve. Large vessels and an anastomotic network of small vessels and capillaries known as the choriocapillaris constitute the richly vascular choroid, which supplies nutrition to the outer part of the retina. The choroid is supplied by the sensory trigeminal nerve and the sympathetic nervous system. Its blood flow is impressively augmented by hypercarbia.

The crystalline lens, located posterior to the iris, refracts rays of light passing through the cornea and pupil to focus images on the retina. The transparent, biconvex lens is largely composed of protein and has an outer cortex and a firm central nucleus. Changes in lens composition are associated with cataract formation. The iris divides the anterior segment of the eye into two chambers: the anterior chamber, bounded anteriorly by the cornea and posteriorly by the iris, and a posterior chamber, bounded posteriorly by the lens and its

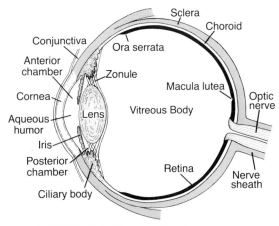

FIGURE 13–1. *Diagram of ocular anatomy.*

supporting zonule. These two chambers communicate through the pupil, which permits the passage of aqueous humor from the posterior to the anterior chamber. The average depth of the normal adult anterior chamber ranges from 2.5 to 3.5 mm.[2] The posterior segment of the eye encompasses the region from the lens to the retina and is occupied by the vitreous.

The retina is a neurosensory membrane composed of ten layers that convert light impulses into neural impulses. These neural impulses are then carried through the optic nerve to the brain. Developmentally, a potential space exists between the outer retinal pigment epithelial layer and the nine inner layers. In the setting of a retinal detachment, this space becomes filled with fluid, leaving the pigment epithelial layer in place but displacing the other nine layers further inward. Although the inner layers of retina receive their blood supply from the central retinal artery, the pigment epithelial cell layer and the rods and cones are supplied by the choroid. Near the central posterior part of the retina is a yellowish area devoid of retinal capillaries, called the macula lutea. At the center of the macula is a small pit, the fovea centralis. Composed largely of color-sensitive cone receptors, the fovea is the thinnest and most sensitive part of the retina.

Located in the center of the globe is the vitreous cavity, filled with a gelatinous substance known as the vitreous humor. This hydrophilic, colorless gel, with an approximate volume of 4.5 mL, accounts for about 80% of the volume of the eyeball.[2] Although largely composed of water, the vitreous also contains a few cells and salts. The vitreous is adherent to the most anterior 3 mm of the retina as well as to large blood vessels and the optic nerve. Under normal conditions, the vitreous contains no blood vessels; it is nourished from aqueous humor and from blood vessels in the retina and the ciliary processes. With age, the regular fibrillar network of the vitreous collapses, leading to erratic liquefaction and pooling of water within the gel. These changes may cause the vitreous to move anteriorly and separate from the retina. Vitreoretinal adhesions may pull on the retina, resulting in holes, tears, and ultimately, retinal detachments. Other retinal pathology may be associated with various conditions that produce retinal ischemia. In this setting, new and abnormal blood vessels grow and adhere to the posterior vitreous. Such neovascularization may result in rupture of the vessel and vitreous hemorrhage.

EXTRAOCULAR MUSCLES

Six extraocular muscles move the eye within the orbit to various positions, accounting for convergence of the eyeball as well as horizontal, vertical, and rotational movements. These muscles are the superior, inferior, medial, and lateral recti and the superior and inferior obliques. The four recti originate from the fibrous ring and dural sheath of the optic nerve at the orbital apex and insert into the sclera posterior to the limbus. Innervation of the superior, inferior, and medial recti is through the oculomotor nerve, whereas the lateral rectus is supplied by the abducens nerve. The superior oblique muscle originates from the sphenoid and passes through the trochlea before its insertion into the posterior superior quadrant of the sclera. It is innervated by the trochlear nerve. The inferior oblique muscle, innervated by the oculomotor nerve, arises from the maxilla and inserts into the posterior inferior portion of the sclera.

EYELIDS

The eyelids consist of four layers (1) the conjunctiva, a semitransparent mucous membrane that, in addition to covering the inner surface of the eyelids, also envelops the anterior sclera as far as the corneal margins; (2) the cartilaginous tarsal plate; (3) a muscle layer composed mainly of the orbicularis and the levator palpebrae; and (4) the skin. The eyelids protect the eye from foreign bodies. Moreover, through blinking, the tear film produced by the lacrimal gland as well as the meibomian and mucous secretions are spread across the surface of the eye, keeping the cornea moist and well nourished. Near the medial margin of each lid is a small elevation, known as the lacrimal papilla, containing the punctum leading into the lacrimal canaliculus. The upper branch of the zygomatic branch of the facial nerve supplies the frontalis and the orbicularis of the upper lid. The lower branch supplies the orbicularis of the lower lid.

LACRIMAL APPARATUS

The lacrimal drainage system, composed of the puncta, canaliculi, lacrimal sac, and nasolacrimal duct, eventually drains into the nose below the inferior turbinate. Blockage of this system may occur, necessitating procedures ranging from lacrimal duct probing to dacryocystorhinostomy, which involves anastomosis of the lacrimal sac to the nasal mucosa.

OCULAR AND ORBITAL BLOOD SUPPLY

Blood supply to the eye and orbit is through branches of both the internal and external carotid arteries. Multiple anastomoses of the superior and inferior ophthalmic veins account for orbital venous drainage, whereas the central retinal vein is mainly responsible for ocular venous drainage. All these veins then empty into the cavernous sinus.

OCULAR PHYSIOLOGY

Although small, the eye is a highly complex organ with several intricate physiological processes. Despite its complexity, the human eye is not the best. Birds, for example, have better visual acuity. (Indeed, some varieties of birds possess two foveas.)[1] Although sensitivity of the human eye increases significantly with dark adaptation, nonetheless many nocturnal animals have a lower threshold to light.

Despite its shortcomings for specific functions, the human eye does provide satisfactory vision in a vast array of circumstances. Humans, for example, have fairly good visual acuity both near and far. Color vision is well developed, and the human eye can adapt to light and dark over an impressive intensity range. Furthermore, the location of the eyes in the front of the head and the decussation of half of the nerve fibers from each retina lead to a retinal correspondence so that excellent stereoscopic vision results.

The physiological functions of the eye most important to the anesthesiologist include the absorption of topical drugs applied to the eye and the formation and drainage of aqueous humor and its influence on intraocular pressure (IOP) in both normal and glaucomatous eyes. These mechanisms related to IOP are most often affected by anesthetic manipulation and directly affect the ability to provide optimal anesthetic conditions and surgical results.

TOPICAL OCULAR ABSORPTION OF DRUGS

Frequently, drugs are instilled into the eye for diagnostic or therapeutic purposes, and systemic effects can occur. These are described extensively in Chapter 17.

Although drugs are absorbed through the cornea and conjunctiva, more substantial and rapid absorption may occur through the mucous membrane of the nose, mouth, and gastrointestinal tracts after these drugs traverse the lacrimal apparatus. Hence, occluding the nasolacrimal duct by applying pressure on the inner canthus of the eye greatly decreases systemic absorption. Digital pressure applied over the duct for 5 minutes is reported to decrease systemic absorption by 67%.[7]

Because the lacrimal apparatus depends on both an active blink reflex and muscle activity, the amount of systemic absorption of eye drops is greatly reduced under general anesthesia. Nonetheless, nasolacrimal duct occlusion is advocated, even with general anesthesia, in patients who might be more vulnerable to the toxic effects of certain ocular medications. In addition, some percutaneous absorption from spillover through the immature epidermis of premature infants can occur.[8]

Pharmacology teaches us that the term *compartment* refers to a fictitious body space within which a drug is always homogeneously distributed and from which exchange to other compartments always occurs at the same rate. Havener[9] reminds us that, with respect to the eye, the concept of compartments of uniform drug distribution is truly fictitious. Here, the rate of metabolic exchange is so swift that even the aqueous humor differs from posterior to anterior chamber. Active transport systems exist in the ciliary epithelium, lens epithelium, and retinal pigment epithelium,[10] as well as in the cornea and other parts of the blood-eye barrier. (Anesthesiologists are generally accustomed to administering drugs that exhibit first-order kinetics whereby the rate of transfer is proportional to the drug concentrations, and the drug half-life is a constant time regardless of the amount of drug present. Active transport systems, however, change drug kinetics from first order to zero order, wherein drug transfer is related to a functional capacity of the body rather than to drug concentration, and thus the half-life of the drug increases when the elimination capacity of the body is saturated.) Fictitious ocular compartments of clinical interest include the cul-de-sac, the anterior chamber, the vitreous space, and various tissues of the eye.[9] For topical medications, the cornea is the barrier to ocular drug entry. For systemic medications, other parts of the blood-eye barrier control drug access.[9]

The cul-de-sac compartment is the space into which topical eye medications enter. Although a single drop of a typical commercial eye drop has a volume ranging from 50 to 75 µl, maximal bioavailability is reached with a drop size of only 20 μl.[11–13] Thus, a single ordinary drop is much too large an amount to be usefully retained. Instilling multiple drops at one time in an attempt to achieve a greater effect accomplishes nothing except exposing the patient to possible toxicity if significant overflow enters the lacrimal excretory system. Additionally, in the normal eye, the tear turnover rate averages 15% per minute.[14] With application of the average drop of ophthalmic drug stimulating lacrimation sufficiently to double the turnover rate, this washout effect accounts for the almost complete disappearance of an instilled drug from the cul-de-sac within 5 minutes. Approximately 80% of a drug applied as an eye drop does not enter the eye, exiting instead through lacrimal drainage from the cul-de-sac.[9] Nonetheless, despite the astonishingly rapid escape of topically applied drugs from the surface of the eye, therapeutic levels are actually not only able to be achieved but persist within the eye for clinically effective periods of time.

Various ocular structures have markedly different permeability, and knowledge of these characteristics guides administration of drugs intended to affect different portions of the eye. For example, penetration of the intact cornea by drugs is based on differential solubility rather than simple diffusion. Because the lipid content of the epithelium and endothelium is 100 times greater than that of the corneal stroma, the former are relatively impermeable to electrolytes but are easily penetrated by lipid-soluble substances.[15] The stroma, however, is relatively resistant to fat-soluble substances but is readily penetrated by electrolytes. Therefore, all medications that readily enter the eye following topical application must have the ability to exist in equilibrium in solution as ionized or nonionized forms (e.g., alkaloids such as homatropine). Substances that are exclusively electrolytes or nonelectrolytes are incapable of penetrating an intact cornea (Fig. 13–2).

The conjunctival epithelium is structurally and physiologically similar to that of the cornea, and their permeability characteristics are similar. Despite its toughness, the sclera does not act as a differential solubility barrier and is actually porous. However, rapid trans-scleral outflow militates against facile intraocular penetration. The thick-walled iris vessels are another part of the blood-eye barrier. The ciliary epithelium is a unique part of the blood-eye barrier, because it actively secretes some ions and allows free passage of others in accordance

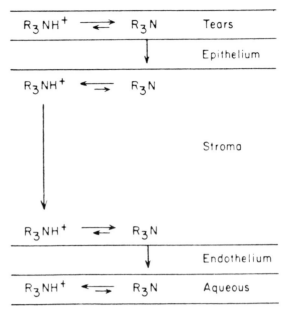

FIGURE 13–2. *Penetration of an alkaloid through the cornea, illustrating differential solubility characteristics. (From Havener WH: Ocular Pharmacology, 5th ed. St. Louis, CV Mosby, 1983, p 20.)*

with the secretion-diffusion theory of aqueous formation (see the following section). On balance, however, the ciliary epithelium blocks entry of most molecules, including protein and most antibiotics, into the aqueous humor.

The penetration of medications into the normal eye may differ dramatically from penetration into a diseased eye. Injury or inflammation disrupts the blood-eye barrier, causing aqueous flare and resulting in enhanced entry of normally excluded molecules, such as antibiotics, into the eye. Surgical manipulation, especially that associated with corneal transplantation, likewise increases drug penetration. The extent of increased permeability is directly related to the amount of epithelial damage present.[16]

In addition to ease of drug penetration, the intraocular concentration depends on its rate of removal. The two chief routes of drug loss are diffusion into the blood and egress through the aqueous humor into Schlemm's canal. Hence, topically applied drugs do not achieve clinically useful concentrations in the posterior globe. Moreover, selective binding of drugs in different parts of the eye may occur. Quantitative pharmacological studies must take into account the phenomenon of uneven intraocular distribution; studies of aqueous concentration of a given drug will not necessarily reflect intraocular penetration or persistence.[9]

FORMATION AND DRAINAGE OF AQUEOUS HUMOR

Two thirds of the aqueous humor is formed in the posterior chamber by the ciliary body in an active secretory process involving both the carbonic anhydrase and the cytochrome oxidase systems. Passive filtration of aqueous humor from the vessels on the anterior surface of the iris accounts for the remaining third. Although the protein content of aqueous humor is as low as 0.02 g/mL, and the glucose, urea, and bicarbonate concentrations are also lower than they are in blood, the concentrations of chloride, sodium lactate, and ascorbate are higher. Aqueous humor has a pH of 7.1–7.2, and its specific gravity is 1.002–1.004. The viscosity is 1.025–1.040.[17] At a state of equilibrium, approximately 2 μL of aqueous humor is formed per minute. At the ciliary epithelium, sodium is actively transported into the aqueous humor in the posterior chamber. Bicarbonate and chloride ions passively follow the sodium ions. This active mechanism results in the osmotic pressure of the aqueous being many times greater than that of plasma.

Aqueous humor flows from the posterior chamber through the pupillary aperture into the anterior chamber, where it mixes with the aqueous formed by the iris. During its passage into the anterior chamber, the aqueous humor bathes the avascular lens, providing essential metabolic materials and removing metabolic wastes. After entering the anterior chamber, the aqueous also bathes the corneal endothelium, fostering healthy corneal metabolism. Aqueous humor then flows into the peripheral part of the anterior chamber and exits the eye through the trabecular meshwork, Schlemm's canal, and the episcleral venous system (Fig. 13–3). A network of connecting venous channels ultimately leads to the superior vena cava and the right atrium. Therefore, obstruction of venous return at any site from the eye to the right side of the heart impedes aqueous drainage and produces an increase in IOP.

MAINTENANCE OF INTRAOCULAR PRESSURE

IOP normally varies between 10 and 22 mmHg and is considered abnormal above 25 mmHg. During anesthesia, an increase in IOP can produce permanent visual loss (see Chapter 14). Therefore, meticulous control of IOP is critical.

Three main factors influence IOP: (1) ex-

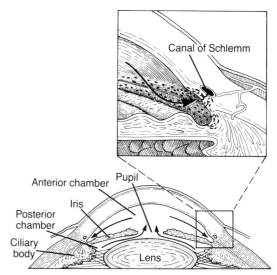

FIGURE 13–3. *Circulation of aqueous humor secreted by the ciliary body in the posterior chamber, passing through the pupil into the anterior chamber, and exiting through the trabecular meshwork into Schlemm's canal.*

ternal pressure on the eye by the contraction of the orbicularis oculi muscle and the tone of the extraocular muscles, venous congestion of orbital veins (seen with coughing and vomiting), and conditions such as orbital tumor; (2) scleral rigidity; and (3) changes in intraocular contents that are semisolid (lens, vitreous, or intraocular tumor) or fluid (blood or aqueous humor).

Sclerosis of the sclera, sometimes seen in the elderly, may be associated with reduced scleral compliance and elevated IOP. Other degenerative changes of the eye associated with aging can also affect IOP; a hardening and enlargement of the lens is the most significant change. These degenerative changes may produce anterior displacement of the lens—iris diaphragm. A resultant shallowness of the anterior chamber angle may ensue, interfering with access of the trabecular meshwork to aqueous humor. Although this process is usually gradual, sometimes rapid lens engorgement occurs, resulting in angle-closure glaucoma.

Changes in the composition of the vitreous that affect the amount of unbound water also influence IOP. Myopia, trauma, and aging produce liquefaction of vitreous gel and subsequent increase in unbound water, which may reduce IOP by facilitating fluid removal. However, under different circumstances, the opposite may occur; that is, the hydration of the more normal vitreous may be associated with increased IOP. Therefore, a slightly dehydrated state should be produced in the surgical glaucoma patient.

Although all the aforementioned factors are important in affecting IOP, the major control of intraocular tension is exerted by the intraocular fluid content, especially the aqueous humor. These critical determinants of IOP are discussed in detail in the following chapter, along with the effects of anesthetics and adjuvant drugs on IOP.

REFERENCES

1. Newell FW: Ophthalmology: Principles and Concepts, 4th ed. St. Louis, CV Mosby, 1978, pp 3–79.
2. Morrison JD, Mirakhur RK, Craig HJL: Anesthesia for Eye, Ear, Nose and Throat Surgery, 2nd ed. London, Churchill Livingstone, 1985, pp 142–150.
3. Beard C, Quickert MH: Anatomy of the Orbit, 2nd ed. Birmingham, Aesculapius, 1977.
4. Mausolf FA: The Anatomy of the Ocular Adnexa. Springfield, Charles C. Thomas, 1975.
5. Warwick R (ed): Wolff's Anatomy of the Eye and Orbit, 7th ed. Philadelphia, WB Saunders, 1977.
6. Bruce RA: Ocular anatomy. *In* Bruce RA, McGoldrick KE, Oppenheimer P (eds): Anesthesia for Ophthalmology. Birmingham, Aesculapius, 1982, pp 3–17.
7. Zimmerman T, Konner KS, Kandarakis AS, et al: Improving the therapeutic index of topically applied ocular drugs. Arch Ophthalmol 1984; 102:551–553.
8. Nachman RL, Esterly NB: Increased skin permeability in preterm infants. J Pediatr 1971; 79:628.
9. Havener WH: Ocular Pharmacology, 5th ed. St. Louis, CV Mosby, 1983, pp 18–43.
10. Reddy VN: Dynamics of transport systems in the eye. Invest Ophthalmol 1979; 18:1000.
11. File RR, Patton TF: Topically applied pilocarpine. Arch Ophthalmol 1980; 98:112.
12. Patton TF, Francoeur M: Ocular bioavailability and systemic loss of topically applied ophthalmic drugs. Am J Ophthalmol 1978; 85:225.
13. Brown C, Hanna C: Use of dilute drug solutions for routine cycloplegia and mydriasis. Am J Ophthalmol 1978; 86:820.
14. Puffer MJ, Neault RW, Brubaker RF: Basal precorneal tear turnover in the human eye. Am J Ophthalmol 1980; 89:369.
15. Kishida K, Otori T: A quantitative study on the relationship between transcorneal permeability of drugs and their hydrophobicity. Jpn J Ophthalmol 1980; 24:251.
16. Berkowitz RA, Klyce SD, Salisbury JD, Kaufman HE: Fluorophotometric determination of the corneal epithelial barrier after penetrating keratoplasty. Am J Ophthalmol 1981; 92:332.
17. Aboul-Eish E: Physiology of the eye pertinent to anesthesia. *In* Smith RB (ed): Anesthesia in Ophthalmology. Boston, Little, Brown, 1973, pp 1–20.

Anesthetics and Intraocular Pressure: Management of Penetrating Eye Injuries

——————— Kathryn E. McGoldrick ———————

DETERMINANTS OF INTRAOCULAR PRESSURE

Normal intraocular pressure (IOP) in humans ranges from 10 to 22 mmHg. This level fluctuates 1–2 mmHg with each cardiac contraction and 2–5 mmHg with diurnal variation. Characteristically, individuals have a higher IOP upon awakening owing to the vascular congestion, pressure exerted on the globe from closed lids, and mydriasis that occur during sleep. Because IOP normally exceeds both tissue pressure (2–3 mmHg) and intracranial pressure (7–8 mmHg), the maintenance of such a relatively high pressure in the eye is demanded by the optical properties of refracting surfaces. The corneal surface should be kept at a constant curvature, and the stroma must be under constant high pressure to maintain a uniform refractive index.[1] However, an abnormally elevated pressure may produce opacities by compromising normal corneal metabolism.

IOP is dependent upon a number of variables, including production and drainage of aqueous humor, fluctuations in choroidal blood volume, scleral rigidity, and extraocular muscle tone along with other sources of extrinsic pressure on the globe. Extrinsic pressure on the eye from virtually any source increases IOP.[2] Hence, an improperly fitting anesthesia mask or an inadvertent touch on the eyelid can elevate IOP. Likewise, expanding intraocular lesions, such as an orbital tumor or a hematoma following retrobulbar block–induced vessel laceration, increase IOP.[3] However, the rates of formation and drainage of aqueous humor are the most important factors determining IOP.

The carbonic anhydrase enzyme system is partially responsible for the formation of aqueous humor through an active secretory process involving a sodium/potassium/adenosine triphosphate pump. (Two-thirds of aqueous humor is formed in the posterior chamber by the ciliary body engaged in this active process; the remaining third is formed by passive filtration of aqueous from vessels on the anterior surface of the iris.)

The difference in osmotic pressure between aqueous humor and plasma is crucial in determining IOP, as illustrated by the equation[1]

$$IOP = K[(OPaq - OPpl) + CP]$$

where K = coefficient of outflow, OPaq = osmotic pressure of aqueous humor, OPpl = osmotic pressure of plasma, and CP = capillary pressure.

Because a small change in plasma solute concentration can dramatically affect aqueous humor production, hypertonic solutions, such as mannitol, are highly effective in rapidly lowering IOP.

Fluctuations in aqueous outflow can also effect impressive changes in IOP. The most important factor influencing aqueous humor outflow is the diameter of Fontana's spaces in the trabecular meshwork, as illustrated by the equation[4]

$$A = \frac{r^4 \times (\text{Piop} - \text{Pv})}{8\eta L}$$

where A = volume of aqueous outflow per unit of time, r = radius of Fontana's spaces, Piop = intraocular pressure, Pv = venous pressure, η = viscosity, and L = length of Fontana's spaces.

When the pupil dilates, IOP increases because Fontana's spaces narrow, and resistance to outflow is increased. Because mydriasis is obviously undesirable in both narrow and wide angle glaucoma, miotics, such as pilocarpine or timoptic, are applied conjunctivally in patients with glaucoma.

The previous equation, depicting volume of aqueous outflow per unit of time, underscores that outflow is sensitive to changes in venous pressure. If venous return from the eye is impaired at any point from Schlemm's canal to the right atrium, IOP increases substantially. This clinical problem results from increased intraocular blood volume and distention of orbital vessels and interference with aqueous drainage. (Whereas changes in either venous or arterial pressure may secondarily affect IOP, excursions in arterial pressure have less importance than do venous fluctuations. In chronic arterial hypertension, ocular pressure returns to normal levels after a period of adaptation brought about by compression of vessels in the choroid as a result of elevated IOP. Hence, a feedback mechanism reduces the total volume of blood, keeping IOP relatively constant in patients with systemic hypertension.)[5]

Vomiting, straining, and coughing dramatically increase venous pressure and IOP as much as 40 mmHg or more. Furthermore, laryngoscopy and tracheal intubation may also elevate IOP, even in the absence of visible reaction to intubation, but especially if the patient bucks or coughs. Although topical anesthetization of the larynx may attenuate the hypertensive response to laryngoscopy,[6] it may not reliably prevent associated increases in IOP. Usually, the IOP elevation from such increases in venous pressure dissipates quickly. However, during anesthesia, even in patients with usually normal IOP, an abrupt and impressive increase in IOP may produce permanent visual loss. If the IOP is already elevated, an additional increase may precipitate acute glaucoma. If penetration of the globe occurs when the IOP is excessively high, blood vessel rupture with subsequent hemorrhage may transpire. IOP becomes atmospheric once the eye

cavity has been entered. Thus, any sudden rise in pressure when the eye is open, as during cataract extraction or penetrating keratoplasty as well as following penetrating trauma, may lead to prolapse of the iris and lens and loss of vitreous. Proper control of IOP is also critical for glaucoma patients. Thus, in addition to preoperative instillation of miotics, other anesthetic goals in managing patients with glaucoma include perioperative avoidance of both venous congestion and overhydration.

EFFECTS OF ANESTHETICS AND ADJUVANT DRUGS ON IOP

CNS depressants, metabolic and respiratory status, temperature, neuromuscular blockers, and various adjuvant drugs all influence IOP.

CNS DEPRESSANTS

Inhalation agents purportedly cause dose-related decreases in IOP. Postulated mechanisms include depression of a CNS control center in the diencephalon,[5] reduction of aqueous humor production, enhancement of aqueous outflow, and relaxation of the extraocular muscles.[7] Virtually all CNS depressants, including barbiturates,[8] neuroleptics, narcotics, tranquilizers, and hypnotics, lower IOP in both normal and glaucomatous eyes. Ketamine was initially reported to increase IOP, but more recent studies have not demonstrated any substantial effect on IOP.[9] However, ketamine's proclivity to cause nystagmus and blepharospasm make it a suboptimal agent for many types of ophthalmic surgery.

Despite its potential to produce pain on injection and skeletal muscle movement, etomidate is generally associated with a significant reduction in IOP.[10] Although premedication with diazepam or fentanyl may diminish the incidence and severity of myoclonus, these drugs cannot totally or reliably eliminate myoclonus, which could be hazardous in the setting of a ruptured globe. Berry and Merin[11] suggest that when it is necessary to take advantage of the cardiovascular stability provided by induction with etomidate in the patient with an open globe, etomidate should be combined with succinylcholine to minimize the time to complete flaccidity.

VENTILATION, METABOLIC STATUS, AND TEMPERATURE

Respiratory acidosis increases both choroidal blood volume and IOP,[12] whereas respiratory alkalosis does the opposite. However, changes in arterial carbon dioxide pressure within a normal physiological range have minimal effect on IOP. Surprisingly, metabolic acidosis reduces choroidal blood volume and IOP, and metabolic alkalosis increases them.

Predictably, hypoxia dilates the choroid blood vessels, leading to increased IOP.

Hypothermia lowers IOP. On superficial assessment, an increase in IOP might be expected with hypothermia because of the associated increase in viscosity of aqueous humor. However, hypothermia results in decreased aqueous humor production and vasoconstriction. Thus, the net result is a reduction in IOP.

NEUROMUSCULAR BLOCKING DRUGS

The nondepolarizing neuromuscular blocking agents are associated with a decrease or with no change in IOP. Curare[13] and pancuronium[14] have been reported to lower IOP, whereas both atracurium and vecuronium are thought to have no intrinsic effect on IOP.[15] In contrast, the depolarizing drug succinylcholine elevates IOP. An average peak increase of approximately 8 mmHg is produced within 1–4 minutes following intravenous (IV) administration. Within 7 minutes, return to baseline IOP usually occurs.[16] The ocular hypertensive effect of succinylcholine has been attributed to several mechanisms, including tonic contraction of extraocular muscles,[7] choroidal vascular dilatation, and relaxation of orbital smooth muscle.[17] The anesthetic and ophthalmic literature attests to the fact that in the presence of a severe, penetrating eye injury, succinylcholine, if given alone without proper pretreatment, can result in herniation of ocular contents.[18, 19] This concern has triggered exploration of methods to attenuate the effect of succinylcholine on IOP or of ways to replace succinylcholine as part of a rapid-sequence induction.

A variety of maneuvers, including prior treatment with acetazolamide,[20] propranolol, and nondepolarizers, have been advocated to prevent succinylcholine-induced increases in IOP. Although some attenuation of the pressure increase may ensue, none of these drugs consistently and completely prevents the ocular hypertensive response.

The efficacy of pretreatment with nondepolarizing muscle relaxants is controversial. In 1968, Miller and colleagues,[21] employing indentation tonometry, reported that pretreatment with small amounts of gallamine or curare prevented succinylcholine-associated increases in IOP. However, in 1978, Meyers and associates,[22] employing the more sensitive applanation tonometer, failed to consistently obliterate the ocular hypertensive response following similar pretreatment therapy. Furthermore, the open globe may possibly react differently from the intact eye in response to drugs.

Smith and coworkers[23] attempted to eradicate succinylcholine-induced increases in IOP by pretreating with lidocaine in doses ranging between 1 and 2 mg/kg. They found, however, that IV lidocaine administered in this fashion did not satisfactorily inhibit the ephemeral increase in IOP following succinylcholine. Nonetheless, Grover and colleagues,[24] in a more recent investigation, noted that Smith's measurements of baseline IOP were obtained following induction with thiopental and hence may not have reflected true baseline values. Grover's group then conducted a similar study but determined baseline IOP in subjects prior to induction of anesthesia. They concluded that 1.5 mg/kg of lidocaine given 1 minute before induction with thiopental prevented an increase in IOP above baseline following both succinylcholine and intubation. Therefore, IV lidocaine may be of value in rapid sequence induction for penetrating eye injuries.

Indu and associates[25] found that patients pretreated with 10 mg of nifedipine sublingually 20 minutes prior to induction did not display the increase in mean IOP above baseline that was seen in a control group following succinylcholine administration and intubation. These investigators proposed, furthermore, that blood pressure control may have been the major factor in attenuating the IOP rise.

ADJUVANT DRUGS: GANGLIONIC BLOCKERS, HYPERTONIC SOLUTIONS, ACETAZOLAMIDE, AND INTRAOCULAR GASES

Ganglionic blockers, such as pentamethonium chloride and tetraethylammonium chloride,[26] produce a dramatic reduction in IOP. Trimethaphan (ARFONAD) also significantly lowers IOP in nonglaucomatous subjects despite mydriasis.

As previously mentioned, IV hypertonic

solutions such as dextran, urea, and mannitol increase plasma osmotic pressure, thereby decreasing aqueous humor formation and IOP.[27] IV administration of acetazolamide likewise lowers IOP by inactivating carbonic anhydrase and thereby interfering with the sodium pump responsible for much of aqueous humor production.

In patients with retinal detachment, the ophthalmologist may inject sulfur hexafluoride (SF_6) into the vitreous to mechanically facilitate reattachment. If nitrous oxide (N_2O) is administered concomitantly, the injected bubble can trigger a rapid and substantial elevation of IOP. In the presence of 70% N_2O, 1 mL of air expands in volume to 2.85 mL within 1 hour. When the poorly diffusible SF_6 is used, the volume increase is even more marked.[28] The associated increase in IOP may compromise retinal blood flow. Therefore, Stinson and Donlon[29] recommend terminating the N_2O 15 minutes before gas injection to prevent significant changes in the size of the intravitreous gas bubble. Furthermore, if a patient requires reoperation and general anesthesia after intravitreous gas injection, N_2O should be avoided for 5 days following air injection and for 10 days following SF_6 injection.[30]

Perfluoropropane (C_3F_8)[31] and octafluorocyclobutane (C_4F_8) may also be employed in vitreoretinal surgery to support the retina. Like SF_6, these gases are relatively insoluble and require discontinuance of N_2O at least 15 minutes prior to injection. Moreover, C_3F_8 lingers in the eye for longer than 30 days.[32]

MANAGEMENT OF "OPEN EYE–FULL STOMACH" SITUATIONS

The challenging situation of the "open eye–full stomach" patient provides an example of conflicting priorities that can obfuscate the planning and execution of anesthesia. Methods and maneuvers used to protect against aspiration of gastric contents must be assessed in consideration of their influence on IOP. The anesthetic management of the patient with a penetrating eye injury who has recently eaten is controversial, and no single approach is ideal. Comprehensive understanding of the effects of various drugs and manipulations on IOP will help the anesthesiologist select the best and safest course for a successful surgical procedure.

Few would debate the management of the patient with a penetrating eye injury once intubation has been accomplished. Rather, controversy is focused on induction techniques, specifically the selection and use of neuromuscular blocking agents for facilitating intubation. Therefore, these blocking agents are discussed later in this chapter, following presentation of the basic, noncontroversial principles of anesthetic management for this complex situation.

PREOPERATIVE PREPARATION AND PERIOPERATIVE GOALS

Penetrating injuries may be the result of intraocular foreign bodies in the anterior or posterior chamber, the lens, or the vitreous humor, or may occur following lacerations of the sclera or cornea. Because penetrating injuries can result in extrusion of intraocular contents, a major anesthetic objective is to prevent additional increases in IOP that can produce further prolapse and loss of intraocular contents. However, any additional damage to the eye following the initial trauma is not necessarily due to anesthetic intervention. In many cases, for example, the patient, prior to induction of anesthesia, may have been crying, coughing, or vomiting or may have been rubbing the eye or squeezing the eyelids closed. All of these maneuvers increase IOP dramatically and may result in irreversible visual damage.

As in all cases of trauma, other injuries should be ruled out, such as skull and orbital fractures, intracranial trauma associated with subdural hematoma formation, and the possibility of thoracic or abdominal bleeding.

Whereas regional anesthesia and performance of an awake intubation are often valuable alternatives for the management of trauma patients who have recently eaten, such options are not available in the case of penetrating eye injuries. Performance of a retrobulbar block is contraindicated in this setting because extrusion of intraocular contents can result. Moreover, although a well-conducted, extremely smooth awake intubation following topical anesthesia might not increase IOP, the overwhelming likelihood is that coughing or straining will occur during intubation, resulting in significantly increased IOP.

Pharmacological aspiration prophylaxis is recommended. An antacid or an H_2 receptor antagonist can be administered to decrease gastric acid production and increase gastric pH. Additionally, metoclopramide is useful to stimulate peristalsis and to facilitate gastric emptying. No attempt should be made to insert a nasogastric tube while the patient is awake, because such a maneuver is guaranteed to trigger a major elevation in IOP.

Stimulation from laryngoscopy and endotracheal intubation may result in an increase in IOP. As mentioned, the ocular hypertensive response to laryngoscopy and intubation may be blunted by using IV lidocaine, 1.5 mg/kg. In addition, sublingual nifedipine may attenuate the IOP response to succinylcholine. Gentle, short-duration laryngoscopy in the presence of adequate skeletal muscle relaxation and anesthetic depth is crucial in assuring minimal changes in IOP.

Other considerations for the open globe patient include avoidance of elevated venous pressure from straining or coughing, which can increase IOP as much as 60 mmHg; appropriate preoxygenation with avoidance, however, of external pressure on the globe from the face mask; application of cricoid pressure to prevent regurgitation; establishing a sufficiently deep level of anesthesia prior to laryngoscopy and intubation to prevent coughing and to avoid a sudden, significant increase in systemic blood pressure; and initiation and maintenance of controlled ventilation following intubation to avoid hypercapnia-associated increases in IOP.

After the patient is intubated, akinesis is mandatory for optimal surgical outcome. Nearly complete suppression of the twitch response elicited by a peripheral nerve stimulator should be maintained until the eye is surgically closed. Furthermore, because surgical results may be jeopardized by postoperative vomiting, intraoperative administration of an IV antiemetic, such as droperidol, and passage of an orogastric tube to decompress the stomach prior to extubation are recommended. Patients with a full stomach must be extubated awake, but IV lidocaine or an appropriate dose of narcotic can be given prior to extubation to circumvent coughing.

SELECTION AND USE OF MUSCLE RELAXANTS

A rapid sequence induction with cricoid pressure and a smooth intubation must be accomplished to protect the airway and prevent significant increases in IOP. The selection and dosage of neuromuscular blocking agent are areas of considerable debate in achieving these universally accepted goals.

Using a barbiturate and an intubating dose of a nondepolarizing muscle relaxant is often described as the method of choice for the emergency repair of a ruptured globe, because pancuronium, in a dose of 0.15 mg/kg, does not increase IOP. This technique has serious disadvantages, however, including the risk of aspiration during the relatively long time (up to 3 minutes) the airway is unprotected. Moreover, a premature attempt at intubation triggers coughing, straining, and a substantial increase in IOP as well as detrimental hemodynamic consequences that may be harmful for adults with coronary artery disease.

A blockade monitor to predict intubating conditions may be unreliable, because muscle groups vary in their response to relaxants. In addition, the long duration of action of pancuronium may mandate postoperative mechanical ventilation. Furthermore, it is not always possible to predict which patients may be difficult to intubate. The rapid return of spontaneous ventilation is often invaluable to assist in the management of a difficult intubation. Clearly, the use of intubating dosages of nondepolarizing agents eliminates this helpful option. Although newer nondepolarizing relaxants, such as vecuronium and atracurium, have shorter durations of action, in equipotent doses these newer drugs have an onset of action as delayed as that of pancuronium. Furthermore, although vecuronium generally has minimal circulatory consequences, intubating doses of atracurium may be associated with histamine release and clinically significant hypotension.

Several studies have assessed the value of extremely large doses of nondepolarizing muscle relaxants to hasten the onset of adequate relaxation for endotracheal intubation. With vecuronium doses of 0.2 and 0.4 mg/kg, Casson and Jones[33] found mean onset times of 95 and 87 seconds, respectively. More recently, Ginsberg and coworkers[34] found comparable though slightly longer onset times. Ginsberg's group reported that the administration of high-dose (400 μg/kg) vecuronium reduces the speed of onset from 208 ± 41 seconds, as seen with the usual intubating dose of 100 μg/kg, to 106 ± 35 seconds. However, this study included factors that could influence the quality of intubating conditions. For example, the doses of diazepam, fentanyl, and thiopental administered prior to intubation varied greatly among patients.

Another innovative approach to hastening the onset of nondepolarizing neuromuscular blockers involves the so-called priming principle. In this concept, approximately one tenth of an intubating dose of nondepolarizing drug is used, followed 4 minutes later by a full intubating dose. Then, after waiting an additional 90 seconds, intubation can supposedly be performed. The rationale is that, theoretically, a large number of cholinergic receptors at the neuromuscular junction can be blocked by a small priming dose of nondepolarizing drug before a significant effect on neuromuscular transmission occurs. When a second, larger dose of nondepolarizing agent is administered, the remaining receptors will, theoretically, be blocked more rapidly than following a single bolus injection of the same total dose. However, studies in this area are characterized by a lack of consistent data. Moreover, priming is not without risk, because aspiration following a priming dose of 0.02 mg/kg of vecuronium has been reported.[35] Although the priming technique may hasten the onset of neuromuscular blockade, it does so at the potential expense of increased morbidity, such as blurring of vision and difficulty with breathing and swallowing, and possible mortality from aspiration.

Another approach involves pretreatment with a nondepolarizing muscle relaxant followed by a barbiturate-succinylcholine sequence. However, as mentioned, the efficacy of pretreatment with small doses of nondepolarizing muscle relaxant to prevent succinylcholine-induced intraocular hypertension is a moot issue. Nonetheless, in a patient with a full stomach, succinylcholine offers the important advantages of rapid onset, short duration of action, and excellent intubating conditions. Given after pretreatment with a nondepolarizing relaxant (e.g., curare 0.06 mg/kg) and an inducing dose of sodium thiopental (4–6 mg/kg), succinylcholine (1.5 mg/kg) causes only slight increases in IOP above baseline.

Libonati and associates[36] at the Wills Eye Hospital in Philadelphia retrospectively reviewed the charts of 100 patients who received anesthesia for repair of open globe injuries. Seventy four received succinylcholine, by either bolus injection or infusion, after pretreatment with a nondepolarizing muscle relaxant. According to the authors, in no case did the ophthalmologist report loss of globe contents. This report, however, has been criticized as a retrospective analysis without a control group for comparison and having as its only end point whether the surgeon complained of extrusion of eye contents. No mention, for example, was made of difficulty with uveal prolapse, bleeding, or reformation of the globe. However, the study is interesting, and

the authors state that in their 10-year experience with approximately 2500 patients who received general anesthesia with succinylcholine to facilitate intubation for penetrating eye injuries, not a single case was associated with extrusion of intraocular contents. Donlon reported a similar 10-year experience at the Massachusetts Eye and Ear Infirmary.[37]

Is a substitute for succinylcholine in rapid-sequence induction for open eye injuries necessary? Edmondson and colleagues[38] compared IOP changes in the absence of eye injury during rapid-sequence inductions using either atracurium or succinylcholine to expedite endotracheal intubation. Although mean IOP was always lower in patients given atracurium, the mean IOP in patients given succinylcholine never increased significantly above baseline levels. This rather surprising finding, the authors pointed out, may be because previous studies reporting elevated IOP following succinylcholine concerned themselves with the effect of succinylcholine in isolation rather than in the context of an actual rapid-sequence induction.

In the early 1990s, succinylcholine appears to remain the best agent for rapid, predictable onset of neuromuscular blockade. The anesthesiologist's first concern must be optimally safe airway management. The search for a nondepolarizing muscle relaxant with succinylcholine's rapid onset and brief duration of action continues. At this time, succinylcholine with pretreatment with a "defasciculating" dose of nondepolarizing agent and with adequate amounts of lidocaine or nifedipine administered in the proper time frame probably remains the most tenable compromise in the open eye–full stomach challenge.

REFERENCES

1. Aboul-Eish E: Physiology of the eye pertinent to anesthesia. *In* Smith RB (ed): Anesthesia in Ophthalmology. Boston, Little Brown, 1973, pp 1–20.
2. Cunningham AJ, Barry P: Intraocular pressure physiology and implications for anaesthetic management. Can Anaesth Soc J 1986; 33:195–208.
3. Donlon JV Jr: Anesthesia for eye, ear, nose and throat. *In* Miller RD (ed): Anesthesia, 3rd ed. New York, Churchill Livingstone, 1990, pp 2001–2023.
4. Hill DW: Physics Applied to Anaesthesia. New York, Appleton-Century-Crofts, 1968, p 41.
5. Adler FH: Physiology of the Eye: Clinical Application, 5th ed. St. Louis, CV Mosby, 1970, p 249.
6. Stoelting RK: Circulatory changes during direct laryngoscopy and tracheal intubation: Influence of duration of laryngoscopy with or without prior lidocaine. Anesthesiology 1977; 47:381–384.
7. Duncalf D, Foldes FF: Effect of anesthetic drugs and

muscle relaxants on intraocular pressure. *In* Smith RB (ed): Anesthesia in Ophthalmology. Boston, Little Brown, 1973, pp 21–33.

8. Joshi C, Bruce DL: Thiopental and succinylcholine: Action on intraocular pressure. Anesth Analg 1975; 54:471–475.

9. Ausinisch B, Rayburn LR, Munson ES, Levy NS: Ketamine and intraocular pressure in children. Anesth Analg 1976; 55:773–775.

10. Thompson MF, Brock-Utne JG, Bean P, et al: Anaesthesia and intraocular pressure: A comparison of total intravenous anaesthesia using etomidate with conventional inhalational anaesthesia. Anaesthesia 1982; 37:758.

11. Berry JM, Merin RG: Etomidate myoclonus and the open globe. Anesth Analg 1989; 69:256–259.

12. Duncalf D, Weitzner SW: Ventilation and hypercapnia on intraocular pressure in children. Anesth Analg 1963; 43:232–237.

13. Agarwal LP, Mathur SP: Curare in ocular surgery. Br J Ophthalmol 1952; 36:603.

14. Litwiller RW, Difazio CA, Rushia EL: Pancuronium and intraocular pressure. Anesthesiology 1975; 42:750.

15. Schneider MJ, Stirt JA, Finholt DA: Atracurium, vecuronium, and intraocular pressure in humans. Anesth Analg 1986; 65:877–882.

16. Pandey K, Badola RP, Kumar S: Time course of intraocular hypertension produced by suxamethonium. Br J Anaesth 1972; 44:191–195.

17. Bjork A, Hallidin M, Wahlin A: Enophthalmus elicited by succinylcholine. Acta Anaesthesiol Scand 1957; 1:41.

18. Lincoff HA, Breinin GM, DeVoe AG: The effect of succinylcholine on extraocular muscles. Am J Ophthalmol 1957; 43:440–444.

19. Dillon JB, Sabawala P, Taylor DB, Gunter R: Action of succinylcholine on extraocular muscles and intraocular pressure. Anesthesiology 1957; 18:44–49.

20. Carballo AS: Succinylcholine and acetazolamide in anesthesia for ocular surgery. Can Anaesth Soc J 1965; 12:486–498.

21. Miller RD, Way WL, Hickey RF: Inhibition of succinylcholine-induced increased intraocular pressure by nondepolarizing muscle relaxants. Anesthesiology 1968; 29:123–126.

22. Meyers EF, Krupin T, Johnson M, Zink H: Failure of nondepolarizing neuromuscular blockers to inhibit succinylcholine-induced increased intraocular pressure—a controlled study. Anesthesiology 1978; 48:149–151.

23. Smith RB, Babinski M, Leano N: The effect of lidocaine on succinylcholine-induced rise in intraocular pressure. Can Anaesth Soc J 1979; 26:482–483.

24. Grover VK, Lata K, Sharma S, et al: Efficacy of lignocaine in the suppression of the intraocular pressure response to suxamethonium and tracheal intubation. Anaesthesia 1989; 44:22–25.

25. Indu B, Batra YK, Puri GD, Singh H: Nifedipine attenuates the intraocular pressure response to intubation following succinylcholine. Can J Anaesth 1989; 36:269–272.

26. Drucker AP, Sadove MS, Unna KR: Ocular manifestations of intravenous tetraethylammonium chloride in man. Am J Ophthalmol 1950; 33:1564.

27. Galin MA, Aizawa F, McLean JM: Intravenous urea in the treatment of acute angle glaucoma. Am J Ophthalmol 1960; 50:379–384.

28. Fineberg E, Machemer R, Sullivan P, et al: Sulfur hexafluoride in owl monkey vitreous cavity. Am J Ophthalmol 1975; 79:67–74.

29. Stinson TW, Donlon JV Jr: Interaction of SF_6 and air with nitrous oxide. Anesthesiology 1979; 51:S16.

30. Wolf GL, Capuano C, Hartung J: Nitrous oxide increases intraocular pressure after intravitreal sulfur hexafluoride injection. Anesthesiology 1983; 59:547–548.

31. Chang S, Coleman DJ, Lincoff HA, et al: Perfluoropropane gas in the management of proliferative vitreoretinopathy. Am J Ophthalmol 1984; 98:180–188.

32. Chang S, Lincoff HA, Coleman DJ, et al: Perfluorocarbon gases in vitreous surgery. Ophthalmology 1985; 92:651–656.

33. Casson WR, Jones RM: Vecuronium induced neuromuscular blockade. Anaesthesia 1986; 41:354–357.

34. Ginsberg B, Glass PS, Quill T, et al: Onset and duration of neuromuscular blockade following high-dose vecuronium administration. Anesthesiology 1989; 71:201–205.

35. Musich J, Walts LF: Pulmonary aspiration after a priming dose of vecuronium. Anesthesiology 1986; 64:517–519.

36. Libonati MM, Leahy JJ, Ellison N: Use of succinylcholine in open eye injury. Anesthesiology 1985; 62:637–640.

37. Donlon JV Jr: Succinylcholine and open eye injury. Part II. Anesthesiology 1986; 64:524–525.

38. Edmondson L, Lindsay SL, Lanigan LP, et al: Intraocular pressure changes during rapid sequence induction of anaesthesia. Anaesthesia 1988; 43:1005–1010.

Pediatric Ophthalmic Surgery: Anesthetic Considerations

———————————————— **Kathryn E. McGoldrick** ————————————————

Ophthalmic surgery is commonly performed on the very young as well as the very old. The most frequent abnormal eye condition among children is strabismus, which accounts for approximately 70% of the pediatric ocular cases performed under general anesthesia. Other pediatric eye conditions that the anesthesiologist encounters include congenital cataracts, congenital glaucoma, ptosis, penetrating trauma, lacrimal disease, retinal detachment, orbital rhabdomyosarcoma, and retinopathy of prematurity. Often, congenital ocular anomalies are associated with serious diseases such as Pierre Robin syndrome, Treacher Collins syndrome, Down's syndrome, glycogen storage disease, and neuromuscular disorders.

Although with adults many ocular operations such as those for cataracts, glaucoma, and retinal detachments may be done equally well under local (retrobulbar or peribulbar block) or general anesthesia, with children the anesthesiologist almost always has to administer general anesthesia to guarantee satisfactory surgical conditions. Important facets of anesthetic management for a variety of pediatric ophthalmic operations are discussed in this chapter.

STRABISMUS

Strabismus surgery is the most common pediatric ocular operation performed in the United States. Approximately 5% of the population have malalignment of the visual axes, which may be accompanied by diplopia, amblyopia, and loss of stereopsis.[1] Treatment modalities include glasses, prisms, and patch therapy. However, surgical correction is the most effective form of treatment, despite the fact that more than one operation may be necessary to achieve final correction.

Eye muscle surgery on patients between 6 and 12 months of age is increasing so that the affected eye can develop normal vision and, hopefully, the two eyes can acquire stereopsis. However, some children still do not have their squints corrected until they are considerably older. The surgery entails a variety of techniques to weaken an extraocular muscle by moving its insertion on the globe (recession) or to strengthen an extraocular muscle by eliminating a short strip of the tendon or muscle (resection).[2]

Infantile strabismus occurs within the first 6 months of life and is often noted in the early neonatal period. Although the vast majority of children with strabismus are healthy, the incidence of strabismus is increased in those individuals with central nervous system (CNS) dysfunction, such as cerebral palsy and meningomyelocele with hydrocephalus. Moreover, strabismus may be the result of oculomotor nerve trauma or of sensory abnormalities, such as cataracts or refractive aberrations.

There are many concerns when caring for young patients (Table 15–1). Many children are fearful of separating from parents and need

TABLE 15–1. Special Concerns with Strabismus Surgery

Postoperative eye patches: child education and awareness
Oculocardiac reflex: prophylaxis and treatment
Forced duction testing and succinylcholine
Malignant hyperthermia
Postoperative vomiting: prophylaxis

more attention than older patients. The correct method for premedication and induction must be chosen carefully for each patient (e.g., no premedication, methohexital per rectum, thiopental IV through a butterfly needle, inhalation induction with or without parents present). Flexibility is necessary, because the induction plan may have to be altered. Other concerns include proper fasting period, fluid management, and use of equipment of the appropriate size. Each child should understand that one or both eyes may be patched after surgery; occluded or diminished vision secondary to patches or ointment may terrify the child as he or she emerges from anesthesia.

Other potential problems are associated with strabismus surgery; for example, there is a high incidence of oculocardiac reflex-induced dysrhythmias and an increased incidence of malignant hyperthermia (MH). MH-susceptible persons often have localized areas of skeletal muscle weakness or other musculoskeletal abnormalities.[3, 4] Studies have explored the incidence of masseter muscle spasm or jaw rigidity as a possible early warning sign of MH. In one study, the incidence of masseter muscle spasm was nearly three times higher in children undergoing strabismus surgery than in the general population.[5] Some workers believe that when masseter spasm does occur, elective surgery should be postponed and muscle biopsy testing performed. A meticulous family history, with emphasis on anesthetic aspects, and intraoperative temperature monitoring are essential for all patients having anesthesia. Many anesthesiologists are now avoiding "routine" succinylcholine administration in strabismus surgery and are intubating under deep inhalation anesthesia or else with the aid of a nondepolarizing muscle relaxant to circumvent the problems secondary to masseter spasm. (MH is discussed further in the next section of this chapter.)

Other aspects of the anesthetic management of strabismus surgery include succinylcholine-induced tonic contracture of the extraocular muscles and an increased incidence of postoperative nausea and vomiting.

In formulating a surgical treatment plan for incomitant strabismus, ophthalmologists often use the forced duction test (FDT) to differentiate between a paretic muscle and a restrictive force impeding ocular movement. To perform FDT, the surgeon grasps the sclera of the anesthetized eye with a forceps near the corneal limbus and moves the eye into each field of gaze, concomitantly assessing tissue and elastic properties. This simple test provides valuable clues to the presence and location of mechanical restrictions of the extraocular muscles.

France and colleagues[6] quantitated the magnitude and duration of interference with the FDT following succinylcholine administration. These investigators demonstrated that quantitation of the force necessary to rotate the globe remained significantly elevated over control for 15 minutes, despite the fact that the duration of rise in intraocular pressure (IOP) and of skeletal muscle paralysis was less than 5 minutes. Because succinylcholine interferes with the FDT, its use is contraindicated less than 20 minutes prior to testing. France suggested performing FDT on the anesthetized patient one of three ways: during the administration of mask inhalation anesthesia, prior to intubation of the trachea, and then using succinylcholine to expedite intubation; after intubation, facilitated by a nondepolarizing neuromuscular blocking drug; or after intubation, under moderately deep inhalation anesthesia, unaided by succinylcholine. However, when deep inhalation anesthesia is elected, atropine 0.02 mg/kg intravenously (IV) should be given before or in the early stage of induction of anesthesia. IV atropine should prevent the decrement in cardiac output that may accompany significant dose-dependent depression of left ventricular function in children.[7, 8] Additionally, IV atropine at this time provides some protection against dysrhythmias resulting from the oculocardiac reflex. For these reasons, many anesthesiologists administer IV atropine routinely to pediatric patients undergoing strabismus surgery.

The oculocardiac reflex, having a trigeminal afferent and vagal efferent limb, is triggered by pressure on the globe and by traction on the extraocular muscles, especially the medial rectus, as well as by traction or pressure on the conjunctiva or on the orbital structures. The reflex may also be elicited by performance of a retrobulbar block,[9] by ocular trauma, and by direct pressure on tissue remaining in the orbital apex.[10] Although the most common manifestation of the oculocardiac reflex is sinus bradycardia, a vast array of cardiac dysrhythmias may occur, including junctional rhythm, ectopic atrial rhythm, atrioventricular block, ventricular bigeminy, multifocal premature ventricular contractions, wandering pacemaker, idioventricular rhythm, asystole, and ventricular tachycardia.[11-12] This reflex may occur during either local or general anesthesia. Hypercarbia and hypoxemia may augment the incidence and severity of the problem.

Studies on the purported incidence of the oculocardiac reflex are characterized by striking variability. Berler's study[9] reported an incidence of 50%, but other sources quote rates ranging from 16 to 82%.[14] Strabismus surgery in children not pretreated with IV atropine may be associated with an incidence as high as 90%. Most studies of oculocardiac reflex in strabismus surgery have involved children anesthetized with halothane. It is not known if the reflex occurs as frequently with other volatile agents or with nitrous oxide-narcotic techniques. However, ketamine anesthesia is also associated with the same high incidence of the reflex.

A variety of maneuvers to obtund or abolish the oculocardiac reflex have been advocated; none has been consistently effective, safe, and reliable. Inclusion of intramuscular (IM) anticholinergic drugs, such as atropine or glycopyrrolate, in the usual premedication regimen is ineffective for oculocardiac reflex prophylaxis.[15] Nearly complete vagolytic blockade requires 0.03–0.05 mg/kg of atropine.[16] Because the peak action of IM atropine occurs approximately 30 minutes following administration, the usual much smaller doses of atropine administered more than 1 hour prior to surgery have provided inconsistent protection against the oculocardiac reflex.

For the young child who is apprehensive about "shots," oral atropine, 0.04 mg/kg given with a sip of water 60–90 minutes preoperatively, is an alternative.[17] However, the oral route is not used often because of its slower absorption and more erratic efficacy.

A retrobulbar injection blocks the afferent limb of the reflex arc, but this regional technique has inherent potential hazards, which include optic nerve damage, retrobulbar hemorrhage, and stimulation of the oculocardiac reflex arc by the retrobulbar block itself.

For pediatric strabismus surgery, most anesthesiologists currently favor routine prophylaxis with IV atropine, 0.02 mg/kg, prior to commencing surgery. Alternatively, IV glyco-pyrrolate, 0.01 mg/kg, can be given, because it may be associated with less tachycardia than atropine in this setting.

Treatment of the oculocardiac reflex, should it appear, depends on its nature and severity. Small decrements in cardiac rate may be acceptable if unaccompanied by significant hypotension. However, if the reflex results in severe sinus bradycardia or hypotension, the surgeon should stop ocular manipulation. Once the heart rate returns to normal, a small dose of atropine, 0.01 mg/kg IV, should be given and its effect noted before resuming surgery. Ventricular dysrhythmias associated with this reflex may require 1–2 mg/kg of IV lidocaine. Extreme caution must be used when giving atropine *during* a dysrhythmia produced by the reflex. Because bizarre, chaotic, and dangerous rhythms have been reported in that setting, atropine should be administered *after* the surgeon has ceased manipulation and the rhythm returns to baseline. With repeated manipulation, bradycardia is less likely to recur, probably secondary to fatigue of the reflex arc at the level of the cardioinhibitory center.[18]

Following prophylaxis with IV atropine, the anesthesiologist begins induction and intubation of the trachea. Anesthesia is commonly maintained with a volatile agent, nitrous oxide (N_2O), and oxygen, although a narcotic N_2O and oxygen technique is also acceptable. The patient is carefully monitored with a precordial stethoscope, electrocardiogram (ECG), blood pressure device, pulse oximeter, fractional inspired oxygen (FIO_2) monitor, and temperature probe. An end-tidal carbon dioxide (CO_2) monitor is also useful, because it detects early malignant hyperthermia. If bradycardia occurs, the surgeon discontinues ocular manipulation, and the patient's ventilatory status and anesthetic depth are quickly assessed. If additional IV atropine is advisable, it is not given while the oculocardiac reflex is active, lest even more dangerous cardiac dysrhythmias ensue.

Vomiting after eye muscle surgery occurs frequently. Abramowitz and associates[19, 20] reported that prophylactic IV administration of 0.075 mg/kg of droperidol, given 30 minutes prior to termination of surgery, was "highly effective" in reducing the frequency and severity of vomiting in pediatric patients undergoing repair of strabismus. Fortunately, because strabismus surgery is commonly performed on an ambulatory basis, no significant prolongation of recovery time was observed with this protocol. More recently, Lerman and coworkers[21] found encouraging results when 75 μg/kg was administered IV at the start of the case, *prior* to manipulation of the extraocular muscles. The proportion of patients who experienced vomiting was dramatically reduced to 10%. Warner and colleagues[22] reported similar results when lidocaine 2 mg/kg IV was given prior to intubation; their series disclosed a 16% incidence of vomiting. Others, however, have not reported such favorable results with lidocaine.[23, 24] Perhaps ondansetron, a selective serotonin antagonist, will prove to be an effective antiemetic for children undergoing strabismus correction.

MALIGNANT HYPERTHERMIA

Initially described in 1960 by Denborough, MH is one of the most dramatic complications of anesthesia. MH is a fulminant hypermetabolic crisis triggered by anesthetic drugs. Although mortality statistics initially hovered around 70%, since the introduction of dantrolene the mortality rate has been impressively lowered to approximately 10%.

An organized, aggressive approach has helped in preventing and treating MH. At the University of Toronto, Drs. Beverly Britt and W. Kalow established an international registry of reported cases that was highly instructive. Furthermore, new information regarding this still incompletely understood phenomenon is shared through international symposia and frequent newsletters, such as those produced by the Malignant Hyperthermia Association of the United States (MHAUS) and the Malignant Hyperthermia Association of Canada.

INCIDENCE

In the past, the incidence of MH was placed at 1/50,000 anesthetic episodes in adults and 1/15,000 in children. However, data collected in Denmark and published in 1985[25] disclosed fulminant MH approximately once in 260,000 general anesthetic exposures. The incidence increased to 1/60,000 when succinylcholine was administered. If nonspecific signs of MH, such as masseter muscle rigidity, were included, the incidence rose to 1/12,000 anesthesia episodes. When additional nonspecific signs of MH, such as fever and unexplained tachycardia, were counted, this incidence increased further to 1/5000 general anesthetics if both an inhalation agent and succinylcholine were used. Thus, variability in the reported incidence of MH is based, in part, on vagaries of definition and on selection of anesthetic agents.

PRESENTATION

MH has many presentations. All forms may become fulminant and result in death. The so-called classic fulminant case is characterized by a rapid rise in body temperature that is associated with muscle rigidity, tachycardia and various other dysrhythmias, rhabdomyolysis, acidosis, hyperkalemia, and, eventually, disseminated intravascular coagulation (DIC). Most of these cases occur during anesthesia, although some may occur in the postanesthetic period. Often, there is a family history of MH or of an unexplained perioperative death. In most instances, therapy for MH is successful if the correct diagnosis is promptly established. Unfortunately, the more fulminant forms are often associated with recrudescence. Therefore, these patients' vital signs and certain laboratory parameters should be carefully monitored, as indicated, for at least 24 hours following the initial episode.

A common presentation of MH is masseter muscle rigidity following succinylcholine. Approximately 50% of these individuals, if given muscle biopsy testing, are noted to be MH-susceptible.[26] However, masseter rigidity following succinylcholine is not uncommon, especially in pediatric patients. Although the incidence in adults is 1/12,000,[25] in pediatric patients at least one study reports[27] the incidence approximates 1% when succinylcholine is used in combination with halothane.

Many believe that masseter muscle rigidity after succinylcholine is a prodrome of MH and that the anesthetic should be immediately discontinued. Usually, if no other symptoms of MH ensue, such as temperature elevation or generalized muscle rigidity, dantrolene treatment is not elected. However, the patient should be closely monitored in a recovery room or intensive care unit for a minimum of 8 hours. Urine myoglobin and blood creatinine phosphokinase (CPK) levels at 6, 12, 18, and 24 hours should be obtained. CPK usually peaks at 10–24 hours after trismus. Although preoperative CPK values are unreliable predictors of MH susceptibility, in the setting of succinylcholine-induced masseter spasm, if the CPK level exceeds 15,000 international units (IU), there is an 88% likelihood of MH susceptibility.[28] If the peak CPK value is 20,000 IU or more, the patient almost invariably proves to be MH-susceptible. Moreover, if patients develop masseter spasm following succinylcholine, even with nonimpressive CPK levels, they should be followed up with neurological evaluation and muscle biopsy. Often, a myotonic syndrome or other myopathy will be detected.

However, masseter muscle rigidity after succinylcholine does not always presage MH, and some experts believe that the anesthetic may be continued with nontrigger drugs and careful monitoring of end-tidal CO_2.

End-tidal CO_2 levels can be invaluable in diagnosing MH early in its course. Likewise, an apparently unexplained tachycardia may often be an early sign of MH. This tachycardia should not be dismissed as merely a manifestation of "light anesthesia" or of hypovolemia. A high index of suspicion is mandatory if MH is to be detected while it is still reversible. Temperature elevation may be a very late sign of MH, and generalized muscle rigidity may never appear.

Because approximately one third of MH cases have occurred during a second or subsequent anesthetic, a previously uneventful anesthetic experience does not imply impunity. However, a personal or family history of MH has great predictive value. More than one aberration in cellular physiology can result in MH, which helps explain apparent vagaries in patterns of inheritance. McPherson and Taylor[29] report a 50% frequency of autosomal dominant inheritance. However, about 20% of families in their study seemed to have either recessive or multifactorial inheritance.

TRIGGERING AGENTS

The extensive list of anesthetic agents that may trigger MH includes depolarizing muscle relaxants and virtually all the potent inhalation anesthetics, such as halothane, ether, cyclopropane, methoxyflurane, enflurane, and isoflurane. Halothane has been the general anesthetic involved in approximately 60% of reported cases, and succinylcholine has been involved in 77%.

Although amide-type local anesthetics were once thought to trigger MH, both amide and ester local anesthetics are now reported to be safe.

Hyperthermia may be induced by nonanesthetic drugs, such as certain psychotropic agents; this condition is called the neuroleptic malignant syndrome (NMS). The signs and symptoms of NMS include fever, rhabdomyolysis, tachycardia, hypertension, muscle rigidity, agitation, and acidosis. The similarity of symptoms and the observation that biopsied muscle from many patients with NMS will exhibit enhanced contractures to halothane and caffeine suggest a link between MH and NMS.[30]

Although the resemblance between NMS and MH is notable, there are significant differences. Whereas MH is acute, NMS tends to occur after longer-term drug exposures. Phenothiazines and haloperidol are common triggering agents for NMS, but sudden withdrawal of drugs used to combat Parkinson's disease can also trigger NMS. In addition, NMS does not seem to be inherited.

Some experts believe that the changes in NMS are a manifestation of dopamine depletion in the CNS by psychoactive agents, because administration of a dopamine agonist is often useful in treatment of NMS.[31] Although a common basis for the two syndromes has not been identified, most anesthesiologists treat patients with a history of NMS as though they were susceptible to MH, until proven otherwise.

MUSCLE DISORDERS AND MALIGNANT HYPERTHERMIA

Diseases that have a strong association with MH include Duchenne's muscular dystrophy and Becker's muscular dystrophy, as well as central core disease; myotonia congenita; NMS; arthrogryposis; and the King-Denborough syndrome, which is characterized by cryptorchidism, hypotonia, webbed neck, lordosis, and pectus deformity. There is some debate whether osteogenesis imperfecta has a strong link with MH. Most anesthesiologists avoid drugs that might trigger MH in all the aforementioned conditions.

Even mild and common muscle problems may have a greater risk of MH. These conditions include inguinal hernia, ptosis, strabismus, generalized muscle bulk, localized muscle weakness, and even a history of muscle cramps, especially if linked with caffeine ingestion.

PATHOPHYSIOLOGY

MH is a disorder of skeletal muscle induced by exposure to certain pharmacological agents. However, the specific site(s) of muscle pathology remain undetermined. The sarcoplasmic reticulum may unload calcium inappropriately, resulting in an increase in cellular calcium.

Furthermore, dantrolene may reverse this rise in intracellular calcium. Much remains to be learned about the pathophysiology of MH.

INTRAOPERATIVE DIAGNOSIS

Increased end-tidal CO_2 should alert the anesthesiologist to the possibility of MH. Arterial blood gases should be drawn; if MH is responsible, dramatic degrees of hypercarbia and acidosis will be found. In cases of MH, arterial carbon dioxide pressure (Pa_{CO_2}) is often above 80 mmHg, and pH is not infrequently in the 6.8–7.1 range.

Other laboratory perturbations include, eventually, hyperkalemia, hypermagnesemia, myoglobinemia with myoglobinuria, elevated pyruvate, lactate, serum CPK, and aldolase.

As previously stated, increases in body temperature may occur relatively late in the course of MH. However, the body temperature of every patient receiving general anesthesia should be carefully monitored continuously.

SCREENING TESTS FOR MH SUSCEPTIBILITY

Testing for MH is another controversial topic. The most reliable and accurate test is the *in vitro* exposure of freshly biopsied muscle to halothane and caffeine. An accentuated contracture response to halothane and caffeine is indicative of MH susceptibility. However, this test needs to be standardized, because some laboratories test the response to caffeine only or to halothane only, whereas others combine the two. Toward the goal of standardization, the Malignant Hyperthermia Association of the United States, in cooperation with the Malignant Hyperthermia Association of Canada, sponsored a workshop in November, 1987, inviting investigators from the 17 North American laboratories currently performing the test to develop uniformity in the performance and reporting of the muscle biopsy test.

Currently in disfavor, the calcium uptake test seemed to yield an inordinate number of false-positive diagnoses. The platelet adenosine triphosphate depletion test is another ambiguous method for diagnosing MH susceptibility.

Serum creatinine phosphokinase levels *per se* are nondiagnostic. About one third of MH-susceptible individuals have normal CPK. Dramatic elevations of CPK may have some predictive value, but exercise, stress, certain drugs, recent muscle injury, and other rela-

tively benign conditions may all be associated with elevated CPK. However, abnormal serum CPK isoenzymes may be helpful in establishing susceptibility, because only the MM isoenzyme is normally found in adult serum. Therefore, in adults, the presence of MB (cardiac) or BB (brain) is considered abnormal.

Klip and colleagues[32] suggested that peripheral blood lymphocytes might provide a relatively noninvasive assay to determine susceptibility. The investigators indicated that halothane induces a significant increase in ionized calcium only in the blood of MH patients. If this test proves reliable in humans, it would be a valuable addition, because the best treatment for MH is prevention. However, at this time, there is no single test that is completely devoid of false positives or false negatives.

TREATMENT OF ACUTE MH

Successful treatment of MH is inextricably linked to preparedness, early detection, and appropriately aggressive therapy. Every anesthetizing area should have readily available a supply of iced IV fluids, dantrolene, cooling blankets, and a written protocol for counteracting MH.

Once the diagnosis of MH is made, inhalation anesthetics and succinylcholine should be immediately discontinued, and the anesthetic tubing from the machine changed, lest any soluble volatile agent remain in the rubber tubing. The soda lime should also be changed. The patient should be vigorously hyperventilated with 100% oxygen. An initial dose of dantrolene 2.5 mg/kg is given IV as rapidly as possible, and bicarbonate, 1–2 mEq/kg, is usually indicated. Additional doses of bicarbonate are titrated to arterial blood gases, and further doses of dantrolene are titrated, depending on the patient's temperature, degree of muscle rigidity, and cardiovascular status.

Dysrhythmia correction commonly follows dantrolene therapy and correction of acid-base and electrolyte status. However, procaine or procainamide may be necessary. Procainamide may be given over a 10-minute interval in a dose of 500 mg–1 g/70 kg, or 7–15 mg/kg, diluted in 500 mL of saline solution. Cardiovascular status must be carefully monitored for signs of myocardial depression.

Rapid correction of hyperthermia is critical, and appropriate methods to lower body temperature include external ice packs; cooling blankets; gastric, wound, and rectal lavage; and rapid infusion of generous volumes of iced saline. Other cooling methods have included peritoneal dialysis and cardiopulmonary bypass. Once the body temperature falls to 38°C, cooling should be discontinued.

Liberal amounts of fluid should be infused, and mannitol and furosemide should be given to maintain urine output. A Foley catheter should be inserted to accurately monitor urine output. Prevention of renal failure secondary to myoglobin casts can usually be accomplished by keeping urinary output above 2 mL/kg/hour.

Temperature, electrocardiogram (ECG), urinary output, and central venous pressure should be continuously monitored. Arterial blood gases and serum electrolytes should be frequently monitored. During and after the MH episodes, hyperkalemia and then hypokalemia, hypercalcemia, and DIC may occur. Over the next several hours, the MH patient will be sensitive to iatrogenic potassium administration, even though previously hyperkalemic plasma levels drop sharply once the temperature of the patient returns to normal. Plasma levels of 2 mEq/L are not unusual. However, potassium replacement should rarely be given, if ever, because potassium may retrigger an MH episode. Previously, digitalis was considered a potential triggering agent, but this view is no longer held.[33] Calcium channel blockers should not be used along with dantrolene.

In the early postepisode period, recrudescence may be a problem. Meticulous monitoring of the patient over several hours is mandatory. There are no absolute, all-inclusive guidelines concerning the dosage and duration of dantrolene therapy after apparent resolution of the acute MH episode. However, in fulminant cases, IV dantrolene, 1–2 mg/kg, probably should be continued every 4–6 hours for at least 24 hours.

In addition to recrudescence, late complications of MH include renal failure, disseminated intravascular consumption coagulopathy, muscle necrosis, neurological deficits, and inadvertent hypothermia. Consultation is available for assistance in managing an MH crisis; the MH "hot-line" number is 209–634–4917.

MANAGEMENT FOR THE MH-SUSCEPTIBLE PATIENT

Known MH-susceptible patients requiring elective surgery should be adequately reassured that the anesthesiologist is fully versed in the anesthetic implications of MH and that appropriate therapeutic modalities and monitoring will be employed. Dantrolene and iced saline must be readily available.

Some who believe that anxiety may predispose to MH favor generous premedication. "Safe" agents include narcotics, benzodiazepines, barbiturates, and antihistamines. However, the phenothiazines should be avoided, because there are similarities between MH and the neuroleptic malignant syndrome.

Except for those patients scheduled for muscle biopsy for MH diagnosis, IV dantrolene pretreatment is recommended in a dose of 2.5 mg/kg over a 15–30 minute interval immediately prior to surgery. Oral dantrolene prophylaxis is no longer thought efficacious.

An anesthetic machine without vaporizers and with a disposable anesthetic circuit and freshly changed CO_2 absorbent is recommended, as is the use of capnography. Of course, continuous monitoring of body temperature is necessary. Arterial and central venous pressure monitoring are employed as indicated by the nature of the surgical procedure.

Regional, local, or major conduction anesthesia is suggested because of their relative safety in this setting. However, if general anesthesia is required, as is usually the case with pediatric patients, a variety of agents may be safely used. These include barbiturates, narcotics, benzodiazepines, N_2O, and most nondepolarizing muscle relaxants. (At worst, N_2O may have some weak triggering properties.) Reversal of nondepolarizing relaxants has been a moot point, but use of neostigmine and atropine is appropriate.[34] All the potent inhalation agents, succinylcholine, and potassium must be avoided.

If intraoperative signs of MH do not appear, most authorities do not advocate continuing dantrolene into the postoperative period. However, at least 8 hours of close postoperative observation are necessary.

CONGENITAL CATARACTS

When lens protein becomes denatured, an opaque, insoluble, proteinaceous precipitate forms, and the resultant opacity is termed a *cataract*. The most effective therapy for bilateral, congenital complete clouding of the crystalline lens is surgical removal as early as possible. Because cataracts severely impede retinal stimulation, they prevent proper visual

TABLE 15–2. Some Causes of Pediatric Cataracts

Idiopathic
Chromosomal disorders
Inborn errors of metabolism
Intrauterine infections
Trauma
Drugs

development. A unilateral complete congenital cataract should also be removed during the first few months of life to prevent deprivation amblyopia. Visual outcome will probably be severely compromised if corrective surgery is delayed beyond 6 months of age.[35]

Although 50% of childhood cataracts are idiopathic, the remainder are associated with chromosomal disorders, inborn errors of metabolism, intrauterine infections, trauma, and certain drugs, such as corticosteroids (Table 15–2). At least 30% of children with congenital cataracts are afflicted with a lesion of another organ system. A partial listing of pediatric syndromes that are associated with cataracts includes trisomy 13 (Patau's syndrome), 18 (Edward's syndrome), and 21 (Down's syndrome); Turner's syndrome; Fabry's disease; galactosemia; glucose-6-phosphate dehydrogenase deficiency; myotonic dystrophy; Albright's hereditary osteodystrophy; Stickler's syndrome; Lowe's syndrome; Hallerman-Streiff syndrome; Smith-Lemli-Opitz syndrome; Pierre Robin syndrome; Goldenhar's syndrome; Kartagener's syndrome; and Werner's syndrome. Germane anesthetic features of many of these entities are discussed in Chapter Sixteen.

One of the most common infectious causes of congenital cataracts is first trimester rubella, when the virus directly invades the embryonic lens. Other congenital infections also associated with neonatal cataracts include cytomegalic inclusion disease, toxoplasmosis, and herpes simplex. Pregnant women who are caring for affected babies should be told that the live virus can be isolated from the nasopharynx, blood, urine, and other body fluids of their patients for several months postnatally. Health care providers should take appropriate precautions.

SURGICAL ASPECTS AND ANESTHETIC MANAGEMENT

Anterior chamber aspiration of the lens is accomplished using an operating microscope with coaxial illumination and either a suction-cutting instrument or a blunt needle and syringe. Optimal surgical conditions include an immobile, maximally dilated pupil that permits adequate observation of the red reflex to assure complete removal of the cloudy crystalline lens. If remnants of the lens remain, low-grade inflammation may ensue. In addition, a uniform IOP should be maintained, because this is a delicate intraocular procedure (Table 15–3).

Although serial doses of mydriatics, such as 2.5% phenylephrine and 1% cyclopentolate, are administered topically in preparation for surgery, additional intraoperative mydriasis is required. Maximal pupillary dilation can be induced by continuous infusion of epinephrine 1:200,000 in a balanced salt solution, delivered through a small-gauge needle placed in the anterior chamber. Almost simultaneously with its administration, the drug is removed by aspirating it from the anterior chamber. The iris usually dilates immediately on contact with the epinephrine infusion, and drug uptake is presumably limited by the intense vasoconstriction of the iris and ciliary body. However, it is theoretically possible for epinephrine to be absorbed by drainage through Schlemm's canal into the venous system or by spillover of the infusion into the conjunctival vessels or drainage to the nasal mucosa.

The extent of systemic absorption of epinephrine is of concern to the anesthesiologist, particularly in view of the drug's dysrhythmogenic proclivity when given concomitantly with potent inhalation agents. However, plasma catecholamine levels during epinephrine infusion into the anterior chamber have not been rigorously studied. Nonetheless, under halothane anesthesia, in both children and adults, Smith and associates[36] were unable to document an increased incidence of cardiac dysrhythmias or signs of systemic effects following instillation of epinephrine 1:1000 (0.4–68 µg/kg) directly into the anterior chamber during cataract surgery. (However, all their patients were given lidocaine, 2 mg/kg, as topical laryngeal anesthesia.) The authors postulated that the globe is not a rich site for systemic absorp-

TABLE 15–3. Special Concerns with Pediatric Cataract Surgery

Associated systemic disease(s)
Avoidance of overly generous use of oxygen in infants less than 44 weeks postconception
Akinesia and proper control of IOP
Adequate mydriasis for surgery
Avoidance of postoperative coughing and vomiting

tion, and therefore general caveats applicable for subcutaneous injection may not be germane for intraocular infusion. In addition, more recent studies[37, 38] have indicated that children appear to have a higher threshold to and lower incidence of exogenous epinephrine-induced dysrhythmias during halothane administration than adults.

As mentioned, the eye must be motionless, and a stable IOP must be maintained to avoid extrusion of intraocular contents. Thus, a sufficiently deep level of anesthesia must be maintained until the wound has been sutured completely closed. Hence, the use of a nondepolarizing muscle relaxant along with a peripheral nerve stimulator has been advocated in these cases. If the child should unexpectedly move when the eye is open, IV thiopental should be given immediately. Succinylcholine should *not* be administered, because it is contraindicated when the eye is surgically open.

Virtually any of the inhalation agents may be administered for cataract surgery. However, because the maximum safe dosage of epinephrine that can be infused into the anterior chamber during general anesthesia has not been firmly established, isoflurane, enflurane, or a balanced technique might theoretically be preferable to halothane. Many of the patients presenting for congenital cataract aspiration are infants only a few days or weeks of age. Consequently, anesthesiologists should be properly concerned about the remote possibility of hyperoxia-induced retinopathy of prematurity (ROP), because the retina is not fully vascularized until 44 weeks postconceptional age. Although ROP is a multifactorial disease, and oxygen is not the only problem, investigators suggest that anesthesiologists should arbitrarily regulate the FIO_2 of oxygen-N_2O or oxygen-air mixtures to maintain an arterial oxygen pressure (PaO_2) of less than 100 mmHg or an oxygen saturation at approximately 95%.

Because proper control of IOP is crucial, and because nondepolarizing neuromuscular blocking drugs are used, ventilation is controlled and carefully monitored through end-tidal CO_2 measurement to avoid hypercarbia. At completion of surgery, any residual neuromuscular blockade is reversed. Upon resumption of spontaneous ventilation, and following IV administration of lidocaine to prevent coughing, the patient's trachea is extubated when he or she is in the lateral position and still rather deeply anesthetized. Postoperatively, the goal is to have a quiet, comfortable

baby who does not engage in maneuvers that trigger wide excursions in venous pressure and, hence, IOP.

CONGENITAL GLAUCOMA

Glaucoma is a condition characterized by elevated IOP, resulting in impairment of capillary blood flow to the optic nerve with eventual loss of optic nerve tissue and function. Congenital glaucoma is usually (80% of cases) inherited in an autosomal recessive pattern and is slightly more common in males (60:40). Primary congenital glaucoma is classified according to age of onset, and 75% of cases are bilateral. (When unilateral, glaucoma is frequently associated with the Sturge-Weber syndrome and, hence, the presence of ipsilateral capillary nevi. These angiomata may also affect the larynx, complicating intubation.) Infantile glaucoma occurs any time after birth until 5 years of age. The juvenile type occurs between the ages of 6 and 30 years. Childhood glaucoma may be associated with various eye diseases or developmental anomalies, such as aniridia, mesodermal dysgenesis syndrome, and retinopathy of prematurity.[39] A small sample of the broad spectrum of diseases that may be linked with glaucoma includes Refsum's syndrome, mucopolysaccharidosis, Hurler's syndrome, Stickler's syndrome, Marfan's syndrome, and von Recklinghausen's disease (neurofibromatosis).

Successful management of infantile glaucoma depends on early diagnosis. Afflicted babies commonly present with epiphora, photophobia, blepharospasm, and irritability. Ocular enlargement, termed *buphthalmos* or "ox eye," and corneal haziness secondary to edema are frequently noted. Buphthalmos is unusual, however, if glaucoma develops after 3 years of age; by then, the eye is much less elastic.

Because infantile glaucoma is usually the result of obstructed aqueous outflow owing to anomalous development of the filtration angle, management frequently requires surgical creation, through goniotomy or trabeculotomy, of a route for aqueous humor to flow into Schlemm's canal. Unfortunately, advanced disease may be refractory to even multiple goniotomies, and a more radical procedure, such as trabeculectomy, or another variety of filtering surgery may be necessary.

Juvenile glaucoma, presenting with a normal-appearing cornea and eye size, is frequently found in conjunction with a family history of open-angle glaucoma and is treated similarly to primary open-angle glaucoma.

In cases of pediatric secondary glaucoma, goniotomy and filtering may be unsuccessful, whereas cyclocryotherapy may be effective in reducing IOP. With this technique, the ciliary body is destroyed with a cryoprobe, cooled to −70°C. This markedly reduces the formation of aqueous humor. Immediately postoperatively, these patients experience considerable pain and may require narcotic analgesics.

The ophthalmologist should examine patients with congenital glaucoma at frequent intervals to measure both corneal diameter and IOP, and to check for cupping of the optic disc and inspect the drainage angle of the anterior chamber. Accurate, reproducible readings of IOP to document response to therapy must be provided. However, the high IOP frequently encountered in infantile glaucoma can be reduced by more than 15 mmHg when surgical anesthesia is achieved. (Although it has been generally accepted that inhalation agents lower IOP in a dose-dependent fashion, a study by Watcha and coworkers[40] failed to demonstrate a dose-dependent effect of halothane on IOP. However, Watcha investigated only a narrow range (0.5–1.0%) of end-tidal halothane concentrations.)

Some anesthesiologists believe that ketamine is a valuable drug to use for examination under anesthesia when infantile glaucoma is part of the differential diagnosis, because ketamine does not spuriously lower IOP. However, even normal infants may sporadically have pressures in the mid-20s. Thus, diagnosis is not based exclusively on the numerical pressure measured under anesthesia. Other diagnostic factors are weighed, including the presence of corneal edema, increased corneal diameter, tears in Descemet's membrane, and cupping of the optic nerve. If these abnormalities are encountered, surgical intervention may be mandatory, even in the presence of an allegedly normal IOP. Although the conditions produced by ketamine may be satisfactory for an examination under anesthesia, ketamine is unsatisfactory for the more exacting operating conditions demanded by goniotomy. The latter is a delicate procedure, and the blepharospasm, nystagmus, sighing, and adventitious movements experienced with ketamine are unacceptable. A formal endotracheal anesthetic should be administered when microscopic glaucoma surgery is necessary (Table 15–4).

The diameter of Fontana's spaces is ex-

TABLE 15–4. Special Concerns with Glaucoma Surgery

Presence of other congenital anomalies
"Appropriate" FIO$_2$ in babies less than 44 weeks postconception
Spurious reductions of IOP by deep inhalation anesthesia
Side effects of ketamine
Akinesia and proper control of IOP
Perioperative instillation of miotics
Avoidance of overhydration as well as hypotension
Side effects of antiglaucoma medication

tremely important in determining aqueous humor outflow, as illustrated by the equation[41]

$$A = \frac{r^4 \times (Piop - Pv)}{8\eta L}$$

where A = volume of aqueous outflow per unit of time; r = radius of Fontana's spaces; Piop = intraocular pressure; Pv = venous pressure; η = viscosity; and L = length of Fontana's spaces.

When the pupil dilates, Fontana's spaces narrow, resistance to outflow is increased, and IOP rises. Because mydriasis is to be assiduously avoided in both narrow- and wide-angle glaucoma, miotics are applied conjunctivally in patients with glaucoma. Moreover, because aqueous outflow is responsive to perturbations in venous pressure, considerable elevation of IOP follows any maneuver, such as coughing, vomiting, or overhydration, that increases venous pressure. Anesthetic goals include perioperative instillation of miotics and avoidance of venous congestion.

In the past, glaucoma patients were not given atropine premedication. However, atropine premedication in the dose used clinically has no effect on IOP in either open- or closed-angle glaucoma. Duncalf and Foldes[42] reported that when 0.4 mg of atropine is given parenterally to a 70 kg person, approximately 0.0001 mg is absorbed by the eye. However, scopolamine has a more pronounced mydriatic effect than atropine; therefore, scopolamine is not recommended in patients with known or suspected narrow-angle glaucoma.[43] *Topical* atropine and scopolamine should be avoided in all patients with glaucoma. IV atropine and neostigmine may be safely used to reverse neuromuscular blockade in patients with glaucoma, because these drugs in conventional dosages have minimal effect on pupil size and IOP.[44] If ketamine is used for an ocular exam under anesthesia, it should follow pretreatment with atropine in order to avoid copious secretions.

Certain antiglaucoma drugs the patient is taking can have systemic side effects and important anesthetic implications. Drugs of potential concern include topical echothiophate iodide, epinephrine, and timolol maleate, as well as oral acetazolamide (see Chapter 17).

"OPEN EYE–FULL STOMACH" SITUATIONS

One of the most challenging situations confronting the anesthesiologist is that of the child with a penetrating eye injury who has recently eaten. The anesthetic management of the "open eye–full stomach" patient is extremely controversial, and no single approach is ideal. Methods employed to protect against aspiration of gastric contents must be balanced against their influence on IOP. Although no simple, clear-cut solution exists, an understanding of the effects of various drugs and manipulations on IOP will assist the anesthesiologist in selecting the best, safest course for a successful surgical result. A child's life must obviously not be jeopardized in favor of his or her eye.

In spite of the excellent protection afforded by the bony orbit and cushioning provided by the retrobulbar fat and eyelids, the incidence of ocular injuries is high, and the resultant damage is often serious. There has been some decrease in injuries since the introduction of better safety measures and goggles in certain sports and workplaces. Nonetheless, childhood eye injuries commonly occur secondary to trauma, fireworks, slingshots, wood-chopping, and sports injuries (Figs. 15–1 and 15–2).

Ocular injuries can be penetrating or non-penetrating. Corneal abrasions are an example of the latter. Penetrating injuries include intra-ocular foreign bodies in the anterior and posterior chambers, the lens, or the vitreous humor, and lacerations of the sclera or cornea. Because penetrating injuries can result in extrusion of intraocular contents, a major anesthetic objective is to prevent additional increases in IOP, which can produce further prolapse and loss of intraocular contents. As in all cases of trauma, other injuries should be suspected, such as intracranial trauma producing a subdural hematoma, skull and orbital fractures, and the possibility of occult abdominal or thoracic bleeding. These conditions should receive prompt and efficient diagnosis and treatment.

Typically, the child with a penetrating eye injury is frightened and crying. Even if food was ingested several hours prior to the injury, fear and agitation will dramatically retard gastric emptying. Thus, the child must be assumed to have a full stomach. However, no attempt should be made to pass a nasogastric tube, which would trigger a potentially disastrous increase in IOP. Antacid aspiration prophylaxis may be given, and if an IV line is present, the child may also receive an H_2-receptor antagonist (which may also be given orally) to decrease gastric acid production and increase gastric pH.[45, 46] Additionally, metoclopramide is useful to stimulate peristalsis and to facilitate gastric emptying. Although some prominent pediatric anesthesiologists are adamantly opposed to the insertion of an IV line while the child is awake and apt to sob and struggle, the injured child has probably already precipitated

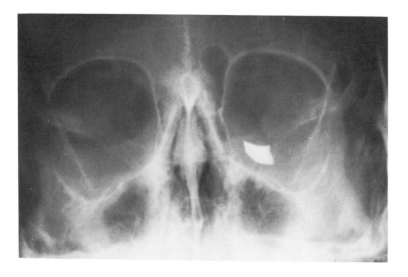

FIGURE 15–1. Plain film showing an intraorbital metallic foreign body in a child. (Photograph courtesy of Jonathan Mardirossian, M.D., Chief of Ophthalmology, St. Agnes Hospital, White Plains, New York.)

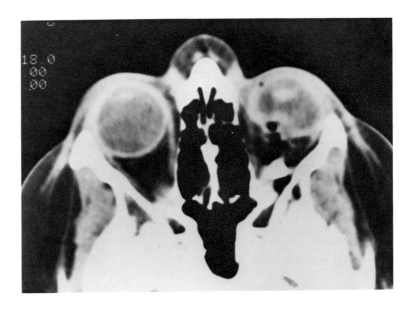

FIGURE 15-2. *CT scan confirming the presence of an intraorbital, rather than an intraocular, metallic foreign body. (Photograph courtesy of Jonathan Mardirossian, M.D., Chief of Ophthalmology, St. Agnes Hospital, White Plains, New York.)*

more damage to the perforated eye by crying and rubbing the eye before hospitalization than is produced by awake venous cannulation. External pressure on the globe (as may be caused by aggressive application of an anesthetic mask) and increased venous pressure (as may result from vomiting secondary to narcotics or from coughing following transtracheal injection) must be avoided.

Using a barbiturate and an intubating dose of a nondepolarizing muscle relaxant is often described as the method of choice for the emergency repair of a ruptured globe, because the nondepolarizing relaxant pancuronium, in a dose of 0.15 mg/kg, has been shown to lower, or at least not increase, IOP. This technique has serious disadvantages, however, including the risks of aspiration and death during the relatively long time—varying from 75 seconds[47] to 2½ minutes[48]—the airway is unprotected. A premature attempt at intubation produces coughing, straining, and a dramatic increase in IOP as well as undesirable cardiovascular side effects, which are more worrisome in adults with coronary artery disease. Also, the long duration of action of pancuronium may make postoperative ventilation a necessity. Although newer nondepolarizing relaxants, such as vecuronium and atracurium, have shorter durations of action, minimal circulatory effects, and no tendency to accumulate, in equipotent doses these newer drugs have an onset of action as delayed as pancuronium's.[49, 50]

Ginsberg and colleagues[51] reported that the administration of high dose (400 µg/kg) vecuronium reduces the speed of onset from 208

± 41 seconds, as seen with the conventional intubating dose of 100 µg/kg, to 106 ± 35 seconds. However, the design of the study did not eliminate factors that could influence the quality of the intubation conditions. For example, the dosages of fentanyl, diazepam, and thiopental given prior to intubation varied greatly among patients.

Another frequently used method for emergency repair involves pretreatment with a nondepolarizing muscle relaxant followed by a barbiturate-succinylcholine sequence. However, the efficacy of pretreatment with small doses of nondepolarizing muscle relaxant to prevent succinylcholine-induced intraocular hypertension remains a controversial issue. Miller and associates,[52] using indentation tonometry, reported that pretreatment with small doses of tubocurarine or gallamine prevented the increase. Using applanation tonometry, however, Meyers and coworkers[53] were unable to consistently block a rise in IOP with similar pretreatment. However, in a patient with a full stomach, succinylcholine offers the important advantages of rapid onset, excellent intubating conditions, and short duration of action. Given after pretreatment with a nondepolarizing relaxant and an inducing dose of sodium thiopental (4–6 mg/kg), succinylcholine causes only slight increases in IOP above baseline.[54] Although the acceptability of this method has been debated, there are no reports in the literature of loss of intraocular contents resulting from a nondepolarizing pretreatment-barbiturate-succinylcholine sequence used in this setting.[55, 56]

Studies by Badrinath and associates[57] indicated that sufentanil premedication (0.05 μg/kg) and pretreatment with a nondepolarizing relaxant plus a high dose thiopental (7 mg/kg) or alfentanil (150 μg/kg) induction effectively block the increase in IOP from succinylcholine and intubation.

For those anesthesiologists who prefer not to start an IV line when the child is awake, intubation during deep halothane anesthesia using cricoid pressure is effective.[58] To avoid the cardiovascular effects of deep halothane anesthesia, once venous access has been established and under application of cricoid pressure, a small dose of a nondepolarizing agent followed by succinylcholine can be administered, and tracheal intubation can be accomplished.

In addition to lacerations, intraocular foreign bodies may also be found in the setting of trauma. Foreign bodies in the anterior and posterior chambers are removed through an incision at the corneoscleral limbus. Foreign bodies in the vitreous are removed through scleral incision. Metal fragments can be removed with a magnet; nonmetallic objects are removed either with small forceps or by a combination of vitrectomy and suction. Sometimes intralenticular foreign bodies are not removed initially but later, after a cataract forms. However, usually early removal is desirable, because foreign bodies may become enmeshed in fibrin, making their later removal difficult. Large foreign bodies, and especially copper objects, can destroy ocular structures, often necessitating enucleation. (Sympathetic uveitis is thought to be an autoimmune sensitivity to uveal pigment, resulting in an inflammatory phenomenon in the *uninjured* eye, which can progress to blindness. Removal of the eye with prolapsed uveal tissue within 10 days of injury eliminates the development of sympathetic uveitis in the contralateral eye, but this must be measured against the possibility of useful vision following careful repair and preservation of the injured eye. Fortunately, the incidence of this dreaded complication has decreased greatly with the use of steroids and antibiotics.)

Surgery is conducted while the patient is unable to move or cough secondary to neuromuscular blockade. A peripheral nerve stimulator is important to indicate satisfactory paralysis. IV droperidol is administered prior to surgery in an attempt to prevent or minimize postoperative nausea and vomiting,[21] and a nasogastric tube may also be passed under anesthesia. When surgery has been completed and spontaneous respiration has returned, the endotracheal tube is removed with the patient awake, in a lateral, head-down position. IV lidocaine in a dose of 1.5–2 mg/kg may be given first to attenuate periextubation bucking and coughing.

A discussion of open eye–full stomach situations should include information on the so-called priming principle.[59, 60] This concept involves using approximately one tenth of an intubating dose of nondepolarizing drug, followed 4 minutes later by an intubating dose. Then, after waiting an additional 90 seconds, intubation can supposedly be performed. However, studies in this area demonstrate wide variability and inconsistency of data. Moreover, priming is not devoid of risk, because at least one case of aspiration following a priming dose of vecuronium has been reported.[61]

Perhaps the wisest and most succinct summary of the management of open eye–full stomach situations is that by Baumgarten and Reynolds,[62] who wrote in 1985:

It may be possible to devise a combination of intravenous anesthetics and nondepolarizing relaxants that totally prevents coughing after rapid intubation. Until this combination is devised and confirmed in a large, controlled double-blind series, clinicians should not apply the priming principle to the open eye–full stomach patient. Use of a blockade monitor to predict intubating conditions may be unreliable, since muscle groups vary in their response to nondepolarizing relaxants. At this time, succinylcholine with precurarization probably remains the most tenable compromise in the open eye–full stomach challenge.

RETINOBLASTOMA

Despite its relative rarity, retinoblastoma is the most frequently encountered pediatric ocular malignancy. With an approximate incidence of 1/20,000 live births, this congenital malignancy usually is diagnosed during the first 3 years of life.[63] Approximately 400 new cases of retinoblastoma are discovered annually in the United States. Less than half of them are of the familial type associated with a deletion of the long arm of chromosome 13.[64] This pleiotropic gene has also been linked with the development of a benign tumor, a retinoma, that was previously considered to be a spontaneously arrested, or regressed, retinoblastoma. The deleted long arm of chromosome 13 (13 q) is also associated with a predisposi-

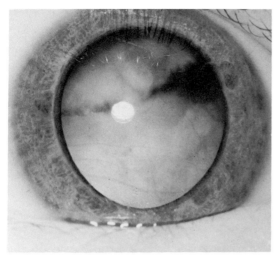

FIGURE 15–3. *An example of leucocoria that proved to be retinoblastoma.*

TABLE 15–6. Differential Diagnosis of Leucocoria

Retinoblastoma	Uveitis
ROP	Incontinentia pigmenti
Juvenile retinoschisis	Nematode endophthalmitis
Coats' disease	Trisomy 13–15
Persistent hyperplastic primary vitreous (PHPV)	

tion later in life to nonocular malignant tumors, usually osteogenic sarcoma, at the site of previous radiation treatment and also in nonirradiated locations. In addition, this chromosomal abnormality has been linked with a tumor of the pineal gland occurring concomitantly with bilateral retinoblastoma. Because some consider the pineal gland to be a primitive organ of sight, the pineal gland lesion has been termed *trilateral retinoblastoma.*[65]

Approximately 30% of retinoblastoma cases are bilateral (Fig. 15–3). These aggressive tumors account for 1% of all cancer-related pediatric deaths; the tumor frequently travels along the optic nerve to the brain and metastasizes to bone, lung, and lymph nodes. Common presenting signs include a white pupillary reflex, strabismus, an apparent ocular inflammation, and glaucoma (Tables 15–5 and 15–6). Treatment may include cryotherapy, photocoagulation, enucleation, chemotherapy, and radiation—either alone or in combination—depending on the grade of tumor and evolving treatment protocols.

Irradiation is a common treatment for retinoblastoma, and frequently infants with retinoblastoma require daily radiation therapy for many weeks. The anesthetic management of these patients is discussed in detail in Chapter

TABLE 15–5. Presenting Signs of Retinoblastoma

Leucocoria	Poor vision
Strabismus	Unilateral mydriasis
Orbital cellulitis	Hyphema
Red eye/glaucoma	Heterochromia iridis

19. Briefly, many satisfactory anesthetic agents and techniques are available and include rectal or IM methohexital; IV or IM ketamine administered after atropine premedication; or a brief inhalation anesthetic, commonly delivered through insufflation or intubation.

If enucleation is required, there may be a relatively high incidence of oculocardiac reflex-induced dysrhythmias associated with this type of surgery. Vigorous traction on the extraocular muscles and deep orbital digital pressure[10] frequently trigger the trigeminovagal arc. The incidence can be effectively reduced by administering IV atropine, 0.02 mg/kg, or glycopyrrolate, 0.01 mg/kg, during the induction period.

Wiggs and Dryja and coworkers[66] developed a diagnostic genetic test that identifies children at risk for developing a form of this cancer. The inheritable form of the tumor is found in 30–40% of retinoblastoma patients, and children from families with a history of hereditary retinoblastoma have had to be examined under anesthesia every 3 months during the first 5 years of their lives. The genetic test developed by Wiggs and Dryja should allow such examinations to focus on children at risk and permit early, vision-saving intervention. Furthermore, the test should eliminate the need to repeatedly examine healthy children under anesthesia.

RETINOPATHY OF PREMATURITY

HISTORICAL BACKGROUND AND POSTULATED ETIOLOGIES

Although Terry[67] first described the pathological condition in 1942, the neologism *retrolental fibroplasia* was coined in 1944 by Harry Messenger, a Boston ophthalmologist who was also a Greek and Latin scholar.[68] More recently, however, the term *retinopathy of prematurity* (ROP) has gained widespread acceptance, because it describes the late cicatricial phase of the disease as well as the earlier acute changes.

In the early 1950s, Patz and colleagues[69]

implicated liberal use of oxygen as the principal cause of ROP. The immature retinal vasculature seems to respond to oxygen in a biphasic fashion, with vasoconstriction of large vessels and vaso-obliteration of capillary beds followed by vasoproliferation when the infant is returned to room air. Deterioration of retinopathy depends on the extent of fibrous traction and the eventual development of traction retinal detachment. Basically, ROP occurs acutely as a vascular retinopathy peripherally and may deteriorate to the cicatricial form when scar tissue places the retina under traction, resulting in detachment and severe visual impairment.

Although oxygen is no longer thought to be the sole factor in the development of ROP, many questions remain unanswered. Hyperoxia-associated vascular pathology may be a direct result of free-radical liberation,[70] and a low-molecular-weight angiogenic factor released from nonperfused retina may promote vasoproliferation.[71, 72] If normal retina can trigger angiogenic activity[73, 74] and if healthy vitreous humor contains a vasoinhibitory element,[75] perhaps proliferation or regression of retinal vessels depends on a shift in the balance between these normally occurring processes, which in turn could be influenced by tissue levels of oxygen.[76]

Approximately 45% of premature infants with a birth weight under 1000 g develop acute retinal changes.[77] Fortunately, 80–90% of this group have spontaneous regression of the acute retinal changes.[78] The remaining 10–20% develop cicatricial changes in the retina that can cause blindness. It is difficult to predict when this devastating cicatricial involvement will occur, and it appears to be influenced by factors other than perinatal oxygen exposure alone.

The National Cooperative Study[79] concluded that birth weight, gestational age, and duration of supplementary oxygen treatment are the most important factors associated with ROP and that these variables are highly interrelated, reflecting functional immaturity (Table 15–7). Furthermore, it is possible that CO_2 level, bright light, and vitamin E deficiency are three additional variables in the pathogenesis of ROP.

Because vitamin E is a known free-radical scavenger, and because transient superoxide free radicals may cause injury to immature retinal vasculature,[70] the possibility that vitamin E may serve a protective function is being vigorously debated. Although many controlled

TABLE 15–7. Factors Implicated in the Pathogenesis of ROP

Low birth weight
Immature gestational age
Duration of supplemental oxygen therapy
? CO_2 levels
? Bright light
? Relative deficiency of vitamin E

clinical studies[80, 81] indicate that vitamin E seems to reduce either the severity or the incidence of ROP, others have demonstrated no difference in the incidence of ROP between patients given IM vitamin E and controls.[82]

Among the known pathogenetic variables, Flynn[83] documented that birth weight was the most significant predictor for risk of proliferative ROP. Babies with a birth weight less than 1000 g had such a high incidence of proliferative ROP that no other exogenous factor, including oxygen, seemed significant. Moreover, sporadic cases of ROP have been reported in premature babies who received little or no supplemental oxygen as well as in full-term infants.[84]

Patz, however, postulates that the rare cases of ROP occurring in babies who received little or no supplemental oxygen can still be explained on the basis of the effects of oxygen.[85] *In utero,* the fetus has a low arterial oxygen tension. However, after birth, with lung expansion and closure of the ductus and the foramen ovale, the arterial oxygen tension in the normal infant (premature or full-term) increases dramatically even without supplemental oxygen. Therefore, it is possible that a sensitive "target organ" such as the immature retina responds to this sudden, significant increase in arterial oxygen partial pressure (Pa_{O_2}) with irreversible retinal arterial and arteriolar vasoconstriction and vaso-obliteration.

Cogan[86] demonstrated that the retina normally is incompletely vascularized temporally even in full-term infants and that the anterior temporal portion does not become fully vascularized until about 4 weeks following birth. All the cases of retinal pathology reported by Brockhurst[84] in full-term infants showed major involvement of the temporal peripheral retina. Hence, the predilection of the disease for the temporal quadrant also gives credence to the concept of oxygen susceptibility of immature retinal vessels, because this is the last zone of the human retina to become vascularized.

Thus, even in the full-term infant, oxygen administration should be confined to specific clinical indications and not given routinely. When supplemental oxygen is needed by an infant whose postconception age is less than 44 weeks, the physician should maintain the Pa_{O_2} within a normal range to minimize the danger of ocular injury. Many find an oxygen-air blender useful in achieving this goal. Transcutaneous oxygen monitors are not always accurate during exposure to surgical stress, N_2O, potent inhalation anesthetic agents, electrical currents in electrocautery, and changes in skin blood flow. The pulse oximeter seems to be more reliable for use in anesthesia, because it reflects deeper tissues and is unaffected by exposure to various anesthetic agents and operating room stresses. Anesthesiologists may be encouraged by the work of Flynn,[87] published in 1984, clarifying the influence of surgery and anesthesia on the development of ROP. Using logistical risk analysis and controlling for such variables as total duration of oxygen exposure, inspired oxygen tensions, hours of mechanical ventilation, and birth weight, Flynn reported that infants requiring surgery and anesthesia had no greater risk of cicatricial ROP than infants who did not have surgery.

A decade ago, the American Academy of Pediatrics[88] recommended that arterial oxygen tension in the newborn be kept between 60 and 100 mmHg. Today, anesthesiologists keep the oxygen saturation at about 95% in infants less than 44 weeks postconception. However, meticulous adherence to these guidelines does not guarantee a safe visual outcome. Even with scrupulous, continuous monitoring of oxygen tension in vulnerable infants, ROP will probably still occur, because ROP is a multifactorial disease. Oxygen therapy is neither a necessary nor a sufficient cause of ROP.[89]

SURGICAL TREATMENT OF RETINOPATHY OF PREMATURITY

Surgical attempts to treat ROP have included photocoagulation, cryotherapy, scleral buckling, closed vitrectomy, and open-sky vitrectomy.

Hirose and Lou[90] made the following statement in 1986:

A major cause of blindness in ROP is retinal detachment or traction fold of the retina resulting from contraction of severe fibrovascular proliferative tissue that develops on the surface of the retina and in the vitreous cavity. Fibrous tissue formation always is preceded by neovascularization in the retina and vitreous, developing at the junction of the vascularized and nonvascularized retina. If we understand that the avascular retina is hypoxic because it is not receiving a sufficient supply of oxygen from the adjacent vascular retina and choroid, and that an angiogenic factor (or factors) is produced that causes a vasoproliferative response in the retina, it is reasonable to consider destroying the avascular retina before fibrovascular response becomes too advanced. For this reason, ablating the avascular retina with photocoagulation or cryotherapy appears plausible.

Among those who reported photocoagulation to be efficacious therapy for acute proliferative ROP include Nagata and Yamagishi,[91] Payne and Patz,[92] and Tabuchi.[93] Many other investigators[94, 95] also found cryopexy to be effective, although it was controversial until recently, because patient selection, method, site, and, particularly, timing of treatment appeared to be extremely important. Published data for the Multicenter Trial of Cryotherapy for Retinopathy of Prematurity[96] showed encouraging preliminary results in the 3-month follow-up of infants treated with cryotherapy. The data supported the efficacy of cryotherapy in reducing by approximately one half the risk of unfavorable retinal outcome from threshold ROP. Although cryotherapy now seems to represent a highly significant treatment advance, an accompanying editorial in the *Archives of Ophthalmology* warns that as-yet-unknown problems may be possible. Tasman[97] explained that, because cryotherapy creates a peripheral chorioretinal adhesion in small eyes, as the eye grows, the area of treated retina that has been firmly anchored may be subjected in some cases to a grave stress leading to retinal breaks and detachment. Hopefully, long-term studies will answer these concerns.

Acute retinal detachment in infants is most commonly of the traction variety, rather than rhegmatogenous or exudative. Often, neovascularization is still present in both the retina and vitreous humor at the time of detachment, and cryotherapy combined with 360-degree scleral buckling may be helpful. The timing of surgical intervention is critical. If the detached retina has been dragged anteriorly toward the lens, scleral buckling will be unsuccessful. With extensive retinal detachment and marked vitreous traction, vitrectomy surgery must be considered. Charles,[98] Lightfoot and Irvine,[99] and Machemer[100] are among those who have reported some success with closed vitrectomy.

Because open-sky vitrectomy allows direct access to the retrolental membrane and offers an excellent view, this technique is well suited to complex cases of ROP. Schepens[101] used this approach as early as 1973, and he and Hirose have reported some success with extremely challenging cases that previously were considered inoperable. The procedure involves trephination of the cornea—preserving it in tissue culture during the vitrectomy—performance of iridotomies and extraction of the lens with a cryoprobe. Following lens extraction, the retrolental membrane and much of the tissue filling the funnel of the totally detached retina are cut and removed. Then, hyaluronic acid is injected, forcing the retina to settle down, and the retinal folds are stretched to become smooth. After iridotomy closure, the corneal button is removed from tissue culture and sutured into its original position with 10-0 nylon. Hirose and Schepens believe the success of open-sky vitrectomy in patients with severe ROP varies greatly, depending on the configuration of the detachment. Total retinal detachments with an open funnel have a better anatomical success rate than those with a closed funnel.

ANESTHETIC MANAGEMENT OF PREMATURE INFANTS

Anesthetic management of premature infants undergoing ocular surgery centers on the judicious administration of either an inhalation agent with N_2O and oxygen, or a balanced technique. Careful control of body temperature and fluid management as well as meticulous monitoring of ECG, blood pressure, temperature, and oxygen saturation are mandatory. Detailed discussion of safe anesthesia techniques for premature infants is presented elsewhere.[102]

Cardiovascular and pulmonary function, anesthetic requirements, hematological parameters, as well as hepatic and renal function are vastly different in premature infants than in older children. For example, the baby born prematurely has relatively noncompliant ventricles, so cardiac output can be augmented only by increasing the heart rate, because stroke volume cannot be increased. If bradycardia (a heart rate less than 120 beats per minute) is not rapidly corrected, a profound drop in cardiac output will ensue.

Control of ventilation involves complex interactions of central ventilatory centers, peripheral chemoreceptors, and peripheral skeletal muscle sensors. When confronted with an hypoxic or hypercarbic challenge, the premature infant is unable to respond appropriately

with sustained hyperventilation. In fact, inappropriate hypoventilation will occur with hypoxemia. In addition to immature central control of respiration, these babies are also prone to diaphragmatic fatigue and may suffer respiratory decompensation on this basis. Thus, a partial listing of causes of apnea in premature infants includes CNS immaturity, hypoxia, diaphragmatic fatigue, hypothermia, and certain diseases, such as respiratory distress syndrome, pneumonia, sepsis, and hypoglycemia. Furthermore, the premature infant with anemia, low levels of 2,3 diphosphoglycerate (DPG) and high levels of hemoglobin F (with its reluctance to unload oxygen to tissues) is especially vulnerable to perioperative hypoxia.

These babies are vulnerable to hypoglycemia during even brief periods of fasting, because they have little in the way of glycogen or fat stores and are not efficient at gluconeogenesis. Also, these infants must be kept warm, because they defend their core temperature at considerable metabolic cost. Metabolic acidosis is produced by cold stress, and this acidosis triggers myocardial depression and hypoxia which, in turn, further exacerbates the degree of metabolic acidosis. Furthermore, hepatic and renal function in premature infants is immature, and their anesthetic requirement is less than that of more mature babies.

The combination of ventilatory depression from residual anesthetic drugs superimposed on immature development of respiratory control centers can easily cause postoperative hypoventilation and hypoxia (Table 15–8). Thus, these infants must be wide awake and vigorously responsive before they are extubated. They must also be carefully monitored postoperatively with 24-hour application of an apnea monitor and ECG, if indicated by patient age and history (apnea-bradycardia episodes) or by intraoperative perturbations. Vigilance and meticulous attention to detail are critical if these fragile babies are to escape

TABLE 15–8. Some Causes of Apnea in Premature Infants

CNS immaturity
Hypoxia
Diaphragmatic fatigue
Hypothermia
Respiratory distress syndrome
Pneumonia
Sepsis
Hypoglycemia

TABLE 16–2. Miscellaneous Multisystem Disorders and Diseases Associated with Cataracts in Children

Alport's syndrome	Noonan's syndrome
Apert's syndrome	Oxycephaly
Atopic dermatitis	Pierre Robin syndrome
Basal cell nevus syndrome	Potter's syndrome
Block-Sulzberger syndrome	Refsum's syndrome
Cockayne's syndrome	Rothmund-Thomson syndrome
Conradi's syndrome	Rubinstein-Taybi syndrome
Crouzon's disease	Smith-Lemli-Opitz syndrome
Frontonasal dysplasia (median cleft-face	Steindert's disease (myotonic dystrophy)
syndrome)	Stickler's syndrome
Generalized lentigo (LEOPARD syndrome)	Syndrome of mitochondrial myopathy of
Hallerman-Streiff syndrome	skeletal and heart muscle
Marinesco-Sjögren's syndrome	Usher's syndrome
Meckel's syndrome	Werner's syndrome

From Martyn LJ, DiGeorge A: Selected eye defects of special importance in pediatrics. Pediatr Clin North Am 34:1517–1542, 1987.

opmental disorders, infectious and inflammatory processes, metabolic diseases, as well as toxic and traumatic insults. In addition, cataracts may occur secondary to intraocular conditions, such as retinopathy of prematurity (ROP), retinal detachment, uveitis, and retinitis pigmentosa.

MENDELIAN INHERITANCE

Many cataracts are hereditary, unassociated with other diseases. Although the most common mode of inheritance is autosomal dominant, autosomal recessive inheritance has also been reported, especially in consanguineous populations. X-linked inheritance of cataracts is known but usually occurs in association with other diseases, such as Fabry's disease or Lowe's syndrome.[4] Hereditary cataracts tend to be of the zonular type and may be either stationary or progressive.[5, 6]

CHROMOSOMAL ABNORMALITIES

Cataracts frequently occur in association with chromosomal defects, especially with trisomy 13 (Patau's syndrome), 18 (Edward's syndrome), and 21 (Down's syndrome). Patients with Down's syndrome often have coronary or cerulean-type cataracts.[7] In Patau's and Edward's syndromes, congenital cataracts often occur in association with other ocular anomalies, such as coloboma and microphthalmia.

CONGENITAL INFECTION SYNDROMES

Frequently, pediatric cataracts are secondary to prenatal infections. Although lens opacities may occur in any of the major congenital infection syndromes, namely, toxoplasmosis, cytomegalovirus infection, syphilis, herpes,[8] and rubella, the rubella syndrome has the most significant cataract formation. The congenital rubella cataract is a dense, pearly, nuclear cataract occupying all or most of the pupillary aperture at birth. Often, there are concomitant ocular signs of congenital rubella infection, including microphthalmos, keratitis, glaucoma, iris atrophy, optic atrophy, and pigmentary retinopathy. Because the rubella virus may persist in the eye for months or even years after birth, cultures of the lens aspirate and aqueous humor can help establish the diagnosis.

Other maternal infections that produce congenital cataracts occasionally include influenza, measles, polio, vaccinia, and varicella zoster[9] (Table 16–3).

METABOLIC DISEASES

Cataracts are a prominent feature of numerous metabolic diseases, especially certain disorders of amino acid, carbohydrate, calcium, and copper metabolism.

The possibility of galactosemia should be a primary consideration in any neonate with cataract(s), and characteristic lens changes should be sought in infants with failure to thrive, hepatomegaly, or direct hyperbilirubinemia. In classic infantile galactosemia with

TABLE 16–3. Maternal Infections Associated with Congenital Cataracts

Rubella	Influenza
Cytomegalovirus	Measles
Toxoplasmosis	Polio
Syphilis	Vaccinia
Herpes	Varicella zoster

galactose-1-phosphate uridyl transferase deficiency, hepatic and cerebral disturbances are caused by excessive accumulation of galactose-1-phosphate. A distinctive cataract is seen, typically of the zonular type, with involvement of the perinuclear layers, often with involvement of the nucleus also. In its early stages, the cataract may have a special "oil droplet" appearance owing to alteration of the refringence of the perinuclear layers. Without intervention, complete opacification of the lens may occur within weeks. Diagnosis is established by measurement of uridyl transferase level in red blood cells. The infant with this condition caused by a mutant recessive gene should receive a galactose-free diet before he or she is 3 months old. With early therapy, the lens changes may be reversible.

In galactokinase deficiency, cataracts may be the sole or initial clinical manifestation. This disorder is much less common than classic galactosemia but is also caused by a mutant recessive gene. Diagnosis is confirmed by measuring the level of the enzyme galactokinase in red blood cells. This condition is also treated by a galactose-free diet.

There is an association between cataracts and hypocalcemia. A variety of lens opacities may be seen in patients with hypoparathyroidism.

Another metabolic disorder important in the differential diagnosis of congenital cataracts is the oculocerebrorenal Lowe's syndrome. In this X-linked disorder, cataract is frequently the presenting sign, with other abnormalities appearing later. These anomalies include mental and growth retardation, hypotonia, metabolic acidosis, aminoaciduria, proteinuria, renal rickets, and a distinctive facies (long with frontal bossing). Although lens changes may be seen frequently in heterozygous female children also, affected male children commonly have obvious dense bilateral cataracts at birth. They may also suffer from associated glaucoma. Interestingly, carrier females in their second decade of life have significantly higher numbers of lens opacities than age-related controls; however, absence of opacities is no guarantee that an individual is not a carrier.

Wilson's disease, a well-known disorder of copper metabolism, is associated with the characteristic Kayser-Fleischer ring, but the lens changes secondary to this disorder are not usually seen in children. The so-called sunflower cataract seen in Wilson's disease patients typically does not appear until later in life.

In diabetes mellitus, cataracts develop secondary to hyperglycemia, accumulation of sorbitol, and the resultant osmotic alterations in the lens. Diabetic cataracts, also referred to as snowflake cataracts, are characterized by white opacities in the anterior and posterior cortex and subcapsular region; vacuoles are sometimes present, and water clefts and separation of sutures may result. Although these lens changes are uncommon in children, some youngsters with juvenile onset diabetes may develop cataracts that progress with remarkable rapidity. Especially during adolescence, some diabetic cataracts may mature in a matter of days, even hours. A harbinger may be the sudden development of myopia, resulting from alterations in the optical density of the lens. Neonatal hypoglycemia,[10] often seen in babies of diabetic and prediabetic mothers, may predispose to the early development of cataracts.

Assorted other metabolic diseases that may be associated with cataracts include some of the sphingolipidoses, mucopolysaccharidoses, and mucolipidoses.

DRUGS AND TOXINS

Of the assorted toxic agents and drugs that may produce cataracts, corticosteroids are of special significance in the pediatric population. The steroid-induced cataracts are posterior subcapsular lens opacities. Their pathogenesis is uncertain, and there is no true consensus regarding the relative importance of dose, duration of treatment, individual susceptibility, and reversibility.

COLOBOMATA

In colobomata, some portion of a structure or tissue is missing. Two major types of ocular colobomata are chorioretinal or fundus coloboma and isolated optic nerve coloboma.

The typical fundus coloboma is caused by malclosure of the embryonic fissure, resulting in a gap in the retina, retinal pigment epithelium, and choroid. These defects may be unilateral or bilateral and usually produce a visual field defect corresponding to the chorioretinal defect.

Colobomata may occur unassociated with other abnormalities, or they may occur in association with microphthalmos, cyclopia, anencephaly, or other major central nervous system (CNS) aberrations. Often, they occur in association with chromosomal abnormalities, especially in the trisomy 13 and 18 syndromes. They may be associated with the CHARGE (congenital heart disease, choanal atresia, mental retardation, genital hypoplasia, and ear anomalies) syndrome or may occur in the VATER (tracheoesophageal fistula, congenital heart disease, and renal anomalies) association.

Isolated colobomata of the optic nerve occur rarely. They may be familial and may also be associated with other ocular pathology as well as with cardiac and other systemic defects.

ECTOPIA LENTIS

Displacement of the lens may be classified topographically as luxation or subluxation. In luxation, the lens is completely displaced or dislocated. In subluxation, some zonular attachments remain, and the lens remains in its plane posterior to the iris, albeit tilted in one direction or another.

The most common cause of lens displacement is trauma, although ectopia lentis may also result from various other ocular diseases, such as intraocular tumor, congenital glaucoma, uveitis, aniridia, or high myopia.

Ectopia lentis may occur as an inherited defect and in association with systemic diseases. Examples of the latter include Marfan's syndrome, homocystinuria, Weill-Marchesani syndrome, hyperlysinemia, and sulfite oxidase deficiency.

Displacement of the lens occurs in about 80% of patients with Marfan's syndrome. Ocular complications such as glaucoma, retinal detachment, and cataract have been reported. Myopia is also common in this autosomal-dominant condition characterized by cardiovascular, skeletal, and ocular abnormalities.

In homocystinuria, the most common biochemical defect of this autosomal recessive condition is deficiency of cystathionine synthase. Skeletal abnormalities, osteoporosis, and abnormal intravascular clotting are other features of the disease. Although one third of homocystinuric individuals have normal intelligence, most are mentally retarded. Ectopia lentis occurs in 90% of patients with homocystinuria, and pupillary block glaucoma may develop. Other abnormal ocular findings may include light-color irides, retinoschisis, retinal detachment, optic atrophy, central retinal artery occlusion, and strabismus.

Other conditions are occasionally associated with ectopia lentis, including Ehlers-Danlos syndrome, Sturge-Weber syndrome, Crouzon's disease, Klippel-Feil syndrome, oxycephaly, and mandibulofacial dysostosis.

GLAUCOMA

Glaucoma in infants and children is usually caused by a developmental abnormality of the filtration angle of the anterior chamber. Frequently, residual mesodermal tissue impedes drainage of aqueous humor through the trabecular meshwork and Schlemm's canal. Long thought to be a recessive condition, primary or simple congenital glaucoma is probably inherited multifactorially. However, glaucoma associated with dominantly inherited goniodysgenesis has been described.

In some children with early onset glaucoma, there is more extensive maldevelopment of the anterior segment of the eye. The terms *mesodermal dysgenesis, anterior cleavage syndrome,* and several named anomalies, including Peter's,[11] Axenfeld's, and Rieger's, are used to describe these serious defects.

Early-onset glaucoma may also be found in conjunction with other ocular anomalies, such as aniridia, cataract, ectopia lentis, and spherophakia. Furthermore, secondary glaucoma may develop in infants with ROP or persistent hyperplastic primary vitreous.

Other major causes of glaucoma in children are trauma, intraocular hemorrhage, ocular inflammatory disease, intraocular tumor, and systemic diseases. A partial list of these systemic disorders includes Sturge-Weber syndrome,[12] von Recklinghausen's disease, Lowe's syndrome, several chromosomal syndromes, and the congenital infection syndromes (TORCH). In children with TORCH, glaucoma may occur as a result of intraocular inflammation. However, in congenital rubella, anomalies of the angle have been reported.

OPTIC NERVE HYPOPLASIA

Optic nerve hypoplasia is a developmental defect characterized by deficiency of optic nerve fibers. The anomaly may be unilateral or bilateral, mild to severe, with a wide range of ophthalmoscopic findings and associated clinical manifestations.

In typical cases, the nerve head is small, with a pale or pigmented crescent or halo between the nerve head and the inner edge of the pigmented retinal epithelium and choroid—hence, the so-called double ring sign of optic nerve hypoplasia.

If present, visual impairment ranges in severity from minimal[13] to moderate reduction in acuity, to unilateral or bilateral blindness. Strabismus or nystagmus secondary to visual impairment is common. Abnormal ocular movements or malalignment may be the presenting sign.

Although optic nerve hypoplasia may occur as an isolated defect in otherwise normal children, the lesion can be associated with aniridia, microphthalmos, coloboma, anencephaly, hydrocephalus, hydranencephaly, and encephalocele. Optic nerve hypoplasia may occur in a syndrome termed *septo-optic dysplasia* or de Morsier's syndrome. There may be associated hypothalamic aberrations and extremely variable endocrine findings.[14, 15] Although an isolated deficiency of growth hormone is most common, multiple hormonal deficiencies, including diabetes insipidus, have been reported.

Although the etiology of optic nerve hypoplasia is unknown, the condition is not familial and no known chromosomal defect has been regularly linked to the disorder. However, it occurs with slightly increased frequency in infants of diabetic mothers,[13] and the prenatal use of drugs such as LSD (lysergic acid diethylamide), meperidine, phenytoin, and quinine has been implicated sporadically.

CRANIOFACIAL ABNORMALITIES

Craniofacial abnormalities with associated ophthalmological complications include the craniofacial dysostoses such as Crouzon's disease, Apert's syndrome, and Goldenhar's syndrome, also known as oculoauriculovertebral dysplasia.

CROUZON'S DISEASE

Crouzon's disease (craniofacial dysostosis) is thought to be transmitted in an autosomal dominant pattern. The striking clinical findings include craniosynostosis, maxillary hypoplasia, hypertelorism, and shallow orbits producing proptosis. Tarsorrhaphy is commonly necessary. The configuration of the skull depends on which sutures close prematurely as well as the time sequence of closure.[16] Hypoplasia of the zygomatic arches and maxilla produce midfacial hypoplasia with a short upper lip and relative prognathism. In addition, with the soft palate against the posterior pharyngeal wall, mouth breathing is necessary, and upper airway obstruction may occur relatively easily. The ocular diseases reported in these patients include cataracts, glaucoma, strabismus, and ectopia lentis (Table 16–4). Deafness has been reported also.

APERT'S SYNDROME

Apert's syndrome is similar to Crouzon's disease, but the former is a manifestation of greater expressivity and penetrance. Other additional features of Apert's include syndactyly; moreover, patients with Apert's have cardiac anomalies and cartilaginous anomalies of the tracheobronchial tree (Table 16–4).

GOLDENHAR'S SYNDROME

The principal features of Goldenhar's syndrome are purportedly caused by developmental anomalies of the first and second branchial arches.[17] However, there is some confusion relative to nomenclature, because structures with other embryological derivatives are often involved. For example, Goldenhar's syndrome refers to the pattern of dysmorphism with vertebral defects (hypoplasia of cervical vertebrae) and epibulbar dermoids or lipodermoids (Figs. 16–1 and 16–2). Other frequently reported features include deafness, malar and mandibular hypoplasia, and malformed lowset ears. Half of the patients have colobomata of the eyelid. Other ocular disorders may include glaucoma, cataracts, and strabismus. Often, the disease is predominantly unilateral and then termed *hemifacial microsomia*.

Approximately 50% of children with Goldenhar's syndrome have congenital heart disease, most commonly tetralogy of Fallot,[18] but ventricular septal defect, patent ductus arteriosus, and coarctation of the aorta are also relatively common. Pulmonary agenesis or hypoplasia has been reported, with the pulmonary involvement occurring on the same side as the facial abnormalities in cases of hemifacial microsomia. Bone anomalies, especially of the vertebral column, occur in approximately 50% of the patients and may include complete or partial synostosis of several cervical vertebrae, occipitalization of the atlas, spina bifida, and anomalous ribs. Renal anomalies and various oral defects, including unilateral hypoplasia of the tongue and palate, as well as cleft lip or palate, may complicate anesthetic management. Airway management may be espe-

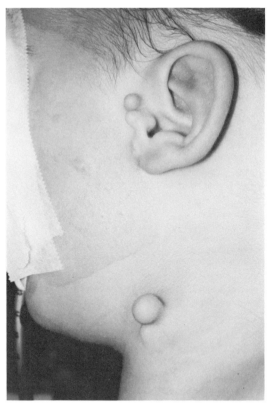

cially demanding; obtaining a satisfactory mask fit may be exceedingly difficult. Cervical spine malformation, in combination with facial hypoplasia and asymmetry, makes endotracheal intubation challenging. The presence of or-

ganic heart disease requires careful selection and titration of anesthetic agents and, depending on the lesion, antibiotic prophylaxis.

With the three aforementioned syndromes, the anesthesiologist should anticipate intubation difficulties (see Table 16–4). The approach to airway establishment may be one of three: awake intubation, either blind or under direct visualization; general inhalation anesthesia followed by intubation, either direct or blind; and tracheostomy, either awake utilizing local anesthesia or with general anesthesia.[16]

DOWN'S SYNDROME

Down's syndrome, also known as trisomy 21 or mongolism, is associated with a vast array of abnormalities, including the combination of a round face and cranium; small, slanted eyes with epicanthal folds; and protruding tongue[19] (Fig. 16–3). In addition, varying degrees of mental and physical retardation are observed, as well as hypotonia (which may improve with 5-hydroxytryptamine therapy)[20] and atlanto-occipital instability or dislocation, chronic upper and lower respiratory infections, funnel chest or pigeon breast, seizures, a history of duodenal atresia or tracheosophageal fistula, and a variety of thyroid abnormalities. Early mortality is primarily secondary to congenital heart defects, which occur in approximately 50% of those afflicted with Down's syndrome. The most common lesions are endocardial cushion defect and ventriculoseptal defect, although lesions such as patent ductus arteriosus,

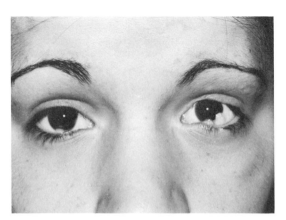

FIGURE 16–2. *Limbal dermoids are frequently associated with Goldenhar's syndrome. (Photograph courtesy of Caleb Gonzalez, M.D., Professor of Ophthalmology, Yale University School of Medicine.)*

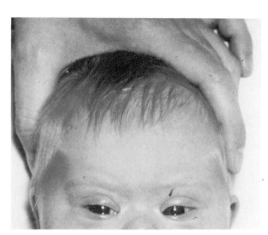

FIGURE 16–3. *An infant with trisomy 21. (Photograph courtesy of Margaret Kenna, M.D., Department of Otolaryngology, Children's Hospital of Pittsburgh, University of Pittsburgh School of Medicine.*

TABLE 16–4. Anesthetic Implications of Assorted Conditions with Ocular Pathology

Syndrome or Disease	Eye Findings	Features Affecting Anesthetic Management
Crouzon's	Glaucoma Cataracts Strabismus Ectopia lentis Hypertelorism Proptosis	Upper airway obstruction Difficult intubation
Apert's	See Crouzon's	Difficult intubation Cardiac anomalies Anomalies of tracheobronchial tree
Goldenhar's	Glaucoma Cataracts Strabismus	Difficult intubation Congenital heart disease
Down's	Cataracts Strabismus Keratoconus	Retardation Airway obstruction Congenital heart disease Seizures Thyroid disorders
Homocystinuria	Ectopia lentis Pupillary block glaucoma Retinoschisis Retinal detachment Optic atrophy Central retinal artery occlusion Strabismus	Severe thromboembolic complications Hypoglycemic convulsions Kyphoscoliosis Osteoporosis
Lowe's	Cataracts Glaucoma	Retardation Osteoporosis Decreased renal excretion of drugs Seizures Hyperchloremic acidosis
Marfan's	Lens subluxation Anomalies of iris and iridocorneal angle Glaucoma Retinal detachment Myopia Cataracts Strabismus	Valvular heart disease Chest deformities Major vascular aneurysms Joint instability Difficult intubation
Myotonia congenita	Cataracts	Avoidance of depolarizing relaxants Avoidance of hypothermia Regional, if possible
Paramyotonia	Cataracts	Avoidance of hypothermia, exercise, potassium, all muscle relaxants, and neostigmine Regional, if possible

Myotonia dystrophica	Cataracts
	Ptosis
	Strabismus
		Avoidance of hypothermia, exercise, potassium, all
		  muscle relaxants, neostigmine, digitalis, dilantin,
		  barbiturates, cholinergics, and anticholinergics
		Cardiac abnormalities
		Tendency to aspirate
		Hypoventilation
		Regional anesthesia, if possible

Riley-Day	Corneal and other damage
	  secondary to absence of
	  lacrimation
		Aspiration pneumonitis
		Abnormal respiratory control
		Postural hypotension
		Paroxysmal hypertension
		Temperature fluctuations

Rubella	Cataracts Microphthalmos Glaucoma Keratitis Iris atrophy Optic atrophy	Retardation and deafness Congenital heart disease Excretion of virus for several months

TABLE 16–4. Anesthetic Implications of Assorted Conditions with Ocular Pathology *Continued*

Syndrome or Disease	Eye Findings	Features Affecting Anesthetic Management
Sickle cell disease	Retinal detachment Vitreous hemorrhage Retinitis proliferans	Anemia Cardiopulmonary disease Vulnerability to hypoxia, acidosis, dehydration, and hypothermia
Sturge-Weber	Vascular malformations Glaucoma Ectopia lentis	Retardation Seizures Airway angiomata
von Recklinghausen's	Ptosis Proptosis Optic glioma or meningioma Optic atrophy Glaucoma	Kyphoscoliosis Possible pheochromocytoma Abnormal response to muscle relaxants
Wagner-Stickler	Vitreous degeneration Chorioretinal degeneration Retinal holes and detachments Cataracts Glaucoma Strabismus	Difficult intubation Mitral valve prolapse Skeletal deformities
Zellweger	Glaucoma Cataract Corneal clouding Vitreous cellularity Retinal pigmentary disorders Optic atrophy Optic nerve hypoplasia	Seizures Hypoprothrombinemia Difficult intubation
Diabetes mellitus	Cataracts Diabetic retinopathy Glaucoma Muscle palsy	"Silent" coronary artery disease Autonomic neuropathy Poor ventricular function Renal impairment Vulnerability to infection, sepsis, and aspiration Stiff joint syndrome

tetralogy of Fallot, and pulmonary vascular disease may occur. When ophthalmic surgery is required, the offending lesions are commonly either strabismus or cataracts, but keratoconus may appear also.

The anesthesiologist must cope with subnormal mentality, airway problems owing to copious secretions and tongue enlargement, and the possibility of major cardiac disease requiring antibiotic prophylaxis (see Table 16–4). Vessel cannulation may be difficult because of hypoplastic peripheral vessels. The effects of sedatives are erratic, and the "usual" dosage should be reduced to avoid complications. Despite nebulous warnings concerning purported dangers of atropine[21–23] in this population, standard dosages of atropine are recommended, because excessive salivation is a feature of this syndrome. During laryngoscopy, the patient's cervical spine should be manipulated only with great care and gentleness. Because the subglottic area may be especially small, an appropriate-sized endotracheal tube that permits an air leak with ventilation should be selected.

HOMOCYSTINURIA

Although rare, homocystinuria is generally considered the second most common inborn error of amino acid metabolism, ranking behind only phenylketonuria in frequency. The incidence of phenylketonuria is about 1:25,000,[24] and that of homocystinuria approximately 1:200,000, except in Ireland, where it is 1:40,000.[25] An error of sulfur amino acid metabolism, homocystinuria is characterized by the excretion of a large amount of urinary homocystine, which can be detected by the cyanide-nitroprusside test. A variety of different genetic abnormalities may be linked with homocystinuria, but the most common is a deficiency of cystathionine β synthase,[26] with accumulation of methionine and homocystine. The disorder is autosomal recessive.

Ectopia lentis has been noted in at least 90% of individuals with homocystinuria. Often, there is subluxation of the lens into the anterior chamber, producing pupillary block glaucoma requiring surgical intervention.

Other ocular findings in homocystinuria may include pale irides, retinoschisis, retinal detachment, optic atrophy, central retinal artery occlusion, and strabismus. Moreover, structural abnormalities of ciliary epithelium and zonules have been documented.

Skeletal manifestations are not unlike those of Marfan's syndrome. Most patients have arachnodactyly, kyphoscoliosis, and sternal deformity. In addition, they may have severe osteoporosis, necessitating gentle positioning on the operating table. Kyphoscoliosis may be associated with restrictive lung disease.

Brown[27] has emphasized that patients with homocystinuria have a high frequency of thromboembolic complications associated with a high mortality (see Table 16–4). An untreated homocystinuric may have as high as 50% perioperative mortality. High concentrations of homocystine irritate the vascular intima, promoting thrombolic nidus formation and increasing the adhesiveness of platelets.[28] Patients with homocystinuria are also at risk for hypoglycemic convulsions secondary to hyperinsulinemia, thought to be triggered by hypermethioninemia.[29] Preoperative measures include a low-methionine, high-cystine diet and vitamins B_6 and B_{12} and folic acid to regulate homocystine levels, and acetylsalicylic acid and dipyridamole to prevent aberrant platelet function, as may be determined by *in vitro* platelet adhesiveness.[30]

Besides appropriate dietary and drug therapy, proper perioperative care of patients with homocystinuria involves prevention of hypoglycemia and measures to maintain adequate circulation. The latter includes the use of dextran 40 and intraoperative wrapping and manipulation of the extremities. Anesthetic agents are selected that foster high peripheral flow by reducing vascular resistance, that maintain cardiac output, and that encourage rapid recovery and early ambulation.[31]

LOWE'S SYNDROME

Lowe's syndrome, also known as the oculocerebrorenal syndrome, is an X-linked recessive disorder associated with cataracts and glaucoma. Other concomitants include mental retardation, hypotonia, renal acidosis, amino aciduria, proteinuria, osteoporosis, and renal rickets, requiring calcium and vitamin D therapy.[32, 33] Histopathological studies of the lens in Lowe's syndrome suggest an early defect in embryogenesis of the lens.

Anesthetic management includes careful attention to acid-base balance and to serum levels of calcium and electrolytes. The administration of drugs excreted by the kidney should be observed carefully, and nephrotoxins should be avoided. The patient with osteoporosis should be positioned on the operating table with extreme gentleness (see Table 16–4).

MARFAN'S SYNDROME

Marfan's syndrome is an autosomal dominant condition characterized by skeletal, cardiovascular, and ocular abnormalities. Patients afflicted with this connective tissue disorder tend to be tall and have long, thin extremities with arachnodactyly and joint hyperextensibility. A high-arched palate and chest deformities, such as kyphoscoliosis and pectus excavatum, are common. Dilation and possible dissection of the aortic root resulting in aortic insufficiency may occur. Dissecting aortic aneurysms of the thoracic or abdominal variety are not uncommon, and disorders of the pulmonary artery or mitral valve, including mitral regurgitation, have been reported. Lung cysts have been documented also.

Most patients with Marfan's syndrome have lens subluxation; displacement of the lens occurs in approximately 80% of these patients. Furthermore, numerous associated iris abnormalities and anomalies of the iridocorneal angle have been noted, including miosis and poor response to mydriatics (attributed to hypoplasia of the dilator muscle of the iris), and hypopigmentation and transillumination of the periphery of the iris. Glaucoma, retinal detachment, and cataracts may develop. Myopia is common (see Table 16–4).

Careful preoperative assessment of cardiovascular status is important, and antibiotic prophylaxis may be appropriate. A high-arched palate and other anatomical variations are probable, so the anesthesiologist should be prepared for a potentially difficult intubation. Laryngoscopy should be carefully performed to circumvent tissue damage and, especially, to avoid hypertension with its attendant danger of aortic dissection. The patient should be carefully positioned to avoid joint and other injuries. Myocardial depressant drugs should be administered with caution. Because the dangers of hypertension in these patients are well known, total avoidance of myocardial depressants is not recommended, but the dose should be cautiously titrated. If pulmonary cysts are present, positive-pressure ventilation may lead to pneumothorax.[34]

CONGENITAL MYOTONIC DISEASES

Any myotonic disease is characterized by delayed relaxation of skeletal muscle after contraction. The three congenital myotonic diseases are myotonia congenita (Thomsen's disease), paramyotonia congenita (Eulenburg's disease), and myotonia dystrophica or atrophica (see Table 16–4). The relationship among these conditions remains unclear, but they probably involve different genetic defects. The most severe disorder is myotonia dystrophica. The ocular problems most frequently encountered in patients with congenital myotonia are cataracts, ptosis, and strabismus.

Myotonia congenita may be inherited in either an autosomal dominant or recessive manner.[35] The disease is characterized by early onset of muscle hypertrophy and is usually associated with a relatively benign course without major systemic involvement. Limited anesthetic risk is linked to this disorder, as long as hypothermia and depolarizing neuromuscular relaxants are avoided. Unfortunately, some children with Thomsen's disease may later develop myotonia dystrophica.[36]

An autosomal dominant disease of unknown pathogenesis, paramyotonia congenita is characterized by myotonia that is precipitated or exacerbated by cold, exercise, potassium administration, depolarizing muscle relaxants, and neostigmine methylsulfate.[37] Therefore, nondepolarizing muscle relaxants are probably best avoided in individuals with paramyotonia congenita, lest reversal with neostigmine be necessary.

Myotonia dystrophica or atrophica is an autosomal dominant disease of unknown etiology. It is an especially debilitating disease associated with endocrine failure (e.g., diabetes mellitus, testicular atrophy) as well as disorders of the cardiovascular, respiratory, and gastrointestinal systems. In addition to the familiar skeletal muscle aberrations, including myotonia, muscle wasting, and weakness, there is diffuse involvement of involuntary muscle.[38, 39]

Myotonia dystrophica represents a significant anesthetic risk. Derangements of swallowing and the possibility of attendant aspiration are worrisome, especially because there may be extensive involvement of the deglutition

mechanism before the patient is aware of any motor dysfunction. Mortality is often caused by aspiration pneumonitis. Furthermore, alveolar hypoventilation and weak cough secondary to diaphragmatic involvement are other concerns.

Cardiac disturbances are common and include assorted dysrhythmias and various degrees of heart block. Sudden death is not unusual. Aberrant responses to digitalis, diphenylhydantoin, and sodium thiopental[40] have been reported. However, Brown and Fisk[41] reported that "contrary to early suggestions, thiopental can be safely used in these patients provided care is taken with doses and rate of injecting when anaesthetizing patients who have myocardial involvement or whose respiratory function is borderline. The nature and dose of premedication should also be borne in mind."

In addition to muscle relaxants, other drugs or factors that can trigger myotonia in these patients include neostigmine, hypothermia, exercise, and alterations in potassium balance. The various inhalation anesthetic agents may cause postoperative shivering and myotonia. Antibiotic drugs with neuromuscular implications, such as neomycin, gentamicin, and kanamycin, should probably be avoided. If possible, local or regional anesthesia should be selected. In addition, antidysrhythmic drugs (digitalis, diphenylhydantoin), cholinergic or anticholinergic agents, and barbiturates should be avoided, if possible, or used with extreme caution.

Because of the clinical overlap among the various myotonias, any drug or technique, known or suspected, to have detrimental effects on any of the three types of congenital myotonia should be avoided, if at all feasible, during anesthetic management.

RILEY-DAY SYNDROME (FAMILIAL DYSAUTONOMIA)

Riley-Day syndrome is a rare autosomal recessive condition seen in Ashkenazi Jewish children. Characterized by low plasma levels of dopamine β oxidase, this disorder has several distinguishing features, including absence of both lacrimation and of response to painful stimuli, excessive drooling and impaired deglutition, motor weakness and aspiration pneumonitis, abnormal respiratory control,[42] erratic temperature swings, postural hypotension, and paroxysmal hypertension secondary to exaggerated response to infused norepinephrine.[43] Absence of lacrimation results in corneal and other ocular injuries.

Because hypotension is associated with this syndrome (see Table 16–4), potent cardiovascular depressants should be avoided or administered in small amounts or concentrations. The inability to respond to pain may be converted to an anesthetic asset when only nitrous oxide and oxygen may be adequate for certain types of surgery. As always, temperature should be continuously monitored, and positional changes should be executed slowly and carefully.

Chronic pulmonary disease manifested by tenacious, viscid secretions, bronchitis, and pneumonitis secondary to chronic aspiration is another perioperative focus for concern. Respiratory depressants should be avoided, and intraoperative suctioning should be performed frequently. Postoperatively, these patients demonstrate abnormal ventilatory responses to hypoxemia and hypercarbia, and inspissated secretions, hypoventilation, and aspiration should be avoided. Use of high humidity gases and extensive pre- and postoperative pulmonary physiotherapy are indicated.

RUBELLA SYNDROME

Maternal rubella in the first 3 or 4 months of pregnancy is associated with a high incidence of patent ductus arteriosus. These infants may also have microcephaly, mental retardation, deafness, cataracts, thrombocytopenia purpura, and hepatosplenomegaly (see Table 16–4). When congenital heart disease is present, the lesion is commonly patent ductus arteriosus, pulmonic stenosis, ventricular septal defect, multiple pulmonary artery coarctations, or a combination of these.

In addition to dense cataracts, other ocular stigmata of congenital rubella infection include microphthalmos, keratitis, glaucoma, iris atrophy or hypoplasia of the iris dilator, synechiae, pigmentary retinopathy, and optic atrophy.

Careful cardiac evaluation is essential preoperatively. Subacute bacterial endocarditis prophylaxis may be indicated, as well as digitalization. Attention to electrolyte status and intraoperative fluid therapy is essential. Myocardial depressants should be given with caution. Furthermore, because these infants may excrete rubella virus for many months following birth, nonimmune hospital personnel who

may be pregnant should not be involved in the care of these babies.

SICKLE CELL DISEASE

Sickle cell disease is an autosomal recessive disorder that occurs most frequently in individuals of African ancestry. Patients with homozygous sickle cell disease have a chronic hemolytic anemia. The disorder is caused by the presence of hemoglobin S, in which a valine molecule is substituted for glutamic acid in the β chain. This substitution causes the hemoglobin S molecule to form polymers at low oxygen tensions, leading to increased viscosity and rigidity of red cells and sickling. These atypical cells lodge in the microcirculation and cause painful vaso-occlusive crises, infarcts, and enhanced vulnerability to infection. Chronic pulmonary disease gradually develops as a result of recurrent pulmonary infection and infarction. Ultimately, these individuals develop pulmonary hypertension, cardiomegaly, and heart failure (see Table 16–4).

Sickle cell disease may be associated with retinitis proliferans, vitreous hemorrhages, and retinal detachment. However, prophylactic laser photocoagulation has been helpful in decreasing the incidence of the aforementioned conditions.

The severity of the anemia depends on the amount of hemoglobin S present. In homozygous SS disease, the hemoglobin S content is 85–90%, the remainder being hemoglobin F. Sickle cell thalassemia (SF) has 67–82% hemoglobin S and is somewhat less severe.

Multiple factors, including anemia, underlying cardiopulmonary disease, and extreme vulnerability to dehydration, hypothermia, hypoxia, and acidosis, place these patients at high risk from anesthesia. Preoperative management should include correction of anemia if hemoglobin is below 7–8 g/100 mL.[44] Whether these patients should receive preoperative exchange transfusions with hemoglobin A is controversial. Transfusion is not without its own risks: isosensitization, hepatitis, acquired immune deficiency syndrome (AIDS), febrile reaction, and even sickle crisis.[45–47] These risks must be weighed against the anticipated benefits for each patient. If the patient's risk of an hypoxic ischemic episode is small (e.g., a child having myringotomy), the risks associated with transfusion may not be warranted. However, for an adult undergoing a pneumonectomy, the risk of an hypoxic or ischemic event is high; then, the decision becomes how much transfusion is necessary. Reasonable goals for preoperative transfusion are (1) a total hemoglobin of between 8 and 12 g/dL and (2) a population of normal hemoglobin AA cells equal to 40–60% of the patient's total red blood cell population.[48] These goals may be achieved by partial exchange transfusion. Transfusion should be with the freshest red blood cells available to maximize oxygen-carrying capacity.

Factors that trigger sickle crises, including dehydration, hypoxia, acidosis, infection, hypothermia, and circulatory stasis, should be avoided. Adequate perioperative volume replacement is critical. Supplemental oxygen and mild hyperventilation are desirable, as well as administration of humidified gases. Following surgery, oxygen therapy and the maintenance of normothermia should be continued for at least 24 hours, because crises may precipitously develop postoperatively.

STURGE-WEBER SYNDROME

The Sturge-Weber syndrome, also known as encephalotrigeminal angiomatosis, is characterized by vascular malformations of the meninges, brain, eye, and skin (Fig. 16–4). Principal manifestations of the disorder include facial nevus flammeus (portwine stain), leptomeningeal angiomas, mental retardation, intracranial calcifications and seizures (see Table 16–4). Ocular stigmata include nevus flammeus involving the eyelids; dilatation and tortuosity of the vessels of the conjunctiva, sclera, and retina; angiomatous lesions of the uveal tract; and glaucoma. Glaucoma usually occurs on the side of the facial nevus flammeus and is not always present in infancy. Long-term monitoring of children with Sturge-Weber syndrome is advisable, because those with vascular anomalies of the eyelids and conjunctiva are most susceptible to the development of glaucoma. Unfortunately, glaucoma in patients with Sturge-Weber syndrome tends to be especially refractory to treatment.

Anticonvulsant premedication and proper sedation, preferably with a benzodiazepine or an appropriate barbiturate, are indicated for these individuals during surgery. Enflurane, with its potential to produce convulsions, should be avoided. The anesthesiologist should be extremely gentle when performing any airway manipulations, because undiagnosed airway angioma may be present.

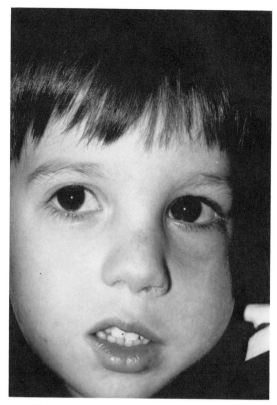

FIGURE 16–4. *A 5-year-old child with Sturge-Weber syndrome and glaucoma. (Photograph courtesy of David S. Walton, M.D., Pediatric Ophthalmologist, Associate Surgeon, Massachusetts Eye and Ear Infirmary.)*

VON RECKLINGHAUSEN'S DISEASE

Von Recklinghausen's disease is an autosomal dominant condition characterized by multiple neurofibromas in the skin and meninges, Lisch nodules (pigmented hamartomas of the iris), and cafe-au-lait spots (six or more exceeding 1.5 cm in diameter). The incidence of the disease is 1:3000, and its pathophysiology is thought to be related to the migration of abnormal neural crest cells to various parts of the body.

Skeletal defects, including severe kyphoscoliosis, are common. With the latter condition, marked reductions in lung volumes and chest wall compliance combined with increased ventilation-perfusion abnormalities and increased pulmonary vascular resistance complicate anesthetic management.

Glaucoma is not common but may occur at any age. More common ocular manifestations include plexiform involvement of the eyelid producing ptosis, neurofibromatous lesions of the conjunctiva and orbital tissues, and optic glioma or meningioma.

Medullary thyroid carcinoma, hyperparathyroidism, and pheochromocytoma may also be associated with von Recklinghausen's disease. In addition to the possibility of severe intraoperative hypertension secondary to occult pheochromocytoma, prolonged neuromuscular blockade has been reported with both depolarizing and nondepolarizing muscle relaxants (see Table 16–4). Moreover, in patients with neuromuscular involvement and muscle atrophy, succinylcholine can induce severe hyperkalemia.

WAGNER-STICKLER SYNDROME

This condition, also known as progressive arthro-ophthalmomyopathy or Stickler syndrome, has an autosomal dominant pattern of inheritance, with great variability of expression. The involvement of ocular, orofacial, and skeletal tissue suggests an underlying connective tissue disease. The most common ocular disorder is degeneration of the vitreous humor, but chorioretinal degeneration, myopia, retinal holes, and retinal detachments are also common. Other ophthalmological problems may include astigmatism, cataracts, glaucoma, and strabismus.

The nonocular features of the disease can be quite subtle and variable and include cleft or high-arched palate, characteristic facies and skeletal abnormalities, as well as mitral valve prolapse and sensorineural hearing loss. Commonly encountered facial characteristics include maxillary hypoplasia, flat nasal bridge and cheeks, long philtrim, malocclusion, and micrognathia. Musculoskeletal abnormalities often noted are loose joints, a marfanoid habitus, arachnodactyly, kyphosis, and scoliosis.[49]

The Wagner-Stickler syndrome may be the most common autosomal dominant connective tissue dysplasia in the North American Midwest, and it is relatively frequent in other parts of the United States and Europe.[50] It is significantly more common than Marfan's syndrome,[51] which has an incidence of 1:20,000.[52] Yet, the Wagner-Stickler syndrome is unfamiliar to many physicians.

Some investigators[53] have implicated degeneration of either collagen or elastin in the pathogenesis of mitral valve prolapse, which occurs in approximately 45% of patients with Wagner-Stickler syndrome.[54] Interestingly, an increased prevalence of mitral valve prolapse occurs in several connective tissue dysplasias, including Marfan's syndrome,[55] the Ehlers-Danlos syndrome,[56] and pseudoxanthoma elasticum.[57]

In caring for a patient with Wagner-Stickler syndrome, the anesthesiologist should be prepared for a potentially difficult intubation because of anatomical features such as micrognathia, malocclusion, and palatal abnormalities (see Table 16–4). Furthermore, although most patients with mitral valve prolapse are essentially asymptomatic, some serious complications have been documented, such as mitral insufficiency, bacterial endocarditis, thromboembolism, dysrhythmias, and sudden death.[58] These patients should be well-hydrated, and tachycardia should be prevented. Although some claim that routine antibiotic prophylaxis for patients with mitral valve prophylaxis is indicated only when a holosystolic murmur is present, others administer antibiotics even if merely a click is heard.

ZELLWEGER SYNDROME

Zellweger syndrome, an autosomal recessive disorder also known as cerebrohepatorenal syndrome, is associated with an abnormality of long-chain fatty acids. These patients have a distinctive craniofacial appearance characterized by high forehead, micrognathia, flat supraorbital ridges, and high-arched palate. Endotracheal intubation in these patients may be challenging (see Table 16–4).

Abnormal neuronal migration and demyelination are major findings, along with hypotonia, seizures, impaired psychomotor development, renal cortical cysts, and hepatosplenomegaly with jaundice and hypoprothrombinemia.

Reported ocular anomalies include glaucoma, vitreous cellularity, cataracts, retinal pigmentary problems, optic atrophy, and optic nerve hypoplasia.

DIABETES MELLITUS

Approximately 5.8 million people in the United States, or almost 3% of the population, have been diagnosed as having diabetes. Probably an additional 5 million people have the disease but have not yet been diagnosed. Diabetes and its complications are listed as the third leading cause of death by disease in the

United States, and the ravages of the disease are believed to cost Americans more than $13.8 billion annually.

Approximately 90% of diabetics have non-insulin-dependent or type II diabetes mellitus (NIDDM). Insulin-dependent diabetes mellitus (IDDM) or type I diabetes requires exogenous insulin to prevent ketosis; it occurs in younger (often juvenile) patients and is more frequently associated with severe end-organ complications.

The renal, neurological, cardiovascular, and ophthalmic complications of diabetes mellitus are well-known. Diabetes is responsible for more than 12% of all new cases of blindness[59] and 20% of all new blindness in individuals between the ages of 45 and 74 years.[60] However, the application of laser photocoagulation and the development of vitrectomy surgery have maintained visual function in many patients who would have otherwise become blind. Laser therapy is capable of reducing visual loss by 50% or more in patients treated adequately and in time.[61]

Ocular problems associated with diabetes include cataracts, muscle palsy, diabetic retinopathy, and neovascular glaucoma. Ischemia to the tissues of the eye is part of the pathophysiology of some of these lesions. Additionally, studies have indicated that disorders of platelet function and microangiopathy are associated with prostaglandins and may be involved in diabetic retinopathy. Lane and colleagues[62] reported that plasma epoprostenol levels were elevated in human diabetics, with a correlation existing between elevation of epoprostenol levels and severity of retinopathy. Diabetic retinopathy characteristically progresses from the relatively early changes of microaneurysm formation, intraretinal hemorrhage, and retinal edema to the proliferative phases with neovascularization of the retina and optic nerve. The proliferative phases are complicated by vitreous hemorrhage and traction retinal detachment. Vitrectomy alone or in combination with photocoagulation, scleral buckling, lensectomy, and gas-fluid exchange has been applied to these pathological entities. Unfortunately, at these more advanced stages of retinopathy, the physiological function of other organ systems is also frequently impaired, increasing anesthetic morbidity. Indeed, a study[63] has shown that variables related to kidney damage were glucose control and, to a lesser degree, duration of diabetes. Variables related to eye disease were, in descending order of significance, duration of diabetes,

glucose control, and age. The frequent association of neovascular glaucoma with proliferative retinopathy mandates the use of antiglaucoma drugs whose systemic actions may further compromise organ systems with pre-existing impaired function.

Organ dysfunction in the diabetic patient is often occult. Therefore, preoperative assessment should focus on the major systemic abnormalities known to afflict diabetics, and intraoperative management must protect organ function, especially of the cardiac, renal, and central nervous systems. The anesthesiologist must be prepared to handle severe perioperative metabolic instability. Profound hypoglycemia secondary to overzealous administration of insulin or insufficient substrate administration can produce severe CNS damage or death. Alternatively, insulin deprivation during severe perioperative catabolic stress and critical illness can result in metabolic decompensation. (Fortunately, eye surgery is usually not associated with significant catabolic stress.) Hyperglycemia with ketoacidosis or nonketotic hyperosmolar crisis can result in critical fluid and electrolyte imbalance, cardiovascular collapse, and serious renal and CNS injury (see Table 16–4).

END-ORGAN DISEASE

To formulate an intelligent perioperative management plan, both end-organ disease in the diabetic patient and the metabolic fluctuations induced by stress and surgery must be understood. The major aberrations encountered in diabetes involve the cardiovascular, renal, gastrointestinal, and endocrine systems. In addition, a few patients manifest the stiff-joint syndrome.

Commonly encountered cardiovascular problems include coronary artery disease, hypertension, cardiac autonomic neuropathy, and impaired ventricular function. Occasionally, unexpected sudden death may occur.

The patient with diabetes mellitus must be considered to be functionally much older than his or her stated age. Atherosclerosis or microangiopathy occurs early. Coronary artery disease is common in patients with long-standing type I diabetes, even when they are only 25 or 30 years of age. Myocardial infarction is five to ten times more common in diabetics than in the general population. Moreover, myocardial ischemia and infarction may be silent in diabetic patients, secondary to denervation of sympathetic afferent fibers associated with autonomic neuropathy. All diabetic adults, with type I or type II, should be considered at high risk for perioperative myocardial ischemia and managed accordingly. A baseline electrocardiogram should be obtained on all adult diabetics, regardless of age and type of surgery scheduled. Anesthetic management is then adjusted appropriate to the results of preoperative evaluation and intraoperative behavior.

It has been reported that 30–60% of diabetics have associated hypertension.[64] Blood pressure must be well controlled prior to surgery to encourage stable intraoperative and postoperative hemodynamic function. Cardiac autonomic neuropathy should be suspected if the patient displays either orthostatic hypotension or an elevated resting heart rate. However, the presence of cardiac autonomic neuropathy does not correlate with age, duration of diabetes, or severity of microvascular complications.[65] In addition to painless myocardial ischemia, another consequence of cardiac autonomic neuropathy is an impaired cardiovascular stress response. Diabetics with autonomic neuropathy may have abnormal hypoxic drive mechanisms centrally or peripherally and, hence, are at greater risk for sudden, unexpected cardiac and respiratory arrest with hypoxia.[66, 67]

When considering cardiovascular function, the anesthesiologist should suspect ventricular dysfunction in patients with chronic diabetes, especially if there is microangiopathy in other systems. Impaired ventricular function may exist even without concomitant coronary artery disease.

Diabetic renal disease, including renal papillary necrosis and glomerulosclerosis, renders the diabetic patient especially vulnerable to perioperative acute renal failure. In addition, the diabetic is at greater risk for urosepsis, which may contribute to systemic sepsis and acute renal failure. Sepsis is a major cause of perioperative complications and death in diabetic patients. When diabetes is poorly controlled, abnormal phagocytic function[68] and depressed cell-mediated immunity[69] may occur.

Another consequence of autonomic dysfunction may be impaired gastric emptying. Although gastroparesis may be asymptomatic, it is also associated with epigastric discomfort, vomiting, and early satiety after food ingestion. Because gastric stasis may increase the likelihood of pulmonary aspiration, a thorough history and a high index of suspicion are essential. Metoclopramide is suggested to facilitate gastric emptying and, hopefully, decrease the incidence of postoperative nausea and vomiting that might predispose to the development of hypoglycemia, dehydration, and other metabolic disturbances. By reducing gastric volume, metoclopramide may also protect against aspiration.

In the occasional patient with juvenile-onset diabetes, fixation of the atlanto-occipital joint with limitation of head extension may make endotracheal intubation difficult or impossible.[70] This problem is frequently associated with short stature and finger-joint contractures and may be caused by abnormal collagen cross-linking by nonenzymatic glycosylation.[71] Stiff-joint syndrome has been reported in approximately 25% of adolescents and young adults with IDDM, and its presence should be sought on preoperative examination[72] so that appropriate airway management may be planned (see Chapter 3).

In diabetics treated with insulin or sulfonyl urea therapy, counter-regulatory responses to hypoglycemia are critical but frequently defective owing to deficient glucagon and epinephrine responses. The diabetic patient taking a β-adrenergic antagonist (as may be prescribed for hypertension) is at increased risk for perioperative hypoglycemic injury.

PERIOPERATIVE MANAGEMENT

Despite the known advantages of "tight" or near euglycemic control in the *chronic* diabetic state, the concept of tight control is inappropriate in the perioperative period. Aggressive attempts to maintain euglycemia may produce dangerous episodes of hypoglycemia. Therefore, the perioperative blood sugar level should be maintained in the 100–200 mg/dL range.

Patients with type I diabetes tend to be more "brittle" than those with NIDDM, and the former should be scheduled as early in the day as possible. Numerous regimens for insulin and substrate infusions have been advocated. However, many experts recommend that type I diabetics be given one third to one half of their normal morning dose of intermediate or long-acting insulin, following a preoperative fasting blood glucose determination. An intravenous (IV) infusion containing 5% dextrose is started and titrated appropriately. Blood glucose levels should be monitored throughout the perioperative period at 1–2 hour intervals. If significant hyperglycemia (greater than 250 mg/dL) develops, small dosages of short-acting (regular) insulin are administered. Alternatively, if the blood sugar level is less than 100 mg, more IV dextrose is given.

Type II diabetics taking daily insulin should have their insulin managed in a manner analogous to the type I diabetics. Those on oral hypoglycemics should avoid taking their hypoglycemic agent on the day of surgery. Some of the oral hypoglycemics, e.g. chlorpropamide (DIABINESE), perhaps should be discontinued earlier, because their long half-life values may predispose patients to hypoglycemia for 2 days after the last dose. The morning-fasting blood sugar level should be determined, and a dextrose infusion initiated. Perioperative blood glucose levels should be monitored frequently, and insulin or dextrose administered accordingly.

Surgical requirements and the presence or absence of end-organ impairment largely determine anesthetic management for the diabetic patient. Fortunately, patients undergoing most types of eye surgery should have minimal surgery-related catabolism. Moreover, the ophthalmic patient is usually able to tolerate oral intake within a relatively brief time following surgery. When oral intake is adequate, the patient may resume his or her usual regimen of control. Because stress exacerbates diabetes, appropriate anxiolytic or analgesic medications should be prescribed.

A retrospective study[73] assessed perioperative risk of nonocular surgery in diabetics. Overall, 15% of patients had significant complications. In these patients, serious cardiac morbidity was predicted by the preoperative presence of congestive heart failure, significant valvular heart disease, and age over 75 years. Noncardiac complications, including infection, renal insufficiency, and cerebral ischemia, occurred in 24% of those patients with diabetic end-organ disease (i.e., retinopathy, neuropathy, or nephropathy), in 29% of those with congestive heart failure or valvular heart disease, and in 35% with peripheral vascular disease. In patients without pre-existing conditions, noncardiac complications (6%) and cardiac complications (4%) were rare. Once again, the type of anesthetic selected was not predictive of risk of complications. This study clearly showed that increased morbidity and mortality occur in diabetic patients with cardiac and end-organ disease.

REFERENCES

1. Martyn LJ, DiGeorge A: Selected eye defects of special importance in pediatrics. Pediatr Clin North Am 1987; 34:1517–1542.

2. DiGeorge AM, Harley RD: The association of aniridia, Wilms' tumor, and genital abnormalities. Arch Ophthalmol 1966; 75:796–798.

3. Kohn BA: Differential diagnosis of cataracts in infancy and childhood. Am J Dis Child 1976; 130:184–192.

4. Krill AE, Woodbury G, Bowman JE: X-chromosomal-linked sutural cataracts. Am J Ophthalmol 1969; 68:867–872.

5. Bateman JB, Spence MA, Marazita ML, et al: Genetic linkage analysis of autosomal dominant congenital cataracts. Am J Ophthalmol 1986; 101:218–225.

6. Francois J: Genetics of cataract. Ophthalmologica 1982; 184:61–71.

7. Ginsberg J, Bofinger MK, Roush JB: Pathologic features of the eye in Down's syndrome with relationship to other chromosomal anomalies. Am J Ophthalmol 1977; 83:874–880.

8. Cibis A, Burke RM: Herpes simplex virus-induced congenital cataracts. Arch Ophthalmol 1971; 85:220–223.

9. Cotlier E: Congenital varicella cataract. Am J Ophthalmol 1978; 86:627–629.

10. McKinnan AJ: Neonatal hypoglycemia—some ophthalmic observations. Can J Ophthalmol 1966; 1:56–59.

11. Kivlin JD, Fineman RM, Crandall AS, et al: Peter's anomaly as a consequence of genetic and nongenetic syndromes. Arch Ophthalmol 1986; 104:61–64.

12. Cibis GW, Tripathi RC, Tripathi BJ: Glaucoma in Sturge-Weber syndrome. Ophthalmology 1984; 91:1061–1071.

13. Petersen RA, Walton DS: Optic nerve hypoplasia with good visual acuity and visual field defects: A study of children of diabetic mothers. Arch Ophthalmol 1977; 95:254–258.

14. Skarf B, Hoyt CS: Optic nerve hypoplasia in children: Association with anomalies of the endocrine and central nervous systems. Arch Ophthalmol 1984; 102:62–67.

15. Costin G, Murphree AL: Hypothalamic-pituitary function in children with optic nerve hypoplasia. Am J Dis Child 1985; 139:249–254.

16. Berry FA, Topkins MJ: Anesthesia for congenital anomalies of the head and neck. In Stehling LC, Zauder HL (eds): Anesthetic Implications of Congenital Anomalies in Children. New York, Appleton-Century-Crofts, 1980, pp 129–143.

17. Warkany J: Congenital malformations and pediatrics. Pediatrics 1957; 19:725.

18. Greenwood RD, Rosenthal A, Sommer A, et al: Cardiovascular malformations in oculoauriculovertebral dysplasia (Goldenhar syndrome). J Pediatr 1974; 85:816.

19. Benda CE: Down's Syndrome: Mongolism and its Management. New York, Grune & Stratton, 1969.

20. Smith RM: Anesthesia for Infants and Children, 4th ed. St. Louis, CV Mosby, 1980, p 537.

21. Priest JG: Atropine response of the eyes in mongolism. Am J Dis Child 1960; 100:869.

22. Berg JM, Brandon MWG, Kirman BH: Atropine in mongolism. Lancet 1960; 2:441.

23. Harris WS, Goodman PM: Hyper-reactivity to atropine in Down's syndrome. N Engl J Med 1968; 279:407.

24. Jervis GA: Phenylpyruvic oligophrenia (phenylketonuria). Res Publ Assoc Res Nerv Ment Dis 1954; 33:547.

25. Wyngaarden JB: Homocystinuria. In Beeson PB, McDermott W, Wyngaarden JB (eds): Cecil Textbook of Medicine, 15th ed. Philadelphia, WB Saunders, 1979, p 2028.

26. Gerritsen T, Waisman HA: Homocystinuria: Cysta-

thionine synthase deficiency. *In* Stanbury JB, Frederickson DS (eds): Metabolic Basis of Inherited Disease, 3rd ed. New York, McGraw Hill, 1972.

27. Brown BR Jr, Walson PD, Taussig LM: Congenital metabolic diseases in pediatric patients: Anesthetic implications. Anesthesiology 1975; 43:197.

28. McDonald L, Bray C, Love F, et al: Homocystinuria, thrombosis, and the blood platelets. Lancet 1964; 1:745.

29. Holmgren G, Falkmer S, Hambraeus L: Plasma insulin content and glucose tolerance in homocystinuria. Ups J Med Sci 1975; 78:215.

30. Harker LA, Slichter SJ, Scott CR, et al: Homocystinemia: Vascular injury and arterial thrombosis. N Engl J Med 1974; 291:537.

31. McGoldrick KE: Anesthetic management of homocystinuria. Anesth Rev 1981; 8:42–45.

32. Richards W, Donnell GN, Wilson WA, et al: The oculo-cerebro-renal syndrome of Lowe. Am J Dis Child 1965; 109:185–203.

33. Morris RC: Renal tubular acidosis: Mechanisms, classification, and implications. N Engl J Med 1969; 281:1405.

34. Steward DJ: Manual of Pediatric Anesthesia. New York, Churchill Livingstone, 1979, pp 246–247.

35. Kim C, Yamada S: Myotonia congenita (Thomsen's disease). Hawaii Med J 1974; 33:15–18.

36. Caughey JE, Myrianthopoulous NC: Dystrophica Myotonia. Springfield, Illinois, Charles C. Thomas, 1963.

37. Thrusch DC, Morris D Jr, Salmon MV: Paramyotonia congenita: A clinical, histochemical and pathological study. Brain 1972; 95:537–552.

38. Watters GV, Williams TW: Early onset myotonic dystrophy. Arch Neurol 1967; 17:137–152.

39. Harvey JC, Sherbourne DH, Siegel CI: Smooth muscle involvement in myotonic dystrophy. Am J Med 1965; 39:81–90.

40. Bourke TD, Zuck D: Thiopentone in dystrophia myotonia. Br J Anaesth 1957; 29:35–38.

41. Brown TCK, Fisk GC: Anaesthesia for Children. London, Blackwell Scientific Publications, 1979, p 289.

42. Filler J, Smith AA, Stone S, et al: Respiratory control in familial dysautonomia. J Pediatr 1965; 66:509–516.

43. Smith AA, Dancis J: Exaggerated response to infused norepinephrine in familial dysautonomia. N Engl J Med 1964; 270:704–707.

44. Gilbertson AA: Anaesthesia in West African patients with sickle cell anaemia, haemoglobin SC disease, and sickle cell trait. Br J Anaesth 1965; 37:614.

45. Howells TH, Hunstman RG, Boys JE, et al: Anaesthesia and sickle-cell haemoglobin. Br J Anaesth 1972; 44:975–987.

46. Schmalzer E, Chien S, Brown AK: Transfusion therapy in sickle cell disease. Am J Pediatr Hematol Oncol 1982; 4:395–406.

47. Murphy SB: Difficulties in sickle cell states. *In* Orkin FH, Cooperman LH (eds): Complications in Anesthesiology. Philadelphia, JB Lippincott, 1983, pp 476–485.

48. Gibson JR: Anesthetic implications of sickle cell disease and other hemoglobinopathies. ASA Refresher Course Lectures 1986; 14:139–158.

49. Liberfarb RM, Hirose T: The Wagner-Stickler syndrome. Birth Defects: Original Article Series 1982; 18:525–538.

50. Herrmann J, France TD, Opitz, JM, et al: The Stickler syndrome (hereditary arthroophthalmopathy). Birth Defects: Original Article Series 1975; 11(6):203–204.

51. Opitz JM, France T, Herrmann J, et al: The Stickler syndrome. N Engl J Med 1972; 286:546.

52. Pyeritz RE, McKusick VA: Marfan syndrome: Diagnosis and management. N Engl J Med 1979; 300:772.

53. Davies MJ, Parker DJ, Bonella D: Collagen synthesis in floppy mitral valve. Br Heart J 1981; 45:345.

54. Liberfarb RM, Goldblatt A: Prevalence of mitral valve prolapse in the Stickler syndrome. Am J Med Genet 1986; 24:387.

55. Brown OR, DeMots H, Kloster FE, et al: Aortic root dilatation and mitral valve prolapse in Marfan's syndrome: An echocardiographic study. Circulation 1975; 52:651.

56. Brandt KD, Sumner RD, Ryan TJ, et al: Herniation of mitral leaflets in the Ehlers-Danlos syndrome. Am J Cardiol 1975; 36:524.

57. Pyeritz RE, Weiss JL, Renie WA, et al: Pseudoxanthoma elasticum and mitral valve prolapse. N Engl J Med 1982; 307:1451.

58. Cheitlin MD, Byrd RC: The click-murmur syndrome: A clinical problem in diagnosis and treatment. JAMA 1981; 245:1357.

59. Klein R, Klein B: Vision disorders in diabetes. *In* Harris MJ, Hammon RF (eds): Diabetes in America. Bethesda, National Institutes of Health, 1985, pp 1–36.

60. Kahn HA, Hiller R: Blindness caused by diabetic retinopathy. Am J Ophthalmol 1974; 78:1.

61. The Diabetic Retinopathy Study Research Group: Photocoagulation treatment of proliferative diabetic retinopathy: Clinical application of Diabetic Retinopathy Study (DRS) findings, Report 8. Ophthalmology 1981; 88:7.

62. Lane LS, Lahav M, Janson P, et al: Abnormalities in plasma platelet factors in patients with diabetes mellitus. Invest Ophthalmol Vis Sci 1982; 22(Suppl):110.

63. Chase HP, Jackson WE, Hoops SL, et al: Glucose control and the renal and retinal complications of insulin-dependent diabetes. JAMA 1989; 261:1155–1160.

64. Peires AN, Gustafson AB: Current therapeutic concepts in diabetic hypertension. Diabetes Care 1986; 9:409–414.

65. Kahn JK, Zola B, Juni JE, Vinik AI: Decreased exercise heart rate and blood pressure responses in diabetic subjects with cardiac autonomic neuropathy. Diabetes Care 1986; 9:389–394.

66. Page MMcB, Watkins PJ: Cardiorespiratory arrest and diabetic autonomic neuropathy. Lancet 1978; 1:14–16.

67. Ciccarelli LL, Ford CM, Tsueda K: Autonomic neuropathy in a diabetic patient with renal failure. Anesthesiology 1986; 64:283–287.

68. Bagdade JD, Nielson KL, Bulger RJ: Reversible abnormalities in phagocytic function in poorly-controlled diabetic patients. Am J Med Sci 1972; 263:451–456.

69. Ploufe JF, Silva J Jr, Fekety R, Allen JL: Cell-mediated immunity in diabetes mellitus. Infect Immun 1978; 21:425–429.

70. Salzarulo HH, Taylor LA: Diabetic "stiff joint syndrome" as a cause of difficult endotracheal intubation. Anesthesiology 1986; 64:366–368.

71. Ammon JR: Perioperative management of the diabetic patient. ASA Refresher Course Lectures 1988; 16:1–15.

72. Grgic A, Rosenbloom AL, Weber FT, Giordano B: Joint contraction—common manifestation of childhood diabetes mellitus. J Pediatr 1976; 88:584–588.

73. MacKenzie CR, Charlson ME: Assessment of perioperative risk in the patient with diabetes mellitus. Surg Gynecol Obstet 1988; 167:293–299.

17

Anesthetic Ramifications of Ophthalmic Drugs

Kathryn E. McGoldrick

Ophthalmic drugs, administered topically, intraocularly, or systemically, may have anesthetic ramifications.

Topical ophthalmic drugs may produce undesirable systemic effects and have deleterious anesthetic implications. Systemic absorption of topical ophthalmic drugs may occur from either the conjunctiva or the nasal mucosa following drainage through the nasolacrimal duct. Although medication tends to be absorbed slowly from the conjunctival sac, absorption is more rapid from mucosal surfaces. Therefore, this danger can be minimized by putting pressure on the inner canthus of the eye, thus occluding the nasolacrimal duct, for a few minutes after each instillation. Finger pressure over the duct for 5 minutes can reduce systemic absorption by 67%.[1] Keeping the eye gently closed for 5 minutes after use of drops can reduce absorption by as much as 65%. Nasolacrimal duct occlusion is important in small children who are highly susceptible to the toxic effects of certain drugs, including belladonna alkaloids. Children have a smaller circulating volume for drug distribution. Some percutaneous absorption from spillover through the immature epidermis of the premature infant may occur.[2] Moreover, systemic absorption may be enhanced in a diseased or postsurgical eye.

Adverse systemic effects after topical eye medication may occur with an overdose in pediatric patients, with elderly patients, with coronary or cerebral artery disease, and with the concomitant use of adrenergic-modifying drugs.

Topical ocular drugs that may cause difficulties include atropine, cocaine, cyclopentolate, echothiophate iodide, epinephrine, phenylephrine, scopolamine, and timolol. In addition, intraocular acetylcholine and sulfur hexafluoride have important anesthetic implications, as do octafluorocyclobutane and perfluoropropane (Table 17–1).

Some drugs given systemically may produce untoward sequelae germane to anesthetic management, including glycerol, mannitol, acetazolamide, and fluorescein.

TOPICAL AGENTS

ATROPINE

Atropine results in mydriasis and cycloplegia. Systemic reactions occur more frequently following topical application in children and elderly patients. These reactions include flushing, thirst, tachycardia, dry skin, temperature elevation, and in geriatric patients, agitation.

Each drop of 1% ophthalmic atropine solution contains about 0.2–0.5 mg atropine.

COCAINE

Cocaine hydrochloride has limited topical ocular use because it may cause corneal damage. However, as the only local anesthetic that produces vasoconstriction and shrinkage of mucous membranes, cocaine is commonly used in a nasal pack during dacryocystorhinostomy. Because cocaine interferes with catecholamine uptake, it has a sympathetic potentiating effect.

TABLE 17–1. Anesthetic Implications of Ocular Drugs

Drug	Concentration(s) (%)	Amount Per Drop (mg)	Potential Problems	Indication(s)
Acetylcholine	1	0.5	Bradycardia, hypotension, increased salivation and bronchial secretions, bronchospasm	Miosis
Atropine	1	0.2–0.5	Flushing, thirst, tachycardia Agitation	Mydriasis Cycloplegia
Cocaine	1–10	0.5–5	Hypertension, dysrhythmias, agitation, hyperthermia, cardiorespiratory arrest, contraindicated in patients taking sympathomimetics	Vasoconstriction
Cyclopentolate	0.5–1 2	0.25–0.5 1	Usually well tolerated CNS toxicity: dysarthria, disorientation, convulsions	Mydriasis, cycloplegia Mydriasis, cycloplegia
Echothiophate	0.03–0.25	0.01–0.1	Prolonged action of succinylcholine, procaine, cocaine, chloroprocaine, and so forth	Antiglaucoma
Epinephrine	0.25–2	0.1–1	Nervousness, hypertension, dysrhythmias, headache, faintness (usually with 2% solution)	Antiglaucoma
Phenylephrine	2.5–10	1.2–5	Usually well tolerated Hypertension, headache, tremulousness, cerebral hemorrhage, myocardial ischemia and infarction	Mydriasis Vasoconstriction Decongestion
Scopolamine	0.5	0.25	CNS excitation and disorientation	Mydriasis Cycloplegia
Timolol	0.25–0.5	0.1–0.25	Systemic, nonselective β blockade	Antiglaucoma
SF_6, C_3F_8, C_4F_8	Not applicable	Not applicable	In the presence of N_2O, may compromise retinal blood flow	Retinal reattachment
Fluorescein	10 or 25	Not applicable	Nausea, vomiting, extravasation, pruritus, headache, urticaria, allergic reactions, hypertension, MI (rare), pulmonary edema (rare), anaphylactic shock (rare)	Diagnostic

Cocaine is well absorbed from mucosal surfaces, although there is a 5–10 minute latency period after application until vasoconstriction is achieved. An ester-linked benzoic acid, cocaine is rapidly hydrolyzed by plasma pseudocholinesterase to benzoyl escogonine. Factors such as echothiophate eye drops, liver dysfunction, and atypical pseudocholinesterase conditions influence the metabolism of cocaine, but with intranasal cocaine, a peak plasma cocaine concentration is generally reached within 1 hour and persists for 4 hours.[3]

One drop of 4% cocaine solution contains approximately 1.5 mg of cocaine. The maximum safe clinical dose is approximately 3 mg/kg and depends on the method, route, site of administration, and rate of metabolism. It is safer to apply repeated small dosages of 4% cocaine intermittently than to apply a single large concentrated dose, provided the maximum safe total dose is not exceeded. Cocaine is commonly applied on pledgets or neurosurgical cottonoids. Direct spraying may cause a greater amount to be absorbed. As a rule, similar dosages can be applied more safely to the nasal mucosa than to the tracheobronchial mucosa, where uptake is especially rapid.

Although the usual maximum dose of cocaine employed in clinical practice is 200 mg for a 70-kg adult, or 3 mg/kg, 1.5 mg/kg is preferable if a volatile anesthetic agent is being used concomitantly, because this lower dose has been shown not to exert any clinically significant sympathomimetic effect in combination with halothane.[4] Although 1 g is considered to be the usual lethal dose for an adult, considerable variation occurs. Furthermore, systemic reactions may appear with as little as

20 mg. Meticulous attention must be paid to the volume used, because there is a narrow range from safety to toxicity to death.

Historically, epinephrine had often been mixed with cocaine to enhance the degree of vasoconstriction produced. This practice is both superfluous and deleterious, because cocaine is a potent vasoconstrictor, and the combination of epinephrine with cocaine may trigger dangerous dysrhythmias. Epinephrine does not enhance the vasoconstrictive efficacy of cocaine, retard the absorption, or prolong the anesthetic effect of cocaine. By blocking the reuptake of endogenous norepinephrine as well as the uptake of exogenous epinephrine, cocaine may sensitize various organs to the effects of epinephrine, thus making a toxic reaction more likely. Cocaine used alone, without epinephrine, to shrink the nasal mucosa does not sensitize the heart to *endogenous* epinephrine during halothane or enflurane anesthesia.[5] However, animal studies have shown that following pretreatment with *exogenous* epinephrine, cocaine facilitates the development of epinephrine-induced dysrhythmias during halothane.[6]

Meyers[7] described two cases of cocaine toxicity during dacryocystorhinostomy, emphasizing that cocaine is contraindicated in hypertensive patients or in patients receiving adrenergic-modifying drugs such as guanethidine, reserpine, tricyclic antidepressants, or monoamine oxidase inhibitors. Additionally, sympathomimetics, such as epinephrine hydrochloride or phenylephrine hydrochloride, should not be given with cocaine.

Signs of cocaine toxicity are referable to the respiratory, cardiovascular, and central nervous systems. Cocaine's effect on the central nervous system (CNS) is biphasic, with initial stimulation followed by depression as inhibitory synapses are stimulated.[8] The patient rapidly becomes excited, anxious, garrulous, and confused. Initially, reflexes are augmented. Headache is common. The pulse becomes rapid and respiration erratic. A chill may herald the sudden onset of hyperthermia. The pupils become dilated, and exophthalmos occurs. Nausea, vomiting, and abdominal pain are common. The patient may complain of something crawling on his or her skin. Delirium, Cheyne-Stokes breathing, convulsions, and unconsciousness occur terminally. Indeed, death may be very rapid following acute cocaine overdosage, and therapeutic maneuvers must be performed quickly.

Before administering cocaine, the physician should carefully search for possible contraindications, including the use of certain concurrent medications. To avoid toxic levels, dosages of dilute solutions should be meticulously calculated and carefully administered. If serious cardiovascular effects occur, intravenous (IV) labetalol may be given to counteract them.[9] Previously, propranolol had been used to control cocaine-induced hypertension.[10] However, a lethal hypertensive exacerbation has been ascribed to unopposed α stimulation.[11] Thus, labetalol offers the advantage of both α and β blockade. IV barbiturates should be given to combat the CNS symptoms of cocaine toxicity. Cooling measures may be required for hyperthermia, including a cooling blanket and ice water or alcohol sponging. In the unfortunate event of cardiopulmonary arrest, the usual resuscitative measures may be attempted.

CYCLOPENTOLATE

Cyclopentolate is a popular short-acting mydriatic with potential CNS toxicity, including dysarthria, disorientation, convulsions, and frank psychotic reactions.[12, 13] This synthetic antimuscarinic agent is also a potent cycloplegic. (Cyloplegia is not attainable without mydriasis and requires higher concentrations or more prolonged application of a given agent.)

Cyclopentolate is commonly used as a 0.5% or 1% solution. Undesirable side effects are purportedly much more likely to follow use of a 2% solution.

ECHOTHIOPHATE IODIDE

Echothiophate iodide is a long-acting anticholinesterase drug still used to treat glaucoma. It may cause cholinergic side effects such as vomiting, hypotension, and abdominal pain. In general, patients on anticholinesterase therapy benefit from preoperative IV atropine to block muscarinic effects and circumvent vagal responses. In the treatment a patient who has received echothiophate iodide within the previous 4 weeks,[14] drugs such as succinylcholine, procaine, cocaine, and chloroprocaine that are metabolized by plasma pseudocholinesterase should be reduced in dosage or avoided entirely. If necessary, succinylcholine can be given in increments of 5 mg, with concomitant monitoring by a peripheral nerve stimulator. A relative overdose of succinylcholine and prolonged apnea can be avoided if the drug is titrated until 95% twitch suppression is achieved.

EPINEPHRINE

Topical 2% epinephrine is used to decrease aqueous secretion, enhance aqueous outflow, and reduce intraocular pressure (IOP) in primary open-angle glaucoma. The usual safe adult systemic dose of epinephrine is 0.5 mg subcutaneously or 0.1 mg IV. One drop of 2% solution contains 0.5–1 mg epinephrine. Occasionally, the 2% solution has been associated with systemic effects such as nervousness, hypertension, pallor, faintness, tachycardia, and other dysrhythmias. Ballin and associates[15] reported an increased frequency of cardiac extrasystoles associated with the use of 0.5 mg of topically applied ocular epinephrine. Lansche[16] reported two cases in which 2.7 mg topical ocular epinephrine triggered, within 1 minute of application, tachycardia, hypertension, headache, faintness, and diaphoresis. These symptoms subsided spontaneously after 15 minutes.

Some believe that epinephrine should not be used in the eye in patients anesthetized with a halogenated hydrocarbon. However, Smith and coworkers,[17] studying patients undergoing cataract surgery by phacoemulsification and aspiration, concluded it is safe to give epinephrine into the anterior chamber in dosages up to 68 μg/kg. The iris with its rich supply of adrenergic receptors may be able to capture the epinephrine with extreme rapidity.

PHENYLEPHRINE

Phenylephrine is a sympathomimetic amine, differing chemically from epinephrine only in lacking an OH in the 4 position on the benzene ring. In addition to being an excellent mydriatic, phenylephrine also produces capillary decongestion. Phenylephrine has a shorter duration of action than belladonna alkaloids, does not cause cycloplegia, and usually does not elevate IOP. A single drop of 10% phenylephrine solution may contain 5 mg of drug. The upper limits of safe use systemically for phenylephrine are 1.5 mg given IV and 10 mg given subcutaneously.

Although systemic effects secondary to topical application of prudent doses are rare, nonetheless severe hypertension, headache, tachycardia, and tremulousness have been documented, as well as reflex bradycardia. Most adverse systemic reactions occur within 1–20 minutes following application[18] and last approximately 20 minutes; they are usually self-limiting. However, hypertension immediately after eye surgery may result in intraocular hemorrhage.

Individuals with coronary artery disease may develop severe ischemia and even myocardial infarction[18] following 10% drops, and those with cerebral aneurysms may suffer cerebral hemorrhage in this setting. The necessity for using 10% drops is dubious, because dose-effect curves indicate that there is little increase in mydriatic effect above a 5% solution.[19] Therefore, the use of only 2½% phenylephrine is recommended in infants and the elderly, as well as for those with severe coronary artery or cerebrovascular disease. Although most reactions are usually brief and self-limiting, if treatment is necessary, small incremental dosages of droperidol or thorazine may be useful. The suggested pediatric limit is one drop of 2.5% solution per eye per hour.

SCOPOLAMINE

Scopolamine produces mydriasis and cycloplegia. Systemic toxicity has been noted after scopolamine eye drops, and such toxicity has a propensity for occurring in small children and the elderly. One drop of 0.5% ophthalmic solution contains approximately 0.2 mg scopolamine. CNS excitation and disorientation, if they occur, can be treated with incremental dosages of physostigmine 0.01 mg/kg IV, repeated once or twice over a 20-minute interval.

TIMOLOL

Timolol maleate, a nonselective β blocker, is a popular antiglaucoma drug. It is commonly used as a 0.25 or 0.5% solution. McMahon and colleagues[20] reported a 23% incidence of adverse reactions affecting primarily the cardiovascular, respiratory, and central nervous systems. Relatively common complaints included fatigue, lightheadedness, disorientation, and a general depression of CNS functions. Cardiovascular perturbations included bradycardia, palpitations, syncope, and congestive heart failure.

Because significant absorption may occur, timolol should be administered with caution, if at all, to patients with known contraindications to systemic β blockers, i.e., asthma, congestive heart failure, and greater than first degree heart block. Life-threatening exacerbation of asthma has been documented in association with timolol drops.[21] Timolol has been implicated in the aggravation of myasthenia gravis[22] and in the production of postoperative apnea in neonates and young infants.[23, 24]

A newer antiglaucoma drug, betaxolol hydrochloride (BETOPTIC), is said to be exclusively a β-1-adrenergic blocker with low potential for systemic effects. Nonetheless, the manufacturers warn against the use of betaxolol in patients with sinus bradycardia, greater than first degree atrioventricular block, cardiogenic shock, or overt cardiac failure.

INTRAOCULAR THERAPY

ACETYLCHOLINE

Acetylcholine may be used following lens extraction to produce miosis. The intraocular use of this drug may produce bradycardia,[25] hypotension, increased salivation, bronchial secretions, and bronchospasm.[26] However, these side effects may be rapidly reversed with IV atropine.

SULFUR HEXAFLUORIDE

For a patient with a retinal detachment, intraocular sulfur hexafluoride (SF_6) may be injected into the vitreous to mechanically facilitate reattachment. If nitrous oxide (N_2O) is given concomitantly, the injected bubble can cause a rapid and dramatic increase in IOP. In the presence of 70% N_2O, 1 mL of air expands in volume to 2.85 cc within 1 hour. When the poorly diffusible sulfur hexafluoride is used, this volume increase is even more impressive.[27] These data are important, because the resultant rise in IOP may compromise retinal blood flow. Stinson and Donlon[28] suggested terminating N_2O at least 15 minutes before gas injection to prevent significant changes in the size of the intravitreous gas bubble. Furthermore, if a patient requires reoperation and general anesthesia after intravitreous gas injection, N_2O should be avoided for 5 days following air injection and for 10 days following SF_6 injection.[29]

PERFLUOROPROPANE AND OCTAFLUOROCYCLOBUTANE

Perfluoropropane (C_3F_8) and octafluorocyclobutane (C_4F_8) may also be employed in vitreoretinal procedures to support the retina.[30] Sim-

ilar to SF_6, these gases are relatively insoluble, and N_2O must be discontinued at least 15 minutes prior to injection. C_4F_8 remains in the vitreous cavity for more than 13 days,[31] and C_3F_8 lingers for longer than 30 days.[32]

SYSTEMIC DRUGS

Various agents, including hypertonic solutions, acetazolamide, and fluorescent dye, given systemically while caring for a patient with ocular disease are of interest to the anesthesiologist.

HYPERTONIC SOLUTIONS

IV hypertonic solutions, such as dextran, urea, mannitol, and sorbitol, elevate plasma oncotic pressure relative to aqueous humor pressure and produce an acute, albeit temporary, reduction in IOP, as shown by the equation

$$IOP = K[(OPaq - OPpl) + CP]$$

where K = coefficient of outflow, OPaq = osmotic pressure of aqueous humor, OPpl = osmotic pressure of plasma, and CP = capillary pressure.

IV mannitol is as effective as urea in reducing IOP and has fewer side effects. Its onset (5–10 minutes), peak (30–45 minutes), and duration of action (5–6 hours) are similar to urea. In addition, both drugs may be associated with an acute intravascular volume overload. Administered immediately prior to or during surgery to lower IOP, mannitol is an inert sugar that accelerates glomerular filtration rate. Because its renal tubular resorption is less than 10%, mannitol causes an obligatory water diuresis with loss of sodium, potassium, and chloride. Recommended dosage should not exceed 1.5–2 g/kg IV over a 30–60 minute interval. Mannitol should be warmed and administered through a filter to avoid infusion of crystals. Serious complications, including renal failure, congestive heart failure, pulmonary congestion, electrolyte imbalance, hypotension, hypertension, and myocardial ischemia, can be associated with rapid infusion of these large doses of mannitol.

The patient's cardiovascular and renal status must be thoroughly evaluated prior to mannitol therapy. The sudden expansion of plasma volume secondary to efflux of intracellular water into the vascular compartment burdens both the heart and kidneys. Marked hypertension and dilution of plasma sodium may ensue.

The resultant sustained diuresis may prompt significant hypotension in volume-depleted patients. Those with prostatic hypertrophy or urethral stenosis may be especially uncomfortable owing to bladder distension and urgency that accompany infusion of large doses of mannitol. A Foley catheter is helpful in this setting.

Glycerin has the advantage of being effective orally. Onset is within 10 minutes of swallowing, with a maximal effect at 30 minutes and a duration of action of 5–6 hours. However, the ocular hypotensive action of glycerin is less predictable than mannitol's, and the associated presence of gastric fluid trapping may cause an increased risk of aspiration.

ACETAZOLAMIDE

Acetazolamide, a sulfonamide derivative, inhibits carbonic anhydrase, thus depressing the sodium pump mechanism responsible for secretion of aqueous humor. IV acetazolamide acts within 5 minutes and exerts its maximum effect at 20–30 minutes. However, acetazolamide has systemic as well as ocular actions. Because renal carbonic anhydrase activity is affected also, bicarbonate diuresis with concomitant impressive losses of water, sodium, and potassium occurs with chronic therapy. Thus, patients on long-term acetazolamide therapy are commonly acidotic, hypokalemic, and hyponatremic. Furthermore, acetazolamide may cause severe acidosis in individuals with chronic lung disease. Acetazolamide should be avoided in patients with serious hepatic or renal impairment or in those who are already significantly hypokalemic or hyponatremic. These electrolyte imbalances can trigger serious dysrhythmias during general anesthesia. Because it is a sulfonamide derivative, acetazolamide may result, rarely, in anaphylaxis, erythema multiforme, Stevens-Johnson syndrome, toxic epidermal necrolysis, and severe bone marrow depression.

A distinct advantage of acetazolamide is its ease of administration. In contrast to the cumbersome volumes of hypertonic solutions required, acetazolamide is easily given in a usual dose of 500 mg dissolved in 10 mL of sterile water.

Topically active carbonic anhydrase inhibitors are currently being investigated and show promise.[33, 34]

FLUORESCEIN ANGIOGRAPHY

Although fluorescein angiography (FA) is more commonly performed in locations other than the operating room, some features of this procedure are of interest to anesthesiologists.

Since its introduction to clinical ophthalmology in 1961 by Novotny and Alvis,[35] the use of FA for the evaluation of structure and pathology of certain ocular vessels has become widespread. FA permits full visualization of the retinal vasculature and any inherent pathology therein. It can also be used to assess the value of photocoagulation therapy to choroidal and retinal vessels in certain ocular and systemic diseases. In addition, angiography of the iris can be performed, although its scope is more limited. By detecting abnormalities of the retinal circulation that would not be visible otherwise, systemic diseases can be diagnosed first by studying the eye with FA. Moreover, FA often is employed to assess the microvasculature of diabetics, hypertensives, sickle cell patients, and patients afflicted with collagen vascular diseases. However, because of their compromised condition, these patients appear to be at an increased risk of developing complications associated with the procedure.[36, 37]

In an aqueous solution of 5 mL of 10% or 3 mL of 25%, fluorescein is given by rapid IV injection, usually into the antecubital vein. The solution is orange-red in the syringe, but upon reaching the eye (which is relatively alkaline) approximately 15–18 seconds later, the color changes to fluorescent green. Fluorescein binds to albumin red cell membranes and other plasma proteins, which causes less of a fluorescence than fluorescein in a free state. When it reaches the ocular circulation, fluorescein is excited by a blue illuminating light (490 nm), and a photographic record of its journey through the eye is made through a yellow-green barrier filter (520 nm).[38] Because fluorescein dye leaks from all vessels except those of the CNS and retina, FA permits a crisp picture and a helpful assessment of the functional integrity of retinal vessels, because any leakage there is abnormal.

The overall incidence of side effects is approximately 4.8%.[39] Mild side effects include nausea, vomiting, extravasation, pruritis, and headaches, most commonly, and urticaria, allergic reactions, and acute hypertension. A few severe side effects have been reported; some patients have died of myocardial infarction,[40, 41] pulmonary edema,[42] and shock following injection of the dye. Fortunately, these catastrophes are rare.

Nausea is the most common side effect, ranging in frequency from 2.43 to 20%. The incidence of a severe reaction to fluorescein injection is approximately 0.6–1%. Cardiovascular complications, the most frequently encountered serious complication, include myocardial infarction, asystole, and circulatory collapse. Pulmonary complications, including laryngeal edema, pulmonary edema, bronchospasm, and anaphylactic shock, are the next most commonly reported serious occurrences, with an incidence of less than 0.5%.[38]

Six deaths have been officially attributed to FA, four of them following myocardial infarction. According to Yannuzzi and associates,[43] the death rate is approximately 1:222,000. The national registry of drug-induced side effects postulates one death a year secondary to the use of fluorescein.

Nausea is clearly the most frequent complication, but other mild adverse reactions include interesting, although rare, phenomena such as discoloration of the skin and conjunctiva and transient blindness. There was no significant difference in the incidence and nature of mild side effects occurring between the 10% and 25% fluorescein solutions.

Despite extensive investigation, the pathophysiological mechanism(s) involved in serious adverse reactions to fluorescein remain undetermined. Those under consideration are listed:

1. vasovagal reaction[42, 44] resulting in compromised coronary perfusion;
2. nonallergic release of histamine unaccompanied by antigen-antibody reactions[41];
3. an immediate hypersensitivity reaction causing release of histamine[41];
4. tachyarrhythmias or hypertensive crises accompanying catecholamine release secondary to anxiety or venipuncture[42, 45];
5. the possible presence of contaminant or trace elements in the dye[46];
6. systemic effect of topical mydriatics[15, 18, 47, 48];
7. direct meningeal irritation[49];
8. any combination of the above.

Premedication with agents such as promethazine (PHENERGAN), prochlorperazine (COMPAZINE), diphenhydramine (BENADRYL), or prednisone[43, 50] has not prevented or diminished the occurrence of complications; such prevention will probably not occur until the etiology of the adverse effects is understood.

REFERENCES

1. Zimmerman T, Konner KS, Kandarakis AS, et al: Improving the therapeutic index of topically applied ocular drugs. Arch Ophthalmol 1984; 102:551–553.

2. Nachman RL, Esterly NB: Increased skin permeability in preterm infants. J Pediatr 1971; 79:628.

3. Johns ME, Berman A, Price JC, et al: Metabolism of intranasally applied cocaine. Ann Otol Rhinol Laryngol 1977; 86:342.

4. Barash PG, Kopriva CJ, Langon R, et al: Is cocaine a sympathetic stimulant during general anesthesia? JAMA 1980; 243:1437.

5. Chung B, Naraghi M, Adriani J: Sympathetic effects of cocaine and their influence on halothane and enflurane anesthesia. Anesth Rev 1978; 5:16.

6. Koehntop DE, Liao J, Van Bergen FH: Effects of pharmacologic alterations of adrenergic mechanisms by cocaine, tropolone, aminophylline, and ketamine on epinephrine-induced arrhythmias during halothane-N_2O anesthesia. Anesthesiology 1977; 46:83.

7. Meyers EF: Cocaine toxicity during dacryocystorhinostomy. Arch Ophthalmol 1980; 98:842.

8. Schenck NL: Cocaine: Its use and misuse in otolaryngology. Trans Am Acad Ophthalmol Otol 1975; 80:343–351.

9. Gay GR, Loper KA: Control of cocaine-induced hypertension with labetalol. Anesth Analg 1988; 67:92.

10. Rappolt RT, Gay GR, Inaba DS: Propranolol in the treatment of cardiopressor effects of cocaine. N Engl J Med 1976; 295:448–449.

11. Ramoska E, Sacchetti AD: Propranolol-induced hypertension in treatment of cocaine intoxication. Ann Emerg Med 1985; 14:1112–1113.

12. Binkhorst RD, Weinstein GW, Baretz RM, et al: Psychotic reaction induced by cyclopentolate: Results of pilot study and a double-blind study. Am J Ophthalmol 1963; 55:1243.

13. Kennerdall JS, Wucher FP: Cyclopentolate associated with two cases of grand mal seizure. Arch Ophthalmol 1972; 87:634.

14. DeRoeth A, Dettbar WD, Rosenberg P: Effect of phospholine iodide on blood cholinesterase levels. Am J Ophthalmol 1963; 59:586.

15. Ballin N, Becker B, Goldman ML: Systemic effects of epinephrine applied topically to the eye. Invest Ophthalmol 1966; 5:125.

16. Lansche RK: Systemic reactions to topical epinephrine and phenylephrine. Am J Ophthalmol 1966; 49:95.

17. Smith RB, Douglas H, Petruscak J, et al: Safety of intraocular adrenaline with halothane anesthesia. Br J Anaesth 1972; 44:1314.

18. Fraunfelder FT, Scafidi AF: Possible adverse effects from topical ocular 10 percent phenylephrine. Am J Ophthalmol 1978; 84:447.

19. Haddad NJ, Moyer NJ, Riley FC: Mydriatic effect of phenylephrine hydrochloride. Am J Ophthalmol 1970; 70:729.

20. McMahon CD, Schaffer RN, Hoskins HD, et al: Adverse effects experienced by patients taking timolol. Am J Ophthalmol 1979; 88:736.

21. Jones FL, Eckberg NL: Exacerbation of asthma by timolol. N Engl J Med 1979; 301:270.

22. Shavitz SA: Timolol and myasthenia gravis. JAMA 1979; 242:1612.

23. Olson RJ, Bromberg BB, Zimmerman TJ: Apneic spells associated with timolol therapy in a neonate. Am J Ophthalmol 1979; 88:120.

24. Bailey PL: Timolol and postoperative apnea in neonates and young infants. Anesthesiology 1979; 51:S16.

25. Babinski M, Smith RB, Wickerham EP: Hypotension and bradycardia following intraocular acetylcholine injection. Arch Ophthalmol 1976; 94:675.

26. Rasch D, Holt J, Wilson M, et al: Bronchospasm

following intraocular injection of acetylcholine in a patient taking metoprolol. Anesthesiology 1983; 59:583.

27. Fineberg E, Machemer R, Sullivan P, et al: Sulfur hexafluoride in owl monkey vitreous cavity. Am J Ophthalmol 1975; 79:67–74.

28. Stinson TW, Donlon JV: Interaction of SF_6 and air with nitrous oxide. Anesthesiology 1979; 51:S16.

29. Wolf GL, Capriano C, Hartung J: Effects of nitrous oxide on gas bubble volume in the anterior chamber. Arch Ophthalmol 1985; 103:418.

30. Peyman GA, Vygantas CM, Bennett TO, et al: Octafluorocyclobutane in vitreous and aqueous humor replacement. Arch Ophthalmol 1975; 93:514–517.

31. Chang S, Coleman DJ, Lincoff H, et al: Perfluoropropane gas in the management of proliferative vitreoretinopathy. Am J Ophthalmol 1984; 98:180–188.

32. Chang S, Lincoff HA, Coleman DJ, et al: Perfluorocarbon gases in vitreous surgery. Ophthalmology 1985; 92:651–656.

33. Podos SM, Serle JB: Topically active carbonic anhydrase inhibitors for glaucoma. Arch Ophthalmol 1991; 109:38–40.

34. Lippa EA, Aasved H, Airaksinen PJ, et al: Multiple-dose, dose-response relationship for the topical carbonic anhydrase inhibitor MK-927. Arch Ophthalmol 1991; 109:46–49.

35. Novotny HR, Alvis DL: A method of photographing fluorescence in circulating blood in human retina. Circulation 1961; 24:82.

36. Acheson R, Serjeant G: Painful crises in sickle cell disease after fluorescein angiography. Lancet 1985; 1:1222.

37. Chazan BI, Balodimos MC, Koncz L: Untoward effects of fluorescein retinal angiography in diabetic patients. Ann Ophthalmol 1971; 3:42–49.

38. Gombos GM, Schechter BA, Gombos DS: Evaluation of the use of fluorescein angiography in clinical ophthalmology. Res Staff Physician 1987; 33:100–107.

39. Butner RW, McPherson AR: Adverse reactions in intravenous fluorescein angiography. Ann Ophthalmol 1983; 15:1084–1086.

40. Cunningham EE, Balu V: Cardiac arrest following fluorescein angiography. JAMA 1979; 242:2431.

41. Amalric P, Bian C, Fenies MT: Incidents et accidents au cours de l'angiographic fluoresceinique. Bull Soc Ophthalmol Fr 1968; 68:968–972.

42. Heffner JE: Reactions to fluorescein. JAMA 1980; 243:2029–2030.

43. Yannuzzi LA, Rohrer KT, Tindel LJ, et al: Fluorescein angiography complication survey. Ophthalmology 1986; 93:611–617.

44. LaPiana FG, Penner R: Anaphylactoid reaction to intravenously administered fluorescein. Arch Ophthalmol 1968; 79:161–162.

45. Tizes R: Cardiac arrest following routine venipuncture. JAMA 1976; 236:1846–1847.

46. Jacob JSH, Rosen ES, Young E: Report on the presence of a toxic substance, dimethyl formamide, in sodium fluorescein used for fluorescein angiography. Br J Ophthalmol 1982; 66:567–568.

47. Wesley RE, Blout WC, Arteberry JF: Acute myocardial infarction after fluorescein angiography. Am J Ophthalmol 1979; 87:834–835.

48. Wilensky JR, Woodward HJ: Acute systemic hypertension after conjunctival instillation of phenylephrine hydrochloride. Am J Ophthalmol 1973; 76:156–157.

49. Wallace JD, Weintraub M, Mattson RH, et al: Status epilepticus as a complication of intrathecal fluorescein. J Neurosurg 1972; 36:659–660.

50. Madowitz JS, Schweiger MJ: Severe anaphylactoid reaction to radiographic contrast media. JAMA 1979; 241:2813–2815.

18

Selection of Techniques for Regional Blockade of the Eye and Adnexa

Kenneth Zahl

This chapter briefly reviews the important anatomy of the ocular and adnexal structures and the various approaches and rationale for regional blockade of the eye. A more detailed consideration of this topic can be found elsewhere.[1]

The terminology used for retrobulbar anesthesia has been confusing since the introduction of *peribulbar* blocking techniques by Kellman, Davis, Mandel, and others. Many have used the term *retrobulbar anesthesia* to include all aspects of regional blockade of the orbit and the eyelids. Retrobulbar anesthesia as described by Atkinson[2] is conventionally thought to mean the injection of anesthetic behind the eye into the muscle cone formed by the extraocular muscles (from the Greek origins of the roots *retros* = behind and *bulbos* = eye). Peribulbar anesthesia has conventionally been used for extraconal injections around the eye but not intentionally into the cone. However, peribulbar anesthesia could be used in place of retrobulbar block, because the retrobulbar injection is given around the eye. To avoid further confusion, the terms retrobulbar and intraconal block are used interchangeably, and periconal block is used instead of peribulbar block.

Perhaps owing to the increased popularity of the periconal block with its inherent safety and ease of learning, more anesthesiologists have learned, or are interested in learning, regional anesthesia techniques, which previously had been the traditional domain of the ophthalmologist. In the last decade there was a controversy over the safety of general endotracheal anesthesia versus regional anesthesia for cataract surgery.[3] However, with the proliferation of extracapsular cataract surgery with intraocular lens implant (over 1 million procedures annually in the United States), the advanced age of the population, and the shift to ambulatory surgery, regional anesthesia is the anesthetic technique of choice most often used for outpatient cataract surgery.

Regional anesthesia of the eye should be approached with caution because of life- or sight-threatening complications. However, anesthesiologists in many hospitals and ambulatory surgery centers where large numbers of cataract operations are performed have completed regional blocks with an equally low, or even lower, incidence of complications compared with other ophthalmologists. In the setting of a busy outpatient ophthalmic surgical suite, case turnover time is greatly decreased by performing an eye block in advance of surgery, which is another reason for the increased demand for anesthesiologists to learn regional techniques of eye blocks.

HISTORICAL CONSIDERATIONS

The history of local anesthesia begins in the field of ophthalomology. Karl Koller, while working with Sigmund Freud, introduced the use of cocaine as a topical anesthetic for minor surgery of the conjunctiva in 1884. Later that year, Knapp probably performed the first regional anesthetic block when he described an intraconal injection of cocaine.[4] Retrobulbar anesthesia with cocaine fell into disrepute later, probably owing to toxic, and often fatal, reactions to the cocaine. By the early 1900s, procaine replaced cocaine for retrobulbar block. Atkinson introduced epinephrine to prolong anesthetic action and later hyaluronidase to promote easier spread of local anesthesia around the eye. He is also credited with describing the classic approach for the retrobulbar block.[3] In 1948 Lofgren synthesized lidocaine, which was widely used until bupivacaine was introduced in the mid-1970s.

ANATOMICAL CONSIDERATIONS

The orbits are pyramidal structures formed by the fusion of many bones of the skull. The orbital rim is composed of three bones: the zygomatic laterally, the maxillary inferomedially, and the frontal bone superiorly. Although there are nine bony openings in the orbit, only several are important for this discussion. The optic canal transmits the optic nerve and artery along with the sympathetic fibers from the internal carotid plexus. The superior orbital fissure lies between the lesser and greater wings of the sphenoid bone. The annulus of Zinn is a fibrous ring that arises from the fissure and forms the apex of the muscle cone (Fig. 18–1). The extraocular muscles, with the exception of the levator and superior oblique muscles, originate from the annulus. The trochlear nerve (cranial nerve IV) and the frontal and lacrimal branches of the first division of the trigeminal (cranial nerve V) nerve exit through the fissure superior to the annulus. The oculomotor (cranial nerve III) and the abducens (cranial nerve IV) nerves enter the muscle cone through the annulus. The superior orbital notch (or foramen in some) transmits the supraorbital nerve and vessels. It is an easily palpable landmark on the superomedial portion of the orbital rim and is used as a guide for the periconal block or block of the superior oblique muscle.

The pyramidal or conical form of the orbit has an approximate volume of 30 mL (Fig. 18–2). Depending on the compliance and speed of injection, 8–10 mL of anesthetic may be given in a periconal fashion. The ciliary ganglion (Fig. 18–3) is usually located 10 mm from

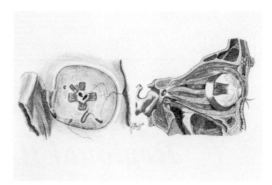

FIGURE 18–1. *The annulus of Zinn arises from the superior orbital fissure and gives rise to the extraocular muscles that form the muscle cone (left illustration). The drawing on the right shows the muscle cone with the lateral rectus divided and the optic nerve (in yellow) within the cone. The optic nerve is in its most relaxed position with eyelid closed. (From Galindo A, Keilson LR, Mondshine RB, Sawelson, HI: Retro-peribulbar anesthesia. In Zahl K, Meltzer MA (eds): Regional Anesthesia for Intraocular Surgery. Ophthalmol Clin North Am 1990; 3:74.)*

the orbital apex and just medial to the lateral rectus muscle. It receives three types of fibers: sensory from the cornea, iris, and ciliary body; short motor divisions of the parasympathetic division to the iris; and sympathetic nerves to the ciliary ganglion (responsible for pupillodilatation). It was once assumed that the muscle cone had to be penetrated to achieve ocular anesthesia (through ciliary ganglion block) and akinesia (through oculomotor and abducens

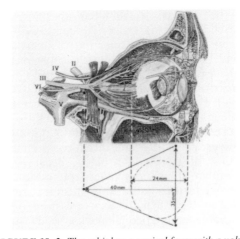

FIGURE 18–2. *The orbit has a conical form with a volume of approximately 30 mL. The average globe has an approximate diameter of 24–25 mm. The average distance from the orbital rim to the apex of the orbit is approximately 40 mm. (From Galindo A, Keilson LR, Mondshine RB, Sawelson, HI: Retro-peribulbar anesthesia. In Zahl K, Meltzer MA (eds): Regional Anesthesia for Intraocular Surgery. Ophthalmol Clin North Am 1990; 3:74.)*

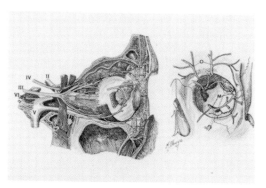

FIGURE 18–3. Nerves in the orbit, including the ciliary ganglions, short and long ciliary nerves. Also included is the final segment of the ophthalmic artery in the upper middle quadrant. The terminal branches of the sensory nerves (ophthalmic O and maxillary M) are represented on the right. (From Galindo A, Keilson LR, Mondshine RB, Sawelson, HI: Retro-peribulbar anesthesia. In Zahl K, Meltzer MA (eds): Regional Anesthesia for Intraocular Surgery. Ophthalmol Clin North Am 1990; 3:74.)

nerve block) of the eye. This was believed to be the anatomical mechanism for the retrobulbar block. Tenon's fascia was once thought to extend from the globe to the muscle cone down to the apex to form a "watertight seal" around the extraocular muscles. Work by Leo Koorneef, a Dutch ophthalmologist, performed while he was a medical student may be used to refute this classic theory.[5] Through careful anatomical, sequential cross section of the eye, he showed that the muscle cone becomes porous at its apex and is often permeated with fat (Fig. 18–4). This probably allows for the

transfer of local anesthetic, and avoidance of intraconal injection, with the periconal technique when sufficient (usually more than 8 mL) volumes are used. In a more recent study, intraconal spread of contrast dye was demonstrated with a simulated periconal blocking technique.[6] The porous nature of the muscle cone also allows for the avoidance of an upper lid block if sufficient volumes of anesthetic are given in the retrobulbar space, as in the Gills-Loyd technique (see intraconal blocks).

The extraocular muscles, except for the superior oblique, originate from the apex of the orbit. All of the four rectus muscles arise from the annulus of Zinn and are innervated in their posterior third on the intraconal surface. The oculomotor nerve innervates the medial, superior, and inferior rectus muscles in addition to the levator palpebrae superioris and the inferior oblique. The abducens nerve innervates the lateral rectus muscle. The superior oblique and levator muscles arise from a point superior and medial to the annulus. The superior oblique is innervated by the fourth, or trochlear, nerve that enters the orbit from without the annulus of Zinn. Often, this muscle continues to function with a conventional retrobulbar injection (with a low volume). This may be diagnosed by unopposed intortion of the eye.

The optic nerve, or cranial nerve II, is often thought of as an extension of the brain and not a true cranial sensory nerve (Fig. 18–5). It is approximately 50 mm in length and somewhat coiled, which allows for free movement of the globe and for mild proptosis (which

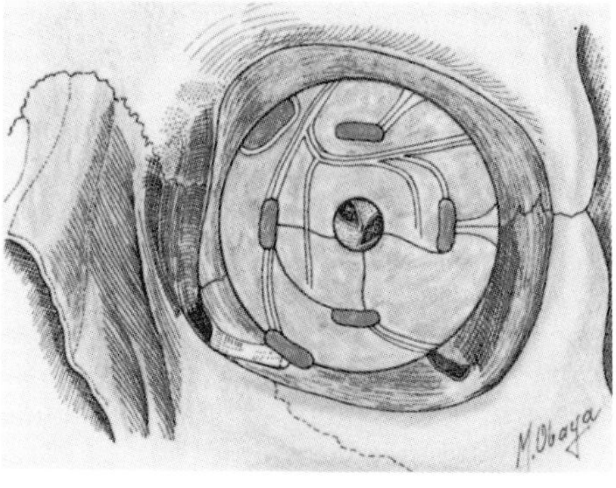

FIGURE 18–4. Schematic representation of the muscles, aponeurosis, and fat at a plane midway between the eye and the tendon of Zinn; the muscle interconnections are porous and loose, allowing easy transfer of fluids between the retro- and peribulbar spaces. (From Galindo A, Keilson LR, Mondshine RB, Sawelson, HI: Retro-peribulbar anesthesia. In Zahl K, Meltzer MA (eds): Regional Anesthesia for Intraocular Surgery. Ophthalmol Clin North Am 1990; 3:74.)

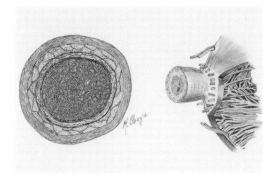

FIGURE 18–5. Optic nerve surrounded by its subarachnoid space, with the central retinal vessels within the nerve fibers. To the right is a schematic representation of the nerve as it enters the posterior pole of the eye with the ciliary nerves, and short arteries and veins. (From Galindo A, Keilson LR, Mondshine RB, Sawelson, HI: Retro-peribulbar anesthesia. In Zahl K, Meltzer MA (eds): Regional Anesthesia for Intraocular Surgery. Ophthalmol Clin North Am 1990; 3:75.)

occurs after intraconal injection). The nerve picks up a pial, arachnoidal, and dural covering while in the optic canal. The dura is fused anteriorly with the sclera and posteriorly with the periorbita in the optic foramen. Cerebrospinal fluid flows within the dura surrounding the nerve to the midbrain; there is a small margin for aberrant needle placement, which explains the complications, such as brain-stem anesthesia, with intraconal block. The anatomy of the eyelids and their innervation are covered in the section on blockade of the orbicularis oculi.

CHOICE OF LOCAL ANESTHETIC

When choosing a local anesthetic, considerations of speed of onset, efficacy, and appropriate duration for surgery and postoperative analgesia have to be considered. Repeated injections, because of a failed block, increase the risk of complications from regional blocks and should be minimized with retrobulbar or periconal anesthesia.

Myoneural toxicity has been described after direct intramuscular injection of the extraocular muscles with bupivacaine, but this is rare. In general, with the volumes and drug concentrations involved, classic systemic toxicity from elevated plasma levels of the local anesthetic is unusual unless an intravascular injection occurs or excessive quantities of local anesthetic are used for a facial nerve block.

Because no drug possesses the ideal properties of both short onset and long duration, a mixture of a short-onset drug (such as lidocaine or mepivacaine) is usually used with a long-duration anesthetic (such as bupivacaine or etidocaine).[7] Local anesthetics are supplied as the hydrochloride salt and are often pH-adjusted toward neutrality to improve onset time.[8] Whereas the active form of the local anesthetic is probably a cation, the anion more readily diffuses across the neural membrane; pH-adjustment increases the concentration of anion and theoretically promotes faster diffusion across the membrane. Studies have demonstrated improved onset time for periconal block when pH-adjusted mixtures of lidocaine/bupivacaine[9] or plain 0.75% bupivacaine[10] are used. Sodium bicarbonate (0.05 mEq) can be added to 10 mL of 0.75% bupivacaine with hyaluronidase 15 units/mL to markedly decrease the onset time and improve efficacy with the first series of injections.[10]

Other adjuvants are commonly used in ophthalmic anesthesia. Hyaluronidase depolymerizes hyaluronic acid, which is prevalent in the connective tissues and decreases the onset time of some nerve blocks. In contrast to other regional blocks (e.g., epidural, peripheral) hyaluronidase helps decrease onset time in retrobulbar anesthesia when used with a mixture of lidocaine and bupivacaine.[11] Many surgeons prefer to use epinephrine-containing solutions of local anesthetics, which may anecdotally decrease the incidence of expulsive choroidal hemorrhage during cataract surgery. Because epinephrine oxidizes lidocaine, these solutions are often marketed with an even lower pH to prolong shelf life, which results in increased onset time.[12] Freshly added epinephrine does not prolong the onset time of pH-adjusted mixtures of lidocaine/bupivacaine.[12] Epinephrine does not extend the duration of local anesthetics, such as bupivacaine, and is not useful for anesthesia *per se.* Therefore, if the surgeon wishes to have epinephrine used, it should be added to the solution just prior to use in a concentration of 5 μg/mL.[12] Warming of local anesthetics to body temperature makes the injection less painful[13] and possibly decreases onset time by promoting faster diffusion.

RETROBULBAR OR INTRACONAL BLOCK

Retrobulbar anesthesia is commonly performed with a blunt 25-gauge needle from the inferotemporal quadrant of the orbit.[2] In the Atkinson method, the patient is instructed to look up and toward the patient's nose. This maneuver theoretically frees the inferior oblique from the course of the needle, but probably does nothing more than hide the needle from the patient. It also places the optic nerve at risk for trauma or a subarachnoid injection. After estimating when to redirect the needle behind the globe, the needle is inserted into the muscle cone (Fig. 18–6). The globe is approximately 25 mm in diameter; therefore, the needle should not be directed behind the globe until this depth has been reached from the most anterior surface of the cornea.

COMPLICATIONS

The classic Atkinson method is no longer widely advocated because of the complications

FIGURE 18–6. *Retrobulbar injection as seen from the lateral approach. The needle is shown entering the lateral rectus muscle of the right eye.*

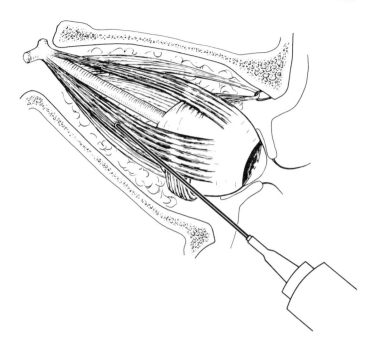

associated from optic nerve penetration. Discussed in greater detail elsewhere in this text, these complications can be classified either as life-threatening, such as respiratory arrest, or as sight-threatening, such as blindness or visual impairment. Respiratory arrest probably occurs from direct spread of local anesthesia[14] to the midbrain and the resultant development of brain-stem anesthesia.[15] Optic nerve damage from direct injection into the nerve has been described.[16]

Retrobulbar hemorrhage, a devastating complication, occurs as often as 1–3% of the time after retrobulbar injection.[17] Retrobulbar hemorrhage is diagnosed by proptosis (with hardness of the globe), chemosis, and the eventual appearance of subconjunctival blood. The suspicion or occurrence of a retrobulbar hemorrhage requires immediate consultation with the patient's ophthalmologist. Intraocular pressure (IOP) becomes elevated with a significant bleed and should be monitored with Schiøtz's tonometer. Central retinal artery pulsations should be followed to rule out the occurrence of a retinal artery occlusion. If absence of flow occurs, a lateral canthotomy should be performed to decompress the orbital pressure.[18] Occasionally, paracentesis of the anterior chamber should be performed to lower IOP if canthotomy does not achieve this. Surgery should be postponed and rescheduled, preferably under general endotracheal anesthesia. As the blood extravasates from the cone, an oculocardiac reflex may occur several

hours later. Consequently, the patient should be monitored for several hours after the hemorrhage. The mechanism for retrobulbar hemorrhage is probably either puncture of the ophthalmic artery or a short ciliary artery. Retrobulbar hemorrhage has not been reported as a complication of the periconal block.

Brain-stem anesthesia probably results from an optic sheath injection.[13] Symptoms include contralateral ophthalmoplegia, ptosis, mydriasis, and even amaurosis; agitation; dysphagia; and respiratory or cardiac arrest. In a prospective study of 6000 patients, Nicoll and colleagues[19] reported that 16 patients developed signs and symptoms of brain-stem anesthesia after retrobulbar block, with eight patients developing a respiratory arrest.

Research in the past decade has suggested that the position of the eye should be modified during retrobulbar injection. Unsold and associates[20] found that the eye was most at risk for optic nerve or ophthalmic artery trauma when in the upward and nasal gaze (Atkinson) position. This study was carried out using computed tomography (CT) scanning of cadavers. The authors recommended performing the injection either in primary gaze or with the eye slightly downward and outward after demonstrating that these positions move the optic nerve sheath farther away from the path of the needle. In Nicoll's study, the incidence of complications was equivalent whether the injection was performed with the eye in the classic Atkinson position or in the neutral gaze.[19]

Atkinson recommended using a blunt needle, but there are no more than anecdotal data and theoretical considerations to justify the blunt instead of the sharp needle. Galindo has introduced a pinpoint needle (Pinpoint Ophthalmica®) that has a dull point that does not cut the tissue.[21] The needle port is on the side of the needle and not at the tip. In his initial study of over 5000 injections with the needle, there have been no serious complications reported. Straus has advocated the use of a curved needle for retrobulbar injection, but there is no large-scale study evaluating the safety of this needle.[22]

Another concern is the length of the standard Atkinson needle, which is 38 mm (1.5 in) and considered too long for the depth of some orbits. In a study of 60 skulls, Katsev and coworkers[23] measured the distance from the inferolateral orbital rim to the optic foramen. The distance ranged from 42–54 mm. Taking into account the size of the optic nerve, the authors concluded that the standard 38-mm needle could perforate the optic nerve where it is fixed exiting the foramen in 11% of the population. Based upon this information, shorter needles of 31 mm (1.25 in) or less should be used for retrobulbar or periconal anesthesia. Because of the high incidence of complications associated with the Atkinson retrobulbar blocking technique,[24] other techniques for regional blockade of the eye have been suggested, such as the Gills-Loyd and periconal blocks.

GILLS-LOYD BLOCK

Gills and Loyd were among the first to modify the retrobulbar block and eliminate the need for a separate facial nerve block with a new approach to the retrobulbar block.[25] They also advocated a transconjunctival approach. The first injection is performed with 1% lidocaine (pH-adjusted with 1 mEq of bicarbonate per 10 mL to decrease onset time and discomfort) and a 27-gauge needle (Fig. 18–7). The lower lid is retracted, and a topical anesthetic is given. To further eliminate discomfort and stinging from the eye drops, a dilute solution of proparacaine (made by adding 1 mL to 15 mL of balanced salt solution) can be used, which is followed with two drops of the full-strength solution. The needle is then inserted through the conjunctiva perpendicular to the face at a point directly below the lateral margin

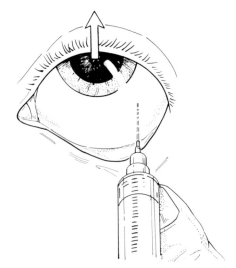

FIGURE 18–7. *The retrobulbar injection is directed in line with the lateral limbal margin with the eye looking upward but not upward and nasally. (Redrawn from Gills JP, Loyd TL: A technique of retrobulbar block with paralysis of orbicularis oculi. Am Intra-ocular Implant Soc J 1983; 9:339.)*

of the limbus. An injection of 3–4 mL is given, and light pressure is applied. This periconal injection blocks the lower lid and the area around the cone.

After 5 minutes, a retrobulbar injection is performed using the same initial approach. A 25-gauge needle is passed deeper along the previous path and redirected into the cone while the patient looks upward (Fig. 18–8). Generally, patients do not complain about, or even notice, the second injection. The patient is asked to look up so any scleral penetration/perforation, which would theoretically pull the eye down, can be detected. Gills believes that by avoiding the inferior temporal approach, the anesthesiologist is less likely to perforate the optic nerve anatomically and, thus, reduce the attendant risks of brain-stem anesthesia or optic nerve trauma.

For the second (intraconal) injection, either 0.5 or 0.75% of pH-adjusted bupivacaine is used (at least 5 mL). Ptosis of the upper lid ensues from block of the levator palpebrae superioris and diffusion of local anesthetic out of the cone. The patient may still have some element of blepharospasm, or squeezing, because the upper lid is not blocked. However, many surgeons can perform an extracapsular cataract extraction rapidly, so this usually is not a problem. Alternatively, a limited van Lint block can be performed to selectively

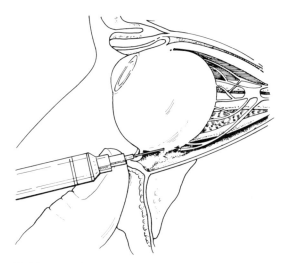

FIGURE 18–8. *Transconjunctival injection is tangential to the globe. The slightest scleral contact will cause the eye to turn downward. Puncture of the globe is less likely than with a transcutaneous injection. (Redrawn from Gills JP, Loyd TL: A technique of retrobulbar block with paralysis of orbicularis oculi. Am Intra-ocular Implant Soc J 1983; 9:340.)*

block the upper lid. Kimbrough and colleagues[26] advocate infiltration of the lower lid as the needle is withdrawn from the cone with a 98% success rate for eyelid paresis.

Postoperative analgesia frequently lasts up to 24 hours and occasionally longer owing to the use of bupivacaine. Facial nerve block is obviated with attendant discomfort during the intraconal injection. Increased dosage of local anesthetic and postoperative paresis of the seventh nerve is avoided also. The block may be performed with little or no sedation and has been proven to be useful and safe. Gills reports no respiratory arrests in over 25,000 injections (personal communication). Retrobulbar hemorrhage is still a concern, however. The techniques for eyelid blocks are reviewed before consideration of periconal anesthesia.

BLOCKADE OF THE ORBICULARIS OCULI

The eyelids are closed by contraction of the orbicularis oculi muscles. As with all other muscles of facial animation, these muscles derive their innervation from cranial nerve VII (the facial nerve). The upper lid is innervated by the temporal branch of the facial nerve, whereas the zygomatic branch supplies the lower lid. In addition to contraction of the orbicularis oculi, contraction of the frontalis

muscle also contributes to eyelid closure; this is demonstrated by looking into a mirror and closing one eye with an index finger placed over the ipsilateral portion of the frontalis muscle. During forceful eyelid closure, contraction of the frontalis muscle is recognized. Akinesia of the eyelids is a necessary anesthetic condition for successful intraocular surgery.[2] Forced closure, or squeezing, of the eyelids may result in increased IOP, which in turn may make surgery difficult and may cause complications such as vitreous loss.

A conventional retrobulbar block (i.e., with 2–4 mL of anesthetic) does not cause paresis of the eyelids, but usually only results in ptosis of the upper lid by paresis of levator palpebrae superioris. However, this alone is an insufficient anesthetic for intraocular surgery. The levator palpebrae derives its innervation from a branch of the oculomotor nerve (cranial nerve III). Blockade of the levator palpebrae does not prevent blepharospasm mediated through contraction of the orbicularis oculi. Owing to the incomplete nature of the muscle cone,[5] especially at the apex, injection of larger volumes of local anesthetic in the retrobulbar space may result in some lid paresis by diffusion of anesthetic into the adnexal areas of the orbit. However, this usually does not allow for more than the performance of brief, superficial corneal surgery.

Van Lint was the first to describe a technique for akinesia of the orbicularis oculi in 1914.[27] Since then, many ophthalmologists have described other techniques for facial nerve blockade.[28–31] Blocking techniques other than the method described by van Lint are performed at more proximal positions along the path of cranial nerve VII and its branches. The Gills-Loyd and periconal blocking techniques obviate the need for separate facial nerve blocks. These latter techniques result in paresis of the eyelids. The mechanism is probably mediated by diffusion of local anesthetic into the eyelids.

VAN LINT'S METHOD

Although Knapp described a retrobulbar injection in 1884, van Lint was the first to describe a technique for temporary akinesia of the orbicularis 30 years later. In the original communication,[27] van Lint observed that it was preferable to make the injection closer to the orbital rim. In this manner, paresis of the terminal branches of the facial nerve would lead to localized akinesia of the orbicularis. In the same article, he pointed out that the injection might be made around the trunk of the nerve, but that this would cause an undesirable paresis of all the branches of the facial nerve. This observation formed the basis for the remainder of the blocking techniques described in this chapter.

In the original communication, the technique described is simple (Fig. 18–9). The needle is introduced 1 cm posterior to the intersection of a horizontal line drawn from the inferior margin of the orbit and a vertical line from the most temporal aspect of the lateral margin of the orbit. The needle is directed toward the bone and deep to the orbicularis muscles. The injections are made as the needle is withdrawn. A 1.5 or 2 in 25-gauge needle is recommended.

There have been modifications of the van Lint block, when anesthetic is directly injected into the eyelids. This technique should be avoided, because it is both painful and may result in bleeding into the lids, which makes opening of the eyelids and insertion of the lid speculum difficult. Others have modified the van Lint technique to inject anesthetic approximately 1 cm away from the lateral orbital rim (see Fig. 18–9). The first injection is made with the needle directed perpendicular to the skull and on the periosteum. The needle is then directed subcutaneously, but directly over the periosteum, in a caudad and cephalad fashion. This modification avoids eyelid edema or bleeding into the lids.

One advantage of the van Lint block is a low risk of a toxic reaction. Paresis is localized to the orbicularis oculi, and blockade of other facial muscles is avoided. The van Lint block is relatively easy to perform and has a high success rate. Disadvantages include pain on injection, eyelid edema, bleeding, and bruising.

O'BRIEN'S METHOD

O'Brien described a method of facial nerve block in 1929.[28] The key landmarks and techniques for the block are described and shown in Figures 18–10 through 18–12. Probably the only advantage of this block is a low risk of an intravascular injection. The principal disadvantage is an incomplete or failed block owing to variations in the course of the upper and lower zygomatic branches of the facial nerve, or ramus communicans from inferior (mandibular and buccal) branches of the facial nerve.

To improve the success rate, Spaeth[29] has advocated a modification of this block. An

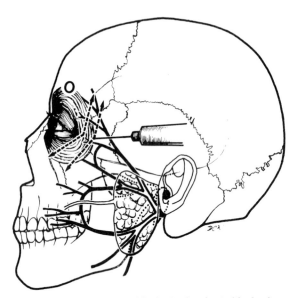

FIGURE 18–9. *van Lint block. In the classic block, the initial injection site begins near the lateral orbital rim. After a skin wheal, the needle is directed perpendicular to contact the periosteum. It is then redirected deep to the lower orbicularis oculi. Anesthetic is injected upon withdrawal of the needle. The needle is redirected cephalad to complete a "V." In the modified van Lint block, the first injection is made approximately 1 cm lateral to the orbital rim. The needle is made to contact the periosteum, and 1 mL of anesthetic is injected. The needle is directed cephalad and caudad in a "V" over the periosteum. Anesthetic may be injected as the needle is advanced or withdrawn. (O, orbicularis ocularis muscle) (From Zahl K: Blockade of the orbicularis oculi. In Zahl K, Meltzer MA (eds): Regional Anesthesia for Intraocular Surgery. Ophthalmol Clin North Am 1990; 3:94.)*

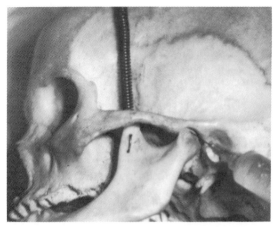

FIGURE 18–10. *O'Brien block. This photograph shows the relationship of the mandibular ramus to the posterior zygomatic process and external auditory meatus. (From Zahl K: Blockade of the orbicularis oculi. In Zahl K, Meltzer MA (eds): Regional Anesthesia for Intraocular Surgery. Ophthalmol Clin North Am 1990; 3:94.)*

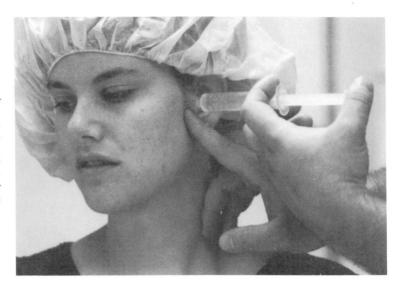

FIGURE 18–11. *O'Brien block. This demonstrates palpation of the condyle of the temporomandibular joint with the index finger anterior to the tragus. The initial injection is given over the posterior zygomatic process and not in the joint capsule. Spaeth recommends redirection of the needle toward the lateral canthus and infiltration of further anesthetic to block lower communicating branches of the seventh nerve. (From Zahl K: Blockade of the orbicularis oculi. In Zahl K, Meltzer MA (eds): Regional Anesthesia for Intraocular Surgery. Ophthalmol Clin North Am 1990; 3:95.)*

additional 5 mL of anesthetic is given after the needle is redirected toward the lateral canthus. Alternatively, larger volumes of anesthetic (i.e., 6–8 mL) than recommended by O'Brien may be given by injecting it as the needle is inserted. This may improve the success rate by promoting better spread of the anesthetic. Facial nerve paralysis has been reported as a complication of the Spaeth modification of the O'Brien block.

ATKINSON'S METHOD

The Atkinson method involves infiltration of a line of anesthetic over the zygomatic arch (Figs. 18–13 through 18–15).[30] The rationale is that all branches of the facial nerve should cross over the arch on the way to the orbicularis. However, in the author's experience, this block is associated with the highest failure rate,

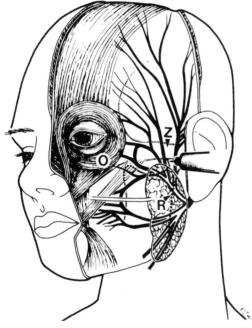

FIGURE 18–12. *O'Brien block. This illustration shows the bony features and course of the facial nerve over the mandibular ramus in relation to the face. (O, orbicularis ocularis; Z, zygomatic process; R, mandibular ramus) (From Zahl K: Blockade of the orbicularis oculi. In Zahl K, Meltzer MA (eds): Regional Anesthesia for Intraocular Surgery. Ophthalmol Clin North Am 1990; 3:95.)*

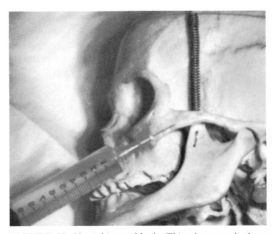

FIGURE 18–13. *Atkinson block. This photograph shows the relationship of the zygomatic arch to the orbit. The needle is positioned in the direction of the injection. (From Zahl K: Blockade of the orbicularis oculi. In Zahl K, Meltzer MA (eds): Regional Anesthesia for Intraocular Surgery. Ophthalmol Clin North Am 1990; 3:96.)*

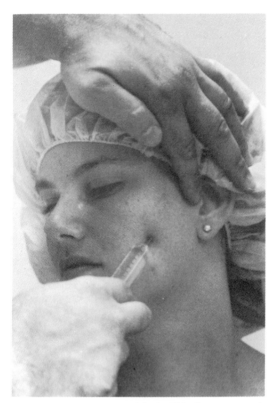

FIGURE 18–14. Atkinson block. This demonstrates the initial injection site for the Atkinson block. The needle is inserted at the inferior portion of the zygomatic arch (usually below the lateral margin of the orbital rim). Anesthetic is injected (5–10 mL) along the arch as the needle is advanced. (From Zahl K: Blockade of the orbicularis oculi. In Zahl K, Meltzer MA (eds): Regional Anesthesia for Intraocular Surgery. Ophthalmol Clin North Am 1990; 3:96.)

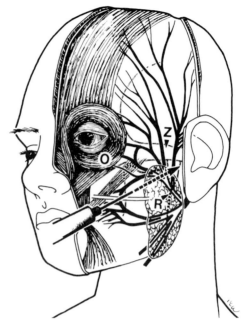

FIGURE 18–15. Atkinson block. This illustration shows the landmarks of the zygomatic arch and orbit, branches of the facial nerve in relation to the face. (O, orbicularis ocularis; Z, zygomatic process; R, mandibular ramus) (From Zahl K, Meltzer MA (eds): Regional Anesthesia for Intraocular Surgery. Ophthalmol Clin North Am 1990; 3:97.)

possibly owing to variations in the course of cranial nerve VII. Postoperative ecchymosis is the other major complication observed. Nevertheless, because this injection also occurs in a relatively safe area in terms of major blood vessels and nerves, toxic reactions should not occur.

NADBATH'S AND REHMAN'S METHOD

Nadbath's and Rehman's method, described in 1963, is the only block that also results in complete hemifacial akinesia, because the injection is performed over the main trunk of the facial nerve.[31] The details of the block are described in Figures 18–16 through 18–18. Because of the close proximity of the injection site to major cranial nerves, such as the vagus, glossopharyngeal, and spinal accessory nerves, complications such as hoarseness, dysphagia,

pooling of secretions, laryngospasm, respiratory distress, and agitation have been described.[32, 33] Complete facial paresis is undesirable in the outpatient setting owing to its misinterpretation as a stroke by family members and the public. In addition, it interferes with food intake and drinking. Long-acting drugs, such as bupivacaine, should be avoided with this block.

SUMMARY OF SEVENTH NERVE BLOCKS

Seventh nerve blocks may be as painful as the retrobulbar block. Because of the complications described earlier, alternate techniques, such as the Gills-Loyd and periconal blocks, are more desirable. Nevertheless, a sound foundation of the anatomy and how to perform these blocks is required if supplementation of these blocks are needed or if retrobulbar anesthesia is preferred.

PERICONAL BLOCK

Davis and Mandel reported and advocated a "peribulbar" or periconal blocking technique

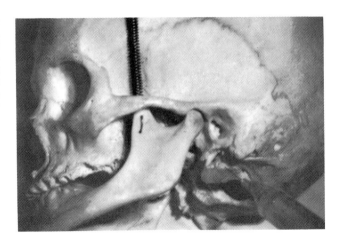

FIGURE 18–16. Nadbath-Rehman block. This photograph shows the relationship of the stylomastoid foramen (located between the mastoid process and stylus) and the external auditory meatus. The needle is positioned in an anterocephalad direction in order to avoid penetration of the jugular foramen. (From Zahl K: Blockade of the orbicularis oculi. In Zahl K, Meltzer MA (eds): Regional Anesthesia for Intraocular Surgery. Ophthalmol Clin North Am 1990; 3:97.)

in 1986.[34] Figures 18–19 and 18–20 illustrate and describe how to perform this block. Periconal blocking is the other end of the spectrum from the retrobulbar block, because the Gills-Loyd block is essentially one half of a periconal block and one half retrobulbar. The muscle cone is never entered. Davis and Mandel have abandoned their two separate, superficial initial lid injections described in their original article and now perform the periconal block, because the anesthetic tends to diffuse back to the lids in any case. The author has modified

their original protocol. For the first injection, 4–5 mL of anesthetic is injected at the inferotemporal position after a slight cephaloposterior trajectory. For the second injection, 4–5 mL of local anesthetic is injected at the superonasal position just below and medial to the supratrochlear notch. A 25-gauge, 1.25 in needle is used and directed just beyond the equator of the globe. During the block, local anesthesia extravasates into the lids to give a *de facto* van Lint block.

Other modifications of the original protocol

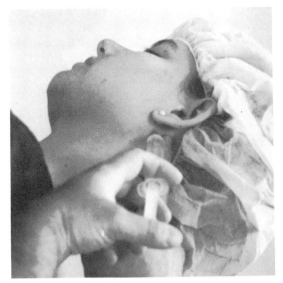

FIGURE 18–17. Nadbath-Rehman block. This photograph demonstrates the injection technique. The index finger rests on the mastoid process, and the needle is inserted between the mastoid process and the posterior border of the mandibular ramus. The needle is advanced in an anterocephalad direction. (From Zahl K: Blockade of the orbicularis oculi. In Zahl K, Meltzer MA (eds): Regional Anesthesia for Intraocular Surgery. Ophthalmol Clin North Am 1990; 3:98.)

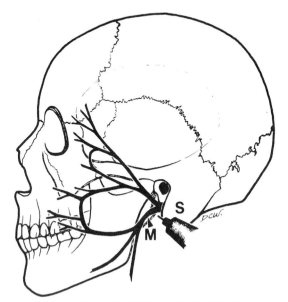

FIGURE 18–18. Nadbath-Rehman block. This illustration demonstrates the exit of the facial nerve from the stylomastoid foramen posterior to the ear. (M, mandibular ramus; S, styloid process) (From Zahl K: Blockade of the orbicularis oculi. In Zahl K, Meltzer MA (eds): Regional Anesthesia for Intraocular Surgery. Ophthalmol Clin North Am 1990; 3:98.)

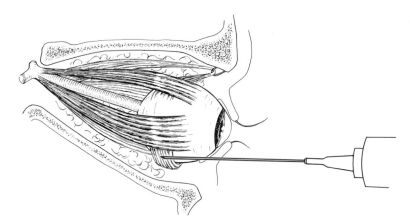

FIGURE 18–19. *Inferotemporal injection with the lateral portions of the right eye removed. The needle does not enter the muscle cone.*

are possible. Pannu of Fort Lauderdale, Florida has described a single injection periconal block with a 25-gauge, 0.5 in needle at the superonasal position (personal communication). With the needle directed to the orbital roof, 10 mL of local anesthetic is slowly injected in a cephaloposterior direction. Davis and Mandel are in the process of evaluating an inferotemporal and inferonasal injection after they discovered some cases of prolonged ptosis of the upper lid (personal communication).

Periconal anesthesia is a safe blocking technique that, to date, has resulted in no life-threatening complications known to Davis, Mandel, or the author. Globe perforation has been reported. The globe should always be displaced away from the needle, especially after the first injection. Significant peribulbar hemorrhage has occurred on three occasions (in approximately 3000 injections) in the author's experience. However, in no case was there a retrobulbar spread, and surgery was not cancelled. Hamilton and associates[35] have reported 5714 peribulbar blocks without brainstem anesthesia or respiratory arrests. The

author has taught a number of anesthesiologists and many ophthalmology residents how to perform this block. No significant complications have been reported back.

Disadvantages of the periconal block include an initially higher failure rate with slow onset of block (during the "learning curve") and increased volume of anesthetic in the orbit with attendant increased forward pressure on the eyeball. However, the avoidance of a retrobulbar hemorrhage, optic nerve damage, blindness, or cardiopulmonary arrest should outweigh those problems. Furthermore, amaurosis occurs rarely, which has advantages for the monocular patient and those undergoing radial keratotomy. pH-adjustment of a lidocaine/bupivacaine mixture or plain bupivacaine with sodium bicarbonate speeds the onset time for akinesia of extraocular muscles.[9, 10] As a matter of practice, this block should be performed 20–30 minutes prior to the start of surgery. Performance of any eye block in a designated block area prior to surgery decreases case turnover time and ultimately increases operating room efficiency and utilization.

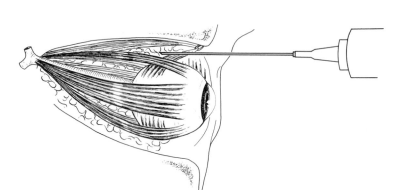

FIGURE 18–20. *Superonasal injection as seen from above with the roof of the orbit removed. The needle is inserted medial to the supraorbital notch (not shown) and just beyond the equator of the globe.*

SUMMARY

The anatomical bases and principles of regional anesthesia for ophthalmic surgery have been reviewed. The retrobulbar block has a low, but appreciable, complication rate. Performing the retrobulbar block with a needle of 31 mm (1.25 in) or less in length with the eye in neutral gaze is recommended to reduce complications. Complications may be as serious as blindness or cardiopulmonary arrest. In the setting of over 1 million intraocular operations performed in the United States annually, any complication rate, however small, results in significant morbidity. Occurrence of these complications should be lower with the Gills-Loyd or a periconal block. The author favors the periconal block, especially for teaching anesthesiologists and ophthalmology residents. Both the Gills-Loyd and periconal blocks have the advantage of avoiding painful seventh nerve blocks, which may be associated with other complications.

REFERENCES

1. Zahl K, Meltzer MA (eds): Regional Anesthesia for Intraocular Surgery. Ophthalmol Clin North Am 1990; 3:1–129
2. Atkinson WS: Anesthesia in Ophthalmology. American Lecture Series. Charles C. Thomas, Springfield, Illinois, 1955, pp 35–39.
3. Lynch S, Wolf G, Berlin I: 2200 cases of cataract surgery under general anesthesia. Anesth Analg 1980; 53:909–913.
4. Knapp H: On cocaine and its use in ophthalmic and general surgery. Arch Ophthalmol 1884; 13:402–406.
5. Koorneef L: New insights in the human orbital connective tissue. Arch Ophthalmol 1977; 95:1269–1273.
6. Zahl K, Nassif J, Som P, Meltzer M: Simulated peribulbar anesthetic injection. Arch Ophthalmol 1991; 2:239–241.
7. Feibel RM: Current concepts in retrobulbar anesthesia. Surv Ophthalmol 1985; 30:102.
8. Galindo A: pH adjusted local anesthetics: Clinical experience. Reg Anesth 1983; 8:35–64.
9. Zahl K, Jordan A, McGroarty J, et al: The use of pH-adjusted bupivacaine/hyaluronidase for peribulbar anesthesia. Anesthesiology 1990; 72:230.
10. Zahl K, Jordan A, McGroarty J, et al: pH-adjusted solutions of lidocaine, bupivacaine and hyaluronidase for peribulbar block. Ophthalmology 1991 (in press).
11. Nicoll JM, Treuren B, Acharya PA, et al: Retrobulbar anesthesia: The role of hyaluronidase. Anesth Analg 1986; 65:1324–1328.
12. Zahl K, Jordan A, McGroarty J, et al: Freshly added epinephrine does not prolong onset time with peribulbar anesthesia. Anesth Analg 1989; 69:2A–S312 (abstract).
13. Bloom LH, Scheie HG, Yanoff M: The warming of local anesthetic agents to decrease discomfort. Ophthalmic Surg 1984; 15:603.
14. Drysdale DB: Experimental subdural injection of local anesthetic. Ann Opthalmol 1984; 16:716.
15. Javitt JC, Addiego R, Friedburg HL, et al: Brain stem anesthesia after retrobulbar block. Ophthalmology 1987; 94:718.
16. Pautler SE, Grizzard WS, Thompson LN, et al: Blindness from retrobulbar injection into the optic nerve. Ophthalmic Surg 1986; 17:334.
17. Morgan CM, Schatz H, Vine AKM, et al: Ocular complications associated with retrobulbar injections. Ophthalmology 1988; 95:660.
18. Kraushar MF, Seelenfreund MH, Freilich DB: Central retinal artery occlusion during orbital hemorrhage from retrobulbar injection. Trans Am Acad Ophthalmol Otol 1974; 78:65.
19. Nicoll JMV, Acharya PA, Ahlen K, et al: Central nervous system complications after 6000 retrobulbar blocks. Anesth Analg 1987; 66:1298.
20. Unsold R, Stanley JA, DeGroot J: The CT-topography of retrobulbar anesthesia. Graefes Arch Clin Exp Ophthalmol 1981; 217:125.
21. Galindo A, Keilson LR, Mondshine RB, Sawelson HI: Retro-peribulbar anesthesia. In Zahl K, Meltzer MA (eds): Regional Anesthesia for Intraocular Surgery. Ophthalmol Clin North Am 1990; 3:71–81.
22. Straus JG: A new retrobulbar needle and injection technique. Ophthalmic Surg 1988; 19:134–139.
23. Katsev D, Drews R, Rose B: An anatomical study of retrobulbar needle path length. Ophthalmology 1989; 94:718–724.
24. Hamilton RC, Gimbel HV, Javitt JC: The prevention of complications in regional anesthesia for ophthalmology. Ophthalmol Clin North Am 1990; 3:111–125.
25. Gills JP, Loyd TL: A technique of retrobulbar block with paralysis of orbicularis oculi. Am Intra-ocular Implant Soc 1983; 9:339–340.
26. Kimbrough RL, Stewart RH, Okereke PC: A modified Gills' block and its effectiveness for lid akinesia. Ophthalmic Surg 1987; 18:14–17.
27. van Lint A: Paralysie palpeprae temporaire provoquee dans l'operation de la cataracte. Ann Ocul (Paris) 1914; 151:420–424.
28. O'Brien CS: Akinesis during cataract extraction. Arch Ophthalmol 1929; 1:447–449.
29. Spaeth GL: A new method to achieve complete akinesia of the facial muscles of the eyelids. Ophthalmic Surg 1976; 7:105–109.
30. Atkinson WS: Akinesia of the orbicularis. Am J Ophthalmol 1953; 36:1255–1258.
31. Nadbath RP, Rehman I: Facial nerve block. Am J Ophthalmol 1963; 55:143–146.
32. Wilson CA, Ruiz RS: Respiratory obstruction following the Nadbath facial nerve block. Arch Ophthalmol 1985; 103:1454–1456.
33. Cofer HF: Cord paralysis after Nadbath facial nerve block. Arch Ophthalmol 1986; 104:337.
34. Davis DB, Mandel MR: Posterior peribulbar anesthesia: An alternative to retrobulbar anesthesia. J Cataract Refractive Surg 1986; 12:182–184.
35. Hamilton RC, Gimbel HV, Strunin L: Regional anesthesia for 12,000 cataract extractions and intraocular lens implantation procedures. Can J Anaesth 1988; 35:615.

CHAPTER 19

Ophthalmic Procedures Performed on an Outpatient Basis

Kathryn E. McGoldrick

Continuing changes in health care have placed the onus of cost containment on the providers. Hospitals and physicians are under increasing pressure from government agencies, industry, insurance companies, and various other organizations to reduce health costs but, concomitantly, to continue to provide the same high standards of care. The provision of health care on an outpatient basis is expanding rapidly. More than 40% of all surgical procedures are now performed in the ambulatory setting. Focusing exclusively on ophthalmologic surgery, in 1977, approximately 95% of all operations were performed on hospital inpatients. However, in 1987 only 10% of all eye surgeries were performed on an inpatient basis.

(Ironically, ambulatory surgery was the oldest form of surgery performed by itinerant surgeons before the advent of organized hospitals. Outpatient surgery in children was first reported in a series of 9000 procedures by Nicoll in 1909, although it had little support until 1970.)

The success of ambulatory surgery depends on the selection of both appropriate patients and surgical procedures that are amenable to an abbreviated clinic stay. Such procedures include those that are relatively brief (i.e., less than 3 hours) and entail minimal blood loss, fluid shifts, and other derangements in the patient's physiology. Ophthalmic surgery involves many procedures that fulfill these stipulations, including examinations under anesthesia, correction of strabismus, radiation treatments, excision of cysts and chalazions, probing of tear ducts, cataract extraction, and various types of surgery to alleviate glaucoma (Table 19–1).

Often, ophthalmic surgery encompasses patients at the extreme ranges of age. The vast majority of patients are either under 10 or over 55 years of age. In this chapter, the anesthetic management of cataract surgery in geriatric patients is discussed. In pediatric patients, strabismus surgery, radiation treatments, and probing and irrigation for congenital epiphora are examples of ophthalmological procedures routinely performed in an outpatient setting, and the suggested anesthetic management of these patients is presented.

TABLE 19–1. Ocular Procedures Amenable to Outpatient Status

Extraocular
Examination under anesthesia
Strabismus repair
Ptosis correction
Lacrimal duct probing and irrigation
Lacrimal tubes
Retinoblastoma (cryotherapy or radiation therapy)
Excision of dermoid cysts
Removal of orbital foreign body
Contact lens fitting
Prosthesis fitting

Intraocular
Cataract aspiration or extraction
Trabeculectomy
Keratoplasty (?)

CATARACT EXTRACTION

Cataract removal and intraocular lens implantation is an increasingly common surgical procedure because of several factors. Perhaps two of the most significant factors are demographics and technology. A rapidly growing population of elderly people and the widespread availability of surgical techniques employing operating microscopes and phacoemulsification devices have increased the demand for this procedure. Because of escalating health care costs, cataract surgery is performed increasingly as an outpatient procedure. The necessity to perform intricate surgery on fragile geriatric patients without overnight hospital admission has been a major challenge for anesthesiologists, resulting in a refinement of anesthetic techniques.

PREOPERATIVE EVALUATION

Once the ophthalmologist has established the diagnosis of surgically remediable cataract disease, the suitability of the patient for outpatient care must be determined. This decision is initially made by the ophthalmologist, who will have assessed the patient's overall medical condition, ability to cooperate, and access to proper postoperative care. Outpatient surgery is not possible if there is no adult responsible for the patient's postoperative care.

Thorough and consistent preoperative teaching is extremely important if outpatient cataract surgery is to be acceptable to, and a satisfactory experience for, the patient. This preoperative instruction is initiated by the ophthalmologist, continued in the anesthetic preoperative interview, and reinforced in the outpatient clinic by the nursing staff. A detailed explanation of preoperative fasting should be emphasized. Preoperative instruction informs patients of the inherent risks, as well as the benefits, of the anesthesia and surgery. At the same time, the repetition of consistent information from numerous sources helps to alleviate anxiety and fear. Because the geriatric patient may have difficulty comprehending technical terminology, instruction should be given clearly, slowly, and patiently using understandable language.

Elderly patients are likely to have illness affecting multiple organ systems; if necessary, multidisciplinary preoperative consultations should be obtained well in advance of the scheduled date of surgery. Approximately 75% of patients over the age of 70 have one or more diseases in addition to the condition being surgically corrected. The most frequent problems in the geriatric population are hypertension, coronary artery disease, chronic obstructive pulmonary disease (COPD), and obesity. Not surprisingly, advanced age is associated with many anesthetic implications (Table 19–2). For instance, large-artery elasticity is reduced, as are cardiac index and conduction velocity. The respiratory system is characterized by a generalized reduction of elasticity and of chest wall compliances; vital capacity and maximal breathing capacity are also decreased. Ventilation-perfusion abnormalities may occur. Renal plasma flow and glomerular filtration rate are diminished, resulting in delayed renal drug clearance. Hepatic drug clearance is reduced. Furthermore, the sympathoadrenal axis is characterized by elevated levels of plasma epinephrine and norepinephrine and reduced autonomic end-organ responsiveness. Protective upper airway reflexes decrease with age, leaving elderly patients susceptible to aspiration.[1] Additionally, elderly patients have an increased incidence of hiatal hernia, suggesting that regurgitation and aspiration of gastric contents may be more likely.[2] However, when Manchikanti and colleagues[3] evaluated acid aspiration risk factors in pediatric (6 months–12 years), adult (18–64 years), and geriatric (more than 65 years) patient groups on the basis of gastric fluid contents, they found that children appeared to be at greatest risk and geriatric patients at least risk.

Nonetheless, even the American Society of Anesthesiologists (ASA) physical status III patients can be acceptable candidates for outpatient anesthesia and surgery provided they are medically well controlled and in optimal condition at the time of surgery. Natof's study[4] disclosed no statistical difference in the com-

TABLE 19–2. Anesthetic Challenges of Advanced Age

Cellular dehydration
Decreased basal metabolic rate
Increased incidence of obesity
Hypertension
Coronary artery disease
Decreased cardiac index and conduction velocity
Delayed renal drug clearance
Diminished hepatic drug clearance
Diminished protective upper airway reflexes
Increased incidence of hiatus hernia
Reduced autonomic end-organ responsiveness
Increased incidence of drug interactions

plication rates of ASA III patients compared to ASA I and II patients. Nonetheless, patients with cardiovascular disease who have a high total risk score according to Goldman and associates' Cardiac Risk Index are not acceptable candidates.[5] Patients with stable angina pectoris or well-controlled congestive heart failure (CHF) are candidates for most outpatient procedures, providing they do not have other complicating diseases and are not physically disabled. Patients with a preoperative diastolic pressure greater than 110 mmHg should be excluded until the hypertension is better controlled. Patients with previously well-controlled hypertension who present in a hypertensive state on the day of surgery are usually allowed to undergo their scheduled operation if their pressure is easily controlled with anxiolytic drugs or a β-blocker such as esmolol.

Patients with stable COPD and those with well-controlled asthma are probably at minimal risk, especially if the procedure can be done using local or regional anesthesia. However, individuals with severe exercise intolerance (ASA IV patients), supplemental oxygen dependence, or a recent acute exacerbation of their pulmonary disease (requiring hospitalization within the last 3 months) should probably be excluded. Although a recent upper respiratory infection may pose no increased risk in otherwise healthy outpatients undergoing minor ambulatory procedures, such a history requires delaying surgery for patients with significant pulmonary disease. Even in patients with normal pulmonary function, elective eye surgery should perhaps be delayed if the patient is coughing.

Diabetes mellitus *per se* may not be a significant risk factor, but patients with concomitant cardiovascular and renal disease may be at increased risk for complications. Because these patients have a high incidence of silent myocardial ischemia, an electrocardiogram (ECG) should be included in the initial evaluation, regardless of the age of the patient. The primary objectives in the perioperative management of an insulin-dependent diabetic are to avoid hypoglycemia and to restore the patient's insulin balance to the preoperative state as soon as possible. To this end, surgery should be scheduled early in the day. Because gastroparesis is a common finding in diabetics, thereby rendering them vulnerable to aspiration, prophylactic use of metoclopramide is recommended. Fasting blood sugar should be established on the morning of surgery, a main-

tenance intravenous (IV) infusion with D5 lactated Ringer's should be started, and half of the patient's usual neutral protamine Hagedorn (NPH) insulin dose given. (Other insulin regimens are also acceptable, but this plan has worked well in our institution.) Blood sugar is checked postoperatively and, if indicated, intraoperatively. Patients are encouraged to resume oral intake as soon as feasible. If the patient is eating well and the postoperative blood sugar is within an acceptable range, the patient should take the remainder of the daily NPH insulin dose.

Taking a thorough drug history is an essential part of the preanesthetic evaluation. Vagaries of absorption, distribution, metabolism, and excretion contribute to the altered response to medication observed frequently in the geriatric population. However, age-related alterations in pharmacokinetics and pharmacodynamics are not the only reasons for untoward drug effects. In addition, there is an increased incidence of drug interactions (seven times greater in the seventh decade than in the third) because of the large number of drugs consumed by elderly persons[6] (Table 19–3).

Although over half of hospitalized geriatric patients experience some transient confusional state postoperatively,[7] this high incidence is decreased in ambulatory surgery geriatric patients, perhaps because of the more rapid return to their usual surroundings as well as the reduced number of medications they receive during their brief stay in the outpatient facility.

Outpatients require the same preoperative evaluation as inpatients with a comparable medical profile and undergoing a similar procedure. Furthermore, the type of anesthesia planned (i.e., regional or general) should not modify the comprehensiveness of the preoperative evaluation or of the perioperative management. In addition to a thorough history and physical examination, appropriate laboratory studies should be performed. Rather than adhering to a rigid catechism of absolute rules for obtaining laboratory data, the physician should order the appropriate tests based on the individual's condition. Levin[8] proposed the following minimal guidelines for adults: hemoglobin for all females regardless of age and for all males over 40. In addition, all patients over 40 should have a preoperative ECG, and a chest radiograph is recommended for all patients over 60. The presence of complicating factors necessitates additional work-up. For example, any patient with diabetes, regardless

TABLE 19–3. Anesthetic Implications of Concurrent Systemic Therapy

Drug	Relevant Features
Acetazolamide	Chronic use results in acidosis, hypokalemia, and hyponatremia
α-Methyldopa	Sedation secondary to reduced CNS levels of norepinephrine, serotonin, and dopamine
	Reduced anesthetic requirement
Clonidine	Acts on α-adrenergic receptors in the medulla
	May cause drowsiness
	? Reduced anesthetic requirement
	If discontinued abruptly, severe rebound hypertension may occur
L-dopa	Hypotension secondary to decreased intravascular volume, reduced renin-aldosterone stimulus, and reduced norepinephrine levels
	Attenuated response to indirect vasopressors
	No concomitant use of droperidol, chlorpromazine, or methyldopa, lest parkinsonian exacerbation occur
	May produce tachycardia and other dysrhythmias
Lithium	May produce nephrogenic diabetes insipidus, tremor, exophthalmos, and salty tears
	Prolongs action of some muscle relaxants
Monoamine oxidase inhibitors	May be fatal if combined with meperidine and possibly other potent analgesics
	Hypertensive crises precipitated by:
	L-dopa
	Sympathomimetic amines that release stored catecholamines (i.e., ephedrine, amphetamine)
	If intraoperative hypotension develops, treat with small amounts of direct-acting vasopressors
	Recommend discontinuation 2 weeks prior to elective surgery, if possible
Reserpine	Depletes norepinephrine stores
	Increased sensitivity to direct-acting vasopressors
	Decreased sensitivity to indirect-acting sympathomimetic amines
Tricyclic antidepressants	Anticholinergic
	Cardiac toxicity, usually dose-related (hypotension, CHF, conduction defects, and dysrhythmias)

of age, should have an ECG; patients on diuretics should have a serum potassium determination; and patients with advanced COPD should have pulmonary function tests.

In summary, physical status, surgical procedure, and proposed anesthetic techniques must be examined individually and collectively before the anesthesiologist accepts or rejects the geriatric outpatient.

ANESTHETIC MANAGEMENT

Historically, the use of general anesthesia was popular in many institutions for cataract extraction. Lynch and coworkers[9] in 1974 reported no major difference in complications such as iris prolapse or vitreous loss between local and general anesthesia for cataract surgery. Since the 1970s, however, regional anesthesia has become predominant for patients undergoing cataract extraction. A variety of factors have influenced this trend, including cost, decreasing duration of the surgical procedure, and enhanced patient acceptance. Currently, in most cases of adult cataract surgery

general anesthesia is reserved only for those special patients with behavioral, motor, or psychiatric disorders or those with some other major contraindication to regional blockade (Table 19–4). Those who require general anesthesia do well provided the eye is kept motionless and a stable intraocular pressure (IOP) is maintained to protect against extrusion of intraocular contents. Thus, a sufficiently deep level of anesthesia is mandatory until the wound has been sutured completely closed; administration of a nondepolarizing muscle relaxant in conjunction with peripheral nerve

TABLE 19–4. Contraindications to Regional Anesthesia for Eye Surgery

Penetrating ocular injury
Inability to lie flat
Tremors
Chronic coughing
Claustrophobia or excessive anxiety
Inability to communicate owing to such problems as deafness or language barrier
Coagulation or bleeding abnormality
Patient's refusal to accept regional blockade

monitoring is advocated. If the patient moves unexpectedly during intraocular surgery, IV thiopental should be given immediately. Succinylcholine should *not* be given and is contraindicated when the eye is surgically open.

Ventilation is controlled and carefully monitored through end-tidal carbon dioxide (CO_2) measurement to avoid hypercarbia. Once surgery is terminated, any residual neuromuscular blockade is reversed. IV lidocaine is suggested approximately 4 minutes prior to extubation to prevent periextubation coughing. Extubation is accomplished in the lateral position (operated eye superior). The postoperative goal is to have a comfortable patient who does not cough or vomit. If postoperative nausea and vomiting occur, droperidol 10 µg/kg is the antiemetic of choice. If the patient is drowsy, however, metoclopramide 0.15 mg/kg IV or small doses of ephedrine, 10–25 mg IV, may be given.

Until recently, execution of regional blocks for ocular surgery was the exclusive province of the ophthalmic surgeon; the anesthesiologist's role was confined to administering IV sedation and providing patient monitoring. Now, however, in many institutions the anesthesiologist performs regional eye blocks in addition to other duties. Regional anesthesia is an effective means to achieve analgesia, akinesis of the globe and orbicularis oculi, and an acceptable level of IOP. Until recently, retrobulbar blockade was the uncontested regional block of choice for cataract surgery, but in the past few years considerable favorable experience with peribulbar injection[10] has been reported.

A partial list[11-23] of complications associated with retrobulbar block includes retrobulbar hemorrhage, stimulation of the oculocardiac reflex, puncture of the globe producing retinal detachment and vitreous hemorrhage, intraocular injection, optic nerve penetration, central retinal artery occlusion, IV or intra-arterial injection, and brain-stem anesthesia. Both retrobulbar and peribulbar blockade are considered contraindicated if a ruptured globe is suspected for fear of prolapsing intraocular contents. Furthermore, patients who are extremely near-sighted are not suitable candidates for retrobulbar block, because they are vulnerable to penetration of the globe. Additionally, the facial nerve injection required with retrobulbar block may be quite painful.

Peribulbar block is considered by many to be easier and less painful than retrobulbar block, because the muscle cone is not entered and the need for seventh nerve block is eliminated. Because the anesthetic is deposited outside the muscle cone, the potential for intraocular or intradural injection is greatly minimized, and the potential for intraconal hemorrhage and direct nerve injury is eliminated. Hamilton and colleagues' experience with peribulbar block shows more than 2000 cases performed without inadvertent brainstem anesthesia or scleral perforation.[10] However, disadvantages of peribulbar block include a higher failure rate (up to 10%) and a longer onset time. Zahl and associates[24] demonstrated more recently that the pH adjustment of a solution of 0.75% bupivacaine and hyaluronidase with sodium bicarbonate hastens the onset time and improves the initial success rate of peribulbar block.

Nonetheless, because a higher volume of local anesthetic is required with peribulbar than with retrobulbar block, vitreous pressure elevation may make surgery more technically difficult. Despite the fact that serious morbidity may occur secondary to retrobulbar block, the incidence of these complications is still extremely low. For example, in a series of 910 patients undergoing retrobulbar block, Petty and coworkers[25] documented 12 cases of major morbidity, including two instances each of globe perforation, cardiovascular collapse, and respiratory arrest secondary to probable intradural injection. In addition, there were three cases of central nervous system stimulation.

Technical aspects of performing both retrobulbar and peribulbar block are discussed elsewhere in this book, and the literature is replete with references.[26, 27]

When the patient arrives in the anesthetizing area, the physician examines the pupil of the affected eye for adequate mydriasis, and then two or three drops of 2% proparacaine solution may be instilled on the conjunctiva for analgesia. Before either retrobulbar or peribulbar block is performed, a cannula is inserted into a peripheral vein, and electrocardiographic, oximetric, and blood pressure monitoring is instituted. An appropriate mixture of bupivacaine, either 0.5% or 0.75%, with lidocaine 2% with 1:200,000 epinephrine and 75–150 international units (IU) hyaluronidase is drawn into a syringe. (Ophthalmologists frequently ask if epinephrine may be safely combined with local anesthetics to effect vasoconstriction and enhance anesthetic duration for cardiac patients. Donlon and Moss[28] reported that release of endogenous catecholamines secondary to suboptimal anesthesia may greatly surpass the relatively minute quantity of exogenous catecholamine injected. They claim that 0.06 mg epinephrine, or 12 mL of 1:200,000, gives some systemic uptake but no undesirable clinical effects.)

The block is then performed according to accepted standards of care. Sedation, if given, is administered so that the patient is calm, cooperative, aware intraoperatively, and *not* obtunded or disoriented. Excessive medication can result in an uncooperative patient and consequent unexpected movements, producing inadvertent loss of intraocular contents during this delicate intraocular surgery. Preoperative monitoring is continued throughout the duration of the procedure to detect, among other aberrations, the occurrence of delayed drug reactions, oculocardiac reflex–induced dysrhythmias, hypo- or hypertension, and hypoxemia. Respiratory arrest secondary to inadvertent brain-stem anesthesia typically does not occur until about 7 minutes after retrobulbar block and is unassociated with seizure activity. Therefore, the patient's oxygenation, ventilation, circulation, and temperature must be appropriately assessed. Monitoring standards are the same for both inpatient and outpatient anesthesia.

Because the patient is awake during the procedure, inappropriate conversation among operating room personnel should be avoided. A mini-drip on the IV infusion discourages the administration of excessive volumes of IV fluids and resultant painful bladder distension. Careful draping of the patient and a flow of supplemental air or oxygen around the patient's face can diminish his or her claustrophobic sensation. Additionally, the operating table should be well-padded and its position adjusted (e.g., hip or knee flexion) to assure maximal patient comfort and intraoperative immobility. Verbal reassurance should be gently dispensed as needed.

Once the operative procedure is completed, the patient is taken to the postanesthesia care unit, where vital signs are assessed frequently. When the patient is ready, fluids by mouth are offered. The patient is gradually encouraged to ambulate and void. Once the patient is satisfactorily assessed for home-readiness by an appropriate professional, he or she is discharged to the care of a responsible adult. Explicit written postoperative instructions should be given to the patient and the accompanying caregiver, and instructions about driving, alcohol or other drug ingestion, and major decision-making for a specified period of time should be given.

A report from the Southern Illinois University School of Medicine studied factors leading to hospital admission of elderly patients following outpatient surgery.[30] Eighteen percent of these patients required hospitalization for hemodynamic stabilization and close observation. This 1989 study indicated that near octogenarians and patients with coronary artery disease were more likely to require hospitalization. Those with coronary artery disease were more likely to have intraoperative rhythm disturbances or sustained hypertension in the recovery phase. Nonetheless, this reported rate of unscheduled admissions seems atypically high.

In the ambulatory surgery population, anesthetic-related deaths occur approximately 0.15/10,000, which is about one tenth of the typical inhospital incidence. Strict adherence to the principles of thorough preoperative evaluation and vigilant perioperative monitoring are essential to ensure the safety of outpatient surgery.

STRABISMUS SURGERY (Fig 19–1)

The anesthesiologist caring for small patients must be concerned about separation anxiety, proper fasting period, fluid titration, and use of appropriate-sized equipment. In addition to the special concerns of pediatric anesthesia, there are many potential problems associated with strabismus surgery in particular. For example, the child should understand that one or both eyes may be patched after surgery; occluded or diminished vision secondary to patches or ointment may terrify the child as he or she emerges from anesthesia. Strabismus surgery is associated with a high incidence of oculocardiac reflex–induced dysrhythmias as well as postoperative nausea and vomiting. An

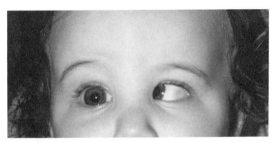

FIGURE 19–1. *A toddler with obvious strabismus. (Photograph courtesy of David S. Walton, M.D., Pediatric Ophthalmologist, Associate Surgeon, Massachusetts Eye and Ear Infirmary.)*

increased incidence of masseter spasm and malignant hyperthermia are seen in the child with strabismus also. (This latter observation is also true of children undergoing ptosis repair, consistent with the impression that malignant hyperthermia (MH)–susceptible persons often have localized areas of skeletal muscle weakness or other musculoskeletal abnormalities.[31, 32]) Another concern involves the effect of succinylcholine on the forced duction testing that is sometimes employed to distinguish between a paretic muscle and a restrictive force impairing ocular movement.

Because succinylcholine interferes with forced duction testing, its use is contraindicated less than 20 minutes prior to testing.[23] Many anesthesiologists are now avoiding the almost routine administration of succinylcholine in strabismus surgery. By intubating either under deep inhalation anesthesia or with the assistance of a nondepolarizing muscle relaxant, the anesthesiologist can obviate both potential masseter spasm and interference with forced duction testing.

Having a trigeminal afferent and vagal efferent path, the oculocardiac reflex is triggered with impressive frequency during surgery of the extraocular muscles. Strabismus surgery in children not pretreated with IV anticholinergics may have a 90% incidence of oculocardiac reflex–induced dysrhythmias. Although most studies of the oculocardiac reflex in strabismus surgery have involved children anesthetized with halothane, ketamine is associated with a similarly high incidence of dysrhythmias. Whether the reflex is as common with other volatile agents or narcotic nitrous oxide (N_2O) techniques has not been established.

Although virtually any dysrhythmia may appear during strabismus surgery, the most common manifestation of the oculocardiac reflex is sinus bradycardia. Numerous maneuvers to attenuate or eliminate the reflex have been proposed. Inclusion of intramuscular (IM) anticholinergic drugs, such as glycopyrrolate or atropine, in conventional premedication doses is ineffective in blocking the oculocardiac reflex,[34] because approximately 0.03–0.05 mg/kg of atropine[35] is required to accomplish this purpose. Moreover, the maximal effect of IM atropine occurs approximately 30 minutes after injection. Therefore, routine (i.e., small) doses of atropine given 1 hour prior to surgery have proven unreliable in preventing reflex dysrhythmias. For the child who is fearful of "shots," oral atropine, 0.04 mg/kg given by mouth 60–90 minutes preoperatively, is an alternative.[36] However, this route affords inconsistent protection owing to erratic absorption patterns. Retrobulbar blockade interrupts the afferent limb of the arc, but this maneuver has many inherent risks.

For pediatric strabismus surgery, most anesthesiologists prefer routine prophylaxis with IV atropine, 0.02 mg/kg, or with IV glycopyrrolate, 0.01 mg/kg, prior to the start of surgery. The latter is claimed to trigger less tachycardia than atropine.[37]

Following prophylaxis with an IV anticholinergic, the anesthesiologist proceeds to induction and tracheal intubation. Anesthesia is commonly maintained with a volatile agent, N_2O, and oxygen, although a narcotic N_2O muscle relaxant and oxygen technique is also acceptable. (Halothane is well tolerated if induction is through a mask. However, once intubation is accomplished, isoflurane should be used, because the latter agent is associated with a more rapid emergence.) The patient is carefully monitored with a precordial stethoscope, ECG, blood pressure device, pulse oximeter, fractional inspired oxygen (FIO_2) monitor, and temperature probe. An end-tidal CO_2 monitor is also extremely valuable, not only as a measure of ventilatory adequacy, but also as a means to detect incipient malignant hyperthermia. If bradycardia occurs, the surgeon stops ocular manipulation, and the anesthesiologist quickly evaluates anesthetic depth and adequacy of oxygenation and ventilation. If additional IV atropine must be used because of worrisome levels of hypotension, for example, the atropine should not be given while the oculocardiac reflex is active, lest even more hazardous dysrhythmias result. Ventricular dysrhythmias produced by the reflex may require 1–2 mg/kg of IV lidocaine.

Vomiting following strabismus surgery is distressingly frequent, perhaps because of an oculogastric reflex. Interestingly, a study by Gibbons and colleagues[38] disclosed that omission of N_2O does not alter the incidence of vomiting in pediatric strabismus surgery when patients are anesthetized with halothane as the principal anesthetic. However, Abramowitz and associates[39, 40] reported that prophylactic IV administration of 75 $\mu g/kg$ of droperidol, given 30 minutes prior to completion of surgery, was highly effective in reducing the severity and frequency (from 85% to 43%) of vomiting in pediatric patients undergoing repair of strabismus. No significant prolongation of recovery time was observed with this protocol. Lerman and coworkers[41] found encouraging results when 75 µg/kg of droperidol was administered IV at the start of the case, *prior* to manipulation of the extraocular muscles. The proportion of patients who experienced vomiting was dramatically reduced to 10%. In addition, Warner and colleagues[42] reported similar results when lidocaine 2 mg/kg IV was given prior to intubation; their series disclosed a 16% incidence of vomiting. However, Christensen and associates[43] in a 1989 study found that IV droperidol, 75 µg/kg immediately after induction, is significantly more effective than lidocaine, 1.5 mg/kg IV, in reducing the incidence of vomiting in unpremedicated children after strabismus surgery. Droperidol did not delay either the time to recovery of full alertness or the time to discharge from the hospital compared with lidocaine (Table 19–5). In the future, perhaps ondansetron will be a valuable drug for both prevention and treatment of nausea and vomiting associated with strabismus surgery.

ANESTHESIA FOR RADIATION THERAPY OF RETINOBLASTOMA

Although rare, retinoblastoma is the most common malignant eye tumor in children and is usually diagnosed and treated during the first 3 years of life (Fig. 19–2). These aggressive tumors account for 1% of all cancer-related pediatric deaths. Treatment may include cryotherapy, photocoagulation, enucleation, chemotherapy, and radiation—either alone or in combination—depending on the grade of the tumor and evolving treatment protocols. Unfortunately, approximately 30% of retinoblastoma cases display bilateral involvement.

Radiation is a common treatment of retinoblastoma. The radiation is usually administered over a 4–6 week interval and divided into 16–24 doses, depending on the age of the patient and the size of the tumor. Hence, these children commonly receive four to five treatments per week for at least 1 month. To provide effective anesthesia affording both immobility and safety in this challenging setting, (1) the patient must be perfectly motionless, but only for periods lasting a few minutes; (2) the patient must be unattended during treatment to protect personnel from radiation exposure; (3) immediate access to the patient in an emergency must be guaranteed; and (4) the radiotherapist must be able to obtain radiograms during treatment to assess target precision.

These demands are best satisfied by administering anesthesia that is both sufficiently deep and sufficiently short-lived and by providing remote monitoring of ventilation and circulation by a precordial stethoscope with lengthened tubing, pulse oximetry, continuous electrocardiographic monitoring, and automatic, noninvasive blood pressure devices.

A wide range of techniques, employing a variety of agents, have been successful in this setting. In the early 1960s, Harrison and Bennet[44] introduced an insufflation technique using a Waters oropharyngeal airway with a sidearm to administer halothane, N_2O, and oxygen to infants undergoing radiotherapy. They reported no complications and rapid recovery. In 1969, Browne and coworkers[45] introduced a slightly different insufflation technique employing a T-piece circuit attached to an orotracheal airway.

In the 1970s, IM ketamine was widely used.[46–48] The usual IM dose is 4–8 mg/kg. However, the chronic use of ketamine often produces tachyphylaxis, necessitating dose modifications. Ketamine may also produce writhing, adventitious body motion, and nystagmus, all of which compromise the accurate delivery of radiation to the proposed small target. Furthermore, ketamine may produce copious oral secretions that may lead to airway obstruction[48] or laryngospasm.[46, 49] The period

TABLE 19–5. Efficacy of Antiemetic Prophylaxis for Strabismus Surgery

Study/Treatment	Percent with Vomiting
Abramowitz (1983)[40]	
Droperidol 75 µg/kg (given approximately 30 minutes before completion)	43
Saline control	85
Lerman (1986)[41]	
Droperidol 75 µg/kg (given before ocular manipulation)	10
Acetaminophen 10 mg/kg PR	60
Codeine 1.5 mg/kg IM	68
Warner (1988)[42]	
Lidocaine 2 mg/kg	16
Lidocaine plus succinylcholine	20
Succinylcholine 1 mg/kg	52
Christensen (1989)[43]	
Droperidol 75 µg/kg	22
Lidocaine 1.5 mg/kg plus droperidol 25 µg/kg	30
Lidocaine 1.5 mg/kg	50

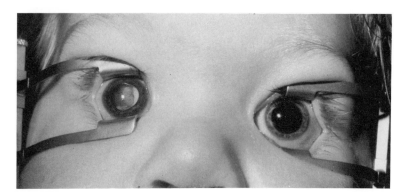

FIGURE 19–2. An infant with retinoblastoma who presented with leucocoria. (Photograph courtesy of David S. Walton, M.D., Pediatric Ophthalmologist, Associate Surgeon, Massachusetts Eye and Ear Infirmary.)

of sedation resulting from ketamine is variable, at best, and, at worst, totally unpredictable. IV ketamine, 1–2 mg/kg, is also an option. An indwelling catheter may be placed and securely taped, thus simplifying the daily IV administration of the selected drug. The catheter's patency can be maintained by flushing four times daily with heparinized (50 μg/mL) saline; the catheter should be removed and a sterile one reinserted every 5 days. If possible, insertion of a Porta-cath is an attractive option. Although the rather high incidence of dysphoric dreaming described by older children and adults is less of a problem in young children following ketamine administration, unpleasant dreams are still a potential threat.

Methohexital (25–30 mg/kg) given rectally has also been used to sedate infants undergoing radiotherapy. However, as with ketamine, tachyphylaxis and prolonged or erratic sedation have been described. Proctitis may accompany repeated rectal doses.[50] The IM route is also an option with methohexital; recommended dose is 10 mg/kg.

In the 1980s, Brett and colleagues[51] described another apparently successful insufflation method using a nasopharyngeal catheter to deliver isoflurane or halothane, N_2O, and oxygen to infants and young children during radiotherapy. Their small patients were placed supine on the treatment table, and anesthesia was induced with either halothane or isoflurane in 70% N_2O and 30% oxygen through a face mask. The concentration of volatile agent was gradually increased until anesthetic depth was sufficient to allow the insertion of an oral airway. To estimate the proper distance to advance the catheter—avoiding entrance to the esophagus, which might cause gastric distension—the distance from the patient's nose to the tragus was measured. A soft, single-orifice 8 or 10 French catheter was then inserted into the posterior pharynx through

either naris and taped to the child's chest. The catheter was attached directly to the gas outflow line of the anesthesia machine, and the FIO_2 was increased to 1.0 using a gas flow of 5 L per minute. The inspired anesthetic concentration given while the patient was unattended varied from 0.7% to 2.0% during isoflurane and from 0.5% to 1.5% during halothane. Once radiation therapy was completed, all patients received oxygen by mask until spontaneous movement was observed. Despite the advantages of this method, Brett[51] noted that patients with an abnormal upper airway (e.g., micrognathia) would be poor candidates for this technique. Also, waste anesthetic gases are difficult to scavenge under these circumstances.

Endotracheal intubation can be used in this setting, but complications from repeated tracheal intubation are possible. Furthermore, endotracheal anesthesia necessitates a greater depth of anesthesia than does insufflation. However, neither of these potential disadvantages contraindicates selection of the endotracheal route.

These unattended patients must be monitored with a pulse oximeter. When remote observation of patients is necessary, the pulse oximeter provides early, clear warning that airway patency may be compromised.

SURGERY OF THE LACRIMAL DRAINAGE SYSTEM

Surgery of the lacrimal drainage system encompasses (1) probing and irrigation for congenital epiphora; (2) silicone tubing intubation for canalicular lacerations and partial or intermittent stenosis of the lacrimal drainage system; (3) removal of the lacrimal sac with or without the emplacement of a Jones Pyrex tube; and (4) dacryocystorhinostomy, the anastomosis of the lacrimal sac to the nasal mucosa. Currently, only probing, irrigation, and silicone tube insertion are commonly done as outpatient procedures. Probing and irrigation for congenital epiphora is popularly viewed as a simple procedure, but numerous methods of anesthetizing patients for this maneuver exist; therefore, the ophthalmologist and anesthesiologist must have a mutual understanding of the technique to be used. Probing can be accomplished in infants without anesthesia or with a relatively light inhalation anesthetic, which may be administered either by mask or by insufflation. If the duct is to be irrigated, the liquid must not enter the pharynx and irritate the larynx, which can be accomplished by having the child sit with the head inclined forward so that any liquid coming through the duct trickles out of the nostril. Another approach is to apply suction to a catheter passed into the nose on the side being irrigated. Gravity drainage with the child's head down in the lateral position may also be employed. Alternatively, especially if the manipulation is expected to be lengthy, the child may be intubated.

Canalicular lacerations and partial stenosis or intermittent obstruction of the lacrimal drainage system are frequently managed with silicone tubing insertion. Canaliculus repair requires the use of the operating microscope. A 0.6-mm silastic tube is placed along the lumen to act as a splint while the torn canaliculus is sutured. This procedure requires the insertion of probes through the puncta, both parts of the canaliculus, the lacrimal sac, and the nasolacrimal duct, removing the probes from beneath the inferior turbinate and tying the ends of the tube together in the nasal cavity. To allow adequate working room for the ophthalmologist, the anesthesiologist must be sure that the nasal passages are patent and unobstructed. An inhalation anesthetic, administered by the endotracheal route, provides satisfactory anesthesia in this setting.

COMPLICATIONS OF PEDIATRIC AMBULATORY SURGERY

In a study by Patel and Hannallah[52] postanesthetic complications were examined in 10,000 pediatric patients at the Children's Hospital National Medical Center (CHNMC) between January 1, 1983, and April 16, 1986. The five most commonly performed procedures were hernia repair, strabismus surgery, myringotomy, adenoidectomy, and dental restoration. Ophthalmologic procedures accounted for 21% of the total operations performed.

At CHNMC, preanesthetic sedation is rarely given. Anesthesia is usually induced by inhalation of N_2O, oxygen, and halothane. If the child is reluctant to accept the mask, IV induction with thiamylal is accomplished. IM ketamine and rectal pentothal or methohexital are administered infrequently. In this study, 59% of the total number of patients were intubated, and prophylactic IV droperidol (75 μg/kg up to a total of 2.5 mg) was frequently administered to those undergoing strabismus surgery.

The overnight admission rate was 0.9%. Protracted vomiting accounted for one third of all overnight admissions. The reasons for overnight admission to the hospital reported in the pediatric literature seem uniform. The results of Patel and Hannallah[52] are in accord with Berry's observations[53] that the most common reasons for hospital admission of pediatric patients from the ambulatory surgery unit are vomiting, fever, croup, and bleeding (Table 19–6). The cited overnight admission rate was lower than the rates reported by Ahlgren and associates (1.7%)[54] and Davenport and coworkers (5.3%).[55] However, it was higher than that reported by Steward (0.1%)[56] and Johnson (0.26%).[57]

These studies confirm the safety of pediatric outpatient anesthesia. Clearly, admission and discharge criteria must be carefully followed to minimize complications that might result in hospital admission. In this context, it is worthwhile to discuss whether premature infants are acceptable candidates for outpatient surgery.

TABLE 19–6. Reasons for Pediatric Overnight Admission*

Reason	Number of Patients	
Protracted vomiting	30	(33%)
Complicated surgery	15	(17%)
Croup	8	(9%)
Parental request	6	(7%)
Fever	6	(7%)
Bleeding	3	(3%)
Sleepiness	2	(2%)
Others	20	(22%)
Total	90	(100%)

*Overall hospital admission rate 90/10,000 patients (0.9%). From Patel RI, Hannallah RS: Anesthetic complications following pediatric ambulatory surgery: A 3-year study. 1988. Anesthesiology 69:1009–1012.

Risk factors linked with prematurity include anemia, aspiration with feeding, episodes of apnea and bradycardia, bronchopulmonary dysplasia, and frequent chest infections with or without wheezing. The so-called sudden infant death syndrome (SIDS) is said to be seven times more likely in those with bronchopulmonary dysplasia. According to Steward,[58] the immaturity of temperature regulation in these infants, as well as the immaturity of central control of respiration and the potential for apnea and bradycardia, predispose these babies to a significantly higher incidence of postoperative complications. No association of apnea with ASA risk category is reported,[59] and preoperative pneumograms have not proven to be reliable in predicting postoperative apnea.[60] However, the incidence and duration of apnea appears to be inversely related to postconceptual age.[60] Many anesthesiologists believe that because the premature infant has significant impairment of respiratory function until at least 1 year of age,[58] outpatient surgery should not be attempted until that age, especially if there is a significant apnea history. Epstein[61] advised that even in a premature infant who has no history of complications, outpatient surgery is not suggested for at least 3–4 months following birth. Coté[62] stated that in his experience with a limited number of infants, the majority of premature infants, even those with a history of apnea, who are more than 46 weeks postconceptional age may be safely anesthetized as outpatients. Nonetheless, these same infants undergoing more complex procedures (e.g., ventriculoperitoneal shunt insertion or revision) are probably at greater risk and would be cared for as inpatients. Although postanesthetic apnea is most likely to occur in infants who are younger than 42 weeks postconceptional age, Downes emphasized that postanesthetic apnea occurs in at least one third of former premature infants who are younger than 60 weeks postconceptional age; therefore, Downes recommended that elective operations be deferred until the infant has reached a postconceptional age of more than 60 weeks.[63]

Unfortunately, the studies that have looked at former premature infants have not been similar in the type of patients studied and the surgical techniques employed. Thus, there are more questions than answers.

Multiple studies of former premature babies under 46 weeks of conceptional age have shown that administration of caffeine reduces or eliminates the problem of postoperative apnea. Welborn and colleagues[64] recommended administration of 10 mg/kg of IV caffeine at the beginning of surgery. However, this group of patients (i.e., those less than 46 weeks postconceptional age) should still be admitted and monitored overnight.

It would be tragic for one of these fragile premature nursery graduates, regardless of postconceptional age, to sustain morbidity, and even possible mortality, in the interests of cost containment.[62] If there is *any* cause for concern, the premature infant should not be scheduled as an outpatient.

REFERENCES

1. Gibbs P, Modell JH: Aspiration pneumonitis. *In* Miller RD (ed): Anesthesia, 2nd ed. New York, Churchill Livingstone, 1986, pp 2023–2050.
2. Janis KM: Anesthesia for the geriatric patient. ASA Refresher Course Lectures 1979; 7:143–154.
3. Manchikanti L, Colliver JA, Marrero TC, et al: Assessment of age-related acid aspiration risk factors in pediatric, adult, and geriatric patients. Anesth Analg 1985; 64:11.
4. Natof HE: Complications associated with ambulatory surgery. JAMA 1980; 244:1116–1118.
5. Goldman L, Caldera DL, Nussbaum SR, et al: Multifactorial index of cardiac risk in noncardiac surgical procedures. N Engl J Med 1977; 297:845–850.
6. Greenblatt DJ, Sellers EM, Shader RI: Drug disposition in old age. N Engl J Med 1982; 306:1081.
7. Vandam LD: To Make the Patient Ready for Anesthesia: Medical Care of the Surgical Patient, 2nd ed. Reading, Massachusetts, Addison-Wesley, 1983.
8. Levin KJ: Laboratory evaluation: What tests and why? *In* Wetchler BV (ed): Problems in Anesthesia: Outpatient Anesthesia. Philadelphia, JB Lippincott, 1988, pp 18–22.
9. Lynch S, Wolf GL, Berlin I: General anesthesia for cataract surgery: A comparative review of 2,217 consecutive cases. Anesth Analg 1974; 53:909.
10. Hamilton RC, Gimbel HV, Strunin L: Regional anesthesia for 12,000 cataract extraction and intraocular lens implantation surgical procedures. Can J Anaesth 1988; 35:615–623.
11. Beltranena HP, Vega MJ, Garcia JJ, et al: Complications of retrobulbar marcaine injection. J Clin Neuro Ophthalmol 1982; 2:159–161.
12. Rosenblatt RM, May DR, Barsoumian K: Cardiopulmonary arrest after retrobulbar block. Am J Ophthalmol 1980; 90:425–427.
13. Hamilton RC: Brain stem anesthesia following retrobulbar blockade. Anesthesiology 1985; 63:688–690.
14. Chang JL, Gonzalez-Abola E, Larson CE, Lobes L: Brain stem anesthesia following retrobulbar block. Anesthesiology 1984; 61:789–790.
15. Drysdale DB: Experimental subdural retrobulbar injection of anesthetic. Ann Ophthalmol 1984; 16:716–718.
16. Lynn JG Jr, Smith RB: Intraoperative complications and their management. Int Ophthalmol Clin 1973; 13:149–175.
17. Ramsay RC, Knoblock WH: Ocular perforation following retrobulbar anesthesia for retinal detachment surgery. Am J Ophthalmol 1978; 86:61–64.

18. Follette JW, Locascio JA: Bilateral amaurosis following unilateral retrobulbar block. Anesthesiology 1985; 63:237–238.
19. Brookshier GL, Gleitsmann KY, Schenk EC: Life-threatening complication of retrobulbar block. Ophthalmology 1986; 93:1476–1478.
20. Nicoll JMV, Acharya PA, Ahlen K, et al: Central nervous system complications after 6000 retrobulbar blocks. Anesth Analg 1987; 66:1298–1302.
21. Meyers EF, Ramirez RC, Boniu KI: Grand mal seizures after retrobulbar block. Arch Ophthalmol 1978; 96:847.
22. Beltranena HP, Vega MJ, Kirk N, et al: Inadvertent intravascular bupivacaine injection following retrobulbar block: Report of three cases. Reg Anaesth 1981; 6:149–151.
23. Cibis PA: General discussion. In Schepens CL, Regan CDL (eds): Controversial Aspects of the Management of Retinal Detachment. Boston, Little Brown, 1965, pp 223–233.
24. Zahl K, Jordan A, McGroarty J, Gotta AW: pH-Adjusted bupivacaine and hyaluronidase for peribulbar block. Anesthesiology 1990; 72:230–232.
25. Petty JM, Davies JM, Strunin L: Retrobulbar block for cataract surgery: Retrospective review of 910 patients. Anaesth Intensive Care 1984; 13:95.
26. Feibel RM: Current concepts in retrobulbar anesthesia. Surv Ophthalmol 1985; 30:102–109.
27. Davis DB, Mandel MR: Posterior peribulbar anesthesia: An alternative to retrobulbar anesthesia. J Cataract Refract Surg 1986; 12:182–184.
28. Donlon JV Jr, Moss J: Plasma catecholamine levels during local anesthesia for cataract operations. Anesthesiology 1979; 51:471–473.
29. Keenan RL: Anesthetic disasters: Incidence, causes, preventability. ASA Refresher Course Lectures, 1987; 221:1–6.
30. Kareti RKP, Callahan H, Draper GA: Factors leading to hospital admission of elderly patients following outpatient eye surgery: A Medicare dilemma. Anesth Analg 1989; 68:S144.
31. Beasley H: Hyperthermia associated with ophthalmic surgery. Am J Ophthalmol 1974; 77:76.
32. Dodd MJ, Phattiyakul P, Silpasuvan S: Suspected malignant hyperthermia in a strabismus patient. Arch Ophthalmol 1981; 99:1247.
33. France NK, France TD, Woodburn JD, et al: Succinylcholine alteration of the forced duction test. Ophthalmology 1980; 87:1282.
34. Mirakur RK, Clarke RSJ, Dundee JW, et al: Anticholinergic drugs in anesthesia—a survey of their present position. Anaesthesia 1978; 33:133.
35. Gavistaki A, Smith RM: Use of atropine in pediatric anesthesia. Int Anesthesiol Clin 1962; 1:97.
36. Joseph MC, Vale RJ: Premedication with atropine by mouth. Lancet 1960; 2:1060.
37. Meyers EF, Tomeldan SA: Glycopyrrolate compared with atropine in prevention of the oculocardiac reflex during eye muscle surgery. Anesthesiology 1979; 51:350.
38. Gibbons P, Davidson P, Adler E: Nitrous oxide does not affect postop vomiting in pediatric eye surgery. Anesthesiology 1987; 67:A530.
39. Abramowitz MD, Epstein BS, Friendly DS, et al: Effect of droperidol in reducing vomiting in pediatric strabismic outpatient surgery. Anesthesiology 1981; 59:A329.
40. Abramowitz MD, Oh TH, Epstein BS: Antiemetic effect of droperidol following outpatient strabismus surgery in children. Anesthesiology 1983; 59:579.
41. Lerman J, Eustis S, Smith DR: Effect of droperidol pretreatment on postanesthetic vomiting in children undergoing strabismus surgery. Anesthesiology 1986; 65:322–325.
42. Warner LO, Rogers GL, Martino JD, et al: Intravenous lidocaine reduces the incidence of post-strabismus vomiting in children. Anesthesiology 1988; 68:618–621.
43. Christensen S, Farrow-Gillespie A, Lerman J: Incidence of emesis and postanesthetic recovery after strabismus surgery in children: A comparison of droperidol and lidocaine. Anesthesiology 1989; 70:251–254.
44. Harrison GB, Bennet MB: Radiotherapy without tears. Br J Anaesth 1963; 35:720.
45. Browne CHW, Boulton TB, Crichton TC: Anaesthesia for radiotherapy: A frame for maintaining the airway. Anaesthesia 1969; 24:428.
46. Cronin MM, Bousfield JD, Hewett EB, et al: Ketamine anaesthesia for radiotherapy in small children. Anaesthesia 1972; 27:135.
47. Bennett JAB, Bullimore JA: Use of ketamine hydrochloride anesthesia for radiotherapy in young children. Br J Anaesth 1972; 45:197.
48. Edge WG, Morgan M: Ketamine and paediatric radiotherapy. Anaesth Intensive Care 1977; 5:153.
49. Balmer HGR, Nunn TJ: Intramuscular ketamine with hyaluronidase. Anaesthesia 1977; 32:636.
50. Hinckle AJ, Weinlander CM: Rectal mucosal injury after rectal premedication with methohexital. Anesthesiology 1984; 61:A436.
51. Brett CM, Wara WM, Hamilton WK: Anesthesia for infants during radiotherapy: An insufflation technique. Anesthesiology 1986; 64:402.
52. Patel RI, Hannallah RS: Anesthetic complications following pediatric ambulatory surgery: A 3-year study. Anesthesiology 1988; 69:1009–1012.
53. Berry FA: Pediatric outpatient anesthesia. ASA Refresher Courses Lectures 1982; 10:17–27.
54. Ahlgren EW, Bennett EJ, Stephen CR: Outpatient pediatric anesthesiology: A case series. Anesth Analg 1971; 50:402–408.
55. Davenport HT, Shah CP, Robinson GC: Day surgery for children. Can Med Assoc J 1973; 105:498–500.
56. Steward DJ: Outpatient pediatric anesthesia. Anesthesiology 1975; 43:268–276.
57. Johnson GG: Day care surgery for infants and children. Can Anaesth Soc J 1983; 30:553–557.
58. Steward DJ: Preterm infants are more prone to complications following minor surgery than are term infants. Anesthesiology 1982; 56:304–306.
59. Liu LMP, Cote CJ, Goudsouzian NG, et al: Life-threatening apnea in infants recovering from anesthesia. Anesthesiology 1983; 59:506.
60. Kurth CD, Spitzer AR, Broennle AM, Downes JJ: Postoperative apnea in preterm infants. Anesthesiology 1978; 66:483–488.
61. Epstein BS: Age limits for ambulatory surgery—do they exist? Lecture at the NYSSA, PGA, December, 1988.
62. Coté CJ: Is the ex-premature a candidate for outpatient anesthesia? Lecture at the NYSSA, PGA, December, 1988.
63. Downes JJ: Ask the experts: At what post-gestational age in a previously premature infant would it be safe to anesthetize a child as an outpatient? Newsletter Soc Pediatr Anesthesia 1989; 2:7–8.
64. Welborn LG, Hannallah RS, Fink R, et al: High dose caffeine suppresses postoperative apnea in former preterm infants. Anesthesiology 1989; 71:347–349.

New Technology: Understanding Ophthalmic Procedures and Their Anesthetic Implications

Kathryn E. McGoldrick
Jonathan Mardirossian

Rapid evolution of science and technology has contributed impressively to strides in ophthalmic surgery in the past few decades. Intraocular gas tamponade has added a new dimension to retinal detachment surgery; vitrectomy has allowed restoration of vision in eyes previously doomed to blindness. Improved operating microscopes, suture materials, and intraocular lenses have revolutionized cataract surgery. Of the estimated 640,000 cataract extractions performed in the United States in 1982, more than 70% involved intraocular lens (IOL) implantations, thus circumventing various problems associated with unilateral cataract management.[1] Just one decade later, more than 1 million such procedures are performed annually.

Neodymium:YAG laser therapy has provided a means of accomplishing iris surgery, vitreolysis for cystoid macular edema, anterior capsulotomy, repositioning of intraocular lenses, and even some posterior segment work. The gentle but powerful excimer laser (the abbreviation for "excited dimers," or the two atoms of an inert gas in an unstable association with halogen atoms) may actually be able to sculpt, or recontour, the cornea. It may then be able to make cuts of incredible minuteness to correct—without scarring—myopia, hyperopia, astigmatism, and blinding corneal scars. Unlike radial keratotomy, which penetrates 90% of corneal thickness, the excimer laser with its highly energetic ultraviolet light photon disturbs only 10%, or 50–60 μm, of corneal tissue.

The prostaglandins dinoprostone and dinoprost, endogenous substances released following ocular irritation, are capable of causing vasodilation, increased vascular permeability, and increased intraocular pressure (IOP).[2] Studies have indicated that disorders of platelet function and microangiopathy are associated with prostaglandins and may be involved in diabetic retinopathy.[3]

Improved anesthetic care has also been part of the technological advances that have enhanced surgical safety and outcome for ophthalmic patients. Anesthesiologists are increasingly aware of the intricacies of intraocular physiology and the effects of anesthetic drugs and manipulations on intraocular dynamics. Sophisticated monitoring equipment has added dimensions of safety to anesthetic armamentarium. New drugs to ameliorate or prevent postoperative nausea and vomiting have helped to protect the results of delicate surgery.

In this chapter, technological advances in ophthalmic diagnosis, surgery, and other treatment modalities are discussed, along with germane features of anesthetic management.

MAGNETIC RESONANCE IMAGING

Magnetic resonance imaging (MRI)—formerly called nuclear magnetic resonance (NMR)—is a relatively recently developed noninvasive diagnostic technique that employs a strong magnetic field and radiofrequency (RF) pulses to generate images. Initial reports indicate effectiveness of the technique in producing high-contrast images. MRI can often see what computed tomography (CT) can not show and is said to excel, for example, in diagnosing brainstem tumors with bone distortion. MRI is employed in some ophthalmic diagnostic work, but its usefulness is somewhat limited to the localization of nonferrous intraocular or intraorbital foreign bodies and lesions of the optic nerve and chiasm. MRI is contraindicated in the evaluation of magnetic intraocular and intraorbital foreign bodies, because the potential for motion of the magnetic foreign body during the test exposes the eye to the risk of additional damage. CT is the preferred test for the evaluation of magnetic foreign bodies.

MRI is contraindicated in patients with cardiac pacemakers, intravascular wires, neurovascular aneurysm clips, and cochlear implants.[4] For example, potential problems with cardiac pacemakers during MRI scanning include possible reed switch closure or damage, pacemaker inhibition or reversion to an asynchronous pacing mode, programming changes, torque on the pacemaker, or development of a voltage across the pacemaker leads.[5, 6] If cerebral vascular aneurysm clips contain ferromagnetic material, these could become displaced while under the influence of the magnetic field.[7]

One of the purported advantages of MRI is that magnetic fields cause no known injury to living organisms. However, the placement of ferromagnetic objects, such as tools, near the scanner is dangerous, because these objects could be attracted toward the center of the magnetic field and cause injury to patients and attending personnel or damage equipment.[8] For example, small items, such as safety pins, may be unexpectedly launched through the air at the scanner and the patient. Larger items, such as intravenous (IV) poles or chairs, can be propelled toward the scanner or tightly adhere.[9]

Patient monitoring during scanning poses problems, because ferrous metal (e.g., iron, cobalt, nickel, and some forms of stainless steel) contained in a wide assortment of monitoring equipment can distort the magnetic field. ECG and other monitoring wires attached to the patient and leaving the scanner act as antennae for stray RF signals.[10] Both these disturbances of MRI function may result in image degradation. Another concern is patient access. The patient, who is placed on the scanner couch and moved into a cylinder opening within the scanner, becomes virtually inaccessible. A cylindric shield used to reduce RF interference is pulled out from the opening, further isolating the patient. It is not unusual for the patient's head to be as much as 25 m from the opening.

Typically, adult patients are placed inside the MRI scanner and monitored by closed-circuit television and a two-way intercommunication system. However, seriously ill or obtunded patients and children may require sedation or ventilatory assistance or general anesthesia and more extensive monitoring. In the imaging suite, equipment to suction, monitor, ventilate, and resuscitate according to the standards adhered to in the operating room must be present.

The influence of the MRI scanner on equipment depends on the strength of the MRI magnetic field, the equipment's proximity to the scanner, the amount of ferromagnetic material it contains, and the design of its electrical circuitry. There is a strong pull by the magnet on the typical anesthesia machine, especially on the gas cylinders, because of the presence of a large amount of ferromagnetic material. Thus, the machine should be outfitted with aluminum tanks. The magnetic pull does not affect the functioning of the anesthetic machines or the oxygen monitor if the machine is kept in the corner of the room approximately 20 ft from the bore. A simple Mapleson D-system interposing a 6-m-long inspiratory limb to administer anesthetic gases, incorporating an aluminum expiratory valve, works nicely.[11]

A brass precordial stethoscope with plastic tubing may be used, although the sounds of RF partially interfere with the quality of the heart sounds. Oscillatory blood pressures can easily be obtained by adding long wide-bore tubing to the cuff and using brass or plastic adapters for the junctions, taking care to keep the dial away from the magnet. A special wireless electrocardiogram (ECG) provides adequate display in the absence of a RF signal, which produces considerable background noise. Only minor modifications, such as using longer tubing and switching the motor to high power, are needed for carbon dioxide (CO_2) monitors that use a suctioning mechanism to sample gases. Any of the commercially available liquid crystal thermometers can be used to determine the skin temperature. Unfortunately, pulse oximetry interferes with the performance of the MRI scanner and is affected by the scanner. Some have suggested correcting this by using a fiberoptic pulse oximeter, but the fiberoptic cable acts as an antenna, carrying stray signals in both directions. Vacanti has postulated that by shielding the cable of the oximeter, the monitor will not distort the image of the MRI scanner.[11] Recently, Ohmeda has produced the MRI-compatible Biox 3700 pulse oximeter, which functions well when the probe is placed on the digit most remote from the bore of the magnet.

A recent advance has been the development of the MRI-compatible Ohmeda Excel 210 anesthesia machine. All ferromagnetic material in the Ohmeda Excel 210 model has been replaced with aluminum or nonmagnetic stainless steel. Recently approved by the Food and Drug Administration and now commercially available, this machine can be used safely in the 1.5-tesla magnetic field. The use of the machine near the magnet does not disturb image quality.

Many anesthetic techniques can be used during MRI. Rectal methohexital (30 mg/kg) or intramuscular (IM) methohexital (10 mg/kg) is often satisfactory. General endotracheal anesthesia may also be administered with any appropriate agent.

In the event of cardiac arrest, resuscitation of the patient in or near the MRI scanner poses problems. ECGs, defibrillators, pacemakers, and perfusion pumps may malfunction. In such circumstances, the magnetic field of a resistive magnet can be turned off quickly. However, several hours are needed to restore a stable magnetic field before routine scans can be continued. Magnetic fields produced by superconducting magnets cannot be turned off, so arrested patients must be removed from the vicinity of the magnet.[10]

VISUAL-EVOKED POTENTIALS AND ELECTRORETINOGRAPHY

Although anesthetic agents affect the results of certain measurements and visual-evoked potentials (VEPs), it is sometimes necessary to assess VEPs in anesthetized patients. For example, VEPs in sedated or anesthetized patients are useful for detecting amblyopia or certain other conditions in uncooperative infants and children. During neurosurgical procedures involving visual pathways, such as trans-sphenoidal and anterior fossa surgery, the VEP monitors the integrity of the visual pathways.[12, 13]

The VEP is elicited by flashes coming from light-emitting diodes that are mounted on goggles over the patient's closed eyes. The resulting evoked potentials have a prominent positive peak with a latency of approximately 100 ms from the onset of the stimuli. This peak, which is called the P1 or P100, is thought to be generated in the striated and parastriated visual cortex and is considered to be a sensitive measure of the integrity of the visual pathways.[14]

Several authors have described the effects of anesthetics on VEP.[15–18] Uhl and colleagues[16] demonstrated that the latency of the P1 in the VEP is longer with increasing concentrations of halothane.[16] Burchiel and associates[17] reported an increased amplitude of the VEP during enflurane anesthesia, whereas Chi and Field[18] demonstrated a marked decrease in amplitude of the VEP at high concentrations of isoflurane. Chi and Field also reported that the latency of the P1 was prolonged at or above 0.9% isoflurane, and they found no consistent influence of nitrous oxide (N_2O) on evoked potentials. In general, cortical-evoked potentials are more sensitive to the effects of anesthetic agents than are the subcortical ones, such as brain-stem auditory-evoked potentials.

Russ and coworkers[19] showed that neuroleptanalgesia with fentanyl, droperidol, and N_2O increased the latency of the P2 (the second prominent peak, with a latency of approximately 170 ms from the onset of stimuli) by 10% without producing significant changes in amplitude. To minimize the effects of isoflurane during monitoring of VEP, its concentration may be decreased and supplemental relaxants or opioids administered, if necessary.

Electroretinography (ERG) is a means of gaining valuable information about the functional state of the retina. ERG appears to be affected by anesthetics also, and these influences must be considered when the ophthalmologist is interpreting the results of ERG testing.

GLAUCOMA

Glaucoma is an insidious, curious, and relentless disease. Despite impressive advances in treatment, glaucoma remains an inscrutable enemy of sight. According to the National Society to Prevent Blindness, more than 62,000 cases of blindness in the United States are attributable to glaucoma. The number of known cases of glaucoma-related blindness rises by 5400 per year. Experts estimate that 2 million Americans have the disease and suffer from some form of visual impairment, and that an additional 1 million cases are undiagnosed. Because glaucoma is exacerbated by the aging process, the prevalence of glaucoma seems likely to increase as the elderly population in America increases. Because there are many forms of the disease, each with its inherent characteristics, the search for a cure or cures is extremely challenging, and thus far, the goal remains elusive. Although there is no way to prevent or cure glaucoma yet, the disease is controllable, particularly if detected early.

Primary open-angle glaucoma (POAG) is the most common form, accounting for up to 80% of all cases of glaucoma in the United States. In POAG, aqueous humor is unable to pass through the trabecular meshwork because of an abnormality in that tissue. POAG is characterized by elevated (above 22 mmHg) IOP, optic nerve damage, and visual field defects. The patient may experience blurred vision or a gradual vision loss, and the disease usually follows a chronic, insidious course. Symptoms may not be evident until the later stages, making POAG the most difficult form of glaucoma to diagnose.

Primary closed-angle glaucoma is characterized by a shallow anterior chamber and a narrow angle that impedes the exit of aqueous humor from the eye. A sharp increase in IOP causes a suddenly painful red eye, blurred vision, and iridescent vision, in which the patient sees halos around lights.

Ocular hypertension is present when the IOP is elevated but there is no optic nerve damage or visual field loss. Often, patients in this category are referred to as "glaucoma suspects," because serious injury, including visual field loss, may eventually occur if the IOP remains elevated over a protracted period.

Secondary glaucomas develop as the result of another major ocular problem that is the identifiable cause of the glaucoma. These etiologies include trauma, inflammation, ocular ischemia, and intraocular hemorrhage.

Developmental or congenital glaucoma may be caused by a membrane blocking the chamber angle or some other structural abnormality. Afflicted infants frequently present with epiphora, photophobia, blepharospasm, irritability, and buphthalmos. Eighty percent of cases of congenital glaucoma are inherited in an autosomal recessive pattern. In addition, congenital glaucoma may be associated with various other eye diseases or developmental anomalies, such as aniridia and retinopathy of prematurity (ROP). (Numerous systemic diseases may be linked with glaucoma, and these include the mucopolysaccharidoses, the Stickler syndrome, and Marfan's syndrome.)

Juvenile glaucoma is similar to POAG and occurs in older children and young adults under 30 years of age.

TREATMENT OF POAG

Adult glaucoma therapy can involve three stages, depending on the individual patient. The first step is drug therapy, which is often an effective way of lowering IOP. Glaucoma medications include four major categories of drugs: adrenergics, anticholinesterases, carbonic anhydrase inhibitors, and cholinergics (Table 20–1). The adrenergics include β blockers (e.g., timolol and betaxolol), which block specific cellular sites involved in aqueous humor formation, and epinephrine, which stimulates specific sites on the cells of the inflow and outflow tissues, causing an increase in outflow of aqueous humor. Carbonic anhydrase inhibitors, such as acetazolamide (DIAMOX), methazolamide (NEPTAZANE), or dichlorphenamide (DARANIDE), are taken orally, unlike the adrenergics, anticholinesterases, and cholinergics, which are administered as topical drops. However, topical carbonic anhydrase inhibitors may soon be available commercially. The carbonic anhydrase inhibitors block an enzyme involved in aqueous humor formation. Cholinergics (e.g., PILOCAR or ISOPTO CARPINE) contract the eye's ciliary muscle and open the outflow channel to facilitate aqueous egress. Cholinergics also con-

TABLE 20–1. Categories of Drugs to Combat Glaucoma

Adrenergics
β Blockers
Epinephrine
Anticholinesterases
Cholinergics
Carbonic anhydrase inhibitors

strict the pupil, reducing the amount of light that enters the eye, and therefore may cause difficulty for older patients with cataracts or other visual impairment. Anticholinesterases (e.g., PHOSPHOLINE IODIDE) likewise constrict the sphincter pupillae muscle and facilitate aqueous humor outflow.

If the patient is at the maximum level of drug therapy and the IOP is still not sufficiently lowered, the next step may be laser treatment. Laser therapy is usually relatively painless and can be performed in the ophthalmologist's office following topical application of one or two drops of a local anesthetic such as proparacaine. Laser light directed at the trabecular meshwork effects an expansion of the pores of this tissue, thus augmenting aqueous humor outflow. This form of treatment is effective in approximately 80% of adults, and its therapeutic efficacy can be permanent in many cases.

If the effects of laser therapy begin to diminish, some patients may require additional laser treatments. For others, a third treatment form, filtration surgery, may be required. During this procedure, the physician surgically creates a valve in the wall of the eye using existing eye tissue, providing the aqueous humor an exit route from the anterior chamber.

Unfortunately, surgically created drainage holes have a tendency to close. To combat this problem, Johns Hopkins University researchers have developed a biodegradable implant that delivers an antiproliferation drug to keep the holes patent. The disk-shaped polymer, about 3 mm in diameter and 1 mm thick, is placed on the surface of the sclera near the holes. As the polymer dissolves, it releases its drug that prevents cellular multiplication. Although the polymer implant is still in the experimental stage, it offers hope to some patients with advanced, refractory glaucoma.

Glaucoma filtering surgery is a delicate intraocular procedure that requires perfect akinesia. Either regional or general anesthesia may be selected. Other anesthetic concerns include proper control of IOP, perioperative instillation of miotics, and avoidance of both overhydration and hypotension. (Hypotension is thought to be especially detrimental because these patients are purportedly vulnerable to retinal artery thrombosis.) In addition, the anesthesiologist must be cognizant of the systemic side effects of antiglaucoma medication (see Chapter 17). Complications of glaucoma surgery include bleeding, infection, chronic inflammation, early or late increase in IOP, possible cataract formation or worsening of pre-existing cataract, and visual loss.

A possible alternative to filtration surgery may involve a special type of laser procedure called a *laser filter*. This procedure eliminates the need for an incision and minimizes the likelihood of postoperative failure. This noninvasive procedure can be performed under local anesthesia in the ophthalmologist's office. Currently, the pulsed-dye laser appears to offer promise in this area. (This unique laser contains dye and therefore can be "tuned" according to the wavelength or color to which a target eye tissue will best respond.)

TREATMENT OF PRIMARY CLOSED-ANGLE GLAUCOMA

Acute angle-closure glaucoma is treated medically with IV mannitol and topical pilocarpine, which constricts the ciliary body.

Chronic angle-closure glaucoma is treated with topical antiglaucoma drugs and, in severe cases, surgery.

TREATMENT OF CONGENITAL AND INFANTILE GLAUCOMA

Unlike POAG, the treatment of congenital and infantile glaucoma is primarily surgical, and surgery should be performed as early as the child's general medical condition permits. Various types of operations can be elected to reduce or control IOP, and these include goniotomy or even trabeculectomy.

Multiple procedures may be required. Even following surgery, long-term medical therapy is often mandatory. Visual prognosis depends on normalization of IOP and prevention of optic nerve damage. Attention must also be directed to correction of associated refractive errors and treatment of amblyopia. Unfortunately, pediatric patients with glaucoma frequently have concomitant complicating factors, such as cataracts, corneal opacities, and retinal and optic nerve abnormalities, that further dim visual prognosis.

The anesthetic management of patients undergoing surgery for congenital glaucoma is discussed in depth in Chapter 15.

CATARACTS

A cataract is an opacity of the crystalline lens secondary to changes in the lens fibers. The word cataract is derived from the Greek word *katarrhegnynai,* meaning "to break down."

Although congenital cataracts are not rare

and may be caused by a variety of chromosomal, hereditary, infectious, inflammatory, metabolic, and nutritional factors, the incidence of cataract disease increases with age. Whereas the overall incidence of cataract-induced visual reduction to 20/30 or less in one study[20] of subjects aged 52–85 years was 15.5%, the incidence of cataract disease defined by the same parameters in the 75–85 year age group was 46%. In the United States alone, approximately 4 million people have a vision-disrupting cataract.

PATHOPHYSIOLOGY

The aging process produces progressive physiological changes in the lens, specifically, increases in density, weight, and size. However, these alterations must be differentiated from the pathophysiological changes that occur with cataract disease, each of which defines a specific type of cataract (Table 20–2). For example, an exaggeration of the normal hardening of fibers in the lens nucleus produces a nuclear cataract, a common variety that accounts for approximately 25% of all senile cataracts.[21]

Cataracts may be further described by their degree of maturity, which is assessed according to the biochemical status of the lens protein. An incipient cataract exhibits increased fluid accumulation between the lens fibers. Whereas an immature cataract still has some transparent protein, a mature cataract is characterized by the complete opacity of all lens protein. In a hypermature cataract, some cortical protein actually becomes soluble.

TABLE 20–2. Pathophysiologic Changes in the Lens

Type of Cataract	Change
Anterior subcapsular	Fibrous metaplasia of lens epithelium
Anterior polar	Subcapsular and capsular cataracts (usually congenital)
Anterior cortical	Liquefaction of lens fibers and development of Morgagni's globules anteriorly in cortex
Nuclear sclerotic	Exaggerated sclerosis of fibers in lens nucleus
Posterior cortical	Liquefaction and globular degeneration of posterior lens cortex
Posterior subcapsular	Posterior migration of epithelial cells under the capsule, forming large, irregular nucleated or bladder cells (commonly associated with drugs and metabolic diseases)

Cataract progression may be accelerated by various systemic conditions, such as poorly controlled diabetes mellitus. The latter condition produces osmotic changes in the lens.

EVALUATION OF CATARACT DISEASE

Cataracts may be either congenital or acquired. Although acquired cataracts are most commonly idiopathic, other causes include systemic disease (diabetes, hypocalcemia), trauma, radiation, drugs (e.g., corticosteroids), toxins (metals), and argon laser therapy.[22]

Cataracts typically cause a progressive loss of vision rather than the more abrupt visual loss frequently noted with primary retinal, vascular, or optic nerve disease. (However, patients with severe juvenile diabetes may develop cataracts over a time course measured in hours.) If cataract disease is suspected, an ophthalmological consultation can determine the presence, nature, and severity of lens opacity and establish the degree of visual compromise.

THERAPY FOR ADULT CATARACTS

Once the diagnosis is established, treatment may be medical, surgical, or both. Medical management is aimed at restricting progression of the disease, for example, by controlling hyperglycemia or restricting steroid use. Other crucial medical elements are optimal refraction, patient education, and regular observation of the patient's condition.

Surgical treatment of cataracts has been performed for at least 3000 years. Indications for surgery depend on the severity and maturity of the cataract, the patient's general health, whether lens-induced glaucoma or uveitis is present, and whether the cataract is interfering with the ability to diagnose or treat disease in the posterior segment. The patient's visual need in relation to visual disability must be weighed, as should the prognosis for visual improvement. The patient should be informed that complications may occur with cataract surgery, including hemorrhage, loss of corneal clarity, chronic inflammation, infection, temporary or permanent blurring of vision owing to retinal edema, retinal detachment, glaucoma, or double vision. These and other complications may occur whether or not a lens is implanted and may result in poor vision, total loss of vision, or loss of the eye. Lens implantation may also result in inability to dilate the pupil and dislocation of the lens. In the future, the intraocular lens may have to be repositioned or surgically removed.

The two surgical approaches to cataract extraction are intracapsular and extracapsular. The former entails removal of the entire lens along with its surrounding transparent capsule. With the latter procedure, the transparent posterior capsule is not removed. Extracapsular extraction is the more popular technique, because it has a lower risk of retinal detachment, allows implantation of a posterior chamber lens, and may have a lower rate of postoperative cystoid macular edema.

Extracapsular cataract surgery consists of two major steps. A 3-mm corneal incision is made, through which is inserted an ultrasonically activated titanium cannula that emulsifies the nucleus and cortex of the lens. This debris is then aspirated from the eye. Next, the incision is enlarged to 7 mm to allow positioning of the intraocular lens. Anterior chamber, iris-plane, and posterior chamber are the three types of intraocular lenses currently available. Of these, the most popular is the posterior chamber lens, which more closely approximates the position of the normal lens.

During cataract surgery, regardless of whether the procedure involves an intracapsular or an extracapsular approach, maximal pupillary dilation is essential. Unfortunately, the iris is sensitive to manipulation and responds by constricting. A mydriatic infusion is helpful in counteracting this response.

The anesthetic management for adult cataract surgery is discussed in Chapter 19.

TREATMENT OF CONGENITAL CATARACTS

The treatment of cataracts in infants and children whose vision is significantly impaired involves (1) surgical removal of lens material to provide an optically clear visual axis; (2) correction of the resultant aphakic refractive error with spectacles, contact lenses, intraocular lens implantation, or perhaps refractive corneal surgery; and (3) treatment of any associated sensory deprivation amblyopia, which may be the most challenging goal to attain in the child's visual rehabilitation. Prognosis is contingent upon a variety of factors, including the presence and nature of any associated ocular anomalies, such as microphthalmia, retinal lesions, optic atrophy, or nystagmus. In addition, affected children may have skeletal, car-

diac, renal, or central nervous system disorders that further complicate their long-term prognosis. However, the possibility of deprivation amblyopia can be reduced by surgically removing congenital cataracts as soon as the neonate's medical condition permits.

Congenital cataracts are characteristically soft and are removed by aspiration rather than extraction. The surgeon makes two incisions in the limbus, one for irrigation and the other for aspiration. The cataract cortex is then sucked out through the capsulotomy. Because the vitreous is a firm gel that is adherent to the lens capsule, in youngsters there is a high risk of vitreous loss if an intracapsular cataract removal is attempted. This delicate intraocular procedure demands maximal pupillary dilation and meticulous anesthetic management, which is presented in detail in Chapter 15.

RETINAL DETACHMENT

Retinal detachments are classified according to their type: traction, exudative, or rhegmatogenous. Traction retinal detachments are the most common type found in the pediatric age group and are usually seen in association with ROP, diabetes, and sickle cell retinopathy. In adults, traction retinal detachment is frequently encountered with either type I or type II diabetes mellitus or with sickle cell retinopathy.

Exudative retinal detachments are seen with a variety of diseases in adults, including tumors (metastatic from the breast or lung), primary melanoma, the rare inflammatory condition known as Harada's disease, uveal effusion syndrome, scleritis, and central serous retinopathy. In pediatric patients, exudative retinal detachment may be associated with conditions such as retinoblastoma, choroidal hemangioma, angiomatosis retinae, and severe renal disease.

Rhegmatogenous retinal detachments, caused by retinal tears, are common in myopic adults, and they may also occur in adults following cataract surgery or following trauma. (Intracapsular cataract extraction has approximately a 2–3% incidence of postoperative retinal detachment, whereas with extracapsular cataract extraction the incidence varies between ½–1%.) Rhegmatogenous retinal detachments are not common in the pediatric age group, but when they do occur they are usually secondary to trauma, such as contusion of the globe. However, pediatric rhegmatogenous retinal detachment may also be secondary to myopia, aphakia, and ROP.

Rhegmatogenous retinal detachment is preceded by a tiny hole or tear in the retina, which may become detached if the vitreous floats the retina off from the pigment epithelium (Fig. 20–1). Symptoms associated with these retinal tears include "floaters" caused by vitreous separation and "flashes," or photopsia, caused by traction of the vitreous pulling on the retina. These small tears may be treated prophylactically by retinal cryotherapy applied through the sclera or with laser photocoagulation. Laser therapy is popular to prevent retinal detachment in this setting. Lasers coagulate tissue protein, causing retinal burns, which seal the retinal breach by forming a chorioretinal scar. The laser wavelength determines which ocular tissue maximally absorbs the laser light energy. Argon green laser energies are useful for peripheral retinal work and some iris lesions. Argon green laser energies should filter out blue wavelengths, which may cause significant damage to the superficial layers of the retina. Krypton red laser energies are useful for macular work. Krypton red's longer wavelengths cause even less damage to superficial retinal layers, an important fact in treatment of the macula. One of the advantages of laser therapy is that it can be conveniently performed in the ophthalmologist's office, following the topical instillation of one or two drops of 0.5% proparacaine. However, if laser treatment involving the macular region is indicated, some suggest performance of a retrobulbar block to ensure reliable akinesia.

Symptoms of full-blown retinal detachment may include showers of black specks, photopsia, and finally a dark shadow or cloud that impinges on the field of vision.

During retinal detachment surgery, the retina is first apposed to pigment epithelium by cryotherapy or diathermy. Then, the scleral buckle is positioned over the retinal tears and sutured in place to cover every retinal tear. Next, the subretinal fluid is drained, if necessary, by perforating the sclera and choroid, and the retina falls back against the scleral buckle, which closes the tears.

Alternatively, a nondrainage scleral buckling procedure involves suturing a compressible scleral buckle in a similar fashion, which then expands postoperatively as the eye becomes hypotonous over the next 12 hours. The increased indentation caused by the expanded buckle pushes the pigment epithelium against the detached retina and closes the holes (Fig. 20–2).

Retinal detachment surgery is predominantly extraocular, although it may briefly become intraocular if the sclera and choroid are perforated. Because a soft eye during detachment surgery is desirable, acetazolamide or mannitol is sometimes administered to lower IOP. Although retinal detachment surgery may be performed under retrobulbar anesthesia, many favor general anesthesia, especially if the detachment is posterior or if the surgery is expected to exceed 2 hours. Rotation of the globe with traction on the extraocular muscles is necessary during detachment surgery, and this maneuver may stimulate the

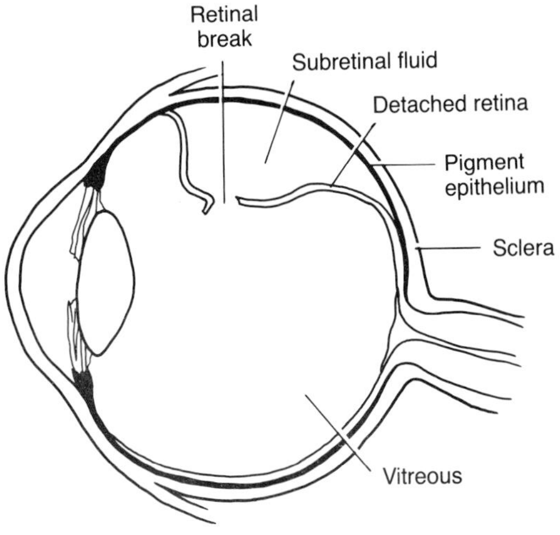

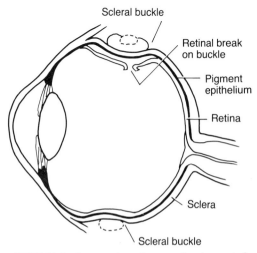

FIGURE 20–1. *Cross-section of an eye showing a retinal break, with the partially detached retina above.*

FIGURE 20–2. *Cross-section of an eye showing an indentation of the sclera with an encircling scleral buckle that has closed the break and reattached the retina.*

oculocardiac reflex. Therefore, the anesthesiologist must carefully monitor and, if necessary, treat any associated dysrhythmias.

In recent years the use of intraocular gases, such as air, sulfur hexafluoride (SF_6), and the perfluorohydrocarbons, has gained popularity as an adjunct to scleral buckling surgery. (Alternatively, silicone oil, functioning as a vitreous substitute, may be injected to effect internal tamponade of retinal breaks.) Many retinologists favor the use of these expanding gases for internal tamponade of the retinal tears in cases in which the tears have not come into complete contact with the underlying scleral buckle. The surface tension of the gas bubble internally occludes the tear, allowing the pigment epithelium pump to evacuate the subretinal fluid. The retina subsequently flattens and comes into contact with the scleral buckle, and the tears become closed.

Owing to blood gas partition coefficient differences, the administration of N_2O intraoperatively enhances the internal tamponade effect of SF_6, only to be followed by a marked reduction in IOP and gas bubble volume postoperatively when N_2O is discontinued. The injected SF_6 bubble, in the presence of concomitant N_2O anesthesia, can produce a dramatic and rapid increase in IOP, reaching a peak within 24 minutes,[23–25] which may be of sufficient magnitude to compromise retinal circulation. Stinson and Donlon[24] recommended discontinuing N_2O approximately 15 minutes prior to gas injection. Wolf and colleagues[25] stated that if a patient requires anesthesia after intravitreous SF_6 injection, N_2O should be omitted for 10 days. If an air bubble rather than SF_6 is injected, N_2O may be administered after the fifth postoperative day. Likewise, octafluorocyclobutane (C_4F_8) remains in the vitreous cavity for more than 13 days,[26] and perfluoropropane (C_3F_8) lingers for longer than 30 days.[27, 28]

Intravitreous gas injection has been a valuable aid to the retina surgeon. Many eyes that previously required reoperation with revision of scleral buckling can now be successfully managed by either an intraoperative or a postoperative intravitreous injection of a small volume of one of these expanding gases. In fact, a postoperative injection can be accomplished after injecting a small bleb of local anesthesia over the pars plana.

In an attempt to bring retinal surgery into the ambulatory setting, pneumatic retinopexy has gained some notoriety recently as a means to achieve primary repair of retinal detachments by exclusive internal tamponade of the retinal tears without the accompanying support and relief of vitreous traction provided by scleral buckling. However, this operation has not become popular because of its selective usefulness and high complication rate, including failure of reattachment, creation of multiple new retinal tears, proliferative vitreoretinopathy, and subretinal accumulation of gas.

Another approach for selected cases has been the safer Lincoff balloon scleral buckling operation. Following application of cryotherapy around the retinal tear, a small balloon catheter, similar to a Fogarty catheter, is placed through a snip incision in the conjunctiva. The deflated balloon tip of the catheter is positioned over the tear, on the outer surface of the globe, under observation with the indirect ophthalmoscope. The balloon is gradually inflated with saline through the catheter, which remains taped to the patient's forehead. The indentation effect is the same as that provided by a permanent scleral buckle. During the next week, the retina reattaches, and the cryotherapy reaction takes hold. The balloon is gradually deflated and removed. Temporary relief of vitreous traction allows for reattachment of the retina, and the cryotherapy, in effect, has welded the retina to the wall of the eye, providing continued attachment of the retina after the balloon scleral buckle has been removed. Unlike pneumatic retinopexy, the Lincoff procedure is a totally extraocular one, because the vitreous cavity is not entered. It has a negligible complication rate and may be performed under either local or general anesthesia.

In more complicated retinal detachments, vitrectomy surgery with a suction-cutting instrument may noticeably improve the success rate in cases such as giant retinal tears (those exceeding 90 degrees where the retina can fold over on itself), in penetrating injuries, and in cases with massive periretinal proliferation.

Scleral buckling results in anatomical reattachment of the retina in 85–95% of cases. A majority of patients require only one operation but, occasionally, multiple surgical procedures may be necessary. The visual results of detachment surgery, however, are less impressive and depend to a large extent on the patient's preoperative visual acuity and whether the macula was involved. When the macula is detached, especially for longer than 24–48 hours, the return of central vision may be limited, even though the retina has been anatomically reattached.

Possible complications of retina surgery include infection, vitreous hemorrhage, glaucoma, corneal defects, cataract, ptosis, diplopia, extrusion of the scleral buckle, loss of vision, and loss of the eye.

SURGERY FOR GIANT RETINAL TEARS

Occasionally, giant retinal tears may be operated on with both the patient and the surgeon in unusual positions to allow gravity to assist in reattaching the retina. The use of an intravitreous injection of air or another gas may also be helpful in achieving the ophthalmic goal. The patient may be strapped to a special table and operated on face-down, or in a steep head-up or head-down tilt according to the site of the lesion. In 1965, Schepens and associates[29] designed and described a power-driven, multipositional operating table. In 1981, Peyman[30] developed an operating table that can rotate 360 degrees around its longitudinal and transverse axes. Supposedly, when this table is used in conjunction with an intravitreous gas injection, a giant break can be tamponaded, regardless of its location.

Fortunately, the patient with a giant tear requiring these specialized approaches tolerates the postural changes quite well. Because this surgery may extend over several hours, general anesthesia is indicated. The endotracheal tube should be meticulously positioned and secured in these cases. If patients are well hydrated prior to turning, only minimal changes in vital signs are usually noted. Most commonly, a slight increase in pulse rate is observed. Furthermore, corrugated rubber extension tubing to attach to the circle system should be readily available to provide the extra length necessary during turning. IV extension tubing should also be employed, and a high pole on which to hang infusion bags during turning should be available.

VITRECTOMY

Vitreous surgery was initially developed in the 1970s and is constantly being refined. By placing a contact lens on the cornea and employing the operating microscope, the surgeon is able to view into the vitreous cavity. Instruments are then inserted into the eye, sometimes after a corneal section (open sky), or more commonly through the pars plana region of the ciliary body. By manipulating various instruments, the surgeon is able to remedy the ocular abnormality, and the vitreous may be removed in order to provide a clearer pathway for light to the retina. (A sterile balanced salt solution is infused as a vitreous substitute.) Among the main indications for vitreous surgery are complicated retinal detachments, intraocular foreign bodies, diabetic membranes, ROP, and proliferative vitreoretinopathy. Possible complications of vitrectomy include retinal detachment, vitreous hemorrhage, infection, glaucoma, corneal clouding and scarring, cataract, ptosis, diplopia, and visual loss.

The principles of anesthetic management are those that apply to any case of intraocular surgery.

OPEN SKY VITRECTOMY

Because open sky vitrectomy allows direct access to retrolental membranes and provides a superb view, this procedure is well suited for treating severe retinal detachment in ROP. Schepens used this approach as early as 1973.[31] Other indications for open sky vitrectomy, besides ROP, include the presence of an extremely large intraocular foreign body, severe massive preretinal retraction (MPR), bullous keratopathy with MPR, retinal incarceration in a corneal or limbal wound, and giant tears extending more than 270 degrees.

Hirose and Schepens (personal communication, 1986) have reported some success with extremely difficult cases of ROP when thick white membranes obscure fundal view and compromise the anterior segment. Previously, these cases had been considered inoperable. The surgeon trephines the cornea, keeping it in tissue culture during the vitrectomy; performs iridotomies at the 12 and 6 o'clock meridians; and extracts the lens with a cryo probe. Following lens extraction, the retrolental membrane and much of the tissue filling the funnel of the totally detached retina are cut and removed. Hyaluronic acid is then injected, forcing the retina to settle down, and concomitantly, the retinal folds are stretched to become smooth. After iridotomy closure, the corneal button is removed from tissue culture fluid and sutured into its original position with 10-0 nylon.

Hirose and Schepens believe the success of open sky vitrectomy in reattaching a totally detached retina in patients with ROP varies greatly, depending on the configuration of the detachment. A much better anatomical success rate has been achieved in total retinal detachment with an open funnel rather than in detachment with a closed funnel. These distinguished retina surgeons believe that open sky vitrectomy has major advantages over closed vitrectomy for treating retinal detachment caused by severe cicatricial ROP. The open technique permits the surgeon to approach the retrolental membrane directly by opening the cornea and removing the lens, thus both facilitating and enabling complete removal of this membrane. The wide exposure of the operative field allows convenient latitude of movement with the surgical instruments and the freedom to interchange them as needed.

Anesthetic management of premature infants undergoing this 3-hour or longer surgical procedure centers on the judicious administration of a volatile anesthetic agent, N_2O, and oxygen, or a balanced technique. Because this is an extremely delicate intraocular procedure, neuromuscular paralysis with a nondepolarizing muscle relaxant is advised for the duration of the intraocular part. IV fluids should be titrated carefully, and meticulous monitoring of ECG, blood pressure, temperature, oxygen saturation, and end-tidal CO_2 is mandatory. The infant's temperature should be maintained at or above 37°C, because hypothermia may result in acidosis, hypoxia, anesthetic overdose, and postoperative obtundation. The trachea is not extubated until the infant is fully awake, because these premature infants have impaired central control of respiration. They respond to hypoxia in a deleterious fashion by reducing their minute ventilation rather than by hyperventilating. Furthermore, the slope of their CO_2 response curve is diminished.

In view of the frequency of apneic or bradycardic episodes in premature infants, apnea monitors and electrocardiographic monitoring are employed for 12 to over 24 hours following surgery, depending on the infant's postconceptional age, history, and perioperative behavior.

Long-term observation and careful evaluation and documentation of visual function as well as anatomical result are needed to assess the efficacy of open sky vitrectomy in this setting. Initial impressions, however, have shown promise.

REFERENCES

1. Stark WJ, Leske ML, Worthen DM, et al: Trends in cataract surgery and intraocular lenses in the United States. Am J Ophthalmol 1983; 96:304–310.

2. Kass M, Podos S, Moses R, et al: Prostaglandin E_1 and aqueous humor dynamics. Invest Ophthalmol Vis Sci 1972; 11:1022–1027.
3. Lane LS, Lahav M, Janson P, et al: Abnormalities in plasma platelet factors in patients with diabetes mellitus. Invest Ophthalmol Vis Sci 1982; 22(Suppl):110.
4. Abrams HL: Cochlear implants are a contraindication to MRI. JAMA 1989; 261:46.
5. Pavlicek W, Geisinger M, Castle L, et al: The effects of nuclear magnetic resonance on patients with cardiac pacemakers. Radiology 1983; 147:149–153.
6. Fetter J, Aram G, Holmes DR Jr, et al: Nuclear magnetic resonance imaging of external and implantable cardiac pacemakers. Chest 1983; 84:345.
7. New PFJ, Rosen BR, Brady TJ, et al: Potential hazards and artifacts of ferromagnetic and nonferromagnetic surgical and dental materials and devices in NMR imaging. Radiology 1983; 147:139–148.
8. Kaufman L, Crooks L, Sheldon P, et al: The potential impact of nuclear magnetic resonance imaging on cardiovascular diagnosis. Circulation 1983; 67:251–257.
9. Geiger RS, Cascorbi HF: Anesthesia in an NMR scanner. Anesth Analg 1984; 63:622–623.
10. Roth JL, Nugent M, Gray JE, et al: Patient monitoring during magnetic resonance imaging. Anesthesiology 1985; 62:80–83.
11. Goudsouzian N: Monitoring general anesthesia for a MRI scan. Anesthesia Patient Safety Foundation Newsletter. 1987; December: 33–35.
12. Feinsod M, Selhorst JB, Hoyt WF, et al: Monitoring optic nerve function during craniotomy. J Neurosurg 1976; 44:29–31.
13. Grundy BL: Intraoperative monitoring of sensory evoked potentials. Anesthesiology 1983; 58:72–87.
14. Chiappa KH, Ropper AH: Evoked potentials in clinical medicine. N Engl J Med 1982; 306:1140–1150.
15. Domino EF: Effects of preanesthetic and anesthetic drugs on visual evoked responses. Anesthesiology 1967; 28:184–191.
16. Uhl RR, Squires KC, Bruce DL, Starr A: Effects of halothane anesthesia on the human cortical visual evoked response. Anesthesiology 1980; 53:273–276.
17. Burchiel KS, Stockard JJ, Myers RR, Bickford RG: Visual and auditory responses during enflurane anesthesia in man and cats. Electroencephalogr Clin Neurophysiol 1975; 39:434.
18. Chi OZ, Field C: Effects of isoflurane on visual evoked potentials in humans. Anesthesiology 1986; 65:328–330.
19. Russ W, Luben V, Hempelmann G: Der Einfluss der Neuroleptanalgesie auf das visuelle evozierte Potential (VEP) des Menschen. Anaesthesist 1982; 31:575–578.
20. Kahn HA, Leibowitz HM, Ganley JP, et al: The Framingham Eye Study. I. Outline and major prevalence findings. Am J Epidemiol 1977; 106:17–32.
21. Straatsma BR, Foos RY, Horowit J, et al: Aging-related cataract: Laboratory investigation and clinical management. Ann Intern Med 1985; 102:82–92.
22. Shapiro A, Tso MOM, Goldberg MF: Argon laser-induced cataract. Arch Ophthalmol 1984; 102:579–583.
23. Fineberg E, Machemer R, Sullivan P, et al: Sulfur hexafluoride in owl monkey vitreous cavity. Am J Ophthalmol 1975; 79:67–74.
24. Stinson TW, Donlon JV Jr: Interaction of SF_6 and air with nitrous oxide. Anesthesiology 1979; 51:S16.
25. Wolf GL, Capuano C, Hartung J: Nitrous oxide increases intraocular pressure after intravitreal sulfur

hexafluoride injection. Anesthesiology 1983; 59:547–548.

26. Chang S, Coleman DJ, Lincoff H, et al: Perfluoropropane gas in the management of proliferative vitreoretinopathy. Am J Ophthalmol 1984; 98:180–188.

27. Chang S, Lincoff HA, Coleman DJ, et al: Perfluocarbon gases in vitreous surgery. Ophthalmology 1985; 92:651–656.

28. Lincoff H, Mardirossian J, Lincoff A, et al: Intravitreal longevity of three perfluorocarbon gases. Arch Ophthalmol 1980; 98:1610.

29. Schepens CL, Freeman HM, Thompson RF: A power driven multipositional operating table. Arch Ophthalmol 1965; 73:671.

30. Peyman GA: A new operating table for the management of giant retinal breaks. Arch Ophthalmol 1981; 99:498.

31. Schepens CL: Clinical and research aspects of subtotal open-sky vitrectomy. Thirty-fifth Edward Jackson Memorial Lecture. Am J Ophthalmol 1981; 91:143.

Ophthalmologic and Systemic Complications of Surgery and Anesthesia

Kathryn E. McGoldrick

There is a low mortality associated with ophthalmic surgery, perhaps owing to thorough preoperative assessment and excellent perioperative monitoring, as well as the limited anatomical extent of the surgery. Most studies investigating ophthalmologic mortality are now obsolete, but a few are mentioned here.

Duncalf and colleagues[1] collected data for 197,653 patients in North America who underwent ophthalmic surgery in 1967. However, this represented a selected sample, because it included the records of only 16% of the ophthalmic surgeons in the geographic region under scrutiny. Of these patients, 70,744 had general anesthesia, with a mortality of 0.65/1000. The remainder were given local anesthesia, with a mortality of 0.62/1000. The two groups of patients were probably not homogeneous. Patients selected for local anesthesia usually have a high average age and a surgical procedure of relatively brief duration, such as cataract surgery. Patients given general anesthesia probably included many children, as well as middle-aged individuals undergoing retinal reattachment surgery.

Petruscak and associates[2] from Pittsburgh reported no intraoperative or recovery room mortality in 17,155 operations over a 5-year span. However, six patients who received local anesthesia and three patients who received general anesthesia died postoperatively within 20 days.

Studies at the Massachusetts Eye and Ear Infirmary[3] presented similar findings, confirm-

ing a low incidence of morbidity as well as mortality. Lang investigated all ophthalmic surgery cases (14,889 procedures) performed at the Massachusetts Eye and Ear Infirmary in a 24-month period between 1977 and 1979. The distribution of cases between local and general anesthesia was about equal, with approximately 7500 cases in each group. Forty-four percent of all adult patients were at least 65, and the average adult (over the age of 18) was 70 years of age. There were two postoperative deaths, both within 48 hours of surgery and anesthesia. One patient (American Society of Anesthesiologists physical status IV) died of septicemia following drainage of an advanced lacrimal gland infection under local anesthesia; a second patient, 36 years old, with severe diabetic complications died suddenly 20 hours after general anesthesia following a severe hypotensive reaction to hydralazine. Two postoperative myocardial infarctions occurred in patients who had cataract extraction under local anesthesia; both patients had a history of a previous myocardial infarction more than 6 months prior to surgery, and both survived. Other nonophthalmic complications of note included urinary obstruction (34 cases) and 18 cases of nonfatal cardiac complications. Only one patient sustained a postoperative cerebrovascular accident, and there were no cases in this series of documented pulmonary embolism—unlike the studies of Kaplan and Reba[4] and Quigley.[5] Patients with urinary obstruction were generally males with prostatic hypertrophy who developed urinary retention associated with bed rest, intravenous (IV) fluids, mydriatics, and anticholinergics. Urinary retention appeared to be unrelated to the use of general anesthesia, although patients in this group who received local anesthesia were significantly older.

Lang concluded: In evaluating the overall performance of an ophthalmology service, mortality should be a rare event. While I hesitate to place a figure on this, services that perform a variety of ophthalmic procedures on all ages of patients should have a mortality rate lower than one in five thousand cases. Studies by Backer et al.,[6] Petruscak,[2] Lynch,[7] and my own[3] support this as a reasonably acceptable standard of practice. In general, the operative experience, properly managed, for most ophthalmology patients, though not devoid of risk, is certainly a relatively safe venture.[3]

Close cooperation and communication among the ophthalmologist, the internist, the anesthesiologist, and the patient leads to operative management that surpasses individual efforts.[8] This teamwork, focusing on careful preoperative evaluation, in conjunction with vigilant perioperative monitoring, is more important than the specific anesthetic agents or methods employed.

In this chapter, assorted complications associated with local or regional anesthesia for ocular surgery are discussed, as are those complications linked with eye surgery under general anesthesia. (Some complications may be associated with both major types of anesthesia.) Then, ocular complications that may occur in patients undergoing anesthesia for nonocular surgery are briefly explored, as are ocular complications that may result from prematurity or oxygen therapy.

COMPLICATIONS ASSOCIATED WITH LOCAL OR REGIONAL ANESTHESIA FOR EYE SURGERY

At our institution, when local anesthesia is elected, the ophthalmologist usually administers the local or regional block, and the anesthetist or anesthesiologist is present to continually monitor the patient's electrocardiogram (ECG), routinely check vital signs, and administer sedation as indicated. If a mature, cooperative patient and a compassionate, communicative surgeon are involved, local anesthesia can be effective for several, if not most,

ophthalmic procedures of reasonable length. Nonetheless, the choice of anesthesia should be individualized. Germane considerations include the nature and duration of the surgical procedure, coagulation status of the patient, the patient's ability to communicate and cooperate, and the preferences of both the patient and the surgeon. Obviously, patients who are deaf or speak only a foreign language and those with psychiatric disturbances, such as claustrophobia, excessive anxiety, or confusion, are poor candidates for local anesthesia. Other relative contraindications include chronic coughing, tremors, and inability to lie flat. Furthermore, retrobulbar blockade is contraindicated in the setting of an open eye injury (Table 21–1).

Local anesthesia is said to be safe for ophthalmic patients with certain types of cardiovascular disease, including those with a history of previous myocardial infarction.[6] Nonetheless, available data have not demonstrated a major difference in complications such as iris prolapse or vitreous loss between local and general anesthesia for cataract surgery.[7] Local anesthesia does not necessarily involve less physiological trespass than general anesthesia and is not *a priori* safer or better. A variety of complications associated with topical, infiltration, and retrobulbar anesthesia are discussed here.

Local anesthesia in conjunction with excessively heavy sedation with a potpourri of narcotics, tranquilizers, and hypnotics is unsatisfactory and should be avoided. This polypharmacology is condemned in view of pharmacological vagaries common in the geriatric population and the attendant risks of respiratory depression, airway obstruction, hypotension, confusion, agitation, obtundation, and prolonged recovery time. This undesirable method is analogous to giving an unintubated patient a general anesthetic, without the associated controllability that general anesthesia

TABLE 21–1. Relative Contraindications to Local Anesthesia

Ruptured globe
Infection at or near injection site
Abnormal coagulation or bleeding profile
Inability to communicate (e.g., language barrier, deafness)
Inability to lie flat
Inability to cooperate (e.g., excessive anxiety, claustrophobia)
Chronic coughing or tremors
Patient refusal

affords. Moreover, undersedation should likewise be avoided, because hypertension and tachycardia are undesirable, especially in patients with coronary artery disease. The goal with local anesthesia is a calm, cooperative, aware patient. Individuals with arthritis or orthopedic deformities must be meticulously positioned and comfortably padded on the operating table. All patients must have adequate ventilation about the face and must be kept warm to avoid shivering and its attendant movement. Continuous electrocardiographic monitoring is essential lest performance of the retrobulbar block, pressure on the orbit, or pulling on the extraocular muscles trigger the oculocardiac reflex arc and produce bradydysrhythmias, tachydysrhythmias, or asystole. In addition, continuous pulse oximetry and capnography have added dimensions of safety unheard of only one decade ago.

Ophthalmologists frequently inquire whether, in cardiac patients, epinephrine may be safely mixed with local anesthetic agents to effect vasoconstriction and prolongation of anesthesia. Donlon and Moss[9] emphasized that release of endogenous catecholamines secondary to suboptimal analgesia may vastly exceed the relatively minute amount of exogenous catecholamine injected. They state that 0.06 mg epinephrine (12 mL of 1:200,000) gives some systemic uptake but causes no untoward clinical effects.

The three main techniques of administering local anesthesia for ocular surgery are topical, infiltration, and regional such as retrobulbar or peribulbar blockade.

Topical Anesthesia

Topical anesthesia may be helpful in facilitating ocular examination, diagnosis, and treatment. Topical anesthesia, for example, may be adequate for removal of corneal foreign bodies.

Topical anesthetics are relatively toxic and should not be injected. However, they act quickly when applied to mucosal surfaces. Because both the rapidity of onset and the duration of anesthetic action increase in proportion to the logarithm of concentration of a given drug until a maximal concentration is achieved,[10] no additional increase in duration is produced by exceeding maximal effective concentration. In fact, administering more than the maximal effective concentration instead produces the possibility of systemic toxicity. Indeed, the optimal concentration of a local anesthetic may be considerably less than the maximal effective concentration, because the former may be less irritating to the eye. In addition, although vasoconstrictors retard the absorption of injected anesthetic solutions, they do not influence the systemic absorption of topical anesthetics from normal mucous membranes, nor do they significantly enhance the duration of topical analgesia.[11]

Popular topical anesthetics are proparacaine, tetracaine, and cocaine. A partial list of topical medications abandoned because of various problems includes solutions of 2% piperocaine, 2% butacaine sulfate, 1% phenocaine, and 0.1% dibucaine.

Solutions of 0.5%–2% tetracaine, a derivative of para-aminobenzoic acid, may be instilled directly into the conjunctival sac. Following instillation, patients may complain of a burning sensation that lasts up to 30 seconds. However, with use of the 0.5% concentration less irritation occurs. The initial discomfort is less pronounced if the patient is instructed to close, rather than rub, the eyes after instillation. However, topical tetracaine may produce corneal toxicity resulting from both chemical and mechanical (i.e., secondary to the patient's rubbing the eye) effects. Healing may be delayed, because tetracaine exerts a deleterious effect on epithelial regeneration owing to inhibition of both mitosis and cellular migration. Because repeated and prolonged application of tetracaine exacerbates epithelial damage, topical anesthesia for the patient's home use to alleviate pain from a corneal abrasion should not be prescribed. True allergy to tetracaine is extremely rare, although an occasional glaucoma patient may develop edematous, erythematous, pruritic lids following repeated use of topical tetracaine for tonometry. In addition to dermatitis of the lids, conjunctivitis may also be noted.

Proparacaine, supplied in a 0.5% solution with addition of 0.2% chlorobutanol and 1:10,000 benzalkonium chloride, has a similar onset, duration (20–25 minutes), and intensity of anesthetic action as tetracaine. However, proparacaine consistently causes less discomfort on instillation than does tetracaine. The incidence of allergic phenomena with proparacaine is low. Patients allergic to tetracaine are not *a priori* allergic to proparacaine, and *vice versa*. Because it is associated with less burning on instillation and causes less punctate epithelial damage, proparacaine is considered by many ophthalmologists to be the topical anesthetic of choice. One to two drops of the

0.5% solution is the usual dose for foreign body removal and tonometry. For "deep" ophthalmic anesthesia, one drop every 5 minutes up to a maximum of five to seven drops is indicated.

Cocaine, an estezoic acid, was the first drug to be successfully employed as a local anesthetic.[12] However, the newer synthetic topical anesthetics have largely replaced cocaine because of its corneal toxicity, its sympathomimetic characteristics, and its addictive potential. Excellent surface anesthesia is obtained by application of 1–4% solution. Rate of onset is similar to that of tetracaine and proparacaine, but the duration of action of 2% cocaine is only 10 minutes, owing to rapid hydrolysis by plasma pseudocholinesterase. Nonetheless, use of two drops of the 4% solution prolongs the anesthetic duration to approach that of tetracaine and proparacaine. However, the epithelial damage produced by cocaine may be serious. Cocaine's corneal toxicity is manifested by grayish corneal pits, irregularities, and not infrequently, large erosions.

Cocaine is the only local anesthetic that inherently produces vasoconstriction and shrinkage of mucous membranes. The usual maximum dose of cocaine employed in clinical practice for procedures such as dacryocystorhinostomy is 3 mg/kg. Although 1 g is thought to be the usual lethal dose for an adult, considerable variation occurs; systemic reactions may appear with as little as 20 mg. Close attention must be paid to the volume used, because there is a narrow range from safety to toxicity to death.

By blocking the reuptake of endogenous norepinephrine and the uptake of exogenous epinephrine, cocaine exerts an indirect sympathomimetic action. (Hence, some pupillary dilation accompanies the use of ocular cocaine, although the pupil retains its ability to converge and to react to light.) Meyers[13] has emphasized that cocaine is contraindicated in hypertensives and in patients receiving adrenergic-modifying drugs such as guanethidine, reserpine, tricyclic antidepressants, and monoamine oxidase inhibitors. Additionally, sympathomimetics, such as epinephrine or phenylephrine, should not be given with cocaine.

Signs of cocaine toxicity are referable to the central nervous system (CNS), respiratory, and cardiovascular systems and were described in Chapter 17. Before administering cocaine, the physician should carefully rule out possible contraindications, including the use of concurrent medications such as adrenergic-modifying drugs and sympathomimetics. To avoid toxic levels, dosages of dilute solutions should be meticulously calculated and carefully administered. If serious cardiovascular side effects occur, IV labetalol should be used to counteract them.[14]

Infiltration Anesthesia

Subconjunctival injections and lid infiltration may be employed to explore surface injuries and remove foreign bodies. However, the ease and apparent safety with which local analgesia can be attained through infiltration agents should not lead to carelessness. The physician must not exceed the maximum allowable dosage and should have appropriate resuscitative drugs and equipment immediately available. Because epinephrine can produce vascular constriction and ecchymosis, it is usually not injected subconjunctivally. In addition, if a ruptured globe is suspected, the ophthalmologist should avoid subconjunctival injections.

Fatal reactions to local anesthetics are seldom secondary to allergy or idiosyncrasy. Rather, they are usually the result of administering excessive quantities of anesthetic or of inadvertent intravascular injection. An accelerated rate of absorption may also result from the presence of lacerated veins or even from normally rich vascularity at the site of injection, from a rapid rate of injection, or from application to mucous membranes or abraded skin. Systemic toxic reactions may also be secondary to a decreased rate of drug detoxification associated with functional impairment of the detoxifying organ and altered metabolic rate of the patient. Other factors that influence toxicity include the use of concurrent medications, the patient's general physical status, acid-base balance (acidosis lowers the toxic threshold), and vagaries of individual sensitivity.

Signs and symptoms of CNS toxic reactions are manifested along a concentration-related spectrum. Drowsiness progresses to loss of consciousness and muscle twitches to generalized tonic-clonic seizures. Cyanosis may appear if ventilation is compromised by seizure activity. Tachycardia and hypertension may occur as a sympathetic response to hypoxia and hypercarbia, but hypotension sometimes develops secondary to the myocardial depressant effects of the local anesthetic.

An inverse relationship exists between the blood levels necessary to generate toxic symp-

TABLE 21–2. Relative Anesthetic Potency of Various Local Anesthetics

Agent	Relative Anesthetic Potency
Procaine	1
Cocaine	2
Lidocaine	2
Mepivacaine	2
Etidocaine	6
Bupivacaine	8
Tetracaine	8

toms and the relative potency of local anesthetic agents. For lidocaine, a level of 4 μg/mL is thought to be the threshold for early symptoms. However, with the more potent agent bupivacaine, toxicity begins to occur in the 2 μg/mL range (Table 21–2).

Although local anesthetics can exert profound effects on the cardiovascular system, in general the cardiovascular system is more resistant than the CNS. As the blood level of a local anesthetic approaches toxic concentration, a decrease in blood pressure may be observed. This initial hypotension is thought to be caused by negative inotropic action rather than by peripheral vasodilation. However, if the situation remains uncorrected, decreased myocardial contractility, depressed conductivity, and reduced heart rate will combine ultimately with peripheral vasodilation to result in circulatory collapse and cardiac arrest (Fig. 21–1). Hypercarbia and acidosis augment the cardiodepressant effect of local anesthetics.

The best therapy for systemic toxic reactions is prevention. The anesthesiologist should aspirate carefully prior to injecting at any site, inject slowly and cautiously, and use the optimum dose, i.e., minimum concentration and volume, for the desired effect. For lidocaine, the maximum suggested dose for infiltration is 4 mg/kg of plain solution and 7 mg/kg of epinephrine-containing solution. For bupivacaine, the maximum suggested dose is 2–3 mg/kg.

If the patient experiences a mild reaction, such as dizziness, tinnitus, circumoral tingling or numbness, blurred vision, slurred speech, nystagmus, or muscle twitches, he or she should be observed closely, because the reaction may become more serious. Oxygen should be administered by face mask or nasal prongs. If convulsions occur, ventilation should be assisted by bag and mask with 100% oxygen, and an appropriate anticonvulsant should be administered. (Diazepam, 5–10 mg, or thiopental, 50–100 mg, can be given I.V.) Convulsions are usually brief, i.e., 60 seconds or less. If they persist, succinylcholine and endotracheal intubation may be necessary to assure an adequate airway and proper oxygenation.

If cardiovascular collapse ensues, all of the measures mentioned earlier may be necessary, as well as mechanical ventilation plus circulatory support with vasopressors and liberal fluid infusion. Closed-chest cardiac compression and resuscitative drugs should be appropriately administered, with attention paid to acid-base status.

Because the possibility of this dramatic range of reactions is present every time local anesthesia is used, venous access must be assured prior to administration of local anesthetics. Care must be exercised in the technique of injection and in dosage calculations. These agents should be given only in geographic sites where adequate resuscitative equipment and properly trained personnel are readily available.

Retrobulbar Blockade

Retrobulbar anesthesia is an extremely practical means to achieve akinesia of the globe and anesthesia of the orbital contents. However, retrobulbar anesthesia should not be administered if a ruptured globe injury is suspected, because this maneuver may trigger prolapse of intraocular contents in that setting. Furthermore, high myopes are not usually considered suitable candidates for retrobulbar blockade, because they are vulnerable to penetration of the globe.

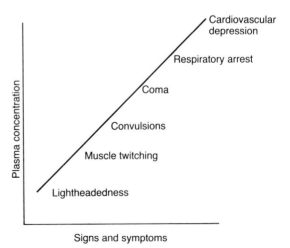

Figure 21–1. Relationship of signs and symptoms of local anesthetic toxicity to plasma concentration.

This technique entails injection of local anesthesia behind the eye into the muscle cone. In the so-called classic approach, the patient is asked to gaze superonasally, and a 1.5 in, 25-gauge needle is introduced through the lower lid, just nasal to the junction of the lateral and inferior rims of the orbit. The needle is advanced approximately 1.5 cm along the inferotemporal wall of the orbit and is directed upward and nasally toward the orbital apex. The plunger is withdrawn to aspirate and, thus, avoid intravascular injection. Approximately 4 mL of anesthetic solution (usually 0.75% bupivacaine mixed with 1.5 or 2% lidocaine plus hyaluronidase, with or without 1:200,000 epinephrine) is then administered. The retrobulbar injection should be followed by gentle massage of the globe to enhance dispersion of the local anesthetic.

A modification[15] of the traditional Atkinson position of turning the globe upward and inward prior to retrobulbar injection has been suggested. Unsöld and coworkers,[16] using computed tomography of a cadaver orbit as the needle is inserted, have shown that in the Atkinson position the optic nerve, the ophthalmic artery and its branches, the superior orbital vein, and the posterior pole of the globe are all brought near the needle tip. Because the nerve is stretched, it may be more vulnerable to needle puncture because it cannot be moved away as easily. Thus, these authors recommend that the globe be positioned in either the primary position or a slightly downward and outward position, and that the needle be directed not toward the orbital apex, as recommended by Atkinson, but slightly lower, toward the inferior part of the superior orbital fissure.

Akinesia of the eyelids is obtained by blocking the branches of the facial nerve supplying the orbicularis. Since first used for ophthalmic surgery by van Lint[17] in 1914, numerous methods of facial nerve block have been described. All block the facial nerve either proximally or distally to its exit point from the skull through the stylomastoid foramen. The van Lint technique may be painful, and some of the other techniques have the advantage of eliminating the "ballooning" or distension of lid tissues commonly encountered with the van Lint approach. These other techniques include the approaches of Atkinson,[18] O'Brien,[19] and Nadbath and Rehman.[20]

A partial list of complications[21-30] associated with retrobulbar block includes stimulation of the oculocardiac reflex arc, retrobulbar hem-

orrhage, puncture of the posterior globe resulting in retinal detachment and vitreous hemorrhage, unintentional intraocular injection, central retinal artery occlusion, penetration of the optic nerve, subdural injection, blindness, and inadvertent brain-stem anesthesia (Table 21–3). Additionally, intravascular injection of local anesthesia may trigger CNS excitation followed by obtundation and cardiovascular collapse.[31, 32] Although the latter complications are commonly associated with injection of local anesthetic into a vein, inadvertent intra-arterial[33] injection may also be associated with CNS toxicity, and the amount of anesthetic involved is much less than with the IV route. Only 1.8 mL of 2% lidocaine injected into an artery of the head or neck region can produce profound toxic reactions.[34] These reactions include virtually instantaneous seizures secondary to ophthalmic artery injection,[33] with retrograde flow into the cerebral circulation.

The possibility of accidental brain-stem anesthesia following retrobulbar blockade should be well known to anesthesiologists and ophthalmologists. This initially insidious, but potentially lethal, complication may occur when accidental access to the cerebrospinal fluid develops secondary to perforation of the meningeal sheaths surrounding the optic nerve. The patency of the pathway under the dural sheath of the optic nerve has been confirmed by contrast radiography[35] and by recovery of lidocaine and bupivacaine from the cerebrospinal fluid of patients who developed respiratory arrest following retrobulbar block.[36] One case report[24] described a typical course involving the gradual onset of unconsciousness and apnea over a 7-minute interval without associated seizures or cardiovascular collapse. (Additionally, transient blindness with paralysis of the third and sixth cranial nerves in the contralateral eye has been occa-

TABLE 21–3. Complications of Retrobulbar Blockade

Retrobulbar hemorrhage
Contraindication in presence of ruptured globe
Stimulation of oculocardiac reflex arc
Puncture of posterior globe, producing retinal
  detachment and vitreous hemorrhage
Intraocular injection
Central retinal artery occlusion
Penetration of optic nerve
Brain-stem anesthesia
IV injection
Intra-arterial injection
Seizures

sionally reported, and this phenomenon is explained by the anesthetic's entering the optic nerve sheath and passing through the optic chiasma to the midbrain. Although the diagnosis of central spread can be confirmed by noting paresis of the extraocular muscles of the contralateral eye, the absence of this symptom does not rule out this possibility.) Because this life-threatening complication occurs unpredictably, the necessity for closely monitored care of all patients having surgery under retrobulbar anesthesia is obvious. Professionals skilled in airway maintenance and in ventilatory and circulatory support should be immediately available whenever retrobulbar blockade is executed.

Peribulbar Block

Various modifications of the technique of retrobulbar blockade have been developed in recent years in an attempt to circumvent some of the disadvantages. For example, peribulbar block is considered by many to be easier, safer, and less painful than retrobulbar block, because the muscle cone is not entered and the need for seventh nerve block is eliminated. Because the anesthetic is deposited outside the muscle cone, the potential for intraocular or intradural injection is minimized, and the potential for intraconal hemorrhage and direct nerve injury is essentially avoided. Davis and Mandel[37] and others have described a two-stage technique of peribulbar anesthesia as follows.

Approximately 0.5 mL of 1% lidocaine is injected into the orbicularis oculi, and an additional 1 mL is injected just beneath the muscle. This first injection is made through an entrance site in the lower eyelid, just above the inferior orbital rim, approximately one fingerbreadth medial to the lateral canthus. The procedure is repeated for the upper eyelid, where entrance is made directly inferior to the supraorbital notch; similar volumes are injected into and just beneath the upper orbicularis oculi.

The second stage is performed with the standard blunt 1¼-in Atkinson 23-gauge retrobulbar needle. Four mL of bupivacaine 0.75% is mixed with 4 mL of lidocaine 1% without epinephrine and 1 mL of hyaluronidase in a 10 mL syringe to which the retrobulbar needle is attached. Immediately beneath the inferior orbicularis oculi, 1 mL of anesthetic solution is deposited. The needle is advanced along the inferior orbit to the equa-

tor of the globe. Following aspiration, an additional 1 mL of solution is deposited at the equator. The barrel of the syringe is then angled over the malar eminence, and the needle is advanced to its full depth in a superior and medial direction. After aspirating, 1–2 mL of local anesthetic is deposited. The needle is withdrawn, and transcutaneous entrance through the superior site is accomplished. One mL of solution is deposited beneath the orbicularis oculi slightly medial to the entrance site. The needle is advanced posteriorly, and 1 mL of solution is deposited at the superonasal equator of the globe. The needle is then passed directly posterior to the superior orbital fissure, and the final 1 mL of solution is injected. (These volumes are approximate and may vary depending on ocular size and orbital configuration.) A folded 4 × 4 is placed over the closed eyelids, and pressure is firmly applied to the lids for approximately 1 minute.

Unfortunately, peribulbar block has a higher failure rate (up to 10%) and a longer onset time than retrobulbar blockade. Complete anesthesia is not obtained for at least 10–12 minutes, although the onset may be hastened by adding sodium bicarbonate to the anesthetic mixture.[38] Because peribulbar anesthesia is primarily a diffusion block, it is helpful to inject a slightly warm solution. Moreover, because a greater volume of local anesthetic is required than with retrobulbar block, increased vitreous pressure may result, thus making surgery more difficult. Reported complications have included peribulbar hemorrhage and perforation of the globe.

OCULOCARDIAC REFLEX

Initially described independently in 1908 by Bernard Aschner and Giuseppe Dagnini, the oculocardiac reflex is elicited by pressure on the globe and by traction on the conjunctiva, orbital structures, and extraocular muscles. It may also be produced by performance of a retrobulbar block[39] as well as by ocular trauma and by direct pressure on tissues remaining in the orbital apex following enucleation.[40] This reflex may appear during both local and general anesthesia, irrespective of depth, but hypercarbia and hypoxemia increase the incidence and severity of this reflex, whose afferent limb is trigeminal and efferent limb is vagal. Although sinus bradycardia is the usual manifestation, other reported dysrhythmias include junctional rhythm, atrioventricular block, ventricular bigeminy, wandering pacemaker, idioventricular rhythm, and asystole.

Investigators differ tremendously in reporting statistics on incidence. Berler's study claimed an overall incidence of 50%,[39] but others cite rates ranging from 16 to 82%.[41, 42] Children having strabismus surgery who are not given appropriate prophylaxis may have a 90% frequency of dysrhythmia. Generally, reports of high incidence involved young subjects who are thought to have more vagal tone.

Several methods to abolish or attenuate the reflex have been promulgated. However, none has proven entirely effective or completely benign. The inclusion of either oral or intramuscular anticholinergic agents, such as atropine, in the "usual" premedication doses is ineffective as prophylaxis.[42–45] The problem is as much one of proper timing as of dosage. However, IV atropine administered within 30 minutes prior to manipulation[42] results in a lower incidence of the reflex, but recommendations continue to differ concerning timing and dosage. Some claim that prophylactic IV atropine is associated with more ominous or refractory dysrhythmias than those commonly triggered by the oculocardiac reflex itself.[46] Atropine may be considered a potential myocardial irritant. Virtually every possible dysrhythmia and numerous conduction defects have been reported following IV atropine, including ventricular tachycardia,[47] ventricular fibrillation,[48] and left bundle branch block.[49] The possible protective value of retrobulbar block is acknowledged, but its disadvantages include stimulation of the reflex arc by the block itself,[39] retrobulbar hemorrhage, optic nerve damage, and inadvertent brain-stem anesthesia.[23]

Many anesthesiologists concur that in adults, routine prophylactic measures, replete with inherent risks, are not usually warranted. If a dysrhythmia transpires, the initial approach includes asking the surgeon to stop manipulation. Then the patient's oxygenation, ventilation, and anesthetic depth are quickly assessed. Frequently, heart rate and rhythm return to baseline within 20 seconds. With repeated manipulation, bradycardia is less likely to recur, probably secondary to fatigue of the oculocardiac reflex at the level of the cardioinhibitory center.[50] However, if the initial occurrence is especially dramatic, or if the reflex prevails or persistently recurs, IV atropine should be given after the surgeon stops ocular manipulation.

Children undergoing strabismus surgery are handled differently. Current recommended practice is to administer atropine 0.02 mg/kg IV prior to commencing surgery.[51, 52] Meyers and Tomeldan[53] are articulate advocates of prophylactic IV anticholinergics for pediatric patients having strabismus repair. These investigators favor glycopyrrolate over atropine, because they claim the former is associated with lesser degrees of tachycardia.

Despite the controversy surrounding incidence and prevention of the oculocardiac reflex, there is consensus that continuous electrocardiographic monitoring by the anesthesiologist is mandatory during eye surgery to detect ominous rhythm disturbances. Continuous pulse oximetry and capnography are invaluable monitors of oxygenation and ventilation—parameters crucial to the patient's global safety and to cardiac rhythm stability.

COMPLICATIONS ASSOCIATED WITH OCULAR DRUGS

Ophthalmic drugs, given topically, intraocularly, or systemically, may have significant anesthetic implications. This topic is discussed in detail in Chapter 17.

In summary, systemic absorption may be enhanced in a diseased or postsurgical eye, and small children and geriatric patients with multisystem disease requiring adrenergic-modifying drugs are especially vulnerable to adverse reactions. Systemic absorption of topical drugs may be impressively reduced by occluding the nasolacrimal duct through pressure on the inner canthus of the eye for 5 minutes and by keeping the eye gently closed for the same length of time following instillation.[54]

Topical ocular drugs associated with potential systemic complications include atropine, cocaine, cyclopentolate, echothiophate iodide, epinephrine, phenylephrine, scopolamine, and timolol. Betaxolol hydrochloride, a known cardioselective β-adrenergic receptor blocking agent, has a package insert stating, "Ophthalmic betaxolol has minimal effect on pulmonary and cardiovascular parameters."[55] However, the insert further states that "caution should be observed in treating patients with a history of cardiac failure."

Because betaxolol has greater lipid solubility and greater plasma protein binding than timolol, there is insufficient active drug in the blood after ocular administration to cause a measurable cardiac effect.[56] Nonetheless, a report[57] of congestive heart failure following proper ophthalmic dosing of betaxolol in a patient with a history of compensated congestive heart failure and sick sinus syndrome treated with digoxin and metolazone should be mentioned. This case reinforces that, as with timolol, caution must be taken with the use of the purportedly oculospecific betaxolol in a patient in whom potential cardiac β blockade presents a significant risk to health.

The intraocular use of substances such as acetylcholine, sulfur hexafluoride, octafluorocyclobutane, and perfluoroprane have previously been discussed, and the attendant implications should be familiar to anesthesiologists and ophthalmologists alike.

Furthermore, drugs given systemically to effect ocular purposes, such as lowering intraocular pressure, or diagnosis include glycerol, mannitol, acetazolamide, and fluorescein. Once again, Chapter 17 discusses germane anesthetic ramifications.

ASPIRATION

Since its description by Mendelson[58] in 1946, the acid aspiration syndrome has been a feared complication of anesthesia. One of the most hazardous situations in anesthesia is the patient who faces surgery with a full stomach. Few conditions demand "emergency" surgery; these include uncontrolled hemorrhage, respiratory obstruction, and acute cranial injury. The indications for immediate ocular surgery are limited. In most types of acute pathology, the patient must be examined thoroughly for other disease or injury, hypovolemia or electrolyte imbalance must be treated, antibiotics and sedatives must be administered, and any other necessary measures to get the patient into optimal, or at least suitable, condition for anesthesia and surgery must be completed. Undue haste could convert an accident into a major catastrophe.

Patients at risk of aspiration are not confined to those individuals who have recently eaten. Well-established risk factors include hiatus hernia, obesity, pregnancy, extreme nervousness, old age, diabetes, and conditions requiring upper abdominal surgery (Table 21–4). The most common factors that precipitate active vomiting during anesthesia are partial respiratory obstruction and anesthesia that becomes "too light." Other factors include strong autonomic stimulation such as peritoneal traction or hypoxia and hypotension, administra-

TABLE 21–4. Risk Factors for Aspiration under Anesthesia

Recent ingestion of food or beverage
Hiatus hernia
Obesity
Pregnancy
Preoperative anxiety
Preoperative pain
Conditions requiring upper abdominal surgery
Partial airway obstruction
Insufficient anesthetic depth
Hypotension
Collagen vascular disease
Increased intracranial pressure
Perioperative obtundation

tion of narcotics, and insertion of an oropharyngeal airway during light anesthesia. The passive phenomenon of regurgitation may be encouraged by Trendelenburg's position, prone position, palpation of the abdomen during light anesthesia, and conditions associated with delayed gastric emptying and, hence, increased intragastric pressure. The latter conditions include pain, anxiety, obstetrical labor, pyloric or intestinal obstruction, metabolic derangements, increased intracranial pressure, and administration of narcotics and parasympathomimetic drugs. (Delaying induction of anesthesia is a common tactic to prevent aspiration, but the decision of how long to wait for a patient to digest gastric contents is difficult and arbitrary. When an accident occurs shortly after a meal, food may remain undigested for more than 18 hours. Because pain and anxiety significantly retard gastric emptying, patients under the influence of these stresses should automatically be assumed to have a full stomach.) In addition, succinylcholine-induced fasciculations are claimed by some to promote regurgitation. Because scleroderma and other collagen vascular diseases are associated with gastroesophageal sphincter incompetence, these patients are at increased risk.

An exact figure denoting the incidence of aspiration under anesthesia cannot be cited. Several investigators have studied the problem of "silent" regurgitation and aspiration. Overall, an incidence of regurgitation between 14 and 26% was found.[59, 60] "Silent" aspiration was documented in 6–8% of cases.[59, 61] More recent studies in 1986 by Olsson[62] reported an incidence of aspiration pneumonitis confirmed by radiographs after anesthesia of 2.2/10,000 anesthetic administrations, with a mortality of 0.2/10,000. Mortality rates had previously been thought to exceed 40% following confirmed aspiration.[63] However, Olsson concluded that today the mortality caused by anesthesia-associated aspiration is much lower.

Morbidity and mortality associated with aspiration vary depending on the volume and chemical nature of the fluid aspirated. Patients at greatest risk are those with at least 25 mL (0.4 mL/kg) of gastric fluid of pH below 2.5 in the stomach. The clinical picture produced by aspiration of gastric contents is a function of the type of material aspirated. Vomiting may produce aspiration of solid particulate matter capable of occluding the tracheobronchial tree and causing lung collapse distal to the blockage. The clinical course depends on the occlusion site and particulate size. Death may occur quickly when the tracheal lumen is blocked. If liquid gastric contents are aspirated, the clinical effects depend on the acidity and volume of the aspirate. Wheezing, rales, and expiratory rhonchi may be noted almost immediately, or these signs and symptoms can be delayed. Likewise, the chest radiograph may be normal for some time after the injury, and the extent of the pneumonitis may not be apparent radiologically for many hours. Nonetheless, tachycardia, dyspnea, cyanosis, hypotension, and pulmonary edema may develop quickly.

Solid matter aspirated into the airway requires prompt removal by bronchoscopy. When liquid is aspirated, suctioning should be performed to reduce pulmonary damage, although mucosal injury occurs within minutes. Small amounts (less than 10 mL) of saline may be used to facilitate airway suctioning. However, attempts to dilute and suction by lavage of the airways is not recommended, because it may only spread the damage.

The initial response to aspiration of liquid with a pH less than 2.5 is an irritative one of intense bronchospasm and transudation of large volumes of fluid from the respiratory epithelium, resulting in profound hypoxemia. Tracheal intubation and mechanical ventilation with positive end-expiratory pressure are often necessary to sustain an acceptable arterial oxygen tension. Aminophylline may be given as a 500-mg IV infusion to treat bronchospasm. Antibiotics are administered only if indicated, i.e., for treatment of the secondary infection that commonly develops following aspiration. Prophylactic antibiotics are indicated only in the setting of aspiration of obviously infected material, such as feces or pus from a pharyngeal abscess. Steroids are not usually recommended.

Aspiration of vomitus or regurgitated material happens at the completion of surgery with nearly the same frequency as it does during induction. Aspiration pneumonitis is not confined to patients having general anesthesia, but may occur even with regional techniques or in any patient whose level of consciousness is impaired by drugs or illness.

Much has been written about the prevention of aspiration during induction by recognizing those patients at greatest risk and performing either an awake intubation with a cuffed endotracheal tube or a skillful rapid sequence induction with Sellick's maneuver (firm pressure on the cricoid cartilage, occluding the esophagus between the trachea and vertebral column) prior to and during intubation. However, an awake intubation is not an option if the patient has a ruptured globe injury, because the associated coughing and straining would trigger a dramatic increase in intraocular pressure (IOP) and prolapse of intraocular contents. In the setting of this type of injury, a nondepolarizing muscle relaxant must be administered prior to giving the appropriate inducing agent and succinylcholine.

Proper airway management is the most important aspect of aspiration prophylaxis, but pharmacological protection is another important avenue. For example, a nonparticulate antacid such as a 0.3 molar solution of sodium citrate, given orally about 15 minutes prior to induction, reduces gastric acidity, although it does not decrease gastric volume. Rao and colleagues[64] reported that a combination of 300 mg cimetidine and 10 mg metoclopramide, given orally more than 2 hours before induction, markedly decreased gastric volume and increased pH. Ranitidine has greater potency and duration of action than cimetidine and also a lower incidence of drug interaction. Alternatively, the H_2 blockers may be given IV 30–60 minutes prior to induction; recommended IV doses are 300 mg cimetidine or 50 mg of ranitidine. Likewise, metoclopramide, the gastric motility-stimulating drug and dopamine antagonist, can be given IV in a 10 mg dose 30–60 minutes prior to induction. Even if there is not sufficient time for these drugs to exert an effect for induction, they probably should be administered if tracheal extubation is anticipated immediately postoperatively.

To reduce the incidence of aspiration at the completion of surgery, a nasogastric tube should be passed and suction applied prior to extubation. Patients at risk should be extubated only when they are fully awake; depression of the glottic reflex lasts at least 2 hours and perhaps as long as 8 hours after extubation, even in patients who seem alert.[65] This, obviously, has implications for postoperative fluid ingestion.

In summary, to reduce the incidence of aspiration pneumonitis, careful preoperative instructions should emphasize the necessity of fasting from solid food for 8 hours prior to elective surgery; also, patients should be questioned thoroughly about ingestion of food and liquids when they arrive for anesthetic induction. High-risk patients should be identified and treated accordingly in terms of anesthetic induction technique. Skillful airway management is essential. In addition, pharmacological prophylaxis against acid aspiration seems reasonable. Lastly, extubation should not be performed until the high-risk patient is wide awake, with reflexes intact.

MALIGNANT HYPERTHERMIA

Malignant hyperthermia is extensively discussed in Chapter 15.

COMPLICATIONS ASSOCIATED WITH ELEVATED INTRAOCULAR PRESSURE

IOP normally varies between 10 and 22 mmHg and is considered abnormal above 25 mmHg. During anesthesia, an increase in IOP can lead to permanent visual loss. If the IOP is already elevated, any additional increase can precipitate an acute episode of glaucoma. If penetration of the globe occurs when the IOP is excessively high, rupture of a blood vessel with subsequent hemorrhage may transpire. Once the eye cavity has been entered, IOP becomes atmospheric, and any sudden pressure increase may result in prolapse of the lens and iris as well as loss of vitreous. Therefore, proper control of IOP is critical for intraocular procedures such as glaucoma drainage surgery, penetrating keratoplasty, open sky vitrectomy, closed vitrectomy, cataract extractions, and repair of penetrating eye injuries.

IOP is significantly influenced by intraocular blood volume, determined mainly by vessel dilatation or contraction in the spongy layers of the choroid plexus. Although swings in both arterial or venous pressure can influence IOP secondarily, excursions in arterial pressure have less impact than do venous fluctuations.

In chronic arterial hypertension, ocular pressure returns to normal after a period of adaptation effected by compression of choroidal vessels as a result of high IOP. Thus, a feedback mechanism decreases the total blood volume, keeping the IOP constant in patients with systemic hypertension.[66] However, if venous return from the eye is impeded at any point from Schlemm's canal to the right atrium, IOP rises markedly as a result of increased intraocular blood volume, distention of orbital vessels, and obstruction of aqueous drainage. Coughing, straining, or vomiting greatly elevate venous pressure and increase IOP by 40 mmHg or more. The harmful implications of these maneuvers cannot be overemphasized. IOP can also be increased by laryngoscopy and tracheal intubation, even without visible reaction to intubation, but especially when the patient coughs. Administration of lidocaine 1.5 mg/kg IV approximately 4 minutes prior to induction may attenuate but not totally eliminate this rise in IOP associated with intubation.[67, 68]

Other preinduction regimens have been suggested to obtund the effect of intubation on IOP. For example, premedicating with sufentanil 0.05 μg/kg and pretreating with a nondepolarizing relaxant plus a high dose (7 mg/kg) thiopental or alfentanil (150 μg/kg) induction effectively block the increase in IOP from succinylcholine and intubation.[69] Clonidine, a centrally acting antihypertensive, given in a dose of 5 mg/kg orally 90 minutes before induction prevents the increase in IOP and attenuates the cardiovascular response to laryngoscopy and intubation.[70]

Fluctuations in aqueous outflow can also dramatically change IOP. The most important factor determining outflow of aqueous humor is the diameter of Fontana's spaces,[71] as illustrated by the equation based on Poiseuille's law:

$$A = \frac{r^4 \times (Piop - Pv)}{8 \eta L}$$

where A = volume of aqueous outflow per unit of time, r = radius of Fontana's spaces, Piop = IOP, Pv = venous pressure, η = viscosity, and L = length of Fontana's spaces.

With mydriasis, Fontana's spaces narrow, resistance to outflow is increased, and IOP rises. Because mydriasis is a threat in both narrow- and wide-angle glaucoma, conjunctivally applied miotics, such as pilocarpine hydrochloride, are often efficacious when applied preoperatively in glaucoma patients. It is clear from the equation that aqueous outflow is also exquisitely sensitive to changes in venous pressure. Because a rise in venous pressure produces an increased volume of ocular blood as well as decreased aqueous outflow, a considerable elevation of IOP occurs. Thus, in addition to preoperative instillation of miotics, other anesthetic recommendations for the patient with glaucoma include perioperative avoidance of venous congestion and overhydration. Hypotensive episodes are best avoided, because these patients allegedly are vulnerable to retinal artery thrombosis.

The anesthesiologist must understand the effects of anesthetic drugs and techniques on IOP. Fortunately, inhalation agents and CNS depressants, in general, including barbiturates, narcotics, neuroleptics, and etomidate, lower IOP. (With etomidate, however, myoclonus may trigger loss of intraocular contents in the setting of an open globe.[72]) It was once thought that ketamine elevated IOP, but ketamine has little, if any, effect on IOP.[73] Hypercarbia and hypoxia elevate IOP, whereas hyperventilation[74] and hypothermia reduce IOP. Most nondepolarizing muscle relaxants lower IOP,[75, 76] and depolarizing relaxants, of course, raise IOP.

Although succinylcholine, given without pretreatment, is contraindicated in patients with penetrating ocular wounds and should not be given for the first time after the eye has been surgically opened, this agent can be used safely in ophthalmologic surgery. Any increase in IOP following succinylcholine is dissipated before surgery is begun. However, succinylcholine should probably not be administered to patients with strabismus who will undergo forced duction testing.[77, 78] (The special challenges of open eye–full stomach patients are discussed in other chapters.)

In summary, methods to prevent untoward elevations of IOP include perioperative instillation of topical miotics in patients with glaucoma as well as avoidance of overhydration and venous congestion. Even in patients with nonglaucomatous eyes, coughing and vomiting should be avoided. Various pharmacological pretreatments, including IV lidocaine, sublingual nifedipine, or oral clonidine, prior to a gentle, brief, "smooth" laryngoscopy and intubation, are helpful. Intraoperatively, proper oxygenation and ventilation are essential. Moreover, patient movement or coughing intraoperatively are to be meticulously avoided. Proper depth of anesthesia and use of nonde-

polarizing neuromuscular blockers in conjunction with monitoring by a peripheral nerve stimulator are crucial. In this context, patient movement or coughing can be a problem with intraocular procedures performed with regional anesthesia as well; oversedating the patient is not the solution, because such patients frequently move unpredictably. Also, snoring that might result from oversedation may cause head movement with the respiratory cycle and further complicate the surgical challenge. With regional anesthesia for ocular procedures, the anesthetic goal is a calm, cooperative, and aware patient.

EMERGENCE PROBLEMS

At extubation, the anesthesiologist is concerned with potentially serious misadventures such as laryngospasm, aspiration, and airway obstruction. Additionally, the ocular anesthesiologist attempts to prevent coughing, retching, and vomiting lest deleterious increases in IOP transpire that could compromise surgical outcome. Because many ophthalmologic procedures, such as strabismus repair, cataract surgery, and trabeculectomy, are now performed on an outpatient basis, the practical consequences of intractable, debilitating nausea and vomiting become obvious.

With the possible exceptions of strabismus, retinal detachment, and cryosurgery, ophthalmic operations are associated with minimal pain. Therefore, the routine administration of narcotic premedication, with its potential emetic effect, is not advocated. Rather, if premedication is given, it should be selected with the objectives of sedation, amnesia, and antiemesis. Rational choices include a benzodiazepine for sedative-hypnotic effect or the phenothiazine promethazine or the antihistamine hydroxyzine for sedative-antiemetic properties.

The oculogastric reflex appears to be a real phenomenon, judging from the frequency of nausea and vomiting following eye muscle surgery. In the early 1980s, Abramowitz and colleagues[79, 80] reported that prophylactic IV administration of 0.075 mg/kg of droperidol 30 minutes prior to termination of surgery was "highly effective" in reducing both the severity and the incidence of postoperative vomiting in pediatric strabismus patients. Furthermore, no significant prolongation of recovery time owing to sedation was noted with this dose of droperidol. Lerman and associates[81] found encouraging results when the same dose of droperidol was administered IV at the start of the case, prior to manipulation of the extraocular muscles. In their series, only 10% of patients experienced vomiting. In addition, Warner and coworkers[82] reported similar results when lidocaine 2 mg/kg IV was given prior to intubation; only 16% of their patients vomited. However, others have not reported such favorable results following lidocaine "prophylaxis."

Coughing on the endotracheal tube may be attenuated by giving IV lidocaine, 1.5–2 mg/kg, a few minutes prior to extubation. Once surgery is completed and the patient is able to breathe spontaneously, he or she may be extubated while still deeply anesthetized—provided no risk factors for aspiration exist—in the lateral position with the operated eye uppermost.

OCULAR COMPLICATIONS OF PREMATURITY AND OXYGEN THERAPY

The intricacies of retinopathy of prematurity (ROP) are discussed in Chapter 15. However, a brief summary is presented here.

In the early 1950s, Patz and colleagues implicated liberal use of oxygen as the principal cause of ROP.[83] For almost three decades, ROP has featured prominently in medical malpractice cases. However, the facts question prior allegations of negligence in the administration of "excess" oxygen.[84]

The immature retinal vasculature seems to respond to oxygen in a biphasic fashion. Initially, vasoconstriction of large vessels and vaso-obliteration of capillary beds occur, followed by eventual vasoproliferation when the infant is returned to breathing room air. The severity of the retinopathy depends on the extent of fibrous traction and whether a traction retinal detachment develops. Furthermore, it is difficult to predict whether vision-threatening cicatricial involvement will occur; that devastating development appears to be influenced by factors other than perinatal oxygen exposure alone. For example, the National Cooperative Study concluded that birth weight, gestational age, and duration of supplementary oxygen treatment are the most important factors associated with ROP and that these variables are highly inter-related, reflecting functional immaturity. In addition, it is possible that carbon dioxide level, bright light, and vitamin E deficiency are other variables that may be involved in the pathogenesis of ROP.

Among the established pathogenetic variables, Flynn[85] showed that birth weight was the most significant predictor for risk of proliferative ROP. Babies with a birth weight less than 1000 g had such a high incidence of proliferative ROP that no other exogenous factor, *including oxygen,* seemed significant. Sporadic cases of ROP have been reported in premature babies who received little or no supplemental oxygen, as well as in full-term infants.[86]

Patz, however, postulated that the sporadic case of ROP that occurs in infants who received minimal or no supplemental oxygen can still be explained on the basis of the effects of oxygen.[87] *In utero,* the fetal environment is characterized by low oxygen tension. After birth, however, the lungs expand and the ductus arteriosus and the foramen ovale close. Hence, the arterial oxygen tension in the infant (premature and full-term) increases dramatically even without administration of supplemental oxygen. Thus, it appears possible that a sensitive "target organ" such as the immature retina responds to this sudden, significant increase in arterial oxygen tension with irreversible retinal arterial and arteriolar vasoconstriction and vaso-obliteration. The retina is immature at birth even in a full-term baby, because the anterior temporal portion does not become fully vascularized until about 1 month following delivery of a full-term infant.[88]

Thus, even in the full-term infant, physicians now administer oxygen only for specific indications rather than giving it routinely. When supplemental oxygen is required in infants less than 44 weeks postconception, physicians maintain the arterial oxygen tension within a normal, rather than supranormal, range to minimize the possibility of visual impairment. However, oxygen is not withheld when it is necessary for the well-being of the infant. *Oxygen is often necessary to prevent brain injury and death.* Moreover, data published in 1984 clarified in an optimistic fashion the influence of surgery and anesthesia on the eventual development of ROP.[89] Employing logistical risk analysis and controlling for such variables as total duration of oxygen exposure, inspired oxygen tensions, hours of mechanical ventilation, and birth weight, Flynn reported that infants requiring anesthesia and surgery had no greater risk of cicatricial ROP than infants not subjected to these stresses.

Today, anesthesiologists and neonatologists generally strive to maintain oxygen saturation, as determined by pulse oximetry, at about 95% in infants less than 44 weeks postconception. However, scrupulous adherence to this guideline does not guarantee a safe visual outcome, nor does deviation from this range necessarily imply negligence. Even with meticulous and continuous monitoring of oxygen tension, in vulnerable infants ROP will probably still occur. ROP is a multifactorial disease that is probably not preventable in extremely low birth weight infants. Oxygen therapy is neither a necessary nor sufficient cause of ROP, and establishment of rigid treatment routines designed to arbitrarily restrict therapeutic oxygen is an undesirable goal.

OCULAR COMPLICATIONS OF ANESTHESIA FOR GENERAL SURGERY

Ophthalmic complications do not occur only in those patients having ocular surgery. Postoperative ocular complications that have been reported following nonocular surgery include corneal abrasion, chemical injuries, thermal injury, minor visual disturbances, and serious visual disturbances, including either transient or permanent blindness. Transient or permanent visual loss has been reported in association with diverse conditions such as acute corneal epithelial edema;[90] central retinal artery occlusion;[91] administration of various pharmacological substances, such as atropine,[92] ketamine,[93] glycine, and amiodarone;[94] performance of attempted stellage ganglion block;[95] Valsalva hemorrhagic retinopathy;[96] retinal ischemia; and acute glaucoma.

Corneal Abrasion

The most common ocular complication of general anesthesia is corneal abrasion caused by the anesthesia mask or surgical drapes. The incidence of corneal abrasion during general anesthesia was reported in one study to be as high as 44%.[97] General anesthesia decreases tear production, an important element in protecting the cornea from drying and subsequent vulnerability to abrasion or ulceration. In addition, ocular injury also may occur as a consequence of anesthesia-induced obtundation of protective corneal reflexes and loss of pain sensation. Taping the eyelids closed, application of protective goggles, and instillation of

petroleum-based ointments (artificial tears) into the conjunctival sac provide protection. However, ointments may be associated with allergic reactions, flammability that may render their use undesirable during surgery of the head and neck, and blurred vision in the early postoperative period.[98] During general anesthesia for surgery caudad to the neck in which the patient is supine, closure of the eyelids with tape with or without ointment should be satisfactory, provided the procedure is less than 3 hours in duration. If the eyelid opens beneath the tape, the tape itself may denude an exposed cornea.

Patients with prominent eyes or exophthalmos (as in Graves' disease) and those with neurological disease, such as Bell's palsy, may be at greater risk of corneal damage, because their eyes do not close easily. These special patients may require surgical closure of the lids with a few sutures. Furthermore, direct eye trauma is best avoided by care in selecting the proper mask size and by being gentle in its subsequent application. The anesthesiologist's hands and instruments should be used with care during laryngoscopy and intubation. Watson and Moran[99] identified two common, but unusual, hazards during laryngoscopy: the end of a plastic (belt style) watchband and the hospital identification card, clipped to the vest pocket of a scrub suit, which comes dangerously close to the patient's eyes during a direct laryngoscopy. Therefore, the eyes should perhaps be protected before laryngoscopy. Additionally, because of the possibility of injury, intraoperative determination of anesthetic depth by eliciting the corneal reflex should not be done.[100]

Pain, tearing, and photophobia are typical symptoms of corneal abrasion. Patients frequently complain of a foreign body sensation, and the pain is characteristically exacerbated by blinking and ocular movement. An immediate consultation by an ophthalmologist is indicated. Treatment consists of the prophylactic application of antibiotic ointment and patching of the injured eye. Although permanent sequelae are possible, healing usually occurs within 24 hours.

Chemical Injury

Liquid disinfectants used to clean reusable anesthetic masks and spillage of solutions during skin preparation may result in chemical damage to the eye. Durkan and Fleming[101] reported on potential eye injury that may result from masks exposed to a disinfecting solution of 2% glutaraldehyde from repeated processing in Cidematic machines that wash, rinse, disinfect, and spin-dry in programmed cycles. It was speculated that, during a cleaning process, heat caused a weak spot in the mask's pneumatic cushion to rupture, exchanging its air with available solution. Identification of the discharged solution collecting in the patient's internal canthus was facilitated by glutaraldehyde's odor. Murray[102] suggested that such a threat can be avoided by (1) careful inspection of every mask treated with liquid chemicals, (2) selection of reusable masks that can be cleaned by ethylene oxide or autoclaving, and (3) use of disposable masks. Otherwise, chemical conjunctivitis may result.

Representatives[103] from the Food and Drug Administration have reported on serious or irreversible corneal damage caused by eye contact with HIBICLENS, a 4% chlorhexidine gluconate solution formulated with a detergent. Because use of chlorhexidine gluconate to prepare facial skin for surgery is a common practice, care should be taken to keep the substance out of the eye and to flush copiously with sterile saline solution or sterile water if contact accidentally occurs. (HIBICLENS also causes sensorineural deafness when it enters the middle ear secondary to the presence of a perforated tympanic membrane.[104, 105] It should not be used in or around the ear if there is a chance that the tympanic membrane is not intact.)

Chemical injury to the eye is certainly preventable. Treatment consists of liberal bathing of the eye with sterile saline or sterile water to remove the offending agent. Postoperatively, an ophthalmologist should examine the eye to document any residual injury.

Thermal Injury

The potential for thermal injury to the cornea or retina from certain laser beams demands that the patient's eyes be protected with moist gauze pads and metal shields and that operating room personnel wear protective glasses.[106]

Mild or Transient Visual Symptoms

Following anesthesia, mild visual disturbances, such as photophobia or diplopia, can occur.[107] Blurred vision in the early postoperative period may reflect residual effects of petroleum-based ophthalmic ointments or ocular effects of anticholinergic drugs administered in the perioperative period. Dhamee and associates[108] reported an incidence ranging between 7 to 14% of benign, transient visual disturbances after gynecological procedures.

Transient visual loss or even ephemeral blindness has been reported perioperatively. For example, Szeinfeld and coworkers[95] reported a case of total reversible blindness following a paratracheal approach to an attempted stellate ganglion block. Apparently, their patient developed inability to speak lasting about 1 minute owing to tongue weakness and approximately 5 minutes of blindness when 1 mL of 0.25% bupivacaine was inadvertently injected into the vertebral artery with subsequent selective vascular distribution into the CNS. The patient's focal symptoms resulted from a highly localized toxic dose, because the Edinger-Westphal nucleus (the motor nucleus of the trigeminal nerve) and the nucleus of the hypoglossal nerve are located beside the midline at the level of the brain stem.

Several interesting reports have documented transient blindness associated with transurethral resection of the prostate (TURP).[109–111] In 1975, Defalque and Miller[109] described a case of temporary blindness without mental changes following overhydration during TURP. Ophthalmologic consultation disclosed normal fundi and pupillary reflexes but absent eyelid reflexes—a picture consistent with cortical blindness. Serum sodium was 110 mEq/L and urine specific gravity 1.001. Over the next 2 hours, the patient diuresed 2 L, and normal vision slowly returned with eventual full recovery. The authors attributed the clinical findings to cerebral edema. However, others have postulated that the visual disturbance is caused by a direct effect of glycine[110, 111] irrigation and subsequent excess absorption rather than to occipital cortical edema. Glycine is considered to be an inhibitory transmitter in the retina, brain stem, and spinal cord.[112] Creel and colleagues[111] obtained electroretinograms from patients experiencing visual impairment associated with the TURP syndrome and documented dropout of oscillatory potentials generated by the retina in those patients who had excessive serum levels of this inhibitory transmitter.

Amiodarone, a drug used for treatment of life-threatening ventricular tachyarrhythmias, has caused usually asymptomatic corneal microdeposits, but occasionally its use may result in visual impairment.[94, 113] Blindness has been reported secondary to the addition of quinine adulterant to heroin.

Hemorrhagic Retinopathy

Retinal hemorrhages, occurring in otherwise healthy persons, secondary to hemodynamic changes associated with turbulent emergence from anesthesia or protracted vomiting are termed Valsalva retinopathy.[114] Fortunately, these venous hemorrhages are usually self-limiting, with complete resolution in a few days to a few months.

The vast majority of these lesions are asymptomatic, because no visual deterioration is noted unless the macula is involved. However, if bleeding into the optic nerve develops, optic atrophy may ensue. If the hemorrhage is massive, the result may be permanent visual impairment.[115] However, some cases of massive hemorrhages may be ameliorated somewhat by vitrectomy.

Retinal Ischemia

The arterial circulation may also be the source of retinal bleeding secondary to extraocular trauma. Fundoscopic examination discloses cotton-wool exudates,[116] a condition known as Purtscher's retinopathy. Therefore, when a trauma patient complains of postanesthetic visual loss, Purtscher's retinopathy should be ruled out. Unfortunately, this entity has a poor prognosis, and the majority of patients afflicted sustain permanent visual impairment.

Retinal ischemia or infarction also may result from direct ocular trauma secondary to pressure exerted by an ill-fitting anesthetic mask, especially in a hypotensive setting, as well as from embolism during cardiac surgery[117] or from the intraocular injection of a large volume of SF_6 in the presence of high concentrations of nitrous oxide.[118] Proper positioning of the patient is important, especially when the patient must be prone or in the jackknife position. When the patient's head is located dependently for surgical position, the anesthesiologist should inspect it frequently by gently raising it from the head rest. This maneuver allows return of circulation to any pressure areas over bony prominences and provides reassurance that external ocular pressure is being avoided and adequate retinal perfusion is being maintained. Otherwise, possible retinal ischemia may develop, especially in the setting of systemic hypotension.

Acute Angle-Closure Glaucoma

Acute angle-closure glaucoma, caused by pupillary block, is a serious multifactorial disease. Risk factors include genetic predisposition,[119] a shallow anterior chamber, increased lens thickness, small corneal diameter, female gender, and advanced age.[120] A study[121] investigated possible precipitating events in persons at risk and found no evidence that the type of anesthetic agent, the duration of surgery, the volume of parenteral fluids, or the intraoperative blood pressure was related to the development of acute angle-closure glaucoma.

Despite its seriousness, acute angle-closure glaucoma may be difficult to recognize. However, physicians should be knowledgeable about this potential complication, because diagnostic delay may deleteriously influence visual outcome. Fazio and associates[121] recommended, therefore, that preoperative evaluation include a thorough ocular history as well as a penlight examination to detect a shallow anterior chamber. (The depth of the anterior chamber is assessed by the distance from the cornea to the iris.) Those patients considered to be at risk should then have preoperative ophthalmic evaluation as well as perioperative miotic therapy. Postoperatively, these patients should be scrupulously watched for red eye or for complaints of pain and blurred vision. Persistent enlargement of the pupils and, especially, unequal enlargement and irregular enlargement (so that the pupil is not round) are the foremost bases for suspicion and for tonometric measurement of IOP.

REFERENCES

1. Duncalf D, Gartner S, Carol B: Mortality in association with ophthalmic surgery. Am J Ophthalmol 1970; 69:610.
2. Petruscak J, Smith RB, Breslin P: Mortality related to ophthalmological surgery. Arch Ophthalmol 1973; 89:106.
3. Lang DW: Morbidity and mortality in ophthalmology. In Bruce RA, McGoldrick KE, Oppenheimer P (eds): Anesthesia For Ophthalmology. Birmingham, Aesculapius Publishing, 1982, pp 195–204.
4. Kaplan MR, Reba RC: Pulmonary embolism as the leading cause of ophthalmic surgical mortality. Am J Ophthalmol 1972; 73:159.
5. Quigley HA: Mortality associated with ophthalmic surgery. Am J Ophthalmol 1974; 77:518.
6. Backer CL, Tinker JH, Robertson DM, et al: Myocardial reinfarction following local anesthesia for ophthalmic surgery. Anesth Analg 1980; 59:257.
7. Lynch S, Wolf GL, Berlin I: General anesthesia for cataract surgery: A comparative review of 2,217 consecutive cases. Anesth Analg 1974; 53:909.
8. Donlon JV: Local anesthesia for ophthalmic surgery: Patient preparation and management. Ann Ophthalmol 1980; 12:1183.
9. Donlon JV, Moss J: Plasma catecholamine levels during local anesthesia for cataract operations. Anesthesiology 1979; 51:471–473.

10. Matsumoto S, Hayashi K, Tsuchisaka H, et al: Pharmacokinetics of surface anesthesia in the human cornea. Jpn J Ophthalmol 1981; 25:355.

11. Adriani J, Zepernick R: Clinical effectiveness of drugs used for topical anesthesia. JAMA 1964; 188:711.

12. Koller K: On the use of cocaine to anesthetize the eye. Arch Ophthalmol 1884; 13:404. (Translated by H Knapp in: On cocaine and its use in ophthalmic and general surgery. Arch Ophthalmol 1962; 68:31.)

13. Meyers EF: Cocaine toxicity during dacryocystorhinostomy. Arch Ophthalmol 1980; 98:842.

14. Gay GR, Loper KA: Control of cocaine-induced hypertension with labetalol. Anesth Analg 1988; 67:92.

15. Feibel RM: Current concepts in retrobulbar anesthesia. Surv Ophthalmol 1985; 30:102–109.

16. Unsöld R, Stanley JA, DeGroot J: The CT-tomography of retrobulbar anesthesia. Graefes Arch Clin Exp Ophthalmol 1981; 217:125–136.

17. van Lint A: Paralysie, palpébrale temporaire provoquée dans l'operation de la cataracte. Ann Ocul 1914; 151:420.

18. Atkinson WS: Akinesia of the orbicularis. Am J Ophthalmol 1953; 36:1255.

19. O'Brien CS: Akinesia during cataract extraction. Arch Ophthalmol 1929; 1:447.

20. Nadbath RP, Rehman I: Facial nerve block. Am J Ophthalmol 1963; 55:143.

21. Beltranena HP, Vega MJ, Garcia JJ, et al: Complications of retrobulbar marcaine injection. J Clin Neuro Ophthalmol 1982; 2:159–161.

22. Rosenblatt RM, May DR, Barsoumian K: Cardiopulmonary arrest after retrobulbar block. Am J Ophthalmol 1980; 90:425–427.

23. Hamilton RC: Brain stem anesthesia following retrobulbar blockade. Anesthesiology 1985; 63:688–690.

24. Chang JL, Gonzalez-Abola E, Larson CE, Lobes L: Brain stem anesthesia following retrobulbar block. Anesthesiology 1984; 61:789–790.

25. Drysdale DB: Experimental subdural retrobulbar injection of anesthetic. Ann Ophthalmol 1984; 16:716–718.

26. Lynn JG Jr, Smith RB: Intraoperative complications and their management. Int Ophthalmol Clin 1973; 13:149–175.

27. Ramsay RC, Knoblock WH: Ocular perforation following retrobulbar anesthesia for retinal detachment surgery. Am J Ophthalmol 1978; 86:61–64.

28. Follette JW, Locascio JA: Bilateral amaurosis following unilateral retrobulbar block. Anesthesiology 1985; 63:237–238.

29. Brookshire GL, Gleitsmann KY, Schenk EC: Life-threatening complication of retrobulbar block. Ophthalmology 1986; 93:1476–1478.

30. Nicoll JMV, Acharya PA, Ahlen K, et al: Central nervous system complications after 6000 retrobulbar blocks. Anesth Analg 1987; 66:1298–1302.

31. Meyers EF, Ramirez RC, Boniu KI: Grand mal seizures after retrobulbar block. Arch Ophthalmol 1978; 96:847.

32. Beltranena HP, Vega MJ, Kirk N, et al: Inadvertent intravascular bupivacaine injection following retrobulbar block: Report of three cases. Reg Anesthesia 1981; 6:149–151.

33. Cibis PA: General discussion. In Schepens CL, Regan CDL (eds): Controversial Aspects of the Management of Retinal Detachment. Boston, Little Brown, 1965, pp 223–233.

34. Aldrete JA, Roma-Salas F, Arora S, et al: Reverse arterial blood flow as a pathway for central nervous system toxic responses following injection of local anesthetics. Anesth Analg 1978; 57:428–433.

35. Reed JW, MacMillan AS, Lazenby GW: Transient neurologic complication of positive contrast orbitography. Arch Ophthalmol 1969; 81:508–511.

36. Kobet KA: Cerebral spinal fluid recovery of lidocaine and bupivacaine following respiratory arrest subsequent to retrobulbar block. Ophthalmic Surg 1987; 18:11–13.

37. Davis DB, Mandel MR: Posterior peribulbar anesthesia: An alternative to retrobulbar anesthesia. J Cataract Refract Surg 1986; 12:182–184.

38. Zahl K, Jordan A, McGroarty J, Gotta AW: PH-adjusted bupivacaine and hyaluronidase for peribulbar block. Anesthesiology 1990; 72:230–232.

39. Berler DK: Oculocardiac reflex. Am J Ophthalmol 1963; 12:56, 954.

40. Kirsch RE, Samet P, Kugel V, et al: Electrocardiographic changes during ocular surgery and their prevention by retrobulbar injection. Arch Ophthalmol 1957; 58:348.

41. Bosomworth PP, Ziegler CH, Jacoby J: Oculocardiac reflex in eye muscle surgery. Anesthesiology 1958; 19:7–10.

42. Taylor C, Wilson FM, Roesch R, et al: Prevention of the oculocardiac reflex in children: Comparison of retrobulbar block and intravenous atropine. Anesthesiology 1963; 24:646–649.

43. Mirakur RK, Clarke RSJ, Dundee JW, et al: Anticholinergic drugs in anaesthesia—a survey of their present position. Anaesthesia 1978; 33:133–138.

44. Blanc VF, Hardy JF, Milot J: Oculocardiac reflex: A graphic and statistical analysis in infants and children. Can Anaesth Soc J 1983; 30:360–369.

45. Joseph MC, Vale RJ: Premedication with atropine by mouth. Lancet 1960; 2:1060.

46. Katz RL, Bigger JT: Cardiac arrhythmias during anesthesia and operation. Anesthesiology 1970; 33:193–213.

47. Horgan J: Atropine and ventricular tachyarrhythmias. JAMA 1973; 223:693.

48. Massumi RA, Mason DT, Amsterdam EA, et al: Ventricular fibrillation and tachycardia after intravenous atropine for treatment of bradycardias. N Engl J Med 1972; 287:336–338.

49. McGoldrick KE: Transient left bundle branch block during local anesthesia. Anesth Rev 1981; 8:36–39.

50. Moonie GT, Rees DI, Elton D: Oculocardiac reflex during strabismus surgery. Can Anaesth Soc J 1964; 11:621–632.

51. Steward DJ: Anticholinergic premedication for infants and children. Can Anaesth Soc J 1983; 30:325–326.

52. Schwartz H: Oculocardiac reflex: Is prophylaxis necessary? In Mark LC, Ngai SH (eds): Highlights of Clinical Anesthesiology. New York, Harper and Row, 1971, pp 109–117.

53. Meyers EF, Tomelden SA: Glycopyrrolate compared with atropine in prevention of the oculocardiac reflex during eye muscle surgery. Anesthesiology 1979; 51:350.

54. Zimmerman T, Konner KS, Kandarakis AS, et al: Improving the therapeutic index of topically applied ocular drugs. Arch Ophthalmol 1984; 102:551–553.

55. Betoptic (betaxolol hydrochloride) package insert. Ft. Worth, Texas, Alcon Laboratories Inc, revised November, 1985.

56. Atkins JM, Pugh BR Jr, Timewell RM: Cardiovas-

cular effects of topical beta-blockers during exercise. Am J Ophthalmol 1985; 99:173–175.

57. Ball S: Congestive heart failure from betaxolol. Arch Ophthalmol 1987; 105:320.

58. Mendelson CL: Aspiration of stomach contents into lungs during obstetric anesthesia. Am J Obstet Gynecol 1946; 30:191.

59. Berson W, Adriani J: "Silent" regurgitation and aspiration during anesthesia. Anesthesiology 1954; 15:644.

60. Turndorf H, Rodis ID, Clark TS: "Silent" regurgitation during general anesthesia. Anesth Analg 1974; 53:700.

61. Culver GA, Makel HP, Beecher HK: Frequency of aspiration of gastric contents by the lungs during anesthesia and surgery. Ann Surg 1951; 133:289.

62. Olsson GL, Hallen B, Hambraeus Jonzon K: Aspiration during anaesthesia: A computer aided study of 185,358 anaesthetics. Acta Anaesthesiol Scand 1986; 30:84.

63. Dines DE, Titus JL, Sessler AD: Aspiration pneumonitis. Mayo Clin Proc 1970; 45:347.

64. Rao TLK, Suseeda M, El-Etv AA: Metoclopramide and cimetidine to reduce gastric pH and volume. Anesth Analg 1984; 63:264.

65. Tomlin PJ, Howarth FH, Robinson JS: Postoperative atelectasis and laryngeal incompetence. Lancet 1968; 1:1402.

66. Adler FH: Physiology of the Eye: Clinical Application, 5th ed. St. Louis, CV Mosby, 1970, pp 249–277.

67. Stoelting RK: Circulatory changes during direct laryngoscopy and tracheal intubation: Influence of duration of laryngoscopy with or without prior lidocaine. Anesthesiology 1977; 47:381.

68. Stoelting RK: Blood pressure and heart rate changes during short duration laryngoscopy for tracheal intubation: Influences of viscous or intravenous lidocaine. Anesth Analg 1978; 57:197.

69. Badrinath SK, Braverman KB, Ivankovich AD: Alfentanil and sufentanil prevent the increase in IOP from succinylcholine. Anesth Analg 1988; 67:S5.

70. Ghignone M, Noe C, Calvillo O, et al: Effects of clonidine on IOP and perioperative hemodynamics. Anesthesiology 1988; 68:707–716.

71. Hill DW: Physics Applied to Anaesthesia. New York, Appleton-Century-Crofts, 1968, p 41.

72. Berry JM, Merin RG: Etomidate myoclonus and the open globe. Anesth Analg 1989; 69:256–259.

73. Peuler M, Glass DD, Arena JF: Ketamine and intraocular pressure. Anesthesiology 1975; 5:575–578.

74. Duncalf D, Weitzner SW: Ventilation and hypercapnia on intraocular pressure in children. Anesth Analg 1963; 43:232.

75. Agarwal LP, Mathur SP: Curare in ocular surgery. Br J Ophthalmol 1952; 36:603.

76. Litwiller RW, Difazio CA, Rushia EL: Pancuronium and intraocular pressure. Anesthesiology 1975; 42:750.

77. Jampolsky A: Strabismus: Surgical overcorrections. Highlights Ophthalmol 1965; 8:78.

78. France NK, France TD, Woodburn JD, et al: Succinylcholine alteration of the forced duction test. Ophthalmology 1980; 87:1282.

79. Abramowitz MD, Epstein BS, Friendly DS, et al: Effect of droperidol in reducing vomiting in pediatric strabismic outpatient surgery. Anesthesiology 1981; 59:A329.

80. Abramowitz MD, Oh TH, Epstein BS: Antiemetic effect of droperidol following outpatient strabismus surgery in children. Anesthesiology 1983; 59:579.

81. Lerman J, Eustis S, Smith DR: Effect of droperidol pretreatment on postanesthetic vomiting in children undergoing strabismus surgery. Anesthesiology 1986; 65:322–325.

82. Warner LO, Rogers GL, Martino JD, et al: Intravenous lidocaine reduces the incidence of post-strabismus vomiting in children. Anesthesiology 1988; 68:618–621.

83. Patz A, Hoeck LE, DeLaCruz E: Studies on the effect of oxygen administration in retrolental fibroplasia: I. Nursing observations. Am J Ophthalmol 1952; 35:1248.

84. Ausman R: Amicus brief—retrolental fibroplasia (ROP). *In* Ausman R, Snyder DE (eds): Medical Library, Lawyer's Edition, Vol 4. Rochester, Lawyer's Cooperative Publishing Co, 1989, pp 727–745.

85. Flynn JT: Acute proliferative retrolental fibroplasia: Multivariate risk analysis. Trans Am Ophthalmol Soc 1983; 81:549.

86. Brockhurst RJ, Chishti MI: Cicatricial retrolental fibroplasia: Its occurrence without oxygen administration and in full-term infants. Graefes Arch Clin Exp Ophthalmol 1975; 195:128.

87. Patz A: Role of oxygen in retrolental fibroplasia. Trans Am Ophthalmol Soc 1968; 66:940.

88. Cogan DG: Development and senescence of human retinal vasculature. Trans Ophthalmol Soc UK 1963; 83:465.

89. Flynn JT: Oxygen and retrolental fibroplasia: Update and challenge. Anesthesiology 1984; 60:397.

90. Richardson RB, McBride CM, Berkely RG, et al: An unusual ocular complication after anesthesia. Anesthesiology 1975; 43:357.

91. Givner I, Jaffe N: Occlusion of the central retinal artery following anesthesia. Arch Ophthalmol 1950; 43:197.

92. Gooding JM, Holcomb MC: Transient blindness following intravenous administration atropine. Anesth Analg 1977; 56:872–873.

93. Fine J, Weissman J, Finestone SC: Side effects after ketamine anaesthesia: Transient blindness. Anesth Analg 1974; 53:72.

94. Ingram DV: Ocular effects of long-term amiodarone therapy. Am Heart J 1983; 106:902–905.

95. Szeinfeld M, Laurencio M, Pallares VS: Total reversible blindness following attempted stellate ganglion block. Anesth Analg 1981; 60:689–690.

96. Boldner PM, Norton MI: Retinal hemorrhage following anesthesia. Anesthesiology 1984; 61:595.

97. Batra YK, Bali M: Corneal abrasions during general anesthesia. Anesth Analg 1977; 56:363.

98. Siffring PA, Poulton TJ: Prevention of ophthalmic complications during general anesthesia. Anesthesiology 1987; 66:569–570.

99. Watson WJ, Moran RL: Corneal abrasion during induction. Anesthesiology 1987; 66:440.

100. Brooks GZ: Ocular injury during anesthesia: Case reports and a review of the literature. Anesth Rev 1978; 5:22–24.

101. Durkan W, Fleming N: Potential eye damage from reusable masks. Anesthesiology 1987; 67:444.

102. Murray WJ: A case of eye injury from a reusable anesthetic mask. Anesthesiology 1988; 68:302.

103. Tabor E, Bostwick DC, Evans CC: Corneal damage due to eye contact with chlorhexidine gluconate. JAMA 1989; 261:557–558.

104. Bicknell PG: Sensorineural deafness following myringoplasty operations. J Laryngol Otol 1971; 85:957–961.

105. Igarashi Y, Suzuki J: Cochlear ototoxicity of chlorhexidine gluconate in cats. Arch Otorhinolaryngol 1985; 242:167–176.

106. Kalhan SB, Cascorbi HF: Anesthetic management of laser microlaryngeal surgery. Anesth Rev 1981; 8:23.

107. Conway C: Neurological and ophthalmic complications of anaesthesia. *In* Churchill-Davidson HC (ed): A Practice of Anaesthesia, 4th ed. Philadelphia, WB Saunders, 1978, p 1021.

108. Dhamee MS, Ghandi SK, Callen KM, et al: Morbidity after outpatient anesthesia—a comparison of different endotracheal anesthetic techniques for laparoscopy. Anesthesiology 1982; 57:A375.

109. Defalque RJ, Miller DW: Visual disturbances during transurethral resection of the prostate. Can Anaesth Soc J 1975; 22:620–621.

110. Ovassapian A, Joshi CW, Brunner EA: Visual disturbances: An unusual symptom of transurethral prostatic resection reaction. Anesthesiology 1982; 57:332–334.

111. Creel DJ, Wang JM, Wong KC: Transient blindness associated with transurethral resection of the prostate. Arch Ophthalmol 1987; 105:1537–1539.

112. Massey SC, Redburn DA: Transmitter circuits in vertebrate retina. Prog Neurobiol 1987; 28:55–96.

113. Mason JW: Amiodarone. N Engl J Med 1987; 316:455–466.

114. DeVoe AG, Norton EWD, Kearns TP, et al: Valsalva hemorrhagic retinopathy: Discussion. Trans Am Ophthalmol Soc 1972; 70:307.

115. Madsen PH: Traumatic retinal angiopathy. Ophthalmologica 1972; 165:453.

116. McLeod D: Reappraisal of the retinal cotton-wool spot. J R Soc Med 1981; 74:682.

117. Gutman FA, Zegarra H: Ocular complications in cardiac surgery. Surg Clin North Am 1971; 51:1095.

118. Stinson TW, Donlon JV: Interaction of SF$_6$ and air with nitrous oxide. Anesthesiology 1979; 51:S16.

119. Drance SM: Angle-closure glaucoma among Canadian Eskimos. Can J Ophthalmol 1973; 8:252.

120. Alsbirk PH: Angle-closure glaucoma surveys in Greenland Eskimos. Can J Ophthalmol 1973; 8:260.

121. Fazio DT, Bateman JB, Christensen RE: Acute angle-closure glaucoma associated with surgical anesthesia. Arch Ophthalmol 1985; 103:360–362.

22

Recovery Room Care and Problems Following Ophthalmic and Otolaryngologic Surgery

Martin Andrew Acquadro

POSTANESTHESIA CARE UNIT MANAGEMENT FOLLOWING OPHTHALMIC SURGERY

Two important goals are safe and successful postanesthetic recovery and the start of safe and successful postsurgical healing. Issues involving the airway, respiration, hemodynamics, (airway, breathing, and circulation), and mental status are of primary importance in postanesthesia care unit (PACU) management. Standard accepted PACU monitoring and discharge criteria, as used at the Massachusetts Eye and Ear Infirmary (MEEI) and shown in Figure 22–1, provide the framework for attention to details that results in successful management.[1]

Following surgical repair, issues such as head position and medications relating specifically to the surgical procedure should not compromise safe standards of PACU management. For example, postoperative management following retinal reattachment includes proper head positioning to promote continuing reattachment and to minimize the mechanical forces tending toward detachment.[2] However, vomiting and the risk of aspiration, or emergence delirium and the possibility of ocular harm to the patient, are the immediate management priority; in these cases, patient positioning may be different than that initially requested by the surgeon.

GENERAL CONSIDERATIONS

Table 22–1 lists a few common ophthalmic surgical postoperative problems. Some procedures with or without complications, listed in Table 22–2, involve specific immediate care that can affect standard PACU management.

Regional anesthesia and sedation for monitored anesthetic care and general anesthesia involve the discharge criteria applicable to other nonophthalmic types of surgery. Complications arising from sedation are often dose-related.[3–5] No standard recommendations can be made, however, regarding the use or nonuse of various anxiolytic and analgesic agents in the perioperative period, because selection of agents and doses administered must be titrated individually. Careful attention to details concerning the patient's history of pre-existing problems and the patient's expectations—along with the clinician's experience—are guiding principles.[1, 4, 5]

Conditions such as asthma, hypertension, coronary artery disease, chronic obstructive pulmonary disease, diabetes mellitus, diminished hearing, blindness involving both eyes, and senile dementia are relatively common causes of postoperative concern in the ophthalmic patient.

Language barriers and physical limitations may influence the choice of anesthesia as well as PACU management. Interpreters, family

M.E.E.I. POST ANESTHESIA CARE UNIT RECORD

Date: _____ In: _____ Out: _____

PRE-Existing Problems: _____

_____

Allergies: _____

Pre-Op. Med. _____

Operative Procedure: _____

Anesthetic Agent: _____

Relaxants: _____

Reversal Agents _____ Intra-op. Problems: _____

Anesthetist _____ ☐ Intubated   ☐ Trach.   ☐ Mask   ☐ Nasal   ☐ Oral airway

Position

Time:														
IV Drugs: gtts │ mgm or mcg.														
Breath sounds														
Temperature														
Rhythm														
SAO$_2$														

Dressing: Dry or see note

Dressing site _____

IV site: _____

O$_2$ Flow _____ % _____

Time on _____ Off _____

Post Anesthetic Care
   Score
Optimal Score = 12

Discharge Score 9-12

240
200
190
180
170
160
150
140
130
120
110
100
90
80
70
60
50

		=													
Airway	Good spontaneous airway	= 2													
	Needs airway support (jaw support, artificial airway or trach.)	= 1													
	Needs & tolerates E.T. tube	= 0													
Respira-tions	Clinically adequate ventilations	= 2													
	Dyspnea or inadequate ventilations	= 1													
	Apneic	= 0													
Color	Pink	= 2													
	Pale, dusky, blotchy, jaundiced	= 1													
	Cyanotic	= 0													
Conscious-ness	Fully awake	= 2													
	Arousable	= 1													
	Unresponsive	= 0													
Blood Pressure	Sys BP ± 20mm Hg Preanesthetic lvl	= 2													
	Sys BP ± 20-40 mm Hg pre-anes. lvl	= 1													
	Sys BP < or > then 40mm Hg pre-anes lvl	= 0													
Cardiac Rhythm	Same as pre-anesthic	= 2													
	Newly abnormal-no therapy required	= 1													
	Newly abnormal-requiring therapy	= 0													
Oximetry	Same as pre-anesthetic	= 0													
	1-2 below pre-anesthetic level	= −1													
	3 or more below pre-anes level	= −2													

FIGURE 22–1. See legend on opposite page

Primary Nurse _____

Associate Nurse _____

Time	PEEP	Resp Rate	Tidal Volume	Insp. Force	T.V. / V.C.	FiO$_2$	pO$_2$	pCO$_2$	pH	Na	K	Hct.	B.S.

TIME	MEDS	RTE	BY

PROGRESS NOTES

Estimated Fluid Deficit

INTAKE			OUTPUT		
Type	OR	PACU	Type	Am't	Time

Total Intake: _____   Total Output: _____   DTV

Discharge Note:· _____

Anesthesiologist: _____

FIGURE 22–1. The postanesthesia care unit record at the Massachusetts Eye and Ear Infirmary includes a summary of the patient's medical history, germane intraoperative information, perioperative fluid therapy, and postoperative vital signs. Discharge criteria are also carefully documented.

TABLE 22–1. PACU Issues Relating to Ophthalmic Surgery

Postoperative Problems	Considerations
Pain	Routine *vs* corneal abrasion, acute angle-closure glaucoma
Nausea/vomiting	Type of surgery, pain, anxiety, oculocardiac reflex
Dysrhythmias	Systemic and eye medications, hypoventilation, OCR
Mental status	Iatrogenic problems, preexisting disease
Hypotension	Diuretics, anesthesia, cardiovascular toxicity of local anesthetics
Hypertension	Eye medications, history of hypertension, bladder distension
Oculocardiac reflex	Ocular traction, orbital pressure, pain
Malignant hyperthermia	1:15,000 pediatric population, 1:50,000 adult population, increased index of suspicion with associated musculoskeletal disorders, strabismus
Bladder distension	Following diuretics
Apnea and bradycardia	In premature infants, overnight monitoring for apnea and bradycardia

members, and adequate psychological support contribute to safe and effective care.

Following general anesthesia, patients at MEEI are routinely placed on an electrocardiographic monitor and pulse oximeter. Their blood pressure, pulse, and respirations are monitored until discharge to the floor or outpatient lounge for further recovery. Following monitored anesthetic care, stable patients are transported immediately to the outpatient lounge or to an inpatient floor. Vital signs are followed. Assessment for discharge is based on fluid intake, ambulation, mental status, and the availability of a responsible party to accompany the patient home.

Hypertension frequently seen postoperatively can be secondary to pain or to preexisting disease, but the potential role of eye medications or a full bladder should not be ignored. Treatments include reassurance, narcotics, acetaminophen, sublingual nifedipine, 10 mg (administered by piercing a hole in the capsule and squeezing the contents of the capsule sublingually), intravenous (IV) labetalol, and bladder catheterization.

Written instructions from the surgeon are provided to the patient, as are follow-up appointments and prescriptions. PACU treatment in the outpatient lounge is generally the same for patients who had undergone general anesthesia or monitored anesthetic care.

HEMORRHAGE

Hemorrhage that may occur preoperatively, intraoperatively, or postoperatively is commonly caused by injury to conjunctival, scleral, anterior ciliary, or vortex blood vessels and capillaries. A pressure dressing to the eye to control postoperative hemorrhage after extensive injury and reoperation is advocated.[6] The pressure induced can elicit the oculocardiac reflex, and cardiac monitoring is recommended.

INTRAOCULAR PRESSURE

Increased intraocular pressure (IOP) can be caused by common PACU problems such as nausea and vomiting or coughing caused by pharyngeal and lower airway irritation seen commonly in patients who smoke. As a general principle, the patient should be extubated without coughing and bucking, because any kind of Valsalva's maneuver can markedly increase IOP. IV lidocaine appears helpful in diminishing the cough reflex.

PRE-EXISTING DISEASES AND COMMON OPHTHALMIC PACU PROBLEMS

When elevated blood pressure occurs, the etiology should be determined. Besides the com-

TABLE 22–2. Procedures that Involve Specific Immediate Care

Procedures and Conditions	Considerations
Cataract surgery Scleral buckling Vitreous injection for detached retinas	Hemorrhage, eye pain, nausea and vomiting, head postion, nitrous oxide, dysrhythmias, ocular pressure, oculocardiac reflex, diuretic and hypertensive effects of medications
Perioperative eye trauma	Oculocardiac reflex, hemorrhage, pain, anesthetic and self-inflicted trauma, nausea and vomiting, hypercarbia
Strabismus surgery	Oculocardiac reflex, nausea and vomiting, malignant hyperthermia vigilance
Conditions associated with increased incidence of malignant hyperthermia	Malignant hyperthermia vigilance

mon etiologies of pain, anxiety, and pre-existing history of hypertension, the medications given in the perioperative period should be considered (Table 22–3). Frequent potential problems in ophthalmic surgery include the use of osmotic diuretics to lower IOP, causing bladder distension, and eye medications that can directly result in elevated blood pressure. Careful questioning of the surgeon, the anesthetist, and the anesthesiologist is necessary at the time of the PACU report to ascertain whether the patient took the usual antihypertensive medications preoperatively and whether any dysrhythmias occurred intraoperatively. Was the dysrhythmia related to the oculocardiac reflex? Are there any changes in the operative site, such as hemorrhage and increased ocular pressure, triggering a postoperative dysrhythmia? Dysrhythmias from the oculocardiac reflex are numerous. They include bradycardia as well as nodal, junctional, and serious atrial and ventricular dysrhythmias.[7]

Patients with ocular disease often have systemic disorders. Therefore, the PACU team must obtain a proper report from the anesthesia team regarding illnesses such as asthma, hypertension, coronary artery disease, endocrine disorders, diabetes mellitus, chronic obstructive pulmonary disease, manifestations of dementia and senility, diminished hearing, his-

tory of anxiety and neurosis, and the status of eyesight in the unoperated eye. Drug interactions affecting multiple organ systems must be understood, particularly in the areas of the central nervous and cardiopulmonary systems. Table 22–3 reviews some of the systemic effects of eye medications and other drugs commonly given in the perioperative period.

NAUSEA AND VOMITING

Nausea and vomiting can be a particularly bothersome complication of anesthesia,[3] resulting in delayed discharge, or in some patients, overnight admission.[1, 5] Nausea and vomiting can cause increased IOP, wound dehiscence, iris prolapse, and intraocular bleeding. Many prophylactic and therapeutic regimens have been proposed, but none has been totally successful.[3] Common factors contributing to nausea and vomiting include movement,[1, 8] narcotics, inhalation agents,[1] hypotension,[9] fear, pain,[1] pharyngeal stimulation,[8] and the surgical procedure itself.[1]

The incidence of postoperative nausea and vomiting varies from 10 to 30% in the general surgical population. It can be 50 to 65% in certain patient populations at higher risk, specifically women undergoing outpatient gynecological procedures and children undergoing strabismus surgery.[10]

In ophthalmic patients, the incidence is higher in those who have had retinal detachment or eye muscle surgery,[4, 11] as well as in female patients,[12] young patients,[12] individuals with a predisposition to nausea and vomiting,[13] and those with a previous history of postoperative emesis.[9] Whether intraoperative use of nitrous oxide triggers postoperative nausea and vomiting remains unresolved.[13]

Although narcotics have been linked with nausea and vomiting in a number of studies, narcotic analgesics may not always precipitate emesis. In fact, relief of pain with the use of narcotics may decrease episodes of nausea.[14] The avoidance or use of narcotics as a supplement to sedation with regional anesthesia in the monitored anesthetic care setting at MEEI is being investigated to see if there is a difference in the incidence of nausea and vomiting associated with anterior segment surgery.

Nausea and vomiting can occur at various times postoperatively. The patient may have no symptoms of nausea and vomiting in the PACU but may develop such symptoms, with or without eye pain, several hours later at home following regional or general anesthesia.

TABLE 22–3. Complications of Medications Used for Ophthalmic Surgery

Drug	Complication
Atropine Scopolamine Pilocarpine	Disorientation, hallucinations
Acetylcholine	Miosis, bronchospasm, increased salivation and bronchial secretions, bradycardia, dysrhythmias
Echothiophate iodide	Respiratory weakness following succinylcholine, prolonged effect of ester-linked local anesthetics
Timolol	Bronchospasm, exacerbation of hypothyroidism and myasthenia gravis, dysrhythmias, bradycardia, hypotension, congestive heart failure
Phenylephrine	Anxiety, tremulousness, dysrhythmias, tachycardia,
Epinephrine	Headache, hypertension
Cocaine	Hypertensive crisis
Acetazolamide	Hypokalemia
Mannitol	Bladder distension, hypotension, hypertension

The trigeminal-vagal oculocardiac reflex is suspected as the cause.

Nonpharmacologic measures to decrease the incidence of nausea and vomiting should not be ignored. These include minimizing stimulation of the oropharynx, careful attention to airway management to avoid gastric distension, and timely removal of an inserted oral airway.[10] Additional measures include minimizing pain and patient movement and avoiding hypotension, hypoxia, and exposure of the patient to other patients who are vomiting.[10]

Of the many regimens proposed to control nausea and vomiting associated with strabismus surgery, one is particularly common. Droperidol 75 μg/kg IV has been shown to reduce the incidence of nausea and vomiting without increasing the discharge time.[15] However, a lower dose of droperidol, which is usually effective in adults, does not have the same efficacy in children undergoing strabismus surgery.[16–18] One study has shown that IV lidocaine 1.5–2 mg/kg prior to tracheal intubation reduces the incidence of postoperative nausea and vomiting to less than 20%.[19] Others, however, have been unable to reproduce such favorable results following lidocaine administration. Metoclopramide also may prove helpful. Benefits of metoclopramide include increased gastroesophageal sphincter tone and an increased rate of gastric emptying.[20, 21]

At MEEI, most patients receive lidocaine 1.5 mg/kg IV, minimal administration of narcotics, droperidol 50 μg/kg IV, metoclopramide 0.1 mg/kg IV, and nasogastric tube suctioning of stomach contents with removal of the nasogastric tube while the patient is asleep. In addition, helpful techniques include gentle surgical manipulation of eye muscles; adequate hydration of the patient with IV crystalloids; and placement of local anesthetics, such as lidocaine and bupivacaine, near the extraocular muscles by the surgeon intraoperatively to minimize afferent impulses and postoperative pain upon awakening.[1]

Table 22–4 reviews some treatments for ophthalmic-related postoperative nausea and vomiting.

EYE PAIN

As previously mentioned, eye pain can be a source of nausea and vomiting. Eye pain and headache can have a number of causes, and a wide spectrum of management options exists. Headache is common following anterior segment surgery. Etiology is often unclear and,

TABLE 22–4. Nausea and Vomiting

Possible Etiologies	Possible Treatments
Opiates (chemoreceptor zone)	Anticholinergics, H-1 antihistamines phenothiazines butyrophenones antidopaminergics
Anxiety	Anxiolytics– benzodiazepines, analgesics–opiates
Pain	Opiates, injectable NSAID
Hypotension with hypoxia of vomiting center	IV volume, O_2
Stomach insufflation	Head and back up, nasogastric tube if tolerated
Oculocardiac reflex	Search for local causes, atropine
Nitrous oxide (controversial)	Antiemetics
Patient movement/ transport	Avoidance of unnecessary motion

paradoxically, can be related to the intraoperative use of narcotics and halogenated agents. Reassurance and acetaminophen are usually quite effective. More localized pain can be related to the use of surgical retractors, surgical wounds, and pressure dressings. Again, reassurance, acetaminophen, and written instructions for the patient to follow are usually sufficient.

Any evidence of proptosis, lid swelling, periorbital ecchymosis, and abnormally severe complaints of eye pain beyond what is reasonably expected require prompt consultation with the patient's surgeon for evaluation and management. Hemorrhage, acute angle-closure glaucoma, and anterior segment ischemia demand immediate attention.

The use of narcotics, intramuscular (IM) or IV, can be especially helpful in managing pain, particularly if pain is suspected to be exacerbating a stormy emergence from general anesthesia in the pediatric, elderly, alcoholic, or emotionally disturbed patient. The PACU team's understanding of pharmacology and emergence phenomena can make the difference between the start of successful surgical healing and disastrous postoperative eye injury. Moreover, patient controlled analgesia (PCA) is an important and accepted way to provide a physiological approach to pain management that many patients now expect in a hospital setting.[22]

A common cause of postoperative eye pain is corneal abrasion. At times it is difficult to determine how the corneal abrasion took

FIGURE 22–5. (A) Head positioning such that the retinal break is dependent may result in internal occluding of the break by vitreous gel. (B) This occluding causes functional closure of the break, so it flattens on the scleral buckle as the subretinal fluid is absorbed. (From Michels RG, Wilkinson CP, Rice TA: Postoperative management. In Michels RG, Wilkinson CP, Rice TA (eds): Retinal Detachment. St. Louis, CV Mosby, 1990, p 892.)

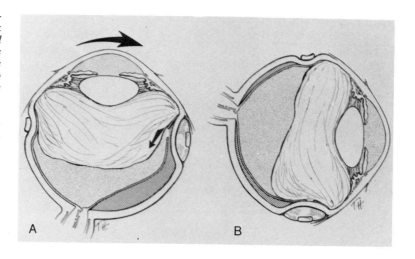

of nausea, and prevention of aspiration. Careful positioning of the head and neck and encouraging the patient to breathe through the mouth, along with steps to minimize nausea and vomiting, are recommended.

Endoscopic procedures, listed in Table 22–6, include laryngoscopy, esophagoscopy, and bronchoscopy. Oropharyngeal procedures, surgery involving the tongue, tonsils, and adenoids, neck operations, and procedures involving the larynx and trachea all have the

possibility of requiring urgent, or even emergent, airway intervention. (Although laser surgery is reported to be associated with less postoperative edema and bleeding, a patient's tissue response to even extremely gentle manipulation cannot always be anticipated.)

Preparation for the complications of bleeding and obstruction from edematous tissue, dislodged tissue, packs that may have been left behind, dental trauma, and mucous plugging is essential. Oral and nasal airways, face

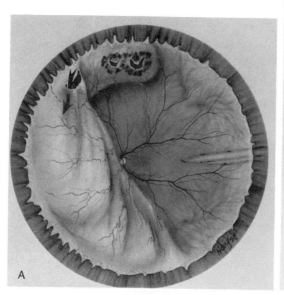
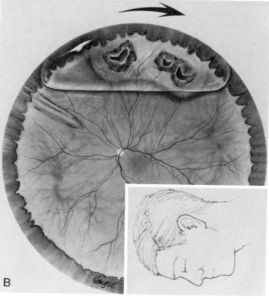

FIGURE 22–6. (A) Prior to injection of gas bubble, the retinal break is not closed and has not flattened onto the scleral buckle. (From Michels RG, Wilkinson CP, Rice TA: Postoperative management. In Michels RG, Wilkinson CP, Rice TA (eds): Retinal Detachment. St. Louis, CV Mosby, 1990, p 894.) (B) Special head positioning causes the gas bubble to be in close contact with the retinal break, thereby causing functional closure of the break and flattening of the break onto the scleral buckle. (From Michels RG, Wilkinson CP, Rice TA: Postoperative management. In Michels RG, Wilkinson CP, Rice TA (eds): Retinal Detachment. St. Louis, CV Mosby, 1990, p 895.)

TABLE 22–5. PACU Concerns Related to Otologic Surgery

Common Otologic Procedures	Considerations
Myringotomy	Head/ear position: facilitation of drainage
Tympanoplasty	Head elevated to minimize eustachian tube edema
Stapedectomy	Dressings monitored for evidence of bleeding or possible prosthesis dislodgment

Mastoidectomies
  Simple
  Modified
  Radical
	Nausea, vertigo, and vomiting; coughing, sneezing, and Valsalva's maneuvers; facial nerve integrity

masks, Ambu bags, intubation equipment, drugs used in advanced cardiac life support as recommended by the American Heart Association, humidified oxygen, and adequate IV lines are necessary for rapid treatment of cardiopulmonary complications. The availability of equipment for transtracheal ventilation is strongly recommended. The immediate availability of equipment that facilitates airway management in a variety of situations is the mark of adequate PACU preparation for the rhinolaryngologic patient.

TABLE 22–6. Endoscopic, Oropharyngeal, and Laryngotracheal Procedures

Common Throat Procedures	Considerations
Laryngoscopy: biopsy, laser; bronchoscopy	Hypercarbia, hypoxia; dysrhythmias; airway difficulties, including difficult intubations, laryngeal trauma, edema, and laryngospasm
Biopsy of tongue; hemiglossectomy	Airway difficulties, copious bleeding, pain, difficulty with speech
Tonsillectomy; adenoidectomy	Hemorrhage, airway obstruction, pain, nausea and vomiting
Laryngectomy; tracheostomy; radical neck dissection	Chronic obstructive pulmonary disease, ethyl alcohol and other substance abuse, nutrition, impaired speech, pain, hemorrhage, pneumothorax and subcutaneous emphysema, nausea and vomiting, high humidity gases for tracheal breathing, complications of tracheal suctioning, impaired speech

Patients with diseases of the head and neck often have associated problems, such as chronic obstructive pulmonary disease, cardiac disease, diabetes, drug and alcohol abuse, and hepatic and renal insufficiency. Therefore, the PACU team must have a thorough report of the patient's history, and the anesthesia care team and the patient's surgeon must be readily available if necessary.

The patient with a rhinolaryngologic problem needs staged cardiopulmonary management. Management starts preoperatively depending on the rhinolaryngologic problem, with or without airway compromise, and continues through intraoperative anesthetic management; assuming the airway problem is corrected or modified as a result of the operative procedure, the patient is then further managed in the PACU. This approach to patient care produces a more cohesive and predictable management plan with fewer surprises postoperatively. Therefore, PACU nurses and anesthesiologists must understand the preoperative problem, the difficulties surrounding airway management intraoperatively, and the altered anatomy as a result of surgery.

The nursing staff should adhere to established nursing policy guidelines for sterile suctioning techniques, particularly regarding tracheostomy care. Avoidance of trauma and infection and promotion of patient comfort and cardiopulmonary stability are important goals.

The problems of neurological complications, including delayed emergence from anesthesia, agitation, and pain, are important, especially if they compromise airway patency and the patient's ability to protect his or her own airway. Hypoxemia, hypercapnea, airway obstruction, and gastrointestinal complications require a comprehensive approach as outlined earlier in this chapter and elsewhere.[10] The precautions followed to minimize aspiration are discussed in previous chapters; in general, anxiety, pain, recent trauma, and recent ingestion of alcohol and fatty food contribute to continued delayed gastric emptying.[25, 26] Because opiate receptors are located throughout the gastrointestinal tract,[27] administration of narcotics may contribute to significant delay in gastric emptying.[28]

A more lengthy period of observation, beyond time spent in the PACU, whether the patient is an inpatient or an outpatient, may alter what is perceived as complications[3]; evidence of airway compromise and injury may be delayed. In general, a more prolonged period of observation in the PACU can be easily justified, especially when the possibility of airway compromise exists.[3]

Many children undergo otorhinolaryngologic surgery, and the high risk of postintubation stridor in this population must be considered; movement of the head and neck intraoperatively is likely to occur. Moreover, the pediatric airway has its smallest diameter at the cricoid ring, and the mucosa of the pediatric larynx is highly vascular and loosely attached, making the subglottic region susceptible to edema.[30] The use of steroids, racemic epinephrine, and humidified oxygen therapy, as well as judicious use of sedation and analgesics under controlled conditions and careful observation, are beneficial treatments for irritated pediatric and adult airways.[1, 30, 31] In pediatric patients with postextubation stridor, inhaled racemic epinephrine, 0.5 mL of 2.25% solution nebulized in 2½ mL of normal saline, can be administered frequently as long as the heart rate remains below 200 beats per minute. In addition, the use of 70% helium and 30% oxygen mixture can be useful if hypoxemia is not an issue. The lower density of helium decreases the work of breathing, especially if airway narrowing is involved.[30] If these measures do not produce a satisfactory response, reintubation is necessary and should be performed with a smaller tube than was used intraoperatively. Extubation is usually feasible 1–3 days later.[30]

Prolonged intubation in adults may result in fluid accumulation in the paranasal sinuses. Only rarely is the fluid purulent. However, sinusitis should be considered in cases of unexplained sepsis. The incidence of glottic and subglottic stenosis associated with intubation is controversial.[30] A tracheostomy is generally not indicated for intubation lasting less than 10 days, and most authorities agree on the desirability of tracheostomy if a patient is to be intubated for longer than 21 days.[30] Oxygen administered to a patient with a tracheostomy should be humidified and, if possible, warmed. Cold, dry gas delivered directly to the tracheostomy site can be irritating and cause inspissation of mucus, resulting in airway obstruction. The importance of sterile technique for tracheal suctioning cannot be overemphasized.

One often overlooked complication is pulmonary edema secondary to airway obstruction. A high index of suspicion is necessary, because the report given to PACU nurses often fails to include mention of perioperative airway obstruction, especially if it was transient.

Postobstructive pulmonary edema can occur, however, in patients who had stridor preoperatively, especially if a mass lesion was the causative agent. This rather unusual complication can also occur following iatrogenic obstruction induced perioperatively, such as with postextubation laryngospasm.

Before being discharged from the PACU, patients should be conscious and able to maintain their airway. The obvious exceptions are those patients who are intubated or who have a surgically established airway. Hemodynamic stability also is essential. Also no active bleeding from either the operative site or drains should be noted.

Ear, nose, and throat (ENT) patients, similar to eye patients, have different and special physical and psychological needs. ENT patients often have surgery performed on their upper airway that may result in feelings of suffocation, discomfort, and pressure. Furthermore, communicating with debilitated, intubated patients who may have undergone laryngectomy or tracheostomy can be difficult and anxiety-provoking for both the patient and the caregiver. These patients require liberal amounts of reassurance and understanding.

Whenever the airway is involved, even relatively minor procedures may evolve into difficult or life-threatening complications, and the PACU team should look beyond the minor nature of the procedure and consider the potentially serious events. Prevention and early detection of complications are crucial to optimal patient care.

Acknowledgment

A special debt is owed the late Dr. Ronald Michels for his permission to reproduce the illustrations in this chapter. He and his future contributions to ophthalmology will be greatly missed.

REFERENCES

1. Donlon JV Jr: Anesthesia and eye, ear, nose, and throat surgery. *In* Miller RD (ed): Anesthesia, 3rd ed. New York, Churchill-Livingstone, 1990, p 2002.
2. Michels RG, Wilkinson CP, Rice TA (eds): Retinal Detachment. St. Louis, CV Mosby, 1990, pp 889–915.
3. Young ML, Conahan TJ: Complications of outpatient anesthesia. Semin Anesthes 1990; 9:62.
4. Wolf GL, Goldfarb H: Complications of ophthalmologic anesthesia. Semin Anesthes 1990; 9:108.
5. Korttila K: Anesthesia potpourri. Semin Anesthes 1990; 9:182.
6. von Noorden GK: Extraocular muscles. *In* Beyer-Machule CK, von Noorden GK (eds): Atlas of

Ophthalmic Surgery, Vol 1. Stuttgart, Georg Thieme Verlag, 1985, pp 437–438.

7. Donlon JV Jr: Anesthesia and eye, ear, nose, and throat surgery. *In* Miller RD (ed): Anesthesia, 3rd ed. New York, Churchill Livingstone, 1990, p 2008.

8. Rosenfeld BA, Miller CF: Commonly encountered recovery room problems. *In* Breslow MJ, Miller CF, Roger MC (eds): Perioperative Management. St. Louis, CV Mosby, 1990, pp 147–163.

9. Meca RS: Postanesthesia recovery. *In* Barash PG, Cullen BF, Stoelting RK (eds): Clinical Anesthesia. Philadelphia, JB Lippincott, 1989, pp 1397–1425.

10. Chaplin S, Feeley TW: Complications in the postanesthesia care unit. Semin Anesthes 1990; 9:98.

11. Mason G, Gacka-Hubler CM: Postanesthesia care of the ophthalmic patient. J Post Anesth Nursing 1986; 1:23.

12. Vance JP, Neill RS, Norris W: The incidence and aetiology of postoperative nausea and vomiting in a plastic surgical unit. Br J Plast Surg 1973; 26:336.

13. Muir JJ, Warner MA, Offord KP, et al: Role of nitrous oxide and other factors in postoperative nausea and vomiting: A randomized and blinded prospective study. Anesthesiology 1987; 66:513.

14. Andersen R, Krohg K: Pain as a major cause of postoperative nausea. Can Anaesth Soc J 1976; 23:366.

15. Christensen S, Farrow-Gillespie A, Lerman J: Post anesthetic vomiting in children undergoing strabismus repair: A comparison of droperidol and lidocaine. Anesth Analg 1988; 67:530.

16. Hardy JF, Charest J, Girouard G, Lepoge Y: Nausea and vomiting after strabismus surgery in preschool children. Can Anaesth Soc J 1988; 33:57.

17. Van Den Berg AA, Lambourne A, Yazli NS, et al: Vomiting after ophthalmic surgery. Anaesthesiology 1987; 42:270.

18. Abramovitz MD, Oh TH, Epstein BS: Antiemetic effect of droperidol following outpatient strabismus surgery in children. Anesthesiology 1983; 59:579.

19. Warner LO, Rogers GL, Martino JD, et al: Intravenous lidocaine reduces the incidence of vomiting in children after surgery to correct strabismus. Anesthesiology 1988; 68:618.

20. Solsnki DR, Suresh M, Ethridge HC: The effects of intravenous cimetidine and metoclopramide on gastric volume and pH. Anesth Analg 1984; 63:599.

21. Manchikanti L, Collins J, Marrero T, et al: Ranitidine and metoclopramide for prophylaxis of aspiration pneumonitis in elective surgery. Anesth Analg 1984; 63:903.

22. Tewes PA, Taylor DR, Bourke DL: Postoperative pain management. *In* Breslow MJ, Miller CF, Rogers MC (eds): Perioperative Management. St. Louis, CV Mosby, 1990, pp 164–179.

23. Isernhagen RD, Michels RG, Glaser BM, et al: Hospitalization requirements after vitreoretinal surgery. Arch Ophthalmol 1988; 106:767.

24. Freeman HM, Tolentino FI: Atlas of Vitreoretinal Surgery, Vol 3. Stuttgart, Georg Thieme Verlag, 1990, pp 201–212.

25. Knieriem K, Stehling L: Aspiration pneumonitis. Semin Anesthes 1990; 9:54.

26. Bannister WK, Sattilaro AJ: Vomiting and aspiration during anesthesia. Anesthesiology 1962; 23:251.

27. Konturek SJ: Opiates and the gastrointestinal tract. Am J Gastroenterol 1980; 74:285.

28. Chase HF: The role of delayed gastric emptying time in the etiology of aspiration pneumonia. Am J Obstet Gynecol 1948; 56:673.

29. Sosis MB: Hazards of laser surgery. Semin Anesthes 1990; 9:90.

30. Quartararo C, Bishop MJ: Complications of tracheal intubation: Prevention and treatment. Semin Anesthes 1990; 9:119.

31. Yao FF, Artusio JF Jr: Anesthesiology, problem oriented management, 2nd ed. Philadelphia, JB Lippincott, 1988, pp 529–535.

Index

Note: Page numbers in *italics* refer to illustrations;
page numbers followed by t refer to tables.

Abscess, peritonsillar, 125–126
  retropharyngeal, 126
Acetazolamide, anesthetic implications of, 228t, 232, 251t
  intraocular pressure and, 185, 186
Acetylcholine, anesthetic implications of, 228t, 231
Achalasia, 58
Acid aspiration syndrome, 280
Acidosis, intraocular pressure and, 185
Acoustic neuroma, 139
Acupuncture anesthesia, 22–23
Adenoidectomy and tonsillectomy, 97–100. See also
  Tonsillectomy, adenoidectomy and.
Adenoma, thyroid, 85
Adenosine, in controlled hypotension, 140
Aging, in preoperative assessment, 70–71
Air embolism, venous, 102, 103–104, 104t
  intraoperative, 166–167, 167t
Airway, adult, 112–113, 113t
  assessment of, intubation and, 24–28
    history in, 24
    physical examination in, 25
  maxillofacial trauma and, 92–93, *93*
  fire in, 167–168
    laser surgery and, 48, 48t, 167–168
  lower, lesions of, anesthetic management in, 46–48
    laser surgery in, 46–48
  pediatric, adult compared to, 113t
    edema of, 112, 113–114, 114t
    general considerations for, 112–113, 113t
    obstruction of, 4–5
      bacterial tracheitis and, 121
      cricothyroidotomy and, 130–131
      epiglottitis and, 117–119, *118*, 118t. See also *Epi-glottitis.*
      foreign body aspiration and, 114–117. See also
        Foreign body, aspiration of.
      laryngeal causes of, 7t
      laryngotracheobronchitis and, 119–121, 120t. See
        also *Laryngotracheobronchitis.*
      nonlaryngeal causes of, 5t
      postobstructive pulmonary edema and, 113–114, 114t
      signs of, 113, 113t
      stridor and, 7, *7*
      tracheostomy and, 121–122
        emergency, 131
  perforation of, surgery and, 166

Airway *(Continued)*
  upper, intubation and, 157
    lesions of, anesthetic management in, 43–46
    obstructed, intubation and. See *Intubation, difficult.*
    problems of, 28
Alcoholism, in maxillofacial trauma, 93
  in preoperative assessment, 69t, 69–70
Alfentanil, in outpatient surgery, 150
  intraocular pressure and, 282
Aminophylline, epinephrine interaction with, 163
  in aspiration under anesthesia, 281
  in foreign body aspiration, 160
Amiodarone, visual loss due to, 286
Anaplastic carcinoma, thyroid, 85
Andy Gump fracture, 91, 92
Anemia, hemolytic, sickle cell disease and, 220–221
Angina, Ludwig's, 126–127
Angiofibroma, nasopharyngeal, juvenile, 106
Angiography, fluorescein, 228t, 232–233
Angiotensin-converting enzyme inhibitor, in controlled
  hypotension, 140
Aniridia, 210, 210t
Antacid, for "open eye–full stomach" patient, 186, 200
Antibiotic, in aspiration under anesthesia, 281
  in congenital myotonic disease, 219
  in epiglottitis, 119
Anticholinergic, as premedication, 147
Anticholinesterase, ophthalmic, topical, 228t, 229–230
Anticonvulsant, in anesthetic toxicity, 164
Antidepressant, tricyclic, anesthetic implications of, 251t
Antiemetic, after stapedectomy, 142–143
  for "open eye–full stomach" patient, 187
  in outpatient surgery, 150
Antisialagogue, in preparation for difficult intubation, 29
  in unanticipated airway difficulty, 34
Apert's syndrome, ocular pathology in, 214, 216t
Apnea, in premature infant, 145, 258
Aqueous humor, 181, *181*
  formation and drainage of, 181, *181*
  intraocular pressure and, 183–184
  outflow of, Fontana's spaces and, 199
  topical drug absorption and, 180
Argon laser, 41t, 41–42. See also *Laser surgery.*
Arthritis, rheumatoid, 2
Aryepiglottic fold, 1, *2*
Arytenoid cartilage, *1*, 2
  dislocation of, 161, 161t
Aspiration. See also *Foreign body, aspiration of.*

Aspiration *(Continued)*
 of gastric contents, intraocular pressure and, 186–188
  muscle relaxants in, 187–188
  preoperative care in, 186–187
 periextubation, 170
 under anesthesia, 280–282
  incidence of, 280–281
  morbidity and mortality in, 281
  prevention of, 281–282
Atkinson method, in facial nerve block, *243*, 243–244, *244*
Atlantoaxial subluxation, 127
 intubation difficulties and, 27, 161
 syndromes associated with, 27
Atracurium, for "open eye–full stomach" patient, 187–188
 in juvenile laryngeal papilloma, 46
 intraocular pressure and, 185
Atresia, choanal, 127–128
 laryngeal, 7–8, 8t
Atropine, in bleeding after tonsillectomy, 124
 in congenital glaucoma, 199
 in epiglottitis, 118
 in foreign body aspiration, 116, 116t
 in intraoperative bradycardia, 162
 in laryngospasm, 159
 in oculocardiac reflex, 279
 in outpatient procedures, as premedication, 147
  for middle ear, 151
  strabismus surgery and, 254
 in retinoblastoma, 203
 in strabismus surgery, 191, 192, 254, 279
 in tonsillectomy and adenoidectomy, 98, 124
 ophthalmic, topical, 227, 228t

Bacterial tracheitis, 121
Barbiturate, for "open eye–full stomach" patient, 187, 188
 juvenile, 201
 in cocaine toxicity, 229
 in Sturge-Weber syndrome, 221
Barotrauma, 165–166
Becker's muscular dystrophy, malignant hyperthermia and, 194
Beckwith-Wiedemann syndrome, difficult intubation and, 25, *25*
Benzodiazepine, in Sturge-Weber syndrome, 221
Betaxolol, complications associated with, 279–280
Bicarbonate, in malignant hyperthermia, 195
Bleeding. See also *Hemorrhage.*
 postoperative, tonsillectomy and, 124–125
Blindness. See also *Vision, loss of.*
 transient, TURP syndrome and, 286
Blood supply, ocular and orbital, 179
Bronchography, 57, 106–107
 propyliodone in, 107
Bronchoscopy, 48–57
 applications of, 48–49
 edema after, 116
 fiberoptic, 51t, 51–57
  general anesthesia for, 51t, *54*, 54–55
   bronchospasm and, 55–56
   cardiovascular complications and, 56
   complications of, 55
   endotracheal tube size and, 54–55
   hypoxemia and, 55
   intraoperative awareness during, 57

Bronchoscopy *(Continued)*
   precautions for, 55
   rapid arousal from, 55
   toxic reactions to, 57
   ventilation characteristics of, 51t, *54*, 54
  history of, 51
  indications for, 51
  local anesthesia for, 51t, 51–54
   aerosolized, 53
   hypoxemia and, 53–54
   laryngeal blockade as, 53
   nasal blockade as, *52*, 52–53
   pharyngeal blockade as, 52–53, *53*
   ventilation characteristics of, 51t
 history of, 48
 in epiglottitis, 118
 in foreign body aspiration, 116, 116t, 160
 outpatient, 153
 rigid, 49–51, 51t
  advantages of, 49
  general anesthesia for, 49–51, 51t
   agents for, 50
   hemodynamics and, 51
   Hopkins lens microscope and, 50
   inhalation, 50, 51t
   minimum alveolar concentration and, 49
   rigid Venturi bronchoscope and, 50, 51t
   side-arm ventilating bronchoscope and, 49–50
   topical anesthesia and, 51
   ventilation characteristics of, 51t
  indications for, 49
  local anesthesia for, 49, 51, 51t
  ventilation characteristics of, 51t
  Venturi, 50, 51t
 ventilating, 49–50
Bronchospasm, during bronchoscopy, 55–56
Bullard laryngoscope, 29, *30*
Buphthalmos, 198
Bupivacaine, anesthetic potency of, 276, 276t
 in anesthetic toxicity, 164
 in cervical plexus block, 21
 in nasal surgery, 17–18
 in peribulbar block, 278

CAD (coronary artery disease), in preoperative assessment, 68–69
Caffeine, in malignant hyperthermia, 195
Calcitonin, hyperparathyroidism and, 86
Calcium channel blocker, in controlled hypotension, 140
Calcium gluconate, in postoperative hypocalcemia, 87
Caldwell-Luc operation, 18, *18*
Cancer. See also *Carcinoma.*
 of head and neck, intraoperative complications of, 169
Carbon dioxide laser, 40–41, 41t. See also *Laser surgery.*
Carcinoma. See also *Cancer.*
 anaplastic, thyroid, 85
 glottic, 65–66, *66*, *67*, 67
 supraglottic, 65–66, *66*, *67*
 thyroid, 85
Cardiac disorder, as complication of tracheostomy, 109, 109t
 diphtheria and, 129
Cardiovascular disorder, during bronchoscopy, general anesthesia and, 56–57
 hyperthyroidism and, 78
 in preoperative assessment, 68–69
 intraoperative, 162–163

Cartilage, arytenoid, *1*, 2
   dislocation of, 161, 161t
  corniculate, at laryngoscopy, 2
  cricoid, *1*, 2
  cuneiform, at laryngoscopy, 2
  laryngeal, *1*, 2
  thyroid, *1*, 2
Cataract, 264–266
  congenital, 196–198
    causes of, 197, 197t
      pediatric syndromes associated with, 197
    surgery in, 197t, 197–198, 266
  evaluation of, 265
  incidence of, 265
  pathophysiology of, 265, 265t
  snowflake, 212
  sunflower, 212
  surgery in, 249–253
    anesthetic management in, 251t, 251–253
    cardiovascular disease and, 250
    chronic obstructive pulmonary disease and, 250, 251
    diabetes mellitus and, 250
    drug interactions and, 250, 251t
    elderly and, 249t, 249–251
    extracapsular, 266
    general considerations for, 249
    intracapsular, 266
    pediatric, 197t, 197–198, 266
    preoperative evaluation in, 249–251
  systemic diseases associated with, 210–212, 211t
    chromosomal abnormalities and, 211
    diabetes and, 212
    drug-induced, 212
    infections and, 211, 211t
    mendelian inheritance and, 211
    metabolic diseases and, 211–212
    toxic agents and, 212
Catecholamine, in sinus surgery, 103, 103t
Central nervous system, anesthetic toxicity in, 163
Cerebrohepatorenal syndrome, ocular pathology and, 217t, 222
Cerebrospinal fluid, postoperative leakage of, 173
Cervical epidural anesthesia, 20–21, *21*
Cervical plexus block, 21–22, *22*
  in thyroid surgery, 81
Cervical spine, mobility of, difficult intubation and, 27
  trauma to, surgery and, 93
Cetacaine spray, 158–159
CHARGE (congenital heart disease, choanal atresia, mental retardation, genital hypoplasia, and ear anomalies) syndrome, 128, 213
Chassaignac's tubercle, 22, *22*
Chemical injury, due to general anesthesia, 285–286
Chemotherapy, intraoperative complications due to, 169
Childhood. See *Pediatrics.*
Chloral hydrate, in delirium tremens, 70
Chlorhexidine, hearing loss due to, 161–162, 173
Choanal atresia, 127–128
Chromosome, abnormal, cataract and, 211
Chvostek's sign, after parathyroid surgery, 87
Ciliary body, 177
Cimetidine, preoperative, 29, 147
Cleft palate, hearing loss and otitis media with, 135
Clonidine, anesthetic implications of, 251t
  intraocular pressure and, 282
Cocaine, dosage for, 164
  epinephrine and, 148, 229
  in lower airway lesion, 47
  in nasal anesthesia, 52

Cocaine *(Continued)*
  in nasal septoplasty, 152
  in sinus surgery, 103, 103t, 152
  ophthalmic, topical, 227–229, 228t
  precautions for, 164
  topical, complications of, 275
    in nasotracheal intubation, 30
  toxicity with, 164, 229, 275
Cochlea, 134
  implant stimulation of, 138
Colobomata, ocular, 212–213
Congenital infection syndromes (TORCH), glaucoma and, 213
Congestive heart failure (CHF), in preoperative assessment, 68–69
Cornea, anesthesia-induced injury to, 285–286
  topical drug absorption and, 180, *180*
Corniculate cartilage, at laryngoscopy, 2
Coronary artery disease (CAD), in preoperative assessment, 68–69
Corticosteroid, in thyroid storm, 79
  pediatric cataract and, 212
Craniofacial dysostosis, 214, 216t
  difficult intubation and, 25, *26*
  ocular pathology and, 214, 216t
Cranium, abnormalities of, ocular pathology and, 214–215, 216t
Creatinine phosphokinase, serum, in malignant hyperthermia, 195
Cricoid cartilage, *1*, 2
Cricoid ring, infant, 5
Cricothyroid membrane, anterior view of, *1*
Cricothyroid muscle, 2
Cricothyroidotomy, *130*, 130–131
Cricothyrotomy, in infant, 117
Cricotracheal membrane, 1, *1*
Croup. See also *Laryngotracheobronchitis.*
  postintubation, 171, 171t
Crouzon's disease, 214, 216t
  difficult intubation and, 25, *26*
  ocular pathology and, 214, 216t
Crying, airway obstruction and, 113, 118
Cryopexy, in retinopathy of prematurity, 205
Crystalline lens, 177–178
Cuneiform cartilage, at laryngoscopy, 2
Curare, intraocular pressure and, 185
Cyanosis, epiglottitis and, 117
Cyclopentolate, in congenital cataract surgery, 197
  ophthalmic, topical, 227, 228t
Cyst, laryngeal, 10–11
Cystic fibrosis, nasal polyps and, 105–106, 106t
Cystic hygroma, 11–12

Dantrolene, in malignant hyperthermia, 195, 196
de Morsier's syndrome, 214
Deafness. See also *Hearing, loss of.*
  sensorineural, progressive, 173
Decadron, in foreign body aspiration, 117
Delirium tremens, in preoperative assessment, 69–70
Depressant, central nervous system, intraocular pressure and, 184
Dexamethasone, in juvenile laryngeal papilloma, 46
  in laryngotracheobronchitis, 120
Diabetes mellitus, cataract and, 212, 250
  end-organ disease and, 223–224
  hypertension and, 224
  juvenile-onset, 224

Diabetes mellitus *(Continued)*
  ocular pathology and, 217t, 222–223
    laser therapy in, 223
  perioperative care in, 224–225
  retinal detachment and, 266. See also *Retina, detachment of.*
  stiff joint syndrome and, 27–28
Diazepam, as premedication, 147
  in anesthetic toxicity, 164
  in delirium tremens, 70
  in endoscopy, 152
  intraocular pressure and, 184
Digitalis, in thyroid storm, 79
Diphtheria, 129
Diplopia, following general anesthesia, 286
Disseminated intravascular coagulation (DIC), in malignant hyperthermia, 193
Down's syndrome, cataract and, 211
  congenital subglottic stenosis and, 9–10
  ocular pathology and, 215, *215,* 217
  surgery and, 97
Droperidol, for "open eye–full stomach" patient, 187
  pediatrics and, 202
  in postoperative vomiting, 254–255, 255t, 283–284
  in strabismus surgery, 192–193
  visual-evoked potentials and, 262
Drug abuse. See also *Alcoholism.*
  in maxillofacial trauma, 93
Duchenne's muscular dystrophy, malignant hyperthermia and, 194
Dysautonomia, familial, ocular pathology and, 216t, 219–220

Ear, 133–143
  anatomy of, 133–135, *134*
    surgical implications in, 141
  congenital hearing loss and, 133–135
  drug-induced damage in, 135
  infection of, 133, 135
  inner, 133–134, *134*
  middle, 133, *134*
    surgery of, *136,* 136–137, 137t
      complications of, 169
      outpatient, 150–151
  pathophysiology of, 133–135
  physiology of, 133–135
  surgery of, 100–103, 135–143
    anatomy and, 141
    controlled hypotension and, 137, 139–141
    general considerations for, 100
    in acoustic neuroma, 139
    in cochlear implantation, 138
    in glomus tumor, 101t, 101–103, 138. See also *Glomus tumor.*
    in Ménière's disease, 137–138
    local anesthesia in, 141, *142*
    mastoidectomy in, *136,* 136–137, 137t
      local anesthesia in, 141, *142*
      recovery room care in, 299–301, 300t
    middle ear and, *136,* 136–137, 137t, 150–151
      complications of, 169
    myringotomy in, 100, 135–136
      local anesthesia in, 141, *142*
      recovery room care in, 299–301, 300t
    otitis media and, 100
    outpatient, 150–151. See also *Outpatient procedure, ear, nose, and throat surgery as.*

Ear *(Continued)*
    postoperative management in, *142,* 142–143
    recovery room care in, 298, 300t
    stapedectomy in, 137
      antiemetics after, 142–143
      local anesthesia in, 141
      recovery room care in, 299–301, 300t
    tympanoplasty in, *136,* 136–137, 137t
      local anesthesia in, 141
      recovery room care in, 299–301, 300t
    tympanostomy tube insertion in, 100
      outpatient, 150–151
    tympanotomy tube insertion in, 100, 135–136
      local anesthesia in, 141, *142*
Eardrum. See *Tympanic membrane.*
Echothiophate iodide, ophthalmic, topical, 228t, 229–230
Ectopia lentis, 213, 217
  Marfan's syndrome and, 218
Edema, after bronchoscopy, 116
  airway, 112
  in laryngotracheobronchitis, 120–121
  postintubation, 171
  pulmonary, postobstruction, 170t, 170–171
    postobstructive, 113–114, 114t
  subglottic, 171
Edwards' syndrome, cataract and, 211
Elderly, cataract surgery in, 249t, 249–251. See also *Cataract.*
Electrolyte balance, intraoperative, 169
Electromyography, intraoperative, 139
Electroretinography, 262
Embolism, air, venous, 102, 103–104, 104t
  intraoperative, 166–167, 167t
Emphysema, as complication of tracheostomy, 108, 109t
  subcutaneous, 165–166
Encephalotrigeminal angiomatosis, ocular pathology and, 217t, 221, *221*
Endoscopy, fiberoptic, flexible, 31–32, *32,* 32t
  outpatient, 152–153
Endotracheal intubation. See also *Intubation.*
  in infancy, 6
  subglottic stenosis due to, 10
Enflurane, epinephrine interaction with, 163
  in congenital cataract surgery, 198
  in hyperparathyroidism, 81–82
  in Sturge-Weber syndrome, 221
  minimum alveolar concentrations of, 49
  visual-evoked potentials and, 262
Ephedrine, in outpatient ophthalmic procedure, 252
Epiglottis, absence of, 8
  adult, 113t, 117
  anatomy of, 2
  anterior view of, *1*
  at laryngoscopy, *2*
  distinguishing features of, 113t
  infant, 113t
  innervation of, 2
  tubercle of, at laryngoscopy, view of, *2*
Epiglottitis, 117–119, *118*
  antibiotic therapy in, 119
  bronchoscopy in, 118
  clinical signs and symptoms of, 117
  cyanosis and, 117
  Haemophilus influenzae type B in, 117
  intubation in, 117–118, 118t, 119
  laryngotracheobronchitis versus, 119, 120t
  management of, 117–119, 118t
  radiographic findings in, 117–118, *118*
  tracheostomy in, 119

Epinephrine, aminophylline interaction with, 163
  cocaine interaction with, 148, 229
  enflurane interaction with, 163
  halothane interaction with, 162–163
  in anesthetic blockade of nasal cavity and septum, 17
  in anesthetic toxicity, 164
  in cervical epidural anesthesia, 21
  in congenital cataract surgery, 197
  in ear surgery, 137
  in epiglottitis, 118
  in foreign body aspiration, 116, 116t, 117
  in intraoperative bradycardia, 162
  in intraoperative dysrhythmia, 162–163
  in juvenile laryngeal papilloma, 46
  in laryngotracheobronchitis, 120
  in nasal anesthesia, 52
  in outpatient surgery, of middle ear, 151
    of sinuses, 152
    ophthalmic procedure and, 253
  in postextubation stridor, 301
  in sinus surgery, 19, 152
  in thyroid surgery, 22
  in tonsillectomy, 19, 99
    adenoidectomy and, 99
  isoflurane interaction with, 163
  topical, in nasotracheal intubation, 30
    ophthalmic, 228t, 230
Epistaxis, 128–129
Esmolol, in hyperparathyroidism, 80–81
  in microlaryngoscopy, 37
  in thyrotoxicosis, 79
Esophagoscopy, 57–58
Esters, toxicity with, 57
Etomidate, in outpatient surgery, 150
  intraocular pressure and, 184
Eustachian tube, 133
  dysfunction of, 135
Extubation, aspiration pneumonitis and, 170
  awake, 170
  complications of, 283–284
  croup and, 171, 171t
  inadvertent, 169
  laryngospasm and, 170
  postobstruction pulmonary edema and, 170t, 170–171
Eye, anatomy of, 176–179, *177*
  blood supply in, 179
  cul-de-sac compartment in, 179
  extraocular muscles in, 178
  eyelids in, 178
  general considerations for, 176
  globe in, 177–178
  lacrimal apparatus in, 178
  orbit in, 176–178
    blood supply of, 179
  anesthesia-induced damage to, 285–286
  nonocular surgery and, postoperative complications of, 285–287
  ophthalmic drugs for. See also names of specific drugs.
    anesthetic implications of, 227–233, 228t
      general considerations for, 227
      intraocular therapy and, 228t, 231
      systemic drugs and, 228t, 231–232
      topical drugs and, 227–231, 228t
    complications associated with, 279–280
  penetrating injury of, full stomach and, 186–188. See also *"Open eye–full stomach" patient.*
    in pediatrics, *200*, 200–202, *201*
  physiology of, 179–182
    aqueous humor and, 181, *181*

Eye *(Continued)*
  general considerations for, 179
  intraocular pressure and, 181–186. See also *Intraocular pressure.*
  "open eye–full stomach patient" and, 186–188
  topical drug absorption and, 179–180, *180*
  surgery of, anesthetic complications of, 272–287
    aspiration and, 280t, 280–282
    emergence and, 283–284
    general anesthesia and, 273–278
    intraocular pressure and, 282–283. See also *Intraocular pressure.*
    local anesthesia and, 273–278
      contraindications to, 273, 273t
      general considerations for, 274
      infiltration, 275–276, *276*, 276t
      retrobulbar blockade and, 267–278, 277t
      topical, 274–275
    malignant hyperthermia and. See *Hyperthermia, malignant.*
    ocular drugs and, 279–280
    oculocardiac reflex and, 278–279
    oxygen therapy and, 284–285
    prematurity and, 284–285
  mortality in, 272–273
  pediatric, 190–207
    congenital cataract and, 196–198
      causes of, 197, 197t
      pediatric syndromes associated with, 197
      special concerns with, 197, 197t
      timing of, 197
    congenital glaucoma and, 198–200, 199t. See also *Glaucoma, congenital.*
    general considerations for, 190
    malignant hyperthermia and, 191, 193–196. See also *Hyperthermia, malignant.*
    "open eye–full stomach" patient and, *200*, 200–202, *201*. See also *"Open eye–full stomach" patient.*
    retinoblastoma and, 202–203, *203*, 203t. See also *Retinoblastoma.*
    retinopathy of prematurity and, 203–207, 204t, 206t. See also *Retinopathy of prematurity.*
    strabismus and, 190–193, 191t. See also *Strabismus.*
  recovery room care in, 291, *292–293*, 294–298
    eye pain and, 296–297, *297*
    general considerations for, 291, 294, 294t
    head position and, 297–298, *298*
    hemorrhage and, 294
    intraocular pressure and, 294
    nausea and, 295–296, 296t
    pre-existing diseases and, 294–295
    record sheet for, *292–293*
    vomiting and, 295–296, 296t
  regional blockade in, 235–247
    anatomical considerations for, *236*, 236–238, *237*
    general considerations for, 235
    historical considerations for, 235–236
    local anesthesia in, 238
    orbicularis oculi blockade and, 241–244
      Atkinson's method for, *243*, 243–244, *244*
      general considerations for, 241, 244
      Nadbath's and Rehman's method for, 244, *245*
      O'Brien's method for, *242*, 242–243, *243*
      van Lint's method for, 241–242, *242*
    peribulbar, 235, 252
    periconal, 244–247, *245*, *246*
    retrobulbar, 238–241, *239–244*

Eye *(Continued)*
  complications of, 238–240, 252
    Gills-Loyd block in, *240*, 240–241, *241*
    needle for, 238, *239*
  systemic diseases associated with defects of, 210–225,
    216t–217t
    aniridia and, 210, 210t
    Apert's syndrome and, 214, 216t
    cataract and, 210–212, 211t
    colobomata and, 212–213
    congenital myotonic disease and, 217t, 219
    craniofacial abnormalities and, 214–215, 216t
    Crouzon's disease and, 214, 216t
    Down's syndrome and, 215, *215*
    ectopia lentis and, 213
    end-organ disease and, 223–224
    glaucoma and, 213
    Goldenhar's syndrome and, 214–215, *215,* 216t
    homocystinuria and, 215, 216t, 217
    Lowe's syndrome and, 216t, 218
    Marfan's syndrome and, 216t, 218–219
    optic nerve hypoplasia and, 213–214
    Riley-Day syndrome and, 216t, 219–220
    rubella syndrome and, 216t, 220
    sickle cell disease and, 217t, 220–221
    Sturge-Weber syndrome and, 217t, 221, *221*
    von Recklinghausen's disease and, 217t, 221–222
    Wagner-Stickler syndrome and, 217t, 222
    Zellweger syndrome and, 217t, 222
Eyelid, anatomy of, 178
  regional blockade of. See *Eye, surgery of, regional
    blockade in.*

Face, chlorhexidine as agent for, 161–162
  maxillofacial trauma and. See also *Maxilla, trauma to.*
    fracture in, 90–92, *92*
  normal anatomy of, 90
  ocular pathology and, 214–215, 216t
  plastic surgery of, 153. See also *Outpatient procedure,
    ear, nose, and throat surgery as.*
  surgery of, recovery room care in, 298–301, 300t
Familial dysautonomia, ocular pathology and, 216t, 219–
  220
Fat embolism, maxillofacial trauma and, 93
Fentanyl, as premedication, 147
  in microlaryngoscopy, 37
  in outpatient surgery, 150
  intraocular pressure and, 184
  visual-evoked potentials and, 262
Fiberoptic bronchoscopy, 51–57. See also *Bronchoscopy,
  fiberoptic.*
Fiberoptic endoscopy, flexible, 31–32, *32*, 32t
  outpatient, 152–153
Fibrosis, cystic, nasal polyps and, 105–106, 106t
Field block, in tonsillectomy, 19, *19*
  of external nose, 15, 16, *17*
Fire, airway, 167–168
  laser surgery and, 48, 48t, 167–168
Fistula, tracheoesophageal, congenital subglottic stenosis
  and, 9–10
Fluorescein angiography, in clinical ophthalmology, 228t,
  232–233
Follicular carcinoma, thyroid, 85
Fontana's spaces, aqueous humor outflow and, 199
  intraocular pressure and, 282
Forced duction test (FDT), 191

Foreign body, aspiration of, 114–117. See also
  Aspiration.
  anesthetic management in, 115–117
  bronchoscopy in, 116
  clinical findings in, 114, 115
  edema and, 116
  endoscopy in, 116
  iatrogenically induced, 159–160
  objects recovered in, 114, 115t
  radiographic findings in, 115, *115*
  urgent, 115–116
Fracture, Andy Gump, 91, 92
  facial, 90–92, *92*. See also *Maxilla, trauma to.*
    difficult tracheostomy and, 157
  laryngeal, 130
Furosemide, in hyperparathyroidism, 86
  in malignant hyperthermia, 196

Galactokinase deficiency, cataract and, 212
Galactosemia, congenital cataract and, 211–212
Gallamine, juvenile "open eye–full stomach" patient
  and, 201
Ganglionic blocker, intraocular pressure and, 185
Gastric emptying, impaired, in diabetes mellitus, 224
Gills-Loyd block, *240*, 240–241, *241*
Glaucoma, 263–264
  angle-closure, acute, anesthesia-induced, 287
  betaxolol in, 231
  congenital, 198–200, 199t, 263, 264
    diseases associated with, 198
    infantile, 198, 199
    intraocular pressure and, 199
    juvenile, 198–199
    secondary, 199
    special concerns with, 199, 199t
  drug therapy in, 263–264
  early onset, 213
  echothiophate iodide in, 228t, 229–230
  epinephrine in, 228t, 230
  infantile, 198, 199, 263, 264
  juvenile, 198–199, 263
  laser surgery in, 264
  pediatric, 198–199, 263, 264
    systemic diseases associated with, 213
  primary, 263–264
  secondary, 263
  surgery in, filtration, 264
    laser, 264
  timolol in, 228t, 230–231
  von Recklinghausen's disease and, 221–222
Globe, anatomy of, *177*, 177–178
Glomus tumor, 138
  anesthetic implications in, 102–103
  general considerations for, 102
  hazards of, 101, 101t
  preoperative evaluation in, 101–102
  surgical bleeding and, 165
  treatment in, 102
Glossopharyngeal nerve, 2–3, 15, *16*
  blockade of, 3–4, *19*, 19–20, 52–53
    in awake intubation, 31
Glottis, carcinoma of, 65–66, *66*, *67*, 67
Glucocorticoid, in hyperparathyroidism, 86
Glycerin, ophthalmic, systemic, 232
Glycopyrrolate, as premedication, 147
  in retinoblastoma, 203
  in strabismus surgery, 192, 254

Glycopyrrolate *(Continued)*
  in tonsillectomy and adenoidectomy, 98
Goiter, etiology of, 77–78
  perioperative management of, 79–82, *80, 81*
Goldenhar's syndrome, ocular pathology and, 214–215, *215,* 216t
Granuloma, vocal cord, 172
Graves' disease, 77–78

H₂ receptor antagonist, as premedication, 147
  preoperative, 29
Haemophilus influenzae type B, in epiglottitis, 117
Halothane, epinephrine interaction with, 162–163
  in congenital cataract surgery, 197
  in controlled hypotension, 139
  in epiglottitis, 118
  in foreign body aspiration, 116, 116t
  in hyperparathyroidism, 81–82
  in juvenile laryngeal papilloma, 46
  in juvenile "open eye–full stomach" patient, 202
  in malignant hyperthermia, 194, 195
  in maxillofacial trauma, 95
  in outpatient strabismus surgery, 254
  in outpatient surgery, 149, 254
  in radiation therapy of retinoblastoma, 255, 256
  in tonsillectomy and adenoidectomy, 98
  intraocular pressure and, 199
  minimum alveolar concentrations of, 49
  visual-evoked potentials and, 262
Hashimoto's thyroiditis, 78
Head, cancer of, intraoperative complications of, 169
  dermatomes of, 15, *16*
  surgery of, vocal cord paralysis and, 172–173
Hearing, loss of, 134–135
    congenital, 134–135
    etiology of, 134–135, 135t
    neonatal, 135
    progressive sensorineural deafness and, 173
    transient, postoperative, 173
Helium, in postextubation stridor, 301
Hemangioma, congenital, 11–12
Hematoma, postintubation, 160
Hemiglossectomy, recovery room care in, 299–301, 300t
Hemolytic anemia, sickle cell disease and, 220–221
Hemorrhage. See also *Bleeding.*
  as complication of tracheostomy, 109, 109t
  retinal, due to general anesthesia, 287
  surgery and, 164–165
Hexafluoride, intraocular pressure and, 186
High frequency jet ventilation (HFJV), in laryngoscopy, 39
High frequency positive-pressure ventilation (HFPPV), in laryngoscopy, 39
Homocystinuria, ocular pathology and, 213, 216t, 217–218
Hopkins lens telescope, 50
Hormone(s), intraoperative imbalances of, 169
  thyroid, replacement therapy with, 84
  thyroxine, 75–77
    in thyroid replacement therapy, 84
Hormone(s), thyroid-stimulating, 76, 77
Hurler's syndrome, carbon dioxide laser surgery in, 40–41
Hydralazine, in controlled hypotension, 140
Hydration, in laryngotracheobronchitis, 120
Hydroxyzine, as premedication, 147
Hygroma, cystic, 11–12

Hyoid, anterior view of, *1*
Hyperparathyroidism, 85–87
Hypertension, diabetes mellitus and, 224
Hyperthermia, in cocaine toxicity, 229
  malignant, anesthetic episodes of, 191, 193–196
    acute, 195–196
    incidence of, 193
    intraoperative diagnosis of, 195
    management for patient susceptible to, 196
    masseter muscle spasm and, 193–194
    muscle disorders and, 194
    neuroleptic malignant syndrome and, 194
    pathophysiology of, 194–195
    presentation in, 193–194
    screening tests for, 195
    tachycardia and, 194–195
    treatment in, 195–196
    triggering agents in, 194
  strabismus surgery and, 191, 193
Hyperthyroidism, 77–83. See also *Thyroid, disease of.*
  anesthetic considerations in, 79–82
  cardiovascular disorder and, 78
  description of, 77
  etiology of, 77t, 77–78
  perioperative management in, 79–82, *80, 81*
  physical findings in, 78
  symptoms of, 78
  thyroid storm and, 78–79, 82
  thyroid surgery complications and, 82–83
  thyrotoxicosis and, 78–79
Hypertonic solution, intraocular pressure and, 186
  ophthalmic, systemic, 231–232
Hypocalcemia, after parathyroid surgery, 87
  after thyroid surgery, 82
  cataract and, 212
  laryngectomy and, 73
Hypoglycemia, postoperative, premature infant and, 206, 206t
Hypoparathyroidism, 87
  after thyroid surgery, 82
Hypoplasia, optic nerve, 213
Hypotension, drug-induced, ear surgery and, 137, 139–141
  Riley-Day syndrome and, 220
Hypothermia, intraocular pressure and, 185
Hypothyroidism, clinical categories in, 83–84
  laryngectomy and, 73
Hypoventilation, postoperative, premature infant and, 206, 206t
Hypoxemia, during bronchoscopy, 53–55
Hypoxia, intraocular pressure and, 185
  postoperative, premature infant and, 206, 206t

Infancy. See also *Neonate; Pediatrics; Premature infant.*
  endotracheal intubation in, 6
  epiglottis in, 113t
  larynx in, 113t
    adult larynx compared to, 4–7
      configuration of, 6
      location of, 5, *5,* 6
      size of, 5
      tissue consistency and, 6–7
    diagnostic laryngoscopy and, 13
    edema and, 6–7
    endotracheal intubation and, 6
    nasal obstruction and, 6
    Pierre Robin syndrome and, 5–6, *6*

Infancy *(Continued)*
  Treacher Collins syndrome and, 5
  upper airway obstruction and, 4–5, 5t
  mandible in, 113t
  strabismus in, 190. See also *Strabismus.*
  tongue in, 113t
  trachea in, 6, 112–113, 113t
Infant, cricothyrotomy in, 117
Infection, maternal, congenital cataract and, 211, 211t
Infiltration anesthesia, complications of, 275–276
Inhalation anesthesia, 161–163
  dysrhythmia and, 162–163
  in congenital myotonic disease, 219
  in thyroid surgery, 84
  in tonsillectomy and adenoidectomy, 98
  potent, malignant hyperthermia and, 194
Insulin, perioperative management in, diabetes mellitus
    and, 224–225
Intraocular pressure, 181–186
  acetazolamide and, 186
  central nervous system depressant and, 184
  complications associated with elevation of, 282–283
  congenital glaucoma and, 199
  determinants of, 183–184
  ganglionic blocker and, 185
  hypertonic solution and, 185–186, 231–232
  intraocular gases and, 186
  juvenile "open eye–full stomach" patient and, *200,*
    200–202, *201*
  maintenance of, 181–182
  metabolic status and, 185
  neuromuscular blocking agent and, 185
  temperature and, 185
  ventilation and, 185
Intubation. See also *Extubation.*
  awake, during esophagoscopy, 58
  complications of, arytenoid dislocation and, 161, 161t
    laryngospasm and, 159
    methemoglobinemia and, 158t, 158–159
    pharyngoesophageal injury and, 160–161, 161t
    rheumatoid arthritis and, 161
  confirmation of, 35
  difficult, 24–35, 156–157
    abscess and, 27
    airway assessment and, 24–28, *26*
    alternatives to, 157
    anterior larynx and, 25–27
    anticipated, 28–31
      equipment in, 29, *30*
      general principles in, 28–29
      patient preparation in, 29
      topical anesthesia in, 29–31
    atlantoaxial subluxation and, 27
    blind nasotracheal intubation and, 32–33
    cervical spine mobility and, 27
    craniofacial dysostosis and, 25, *26*
    flexible fiberoptic endoscopy in, 31–32, *32*, 32t
    hypoplastic mandible and, 25–26, *26*
    incidence of, 24, 156
    large tongue and, 25, *25*
    lighted stylet in, 33
    microsomia and, 25
    nasotracheal, 157, 160
    neck manipulation and, 27
    obesity and, *25*
    preparation for, 157
    prevertebral soft tissue swelling and, 28
    prognostic signs of, 24–28, *25*, *26*, 156–157
    retrograde tracheal intubation in, 33

Intubation *(Continued)*
    stiff joint syndrome and, 27–28
    tactile intraoral endotracheal tube placement in, 32
    tumor and, 27
    unanticipated, 33–35
    upper airway problems and, 157
  emergency, 117
  endotracheal, in infancy, 6
    subglottic stenosis due to, 10
  failed, 34
  fire hazard in, 99
  general considerations for, 24
  history of, 24
  hyperparathyroidism and, 80–81
  in anesthetic toxicity, 164
  in bleeding after tonsillectomy, 124
  in craniofacial abnormalities, 215
  in epiglottitis, 117–118, 118t, 119
  in foreign body aspiration, 160
  in juvenile "open eye–full stomach" patient, 201, 202
  in laryngeal trauma, 130
  in laryngeal web, 10
  in laryngectomy, 72
  in laryngotracheobronchitis, 119, 121
  in maxillofacial trauma, 94, 95
  in penetrating eye injury, full stomach and, 186–188
    muscle relaxants in, 187–188
    preoperative care in, 186–187
  in radiation therapy of retinoblastoma, 256
  in tonsillectomy and adenoidectomy, 98
  inadvertent dislodgment of, 169
  laryngeal injury due to, 160–161
  lidocaine during, 51
  nasal, complications of, 160
    difficult, 157
  nasotracheal, blind, 32–33
    difficult, 157, 160
    topical anesthesia for, 30
  oral, complications of, 160
  pharyngoesophageal injury due to, 160–161
  recovery room care after, 301
  subglottic stenosis and, 172–173
  tracheal, injury and, 173
    retrograde, 33
    vocal cord paralysis and, 3
  vocal cord granuloma and, 172
  vocal cord paralysis and, 172–173
Isoflurane, epinephrine interaction with, 163
  in congenital cataract surgery, 198
  in controlled hypotension, 139
  in hyperparathyroidism, 81–82
  in tonsillectomy and adenoidectomy, 98
  visual-evoked potentials and, 262

Jaw, mobility of, maxillofacial trauma and, 92–93, *93*
Jet ventilation, high frequency, in laryngoscopy, 39
  in microlaryngoscopy, 38–39
  transtracheal, percutaneous, 34–35
  Venturi, 38–39
    in juvenile laryngeal papillomas, 46
    in laser surgery, 45, 46
Job-Basedow's syndrome, 78
  Juvenile laryngeal papilloma, laser surgery in, 45–46
Juvenile nasopharyngeal angiofibroma, 106

Ketamine, as premedication, 147
  in infantile glaucoma, 199
  in maxillofacial trauma, 95
  in outpatient surgery, 254
    for strasbismus, 150
  in radiation therapy of retinoblastoma, 255–256
  in thyroid surgery, 84
  intraocular pressure and, 184, 283
King-Denborough syndrome, malignant hyperthermia
    and, 194

Labetalol, in cocaine toxicity, 229
  in controlled hypotension, 140
  in hyperparathyroidism, 81
Lacrimal apparatus, 178
  surgery of, 257
Laryngeal web, 10
Laryngectomy, 72–73
  recovery room care in, 299–301, 300t
  regional anesthesia for, 20, 22
Laryngocele, 10–11
Laryngomalacia, 8, 8t
Laryngoscopy, 29, *30*
  anesthesia in, 19
    childhood and, 13
    infancy and, 13
  difficult. See *Intubation, difficult.*
  in laryngotracheobronchitis, 119
  in neonate and infant, 13
  intraocular pressure and, 187
  recovery room care in, 299–301, 300t
  view of larynx at, *2*
Laryngospasm, 4
  intubation-induced, 159
  periextubation, 170
Laryngotracheobronchitis, 119–121, 120t
  diagnosis of, 119–120, 120t
  edema in, 120–121
  epiglottitis versus, 119, 120t
  general considerations for, 119
  intubation in, 121
  management of, 120–121
  postintubation, 171, 171t
  viral etiology of, 119, 120t
Laryngotracheoesophageal cleft, 10
Larynx, adult, 4–7, 113t
  infant larynx compared to, 4–7
    configuration of, 6
    location of, 5, *5*, *6*
    size of, 5
    tissue consistency and, 6–7
  anatomy of, *1*, 1–4, 65, *66*
    anterior view in, *1*
    at laryngoscopy, view of, *2*
    cartilage in, *1*, 2
    muscle in, 2
    nerve block and, 3–4
    nerve supply in, 2–3
  anterior, difficult intubation and, 26–27
  at puberty, 6
  carcinoma of, epidemiology of, 65–66, *66*
    general considerations for, 65–66
    laryngectomy in, 72–73
    microlaryngoscopy in, 71–72
    neck dissection in, 74–75. See also *Neck, surgery of.*
    preoperative assessment in, 66–71
      aging and, 70–71

Larynx *(Continued)*
    airway disease and, 66–68
    alcoholism and, 69t, 69–70
    cardiovascular status and, 68–69
    liver disease and, 69t, 69–70
    pulmonary disease and, 66–68
  radiation therapy in, 64, 75
  congenital anomaly of, 7–13, 8t
    congenital hemangioma as, 11–12
    cystic hygroma as, 11–12
    laryngeal atresia as, 7–8, 8t
    laryngeal cyst as, 10–11
    laryngeal papilloma as, *12*, 12–13
    laryngeal web as, 10
    laryngocele as, 10–11
    laryngomalacia as, 8, 8t
    laryngotracheoesophageal cleft as, 10
    lymphangioma as, 11–12, *12*
    subglottic stenosis as, 9–10
    vocal cord paralysis as, 8–9
  distinguishing features of, 113t
  gender differences in, 6
  infant, adult larynx compared to, 4–7
    configuration of, 6
    location of, 5, *5*, 6
    size of, 5
    tissue consistency and, 6–7
  obstruction of, 112–113
  intubation-induced injury to, 160–161
  outpatient surgery of, 152–153. See also *Outpatient
    procedure, ear, nose, and throat surgery as.*
  papilloma of, *12*, 12–13, 45–46
  pediatric, laryngoscopy and, 13
    papilloma of, laser surgery in, 45–46
  physiology of, 4
  recurrent nerve in, postoperative damage to, 82
  spasm in, 4
    intubation-induced, 159
    periextubation, 170
  surgery of, laryngectomy in, 72–73
    recovery room care in, 299–301, 300t
    regional anesthesia for, 19–20, *19–20*, 22, *22*
  trauma to, 129–130, 130t
Laser-guard device, 45
Laser microsurgery, risk of, 13
Laser surgery, 39–48
  airway fire and, 48, 48t, 167–168
  anesthesia management in, 43–48
    general consideration for, 43
    intraoperative management and, 43–48
      juvenile laryngeal papillomas and, 45–46
      lower airway lesions and, 46–48
      metallic tapes in, 45
      safety precautions in, 45, 45t
      tubes for, 43–45, *44*, 167–168
      upper airway lesions and, 43–45, *44*
      Venturi ventilation technique in, 45, 46
    preoperative considerations for, 43
  argon, 41t, 41–42
  carbon dioxide, 40–41, 41t
  features of, 41t
  history of, 39
  in glaucoma, 264
  in ocular pathology of diabetes mellitus, 223
  neodymium: yttrium-aluminum-garnet, 41t, 42, *42*
  ocular damage caused by, 41, 42, 42t
  outpatient, 153. See also *Outpatient procedure, ear,
    nose, and throat surgery as.*
  pediatric, complication rate in, 156

Laser surgery *(Continued)*
  potassium-titanyl-phosphate, 41t, 42, 42t
  principles of, 40
  ruby, 42–43
  safety concerns in, 39–40, *40*, 43, 48, 48t
  thermal injury due to, 286
L-dopa, anesthetic implications of, 251t
LeFort fracture, 91–92, *92*
Lens, crystalline, 177–178
  displacement of, 213
  ectopia of, 217
  in Lowe's syndrome, 218
  subluxation of, 213, 215
    Marfan's syndrome and, 218
Leucocoria, differential diagnosis of, *203*, 203t
Lidocaine, anesthetic potency of, 276, 276t
  during intubation, 51
  in anesthetic toxicity, 163, 164
  in cervical epidural anesthesia, 21
  in cervical plexus block, 21
  in congenital cataract surgery, 198
  in emergency tracheostomy, 131
  in esophagoscopy, 57–58
  in extubation, 284
  in foreign body aspiration, 116, 116t
  in laryngeal blockade, 95
  in lower airway lesion, 47
  in microlaryngoscopy, 37, 71
  in middle ear outpatient surgery, 151
  in nasal anesthesia, 52
  in nasal septoplasty, 152
  in nasal surgery, 17–18
  in "open eye–full stomach" patient, juvenile, 202
  in outpatient adenoidectomy, 151–152
  in outpatient ophthalmic procedure, 252
  in outpatient surgery, 150
    sinus and, 152
  in peribulbar block, 278
  in pharyngeal anesthesia, 52–53
  in postoperative vomiting, 255, 255t
  in sinus surgery, 18, 152
  in strabismus surgery, 192–193
  in tonsillectomy, 19
    adenoidectomy and, 99
  in tracheal intubation, 20
  in tracheostomy, 108
  intraocular pressure and, 185, 187
  topical, in nasotracheal intubation, 30–31
  toxicity with, 57
Lightwand, 33
Lincoff balloon scleral buckling operation, 268
Lip, carcinoma of, 64. See also *Oral cavity, carcinoma of.*
Liver disease, in preoperative assessment, 69t, 69–70
Lowe's syndrome, cataract and, 212
  ocular pathology and, 216t, 218
L-thyronine, in thyroid replacement therapy, 84
Ludwig's angina, 126–127
Lugol's solution, in hyperparathyroidism, 78
Lymphangioma, congenital, 11–12, *12*

Magnetic resonance imaging, 261–262
Malignant Hyperthermia Association of Canada, 193
Malignant Hyperthermia Association of the United
  States (MHAUS), 195
Mallinckrodt Laser-Flex endotracheal tube, 44, *44*, 168
Mandible. See also *Face.*

Mandible *(Continued)*
  distinguishing features of, 113t
  hypoplastic, difficult intubation and, 25–26, *26*
  trauma to, 91, *91*
Mannitol, in malignant hyperthermia, 196
  ophthalmic, systemic, 231–232
Marfan's syndrome, ectopia lentis and, 213
  ocular pathology and, 216t, 218–219
Masseter muscle, spasm of, 191, 193–194
Mastoidectomy, *136*, 136–137, 137t
  local anesthesia in, 141, *142*
  recovery room care in, 299–301, 300t
Maxilla, trauma to, *92–94*, 92–95
  airway evaluation and, 92–93, *93*
  anesthesia in, *94*, 94–95
  facial fracture and, 90–92
    usual lines of, 91–92, *92*
  medical problems concurrent with, 93
  normal anatomy and, 90
  preoperative evaluation in, 94
  surgical problems concurrent with, 93–94
Mendelian inheritance, cataract and, 211
Ménière's disease, 137–138
Meningitis, postoperative, 173
Metabolic disease, cataract and, 211–212
  metabolic acidosis as, intraocular pressure and, 185
Methemoglobinemia, 158t, 158–159
Methimazole, in hyperparathyroidism, 78
Methohexital, as premedication, 147
  in outpatient surgery, 150
  in radiation therapy of retinoblastoma, 256
  magnetic resonance imaging and, 262
Methyldopa, anesthetic implications of, 251t
Methylene blue, in methemoglobinemia, 158–159
Metoclopramide, as premedication, 147
  for "open eye–full stomach" patient, 186
    juvenile, 200
  in outpatient ophthalmic procedure, 252
Microlaryngoscopy, 37–39, 71–72
  intraoperative management in, 38–39
  intubation in, 37–38
  laryngeal tumor and, 37, *38*
  local versus general anesthesia in, 37
  outpatient, 153
  preoperative evaluation in, 37–38, *38*
  risk factors in, 37
Microsomia, difficult intubation and, 25
  hemifacial, 214
Midazolam, as premedication, 147
  in endoscopy, 152
  in lower airway lesion, 47
  in outpatient surgery, 150
Mithramycin, hyperparathyroidism and, 86
Mongolism. See *Down's syndrome.*
Monoamine oxidase inhibitor, anesthetic implications of, 251t
Morbidity, in ophthalmic surgery, 272–273
Morphine, in tonsillectomy and adenoidectomy, 99
Mortality, in ophthalmic surgery, 272–273
Multiple endocrine neoplasia, 87
Muscle relaxant, for "open eye–full stomach" patient, 187–188
    juvenile, 201–202
  in ear surgery, 137
  in laryngospasm, 159
  in laser surgery, 153
  in outpatient surgery, 150
  intraocular pressure and, 185
  nerve integrity and, 168–169

Muscle relaxant *(Continued)*
  nondepolarizing, 187–188
Muscle(s), cricothyroid, 2
  disorders of, malignant hyperthermia and, 194
  extraocular, anatomy of, 178
  eye, masseter muscle spasm and, 191, 193–194
    surgery of, 190
  laryngeal, 2
Muscular dystrophy, Becker's, malignant hyperthermia and, 194
  Duchenne's, malignant hyperthermia and, 194
Mydriatic, in congenital cataract surgery, 197
Myocardial infarct, maxillofacial trauma and, 93
Myocardial sensitization, 162
Myotonia congenita, ocular pathology and, 217t, 219
Myotonia dystrophica, ocular pathology and, 217t, 219
Myotonic disease, ocular pathology and, 217t, 219
Myringotomy, 100, 135–136. See also *Ear, surgery of.*
  local anesthesia in, 141, *142*
  recovery room care in, 299–301, 300t
Myxedema coma, 84

Nadbath-Rehman method, for facial nerve block, 244, *245*
Nadolol, in hyperthyroidism, 80
Narcotics. See also names of specific agents.
  in outpatient surgery, 150
  postoperative, thyroid surgery and, 84, 85
Nasal cavity, anesthesia of, 17, 18, *18*
Nasal polyp, 105–106
Nasopharyngoscope, flexible, 8
Nasopharynx, juvenile angiofibroma of, 106
Nausea, ear surgery and, 298
Nd:YAG laser. See also *Laser surgery.*
  in lower airway lesion, 46–48
Neck, cancer of, intraoperative complications of, 169
  dermatomes of, 15, *16*
  hematoma of, postoperative, 82
  innervation of, 15, *16*
  oral laryngeal carcinoma and, 64
  surgery of, intraoperative dysrhythmia and, 162t, 162–163
    major, 75–87
      parathyroid disease and, 85–87
      thyroid disease and, 75–85. See also *Thyroid, disease of.*
    metastases and, 74–75
    outpatient, 153. See also *Outpatient procedure, ear, nose, and throat surgery as.*
    recovery room care in, 298–301, 300t
    regional anesthesia for, 20–22, *21*, *22*
Neodymium: uttrium-aluminum garnet laser, 41t, 42, *42*. See also *Laser surgery.*
Neonate. See also *Pediatrics.*
  larynx in, 5
    congenital anomaly and, 7–13. See also *Larynx, congenital anomaly of.*
    diagnostic laryngoscopy and, 13
  premature. See *Premature infant.*
  strabismus in, 190
Nerve(s), cervical plexus block and, 21–22, *22*
    in thyroid surgery, 81
  facial, 133
    in ear surgery, 137, 139
  glossopharyngeal, 2–3, 15, *16*
    blockade of, 3–4, *19*, 19–20, 52–53
      in awake intubation, 31

Nerve(s) *(Continued)*
  glossopharyngeal, blockade of, 52–53
  infraorbital, blockade of, 17
  infratrochlear, blockade of, 17
  intraoperative injury to, 168–169
  laryngeal, 2–3, *94*, 94–95
    blockade of, *94*, 94–95
    glossopharyngeal nerve as. See *Nerve(s), glossopharyngeal.*
    inferior, 3
      nerve block and, 4
    superior, 3
      nerve block and, 3–4
  maxillary, 15, *16*
    blockade of, 18, *18*
  neck, 15, *16*
  olfactory, 15, *17*
    blockade of, 15, *16–18*, 17–19
  optic, hypoplasia of, 213
    regional blockade of, 235–247. See also *Eye, surgery of, regional blockade in.*
  peribulbar block and, bupivacaine in, 278
    complications of, 278
  pharyngeal, 15, *16*
  retrobulbar block and, Atkinson method in, *243*, 243–244, *244*
    complications of, 276–278, 277t
  tonsil, 19
  trigeminal, 15, *16*
  vagus, 3, 15, *16*
Neurofibroma, von Recklinghausen's disease and, 221
Neuroleptic malignant syndrome, 194
Neurological function, aging and, 71
Neuroma, acoustic, 139
Neuromuscular blocking drug, intraocular pressure and, 185
Neuropraxia, 3
Nifedipine, intraocular pressure and, 185
Nitroglycerin, in controlled hypotension, 140
Nitrous oxide, in ear surgery, *136*, 136–137
  in foreign body aspiration, 116, 116t
  in juvenile laryngeal papilloma, 46
  in middle ear outpatient surgery, 151
  in middle ear surgery, 169
  in outpatient surgery, 149
  in retinal detachment surgery, 268
  in sinus surgery, 103, 103t
  in thyroid surgery, 84
  in tympanic membrane rupture, 169
  intraocular pressure and, 186
  sulfur hexafluoride and, 231
  visual-evoked potentials and, 262
Norton endotracheal tube, 44
Norton tube, 168
Nose. See also *Nasal entries.*
  external, blockade of, 15, *16–18*, 17–19
  innervation of, 15, *17*
  intubation of, blind, 32–33
    complications of, 160
    difficult, 157, 160
    topical anesthesia for, 30
  local anesthetics used in surgery of, 17–18
  outpatient surgery of, 152. See also *Outpatient procedure, ear, nose, and throat surgery as.*
  surgery of, 104–106
    general considerations for, 104–105
    juvenile nasopharyngeal angiofibroma and, 106
    local anesthesia in, 104–105
    nasal polyps and, 105t, 105–106

Nose *(Continued)*
  recovery room care in, 298–301, 300t
  vasoconstriction of, 18
Nucleus Mini-22 device, 138

Obesity, intubation difficulty and, *25*
O'Brien method, for facial nerve block, *242*, 242–243, *243*
Octafluorocyclobutane, in retinal detachment surgery, 268
  intraocular, 228t, 231
  intraocular pressure and, 186
Oculocardiac reflex, 192
  in retinoblastoma, 203
  ophthalmic surgery and, 278–279
Oculocerebrorenal syndrome. See *Lowe's syndrome.*
Oculogastric reflex, 283–284
"Open eye–full stomach" patient, 186–188
  intraocular pressure and, in juvenile, *200*, 200–202, *201*
  juvenile, *200*, 200–202, *201*
  muscle relaxants for, 187–188
  preoperative care for, 186–187
  priming principle for, 202
Ophthalmic. See *Eye.*
Oral cavity, carcinoma of, epidemiology of, 64, *65*
  preoperative assessment in, 66–71
    aging and, 70–71
    airway disease and, 66–68
    cardiovascular status and, 69t, 69–70
    liver disease and, 69t, 69–70
    pulmonary disease and, 66–68
  outpatient surgery of, 151–152. See also *Outpatient procedure, ear, nose, and throat surgery as.*
  radiation therapy in, 75
Orbit, anatomy of, 176–178
  blood supply to, 179
  fracture of, 176
  lesions of, 176
Oropharynx, carcinoma of, epidemiology of, 64–65
  microlaryngoscopy in, 71–72
  neck dissection in, 74–75. See also *Neck, surgery of.*
  preoperative assessment in, 66–71
    aging and, 70–71
    airway disease and, 66–68
    alcoholism and, 69t, 69–70
    cardiovascular status and, 68–69
    liver disease and, 69t, 69–70
    pulmonary disease and, 66–68
  radiation therapy in, 75
Otitis media, 100
  mastoidectomy in, *136*, 136–137, 137t
  myringotomy and tympanotomy tube placement in, 135–136
  tympanoplasty in, *136*, 136–137, 137t
Outpatient procedure, ear, nose, and throat surgery as, 144–153
  anesthetic management in, 147
    general, 149–150
    local, 148
    monitoring in, 147–148
    premedication in, 147
    regional, 148–149
  cancellation of, 146–147
  complications of, 144–145
  discharge criteria in, 146
  general considerations for, 144

Outpatient procedure *(Continued)*
    patient selection in, 145
    postoperative care in, 145–146
    procedures appropriate for, 144–145
    sociological concerns in, 145–146
  ophthalmic, 248t, 248–258
    anesthesia for radiation therapy in retinoblastoma and, 255–256, *256*
    cataract extraction and, 249–253. See also *Cataract, surgery in.*
    general considerations for, 248
    lacrimal drainage system surgery and, 256–257
    pediatric complications of, 257t, 257–258
    strabismus surgery and, *253*, 253–255
Oxygen, in anesthetic toxicity, 164
  in cricothyroidectomy, 131
  in emergency tracheostomy, 131
  in epiglottitis, 118
  in foreign body aspiration, 116, 116t
  in juvenile laryngeal papilloma, 46
  in laryngotracheobronchitis, 120
  in retinopathy of prematurity, 204t, 204–205
  in venous air embolism, 167
  ocular complications of, 284–285

Pancuronium, for juvenile "open eye–full stomach" patient, 201
  for "open eye–full stomach" patient, 187–188
  intraocular pressure and, 185
Papillary carcinoma, thyroid, 85
Papilloma, laryngeal, *12*, 12–13
  juvenile, laser surgery in, 45–46
  vocal cord, outpatient surgery of, 153. See also *Outpatient procedure, ear, nose, and throat surgery as.*
Para-aminobenzoic acid (PABA), toxicity with, 57
Paramyotonia, ocular pathology and, 217t, 219
Paranasal sinus, surgery of, 103–104
Parathyroid gland, 85–87
  hyperparathyroidism and, 86–87
  hypoparathyroidism and, 87
  multiple endocrine neoplasia and, 87
  parathyroid hormone and, 85–86
  physiology of, 85–86
  surgery of, 86–87
  vitamin D and, 86
Parathyroid hormone (PTH), 85–86
Parathyroidectomy, 86–87
Patau's syndrome, cataract and, 211
Patent ductus arteriosus, 220
Peanut, aspiration of, 114, 117. See also *Foreign body, aspiration of.*
Pediatrics. See also *Infancy; Neonate.*
  airway in, 112–113, 113t. See also *Airway, pediatric.*
  atlantoaxial subluxation in, 127
  cataract in, 196–198
    causes of, 197t
    surgery for, 266
    syndromes associated with, 197
    systemic diseases associated with, 211
  choanal atresia in, 127–128
  eye surgery in, 190–207. See also *Eye, surgery of, pediatric.*
  juvenile laryngeal papillomas of, laser surgery in, 45–46
  laryngeal obstruction in, 7, 7t
  outpatient procedures in, 257t, 257–258
  overnight hospital admissions in, 257t, 257–258

Pediatrics *(Continued)*
  premedication in, 147
  tracheostomy in, 108
    airway obstruction and, 122
    complication rate in, 156
    mortality rate in, 156
Percutaneous transtracheal jet ventilation (TTJV), in
    failed intubation, 34
Perfluoropropane, in retinal detachment surgery, 268
  intraocular, 228t, 231
  intraocular pressure and, 186
Peribulbar block, bupivacaine in, 278
  complications of, 278
Peritonsillar abscess, 125–126
Pharyngitis, postintubation, 160
Pharyngolaryngoesophagectomy, with gastric
    interposition, 73–74
Pharynx, carcinoma of, 64–65. See also *Oropharynx,
    carcinoma of.*
    pharyngolaryngoesophagectomy in, 73–74
  infection of, 125–127
    general considerations for, 125
    Ludwig's angina as, 126–127
    quinsy as, 125–126
    retropharyngeal abscess as, 126
  sensory innervation of, 15, *16*
  surgery of, regional anesthesia in, *19*, 19–20
Phenylephrine, in congenital cataract surgery, 197
  ophthalmic, topical, 228t, 230
Photocoagulation, in retinopathy of prematurity, 205
Photophobia, following general anesthesia, 286
Pierre-Robin syndrome, 5, *6*
Plasma iodide, 75
Plastic surgery, outpatient, 153
Plummer-Vinson syndrome, 65
Pneumonia, as complication of tracheostomy, 109, 109t
Pneumonitis, aspiration, 160
  periextubation, 170
Pneumothorax, as complication of tracheostomy, 108,
    109t
  intraoperative, 166
  maxillofacial trauma and, 93–94
Polypectomy, nasal, 152
Polyvinylchloride (PVC), tube, in laser surgery, 43–45
Posterior commissure, 1, *2*
Potassium iodide, in hyperparathyroidism, 78
  in hyperthyroidism, 80
Potassium replacement, in malignant hyperthermia, 196
Potassium-titanyl-phosphate laser, 41t, 42, 42t. See also
    Laser surgery.
Pregnancy, cataract and, systemic diseases associated
    with, 211, 211t
  congenital cataract and, 197
  rubella in, patent ductus arteriosus and, 220
  thyrotoxicosis in, 79
Premature infant, apnea in, 206, 206t, 258
  ocular complications in, 284–285
  retinopathy of prematurity in, 203–207, 204t, 206t. See
    also *Retinopathy of prematurity.*
Prevertebral soft tissue swelling, 28
Procainamide, in malignant hyperthermia, 195
Progressive arthro-ophthalmomyopathy, 217t, 222
Progressive sensorineural deafness, postoperative, 173
Promethazine, as premedication, 147
Proparacaine, in outpatient ophthalmic procedure, 252
  topical, complications of, 274–275
Propofol, in outpatient surgery, 150
Propranolol, in cocaine toxicity, 229
  in hyperparathyroidism, 78, 80–81

Propranolol *(Continued)*
  in hyperthyroidism, 80
  in thyrotoxicosis, 79
  intraocular pressure and, 185
Propyliodone, in bronchography, 107
Propylthiouracil (PTU), in hyperthyroidism, 78
  in thyrotoxicososis, 79
Prostaglandin, in controlled hypotension, 140
Prostate, TURP syndrome and transient blindness with,
    286
Pseudo-Ludwig's angina, 126
Puberty, larynx at, 6
Pulmonary disease, aging and, 70
  carcinoma and, 66–68
  Riley-Day syndrome and, 220

Quinsy, 125–126

Radiation therapy, in head and neck carcinoma, 75
  in retinoblastoma, 255–256, *256*
Radioactive iodine, in hyperthyroidism, 79
Ranitidine, as premedication, 147
  preoperative, 29
Regional anesthesia, acupuncture as, 22–23
  in laryngeal surgery, *19*, 19–20, *20*
  in nasal surgery, 15, *16–18*, 17–19
  in neck surgery, 20–22, *21*, *22*
  in pharyngeal surgery, *19*, 19–20
  in thyroid surgery, *21*, 22
Renal function, aging and, 70
Reserpine, anesthetic implications of, 251t
Respiratory acidosis, intraocular pressure and, 185
Retina, 178
  detachment of, 266–269, *267*
    rhegmatogenous, *267*, 268–269
    surgery in, *267*, 267–269
      complications of, 269
      intraocular gases in, 268
      Lincoff balloon scleral buckling in, 268
      scleral buckling procedure in, *267*, 267–268
      vitrectomy as, 268–270. See also *Vitrectomy.*
  giant tears in, 269
  hemorrhage in, due to general anesthesia, 287
  ischemia of, due to general anesthesia, 287
Retinoblastoma, 202–203, *203*, 203t
  anesthetic management in, 203
    radiation therapy and, 255–256, *256*
  familial, 202–203
  genetic test in, 203
  incidence of, 202
  oculocardiac reflex in, 203
  presentation in, 203, 203t
  trilateral, 203
Retinopathy of prematurity, 203–207, 204t, 206t
  anesthetic management in, 206t, 206–207
  historical background in, 203–205
  incidence of, 204
  open sky vitrectomy in, 269–270. See also *Vitrectomy.*
  oxygen therapy in, 204t, 204–205
  postulated etiologies in, 203–205, 204t
  surgery in, 205–206
Retrobulbar block, Atkinson method of facial nerve
    block in, *243*, 243–244, *244*
  complications of, 276–278, 277t
Retropharyngeal abscess, 126

Rheumatoid arthritis, 2
Riley-Day syndrome, ocular pathology and, 216t, 219–220
ROP. See *Retinopathy of prematurity.*
Rubella syndrome, ocular pathology and, 216t, 220
Ruby laser, 42–43. See also *Laser surgery.*

Sanders rigid Venturi bronchoscope, 50, 51t
Saunders jet bronchoscopic ventilation technique, 71
Schwartz-hyoid maneuver, in anterior larynx identification, 26
Sclera, sclerosis of, 181
Sclerosis, of sclera, 181
Scopolamine, in congenital glaucoma, 199
   topical, 228t, 230
Septo-optic dysplasia, 214
Septoplasty, nasal, 152
Septum, anesthesia of, 17, 18, *18*
Sickle cell disease, ocular pathology and, 217t, 220–221
Silicone tube, in laser surgery, 43–44
Sinus, frontal, blockade of, *16–18*, 18–19
   maxillary, blockade of, 18, *18*
   surgery of, 103t, 103–104
      air embolism and, 103–104, 104t
      bleeding and, 103
      cocaine in, 103
      intranasal anatomy and, 103
      outpatient, 152. See also *Outpatient procedure, ear, nose, and throat surgery as.*
      postoperative complications of, 104
Sinusitis, outpatient surgery in, 152
Sipple syndrome, 87
Smoking, carcinoma and, 64, 65, 67–68
Sodium citrate, as premedication, 147
Sodium iodide, in thyrotoxicosis, 79
Sodium nitroprusside, in controlled hypotension, 139–140
   juvenile nasopharyngeal angiofibroma and, 106
Sodium thiopental, in outpatient surgery, 150
Sore throat, after surgery, 146
Sphenopalatine ganglion block, 17, *18*
Spinal anesthesia, transient hearing loss and, 173
Stapedectomy, 137
   antiemetic after, 142–143
   local anesthesia in, 141
   recovery room care in, 299–301, 300t
Stenosis, subglottic, 173
   congenital, 9–10
   tracheal, postoperative, 173
Steroid, in foreign body aspiration, 116, 116t
   in laryngotracheobronchitis, 120
Stickler syndrome, ocular pathology and, 217t, 222
Stiff joint syndrome, difficult intubation and, 27–28
Strabismus, general considerations for, 190
   surgery in, 190–193, 191t
      antiemetic prophylaxis in, 254–255, 255t
      forced duction test and, 191
      malignant hyperthermia and, 191, 191t. See also *Hyperthermia, malignant.*
      masseter muscle spasm and, 191
      oculocardiac reflex and, 191–192
      outpatient, *253*, 253–255
      special concerns with, 190–191, 191t
      vomiting after, 192–193
Stridor, 7, *7*
   in airway obstruction, 7, *7*, 113, 113t

Stridor *(Continued)*
   laryngomalacia, 8, 8t
   postintubation, 301
Stroke, maxillofacial trauma and, 93
Sturge-Weber syndrome, ocular pathology and, 217t, 221, *221*
Stylet, lighted, difficult intubation and, 33
Subluxation, atlantoaxial, 127
      intubation difficulties with, 27, 161
      syndromes associated with, 27
   lens. See also *Ectopia lentis.*
      Marfan's syndrome and, 218
Succinylcholine, echothiophate iodide and, 229–230
   for "open eye–full stomach" patient, 188, 201, 202
   in anesthetic toxicity, 164
   in bleeding after tonsillectomy, 124
   in foreign body aspiration, 116, 116t
   in juvenile laryngeal papilloma, 46
   in laryngospasm, 159
   in outpatient surgery, 150
      strabismus and, 254
   in strabismus surgery, 191, 254
   intraocular pressure and, 184, 185, 283
   malignant hyperthermia and, 193
   masseter muscle spasm and, 193–194
Sufentanil, in lower airway lesion, 47
   in outpatient surgery, 150
   intraocular pressure and, 282
Sulfur hexafluoride, intraocular, 228t, 231
Symbion cochlear implant, 138

Tachycardia, in malignant hyperthermia, 194–195
Tetracaine, in nasal anesthesia, 52
   topical, complications of, 274–275
      in nasotracheal intubation, 30
   toxicity with, 57
Thermal injury, due to laser surgery, 286
Thiopental, in anesthetic toxicity, 164
   in bleeding after tonsillectomy, 124
   in congenital myotonic disease, 219
   in elevated intraocular pressure, 282
   in foreign body aspiration, 116, 116t
   in lower airway lesion, 47
   in thyroid surgery, 84
Throat, surgery of, outpatient, 144–153. See also *Outpatient procedure, ear, nose, and throat surgery as.*
   recovery room care in, 298–301, 300t
Thyrohyoid membrane, anterior view of, *1*
Thyroid, anterior view of, *1*
   carcinoma of, 85
   cartilage in, *1*, 2
      infant, 6
   disease of, 75–85
      hyperthyroidism as, 77–83. See also *Hyperthyroidism.*
      hypothyroidism as, 83t, 83–85
      multiple endocrine neoplasia and, 87
      neoplasm as, 85
      scintigraphy in, 77
      thyroid function and, 75–76, 76t
         tests for, 76–77, 77t
      ultrasonography in, 77
   hormones of, replacement therapy with, 84
   surgery of, complications of, 82–83
      perioperative management and, 79–82, *80*, *81*
      postoperative thyroid replacement therapy and, 84

Thyroid *(Continued)*
  regional anesthesia in, *21*, 22
Thyroid hormone, replacement therapy with, 84
  thyroid-stimulating, 76, 77
  thyroxine, 75–77
    in thyroid replacement therapy, 84
Thyroid-stimulating hormone (TSH), 76, 77
Thyroid storm, intraoperative, 82
  medical management in, 78–79
  postoperative, 82
Thyroidectomy, vocal cord paralysis and, 3, 172–173
Thyroiditis, 78
Thyrotoxicosis, medical management of, 78–79
  thyroid surgery in presence of, 22
Thyroxine, 75–77
  in thyroid replacement therapy, 84
Timolol, ophthalmic, topical, 228t, 230–231
"To-and-fro" stridor, 7, *7*
Tongue, adult, 113t
  carcinoma of, 64, 65t. See also *Oral cavity, carcinoma of.*
  distinguishing features of, 113t
  large, difficult intubation and, 25, *25*
Tonsillectomy, adenoidectomy and, 97–100
    complications of, 97
    contraindications for, 97
    incidence of, 97
    indications for, 97
    induction and intraoperative management in, 98–100
    outpatient, 151–152
    postoperative care in, 99–100
    preoperative preparation in, 97–98
    recovery room care in, 299–301, 300t
  mortality rate in, 164–165
  postoperative bleeding and, 124–125, 164–165
  regional anesthesia for, 19, *19*
Tonsils, innervation of, 19
Topical anesthesia, complications of, 274–275
  in difficult intubation, 29–31
  in laser surgery of lower airway lesions, 47
  in microlaryngoscopy, 71
  rigid bronchoscopy and, 49
  spray systems for, 30
TORCH (congenital infection syndromes), glaucoma and, 213
Trachea, adult, size of, 53
  anterior view of, *1*
  at laryngoscopy, view of, *2*
  distinguishing features of, 113t
  infant, 6, 112–113, 113t
  intubation of. See also *Intubation.*
    injury and, 173
    regional anesthesia for, *19*, 20, *20*
    retrograde, 33
    vocal cord paralysis and, 3
  postoperative complications of, 173
Tracheitis, bacterial, 121
Tracheoesophageal fistula, congenital subglottic stenosis and, 9–10
Tracheostomy, 107–109
  anesthesia in, 108
  complications of, 108–109, 109t
  congenital hemangioma and, 11
  emergency, 131
  esophageal erosion and, 109, 109t
  extubation in, 119
  general considerations for, 117, 119
  in childhood, 108
  in diphtheria, 129

Tracheostomy *(Continued)*
  in epiglottitis, 119
  in laryngeal trauma, 130
  in laryngotracheobronchitis, 121
  indications for, 107–107t
  laryngeal papilloma and, 12–13
  laryngeal web and, 10
  local anesthesia for, 108
  microlaryngoscopy and, 38
  pediatric, 108
    airway obstruction and, 122
    complication rate in, 156
    mortality rate in, 156
    regional anesthesia for, 20
    short-term complications of, 173
    surgical techniques in, 108
    tube displacement in, 109, 109t
    tubes for, 107
Trauma, laryngeal, 129–130, 130t
  mechanical, 165–166
Treacher Collins syndrome, 5
  tactile intraoral endotracheal tube placement in, 33
Tricyclic antidepressant, anesthetic implications of, 251t
Trimethaphan, in controlled hypotension, 140
Trisomy 13. See *Patau's syndrome.*
Trisomy 18. See *Edwards' syndrome.*
Trisomy 21. See *Down's syndrome.*
Trousseau's sign, after parathyroid surgery, 87
TSH. See *Thyroid-stimulating hormone.*
TTJV. See *Percutaneous transtracheal jet ventilation.*
Tubocurarine, for juvenile "open eye–full stomach" patient, 201
Turner's syndrome, hearing loss and otitis media with, 135
TURP (transurethral resection of prostate) syndrome, transient blindness and, 286
Tympanic membrane, 135, 136
  intraoperative rupture of, 169
Tympanoplasty, *136*, 136–137, 137t
  local anesthesia in, 141
  recovery room care in, 299–301, 300t
Tympanostomy tube, insertion of, 100
  outpatient, 150–151
Tympanotomy tube, insertion of, 135–136
  local anesthesia in, 141, *142*

Uveal tract, 177, *177*
Uveitis, sympathetic, 202

Vagus nerve, 15, *16*
  in laryngeal innervation, 3
Valium, in endoscopy, 152–153
Vallecula, 1, *2*
van Lint method, for facial nerve block, 241–242, *242*
Vasoconstrictor, in sinus surgery, 103
Vasopressor, in anesthetic toxicity, 164
VATER (tracheoesophageal fistula, congenital heart disease, and renal anomalies) syndrome, colobomata and, 213
Vecuronium, for "open eye–full stomach" patient, 187–188, 201, 202
  in juvenile laryngeal papilloma, 46
  intraocular pressure and, 185
Venous air embolism, 102, 103–104, 104t
  intraoperative, 166–167, 167t

Venturi bronchoscope, complications of, 56
  rigid, 50, 51t
Venturi effect, 50
Venturi jet ventilation, 38–39
  in juvenile laryngeal papilloma, 46
  in laser surgery, 45, 46
Vertigo, 134
Vestibular fold, at laryngoscopy, *2*
Viral infection, in bacterial tracheitis, 121
  in laryngotracheobronchitis, 119, 120t
Vision, loss of, following anesthesia, 286
  transient, TURP syndrome and, 286
Visual-evoked potential, anesthetic implications of, 262
Vitamin D, production of, 86
Vitamin E, in retinopathy of prematurity, 204, 204t
Vitrectomy, in diabetic retinopathy, 223
  in retinal detachment, 268–270
  in retinopathy of prematurity, 205–206
Vitreous humor, 178
  degeneration of, Wagner-Stickler syndrome and, 222
Vocal cord, adult, 5
  false, 1, *2*
  infant, 5
  paralysis of, after thyroid surgery, 82
    bilateral, 3
    causes of, 3, 9
    congenital, 3, 8–9
    postintubation, 160–161
    postoperative, 172–173

Vocal cord *(Continued)*
    surgery as cause of, 3
    thyroidectomy and, 3
  postoperative granuloma of, 172
  true, 1, *2*
Vocal fold, at laryngoscopy, *2*
Vomiting, after eye muscle surgery, 192–193
  during anesthesia, 280t, 280–282. See also *Aspiration.*
  ear surgery and, 298
Vomitus, aspiration of, 159
von Recklinghausen's disease, ocular pathology and, 217t, 221–222

Wagner-Stickler syndrome, ocular pathology and, 217t, 222
Web, laryngeal, 10
Wermer's syndrome, 87
Wheeze, expiratory, 7
Wilson's disease, cataract and, 212

Xomed laser shield silicone endotracheal tube, 44, *44*
Xomed tube, 168

Zellweger syndrome, ocular pathology and, 217t, 222